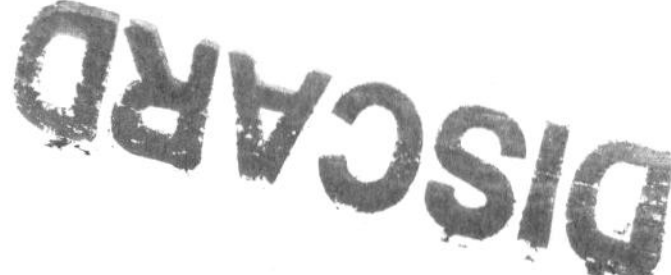

Laboratory Procedures *for* Medical Office Personnel

Laboratory Procedures *for* Medical Office Personnel

Craig A. Stepp, JD, MT(ASCP), CLS

Professor of Laboratory Science, Fresno City College, and Clinical Laboratory Scientist, St. Agnes Medical Center, Fresno, California; Member of the California Association of Medical Laboratory Technologists; Attorney in private practice, Fresno, California

FORMERLY Supervisor, Pathological and Clinical Services Laboratory and Sierra Community Hospital Clinical Laboratory, Fresno, California

MaryAnn Woods, PhD, RN, CMA

Professor, Health Sciences and the Arts Division, and Director of the Medical Assistant-Clinician Program, Fresno City College, Fresno, California; Member of California Certifying Board for Medical Assistants; Member of California Association for Medical Assistant Instructors

W.B. SAUNDERS COMPANY

A Division of Harcourt Brace & Company

Philadelphia London Toronto
Montreal Sydney Tokyo

W.B. SAUNDERS COMPANY
A Division of Harcourt Brace & Company

The Curtis Center
Independence Square West
Philadelphia, PA 19106

Library of Congress Cataloging-in-Publication Data

Stepp, Craig A.
Laboratory procedures for medical office personnel / Craig A. Stepp, MaryAnn Woods. — 1st ed.
p. cm.
ISBN 0-7216-5275-1
1. Diagnosis, Laboratory. 2. Medical assistants. I. Woods, MaryAnn. II. Title.
[DNLM: 1. Diagnosis, Laboratory—methods. 2. Technology, Medical. 3. Health Personnel. QY 25 S837L 1998]
RB37.S696 1998
616.07'56—dc21
DNLM/DLC

97-6736

LABORATORY PROCEDURES FOR MEDICAL OFFICE PERSONNEL ISBN 0-7216-5275-1

Printed in the United States of America

Last digit is the printed number: 9 8 7 6 5 4 3 2 1

Because of our years of teaching, and the experiences this employment has given us, we felt a real need for a text that could be used as a curriculum for students and as a learning resource and reference. For this reason we wish to dedicate this book to you, the student, for you are the reason it was written.

Preface

Laboratory Procedures for Medical Office Personnel is designed to provide the basic principles and methods for laboratory skills. The underlying pedagogy consists of a textbook/procedure-technique approach designed to help the student in perfecting the newly learned techniques and to aid the instructor in establishing an outline for study and learning competencies. The *Student Review* gives the student a combination of reinforcement exercises for each chapter, combined with case studies and critical thinking situations that will encourage the student to make decisions based on learned knowledge. The *Instructors' Guide* is designed to assist the instructor by explaining how the textbook is structured to meet the criteria of the competency-based curriculum, aiding in lecture organization, and offering suggestions in the presentation of many concepts and procedures.

Because of the explosion of advancements and new methodologies in this area, it is no longer practical to expect an individual to gain the necessary knowledge without formal instruction. We have directed our efforts toward meeting the needs of students studying medical laboratory procedures. This text also serves as a quick reference of testing procedures for nurses, physicians, laboratory technicians, and hospital personnel. The nonprofessional who is interested in becoming acquainted with current laboratory testing techniques will also find the book rewarding and helpful.

The textbook presents medical and clinical laboratory procedures and techniques that are significant to medical and laboratory assistants as well as to other health care professionals. The text familiarizes students with the various duties and responsibilities performed by laboratory personnel, starting with the initial physician's order and continuing through sample collection and processing, testing, reporting, maintenance, quality control, and quality assurance.

The student is provided with a basic knowledge in procedures by being given an overview of the anatomy/physiology involved and the main reasons why certain tests are ordered. Students will then be able to build on this basic foundation. The book is designed as a classroom teaching text for programs requiring a laboratory component, yet its organization incorporates self-teaching features that allow students to work through chapters at their own pace without outside guidance. We have tried to take into account the needs of both the instructor who employs the traditional lecture and demonstration method and students who must proceed at their own pace through independent study.

The material is presented at a level suitable for the average student. No previous knowledge of anatomy, physiology, or biology is necessary (although completion of a basic biology course is helpful).

The book is divided into six units, and each unit covers one major division of the laboratory. The units are then divided into chapters with similar formats and organized as follows:

Chapter outline and learning objectives

Textual material

Quality and quantity controls for the specific test

Specimen collection

Testing procedures with descriptive commentary

Testing outcomes

Reporting the test results

Student achievement and evaluation guidelines

Each chapter begins with learning objectives, which indicate the direction of the chapter material and provide concrete ways for students to assess mastery. Full-color photographs and diagrams depicting laboratory data are included throughout to help the student read and report quickly and accurately on the testing data. Each chapter concludes with a chapter review in which students are asked to apply the principles discussed and demonstrated.

It is our hope that students will continue to use this text as a reference guide when they enter the workplace. The material is presented in a way that facilitates quick reference to a given procedure or test result. We hope that using this text will be as fascinating to you as writing it was for us.

Craig A. Stepp, JD, MT(ASCP), CLS

MaryAnn Woods, PhD, RN, CMA

Acknowledgments

We wish to express our appreciation to the individuals who contributed information used in the development of this book:

Hilaria Fiorini, MT, CLS in Therapeutic Drug Monitoring

Alan Barbour, PhD, CLB in Toxicology

Joyce Gordon, MT, CLS in Blood Chemistry

Wilma Orr, MT, CLS in Special Procedures

The staff at St. Agnes Medical Center Clinical Laboratory in photography

Dr. Tschang and the Bacteriology staff in photography

Dr. Jerry Nelson and his Clinical Laboratory staff in photography

Ron Halder for photography procedure set-up

Kathleen Thompson, RNFA, for writing chapter review questions

Of course, this project would have never reached completion without the guidance, support, and encouragement of the W.B. Saunders staff. We are deeply grateful to Helaine Barron, whose letters and phone calls kept us focused and on target. Helaine spent countless hours developing this book and worked hard to give it a special touch of elegance.

Reviewers

Special thanks go to the following people who graciously gave their time and expertise to review various chapters of this book.

Rev. Dr. Geneva M. Burch
Department of Science and Math
West Virginia Northern Community College
Benwood, West Virginia

Pamela Burton, CMA, LRT, CPT (ASPT)
Allied Health and Life Science Department
Sellersburg, Indiana

Agnes Cannella, BS (MT)
South College and St. Joseph's Hospital Clinical Laboratory
Savannah, Georgia

Mary Chiaravalloti, RN, CMA
Department of Medical Assisting
Bryant & Stratten
Buffalo, New York

Barbara M. Dahl, CMA
Department of Medical Assisting
Whatcom Community College
Bellingham, Washington

Bonnie Lou Diester, MA, MS, BSN, AAS
Chair, Department of Medical Assisting
Broome Community College
Binghamton, New York

Christine L. Fessler, BSTE, CMA, CPT (ASPT)
Director of Education
Akron Medical-Dental Institute
Cuyahoga Falls, Ohio

Eugenia Fulcher, MEd, BSN
Department of Medical Assisting
Swainsboro Tech
Swainsboro, Georgia

Rona Goldman, CMA-AC, CCVT
Medix School
Towson, Maryland

Michelle Green, MPS, BS, AAS
Physical and Sciences Department
Alfred State College
Alfred, New York

Melisse Gross, Instructor
Diploma Program
Department of Long Term Care and Allied Health
Vancouver Community College
BC Women's Hospital
Vancouver, British Columbia, Canada

Jeanne Howard, EPCC, AAS
Department of Medical Assisting Technology
El Paso Community College
El Paso, Texas

Sally Ann Murdock, MS, BSN
Department of Medical Assisting
San Diego Mesa College
San Diego, California

Lisa Nagle, CMA
Department of Medical Assisting
Augusta Technical Institute
Augusta, Georgia

Bev Philpott, BSc
Department of Health Science
Kirkwood Community College
Cedar Rapids, Iowa

Brief Contents

Procedure Symbols

Following proper safety methods to protect yourself and your co-workers in the laboratory is essential. In this text each procedure is headed with one or more symbols to alert you to the proper method of protecting yourself when performing that procedure. These symbols are:

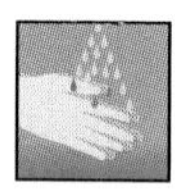

1. Wash hands before and after performing the procedure.

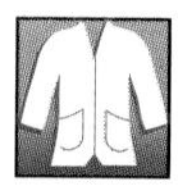

2. Wear a lab coat.

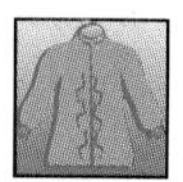

3. Wear a barrier gown.

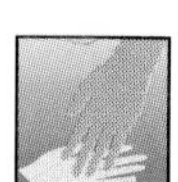

4. Wear gloves.

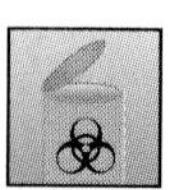

5. Dispose of bioharzardous materials in the biohazardous waste container.

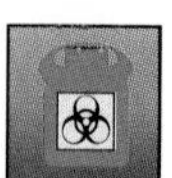

6. Dispose of needles and other sharp instruments in the sharps container.

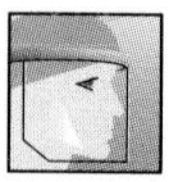

7. Wear face protector (goggles, mask, or shield).

Contents

Unit VI
Microbiology 307

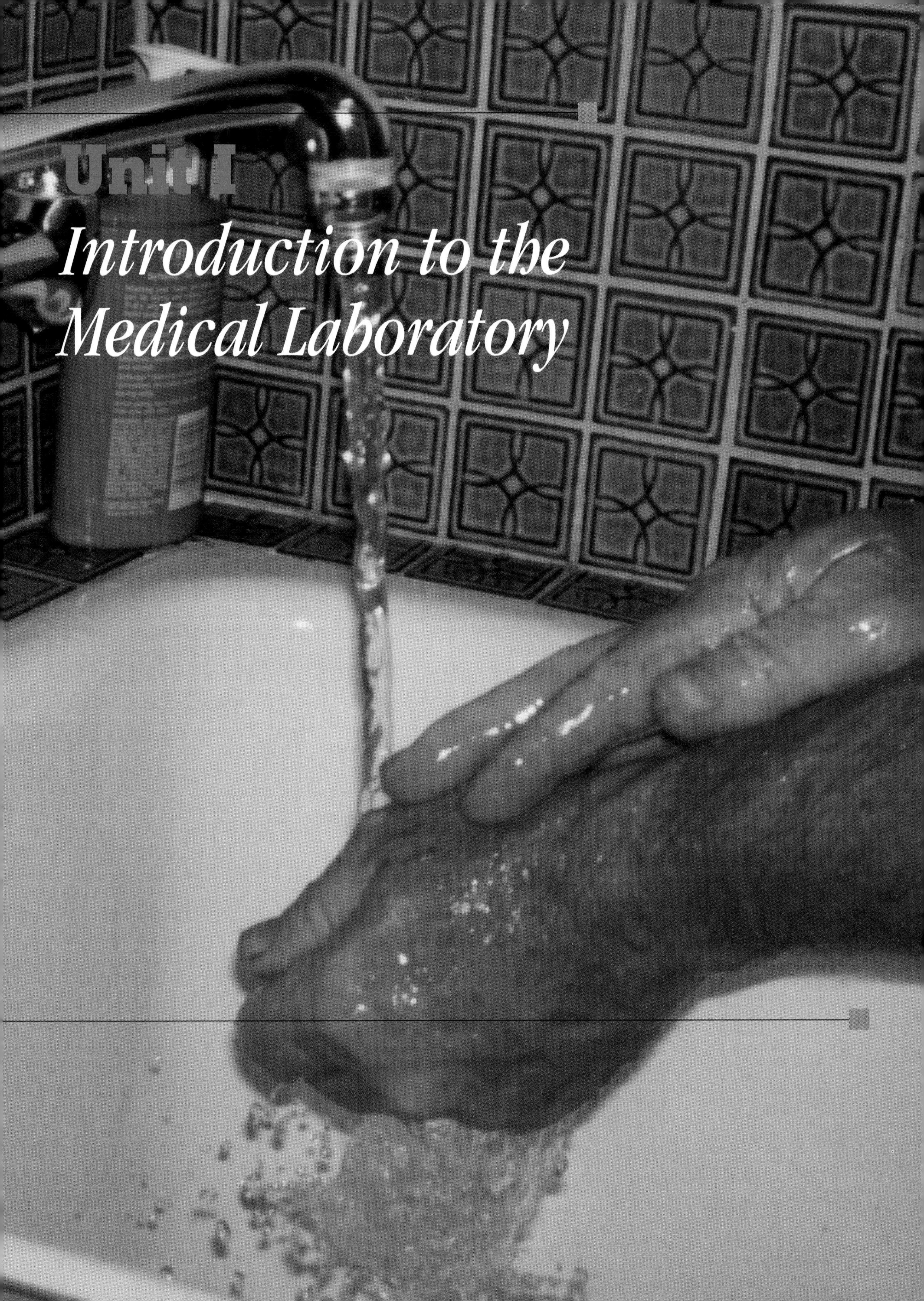

Unit I

Introduction to the Medical Laboratory

Vocabulary

aerobic: requiring oxygen for the maintenance of life

anaerobic: able to grow and function without air or oxygen

assay: an analysis of the purity or effectiveness of any biological substance, including drugs

biopsy: excision of a small sample of tissue from the body for diagnostic or therapeutic purposes

coagulation: the process of transforming a liquid into a solid

cytology: the study of cells and their formation

feces: the end product of digestion; bowel movement

gastric: pertaining to the stomach

hematology: the study of the characteristics, formation, and effects of blood

histology: the science dealing with the microscopic identification of cells and tissue

laboratory: a facility for the biological, microbiological, serologic, chemical, immunohematologic, hematologic, biophysical, cytologic, pathological, or other examination of materials derived from the human body for the purpose of providing information for the assessment, diagnosis, prevention, or treatment of any disease or condition affecting the health of human beings

occult: hidden or difficult to observe directly

pathology: the scientific study of the characteristics, causes, and effects of disease

sensitivity: susceptibility to a drug or an antigen

serology: the laboratory medicine that studies blood serum for evidence of infection by evaluating antigen-antibody reactions in vitro

toxicology: the scientific study of poisons, their detection, their effects, and methods of treatment for the conditions they produce

Chapter Objectives

After reading this chapter, you should be able to:

1. Define the vocabulary terms.
2. Identify the two major areas in the laboratory and list the departments included in each area.
3. Name one agency that grants the technologist title.
4. Identify one agency that grants the technician title.
5. Outline the role of the medical assistant in the medical laboratory.
6. List the assay tests that are most frequently performed on a patient.

Chapter 1
The Medical Laboratory

Rapid scientific advances in diagnostic and treatment instrumentation within health care settings have led to numerous changes within the clinical **laboratory.** Almost every patient who is admitted to a hospital or seen in a physician's office also becomes a patient in the clinical laboratory. In the past few years, rapid advances in clinical laboratory automation and procedures have spurred tremendous growth in the clinical laboratory, at a rate that has exceeded hospital growth. Sophisticated technology and automation have added new dimensions to the diagnosis and treatment of disease.

The clinical laboratory department is composed of two major areas. In the clinical pathology area, blood and other types of body fluids and tissues, such as urine, cerebrospinal fluid (CSF), **biopsy** specimens, and **gastric** secretions, are analyzed. The area of anatomic pathology is concerned with autopsy and cytologic examinations, as well as surgical pathology procedures. The clinical laboratory primarily offers patient services, but is also involved in research, development, and teaching in order to maintain the high quality of laboratory services.

In the laboratory, specimens are tested, analyzed, and evaluated. Precise measurements are made, and the results are then calculated and interpreted. Tests are performed manually (by hand) or through automation (by using specialized instruments). These tests are performed by professionally trained medical technologists, medical laboratory technicians, and other trained allied health personnel.

Laboratory Staffing

Certified Medical Technologist

The *certified medical technologist* has a baccalaureate degree and additional formal training in a laboratory. To become certified, an individual must pass an examination given by a national certifying agency.

Certifying Agencies and Titles Granted

- American Society of Clinical Pathologists
  MT-(ASCP) Medical Technologist
- American Medical Technologists
  MT(AMT) Medical Technologist
- Department of Health and Human Services
  CLT(HHS) Clinical Laboratory Technologist
- National Certification Agency for Medical Laboratory Personnel
  CLS(NCA) Clinical Laboratory Scientist
- International Society for Clinical Laboratory Technology
  RMT(ISCLT) Registered Medical Technologist

Certified Medical Laboratory Technician

The *certified medical laboratory technician* has completed a specialized training program that is 1 to 2 years in length and has passed an examination given by one of the national certifying agencies. The training program must meet the standards set by the National Accrediting Agency for Clinical Laboratory Sciences (NAACLS).

Certifying Agencies and Titles Granted

- American Medical Technologists
  MLT(AMT) Medical Laboratory Technician
- American Society of Clinical Pathologists
  MLT-AD(ASCP) Medical Laboratory Technician, Associate Degree
- American Society of Clinical Pathologists
  MLT-C(ASCP) Medical Laboratory Technician, Certificate
- National Certification Agency for Medical Laboratory Personnel
  CLT(NCA) Clinical Laboratory Technician
- International Society for Clinical Laboratory Technology
  RLT(ISCLT) Registered Laboratory Technician

Certified Medical Assistant

The medical assistant attends a 1- to 2-year training program at a community college, vocational-technical school, or a private institution. Upon course completion, the medical assistant is well advised to seek certification through a credentialing process. Before working in a laboratory, the assistant may be required to complete additional specialized courses. These may be offered at an institution of higher learning or through a medical laboratory as part of on-the-job training. In the laboratory setting, the *certified medical assistant* performs the same duties as the laboratory assistant/phlebotomist.

Certifying Agencies and Titles Granted

- American Association of Medical Assistants (AAMA)
  CMA Certified Medical Assistant
- Accrediting Bureau of Health Education Schools (ABHES)
  RMA Registered Medical Assistant
- California Certifying Board for Medical Assistants
  CCMA-C(CCBMA) California Certified Medical Assistant-Clinical

Laboratory Assistant/Phlebotomist

The *laboratory assistant/phlebotomist* is a multiskilled professional who has received specialized training in the collection and preparation of laboratory specimens.

Under the direction of a technically certified supervisor, this individual must demonstrate proficiency in performing the duties of the position before being authorized by the employer or the agency to assume full responsibility.

GUIDELINES

Responsibilities of the Laboratory Assistant/Phlebotomist

- Collect adequate blood specimens by correct venipuncture technique or microtechnique from adults, children, and infants.
- Correctly label, process, and store all specimens according to departmental policy.
- Start glucose tolerance procedures and collect remaining specimens at the required times; draw other timed specimens as indicated.
- Perform automated testing of given laboratory specimens.
- Assist, as directed by supervisor, in testing procedures.

Laboratories operate under the direction of a *pathologist,* a physician specially trained in the nature and cause of disease, or *a clinical laboratory scientist* with a doctorate degree.

Medical laboratories are located in either hospitals or nonhospital facilities. Nonhospital facilities include physician's offices, clinics, public health departments, health maintenance organizations (HMOs), and private *reference laboratories.*

The laboratory is divided into various departments, which may include **hematology,** chemistry, microbiology, specimen collection and processing, blood bank, coagulation, **serology, histology,** cytology, toxicology, urinalysis, and special chemistry. The laboratory in the physician's office usually performs procedures in hematology, chemistry, microbiology, serology, and urinalysis.

PROCEDURE 1–1

Laboratory Personnel Interview

Principle

To learn about laboratory operations and the roles and responsibilities of laboratory workers

Procedural Steps

1. Choose an individual that works in your laboratory training facility or in one of the laboratories located in your community. Meet with this person and ask him/her the following questions.
   a. How long have you worked in the laboratory?
   b. Where did you receive your laboratory training?
   c. Are you required to be licensed or certified?
   d. How many people are employed here? What are their areas of expertise?
   e. What are your responsibilities in the laboratory?
   f. Does your laboratory have a procedure or protocol book? May I see it? (Look at the book and write a paragraph on what it contains and how it is organized.)
   g. What is this laboratory's procedure for processing tests?
   h. Is this laboratory divided into testing areas?
   i. What percentage of the tests performed are done by computer or automation?
   j. Question of your choice:
   k. Question of your choice:
2. Using the information you received and observed, write a two-page report on the laboratory you visited. Include your impressions and opinions.

Clinical Pathology Laboratory

Clinical Chemistry

The clinical chemistry section is one of the largest areas in the clinical laboratory.

TEST

Essential Clinical Laboratory Tests

- Blood gases
- Blood glucose
- Blood urea nitrogen (BUN)
- Enzyme analysis
- Serum creatinine
- Serum electrolytes (sodium, potassium, bicarbonate, chloride)
- Serum iron and iron-binding levels
- Serum lipids (triglycerides, cholesterol)
- Quantitative measurement of serum proteins

The clinical chemistry section usually has a **toxicology** area for drug analysis and an area for the analysis of hormones. Other procedures generally conducted in this section are bilirubin level and liver function analysis and cerebrospinal fluid and gastric fluid analyses.

This section has become highly automated, and most of the clinical procedures require a smaller volume of blood for each analysis than in the past. Automation has greatly increased the efficiency and quality assurance within the clinical chemistry section (Fig. 1–1).

Figure 1–1. *Working in the chemistry laboratory.*

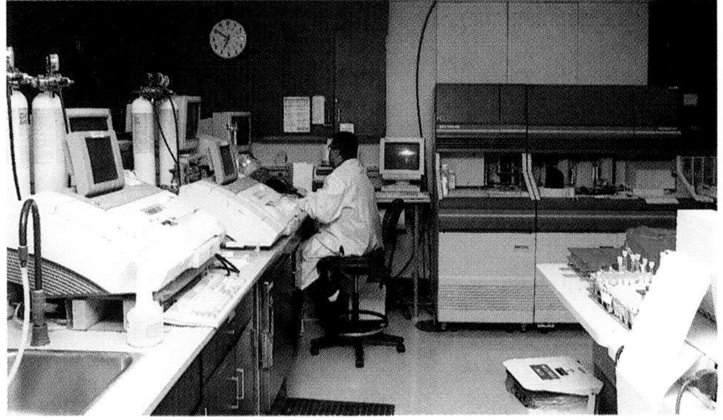

Hematology

In the hematology section of the laboratory, **assays** are conducted to identify diseases of blood-forming tissues. Body changes can be evaluated through changes in the blood. Frequently, coagulation studies, clinical microscopy, and urinalysis are subdivisions within the hematology section. Hematologic results are extremely valuable diagnostic tools and are often integral parts of a patient's examination. Most health care facilities require that the hematologic assay referred to as the complete blood count (CBC) be run on every individual admitted as a patient to the health care facility. In fact, most physicians require that a CBC be done as part of every complete physical examination.

TEST

Components of the CBC

- Red blood cell count (RBC)
- White blood cell count (WBC)
- Hemoglobin (Hgb or Hb)
- Hematocrit (Hct or Crit)
- Differential white count (Diff)
- Erythrocyte indices (MCV, MCH, and MCHC)
- Platelet count

TEST

Other Assays Relating to Hematology

- Erythrocyte sedimentation rate (ESR)
- Eosinophil count
- Reticulocyte count
- Body fluid cell count
- Malarial smears

As most laboratories are now fully automated, blood specimens can now be assayed for various hematologic parameters simultaneously, and the results can be electronically computed.

Also in the hematology section, screening tests and confirmatory assays for **coagulation** (clotting) are performed. The two most common coagulation assays are prothrombin time (PT) and partial thromboplastin time (PTT). The platelet count and the fibrinogen assay are used to detect coagulation problems.

When a patient is seen in a health care facility, a urinalysis is performed on a random urine sample (see Unit II). The clinical microscopy and urinalysis area uses microscopic and chemical procedures to screen urine specimens for abnormalities. Assays performed on a urine specimen include the physical and chemical examination of urine. A microscopic examination is also performed to determine the presence or absence of crystals, casts, and white and red blood cells.

Clinical Microbiology

The principle tasks performed in the microbiology section of the laboratory are identifying and culturing bacterial pathogens and their toxins. In this section, bacterial **sensitivity** to a particular antibiotic is evaluated. When a physician wishes to have this type of an evaluation done, a culture and sensitivity test is requested.

ANALYZE

Classification Methods for Bacterial Pathogens

- Appearance after Gram staining
- Shape of the microorganisms (cocci, bacilli, spirochete)
- Whether it is **aerobic** or **anaerobic**

In addition to bacterial pathogens, the clinical microbiology section also analyzes pathogenic parasites, fungi, and viruses.

ANALYZE

Major Methods for Analysis

- Growth patterns of cultured microorganism
- Sensitivity of an organism to antibiotics
- Biochemical properties of an organism

Tests for **occult** blood in **feces,** urine, and other human secretions are frequently performed in the clinical microbiological section.

Specimens being tested and analyzed in the clinical microbiology section are highly infectious, and are frequently considered to be biohazardous. Thus, extreme caution must be exercised when collecting, processing, or disposing these specimens (Fig. 1–2).

Immunohematology-Serology

In the immunohematology-serology section of the laboratory, the major tasks include determining antigen-antibody reactions and blood banking.

TEST

Common Serologic Tests

- Venereal Disease Research Laboratory (VDRL)
- Rapid plasma reagin (RPR)
- Fluorescent treponemal antibody absorption (FTA-ABS)
- Cold agglutinins
- Febrile agglutinins
- Rubella
- Anti-streptolysin O titer (ASO titer)
- Anti-DNase B
- Fungus antibody tests
- Monospot

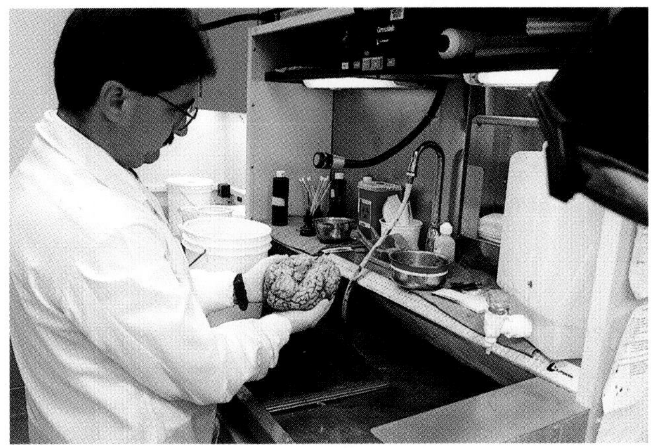

Figure 1–2. *Working in the anatomic pathology laboratory.*

The blood banking section assumes responsibility for providing blood products to a recipient when ordered. These products include whole blood, packed red blood cells, platelets, and fresh frozen plasma (FFP). Procedures performed in this section include the grouping and typing of donor and recipient blood, Rh antibody titer factoring, direct antiglobulin testing (Coombs' test), and hepatitis B surface antigen.

Anatomic Pathology Laboratory

Usually found in large laboratories, the anatomic **pathology** section has responsibility for forensic pathology, autopsy, **cytology,** histology, and DNA probe analysis. The major function of this section is to analyze body tissues for the cause and effect of disease. It is in this area that forensic medical procedures, such as DNA fingerprinting, are performed. Chromosomal analysis, genetic testing, and paternity determinations are also performed in this section. These tasks require competence in preparing specimens of peripheral blood, bone marrow, solid tissue, and amniotic fluid.

As the technology in this section is growing so rapidly, it is likely that, in the near future, all laboratories will be performing analyses in this area.

Summary

This chapter describes how different laboratory personnel, each with a specific specialty, work together to provide diagnostic treatment information that is often critical to a patient's health. Whatever the role you choose, working in a laboratory will always involve commitment and dedication.

Chapter Review

True or False

Circle T or F to indicate the correct answers to the following:

T F 1. One major area of the laboratory is the clinical laboratory department.

T F 2. The certified medical technologist has an associate degree.

T F 3. In the laboratory, the certified medical assistant performs the same duties as the laboratory assistant.

T F 4. A pathologist is a physician specially trained in diagnosing diseases.

Fill in the Blanks

Complete the following statements:

5. The chemistry section of the laboratory usually has a toxicology area for the analysis of ______________ and ______________ .

6. The most common coagulation assays are the ______________ and ______________ .

7. Assays performed on a urine specimen include the ______________ , ______________ , and ______________ .

8. Components of the complete blood count are ______________ , ______________ , ______________ , ______________ , and ______________ .

Multiple Choice

Circle the letter that represents the single best answer:

9. Common serologic testing may include:
   a. VDRL
   b. Rubella
   c. RPR
   d. a and b
   e. a, b, and c

10. Blood products include:
    a. Whole blood
    b. Packed RBCs
    c. Platelets
    d. Fresh frozen plasma
    e. All of the above

Vocabulary

AIDS: acquired immunodeficiency syndrome
asepsis: the absence of viable pathogenic organisms
asymptomatic: without signs or symptoms
autotrophs: organisms that are capable of producing needed nutrients as long as water, carbon dioxide, inorganic salts, and a source of energy are available
benign: noncancerous; not life-threatening
caustic: any substance that is destructive to living tissue
edema: an interstitial collection of fluid
germicidal agent: a drug that kills pathogenic microorganisms
HBV: hepatitis B virus
HIV: (human immunodeficiency virus) a virus that causes acquired immunodeficiency syndrome (AIDS) and that is transmitted through sexual contact and exposure to infected blood or blood components
infectious organisms: pathogenic microorganisms that invade the body, causing disease by local cellular injury
pathogenic: pertaining to an agent that causes or is capable of causing disease
pathogens: any disease-producing agent or microorganism
phagocytosis: the process by which certain cells surround, engulf, and digest microorganisms and cellular debris
reservoir host: a host that harbors infectious organisms, without sustaining injury or illness to self, and that may serve as a carrier of disease to others
septicemia: disease associated with toxins in the blood; blood poisoning
suppuration: the production of pus and purulent matter
UL: Underwriters' Laboratory
volatile: capable of boiling at a low temperature or evaporating quickly at room temperature

Chapter Objectives

After reading this chapter, you should be able to:

1. Define the vocabulary terms.
2. List the safety guidelines for proper use of electrical equipment.
3. Describe the information that Material Safety Data Sheets (MSDS) must include.
4. List the guidelines for minimizing chemical hazards in the laboratory.
5. Identify your local emergency phone numbers.
6. List the emergency equipment that should be readily available in the laboratory.
7. Outline the chain of infection.
8. Describe the types of hepatitis.
9. List the circumstances under which you are expected to wash your hands.
10. Identify the precautions to be observed when handling laboratory specimens.
11. List the precautions that should be observed when disposing of infective waste.
12. Demonstrate correct handwashing technique.

Chapter 2
Safety in the Laboratory

Safety rules are usually based on common sense. Most accidents occur when these rules are neglected, overlooked, or ignored. Accidents generally occur when safety is compromised because of haste and resultant shortcuts. These shortcuts can lead to personal injury and equipment damage. When an accident occurs, it must be reported to your supervisor immediately. Trying to cover up the incident can lead to serious, even disastrous results.

The U.S. Public Health Service's Centers for Disease Control (CDC) did considerable research on personal and environmental laboratory safety. From this research, a recommended set of safety regulations for the workplace, known as Standard Precautions, were established and the Occupational Safety and Health Administration (OSHA) was given the task of enforcing these precautions. According to the Standard Precautions regulations, all human blood and certain human body fluids are treated as if they are known to be infectious for human immunodeficiency virus (HIV), hepatitis B virus (HBV), and other blood-borne pathogens. The OSHA-organized Standards *must* be observed when dealing with all patients, regardless of their known or suspected diagnosis.

The major areas of greatest concern in the laboratory are divided into three classifications that are described as "laboratory hazards." These hazard areas are physical, chemical, and biological.

Laboratory Hazards

Physical Hazards

Physical hazards include fires resulting from electrical malfunction or alcohol lamps. All personnel must be familiar with the location of fire extinguishers and fire escape routes. All electrical equipment must be kept in proper repair, and manufacturer's instructions for use of the equipment must be followed.

GUIDELINES

Electrical Safety Regulations

- Use only grounded plugs that have been approved by Underwriters' Laboratory **(UL).**

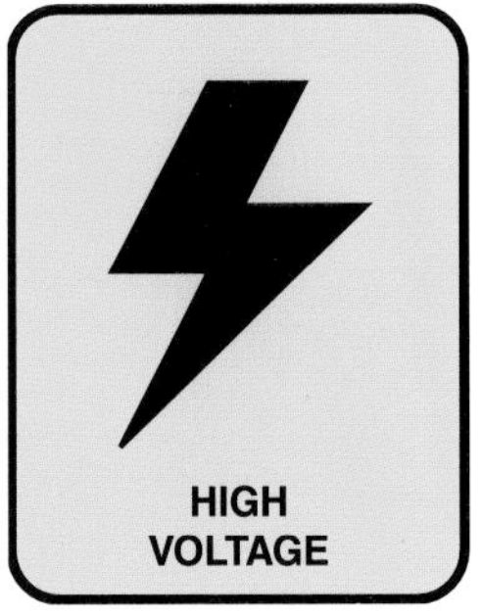

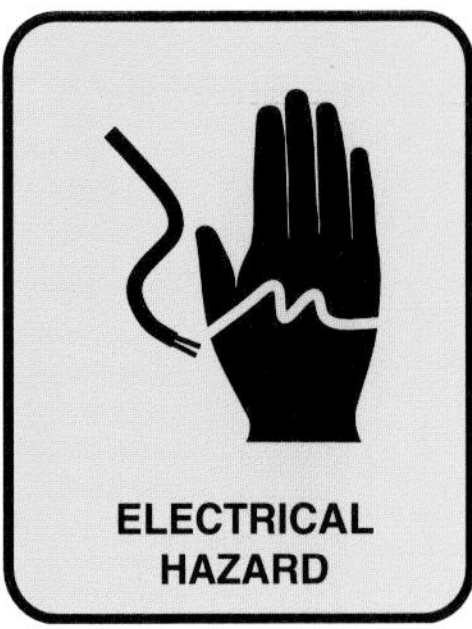

Figure 2–1. *High voltage and electrical hazard labels.*

- Never use extension cords.
- Avoid electrical circuit overloading.
- Inspect all cords and plugs periodically for damage.
- Use a surge protector on all sensitive electronic devices.
- Before servicing, UNPLUG the device from the electrical outlet.
- Use signs and/or labels to indicate high voltage or electrical hazards (Fig. 2–1).

Chemical Hazards

OSHA regulates and enforces safety and health procedures in the workplace. One of its major concerns is a safe working environment for those who produce and work with chemical substances. Chemical hazards include contact with corrosives, **caustics,** flammable materials, and toxic or carcinogenic substances. Caution should be exercised when handling any chemicals and specimens so as to avoid spills and splashes. Figure 2–2 shows warning labels that are used to identify areas in which specific substances are used. OSHA requires vendors of hazardous chemicals to provide Material Safety Data Sheets (MSDS) to all its customers. These sheets contain information on the proper storage, handling, and disposal of a given product, and also describe any health or safety risk associated with the use of the product. Each laboratory is required to maintain a notebook containing the MSDS for all chemicals used in that laboratory (Fig. 2–3).

GUIDELINES

Chemical Safety Regulations

- If the skin or eyes come in contact with any chemicals, immediately wash the area with water for at least 5 minutes.
- Store flammable or **volatile** chemicals in a well-ventilated area.
- After use, immediately recap all bottles containing toxic substances.
- Label all chemicals with the required MSDS information.

Biological Hazards

Biological hazards are those involving specimens and reagents that are capable of transmitting disease or that contain **pathogenic** bacteria.

GUIDELINES

Biological Safety Regulations

- Disinfect the laboratory work area before and after each use when dealing with biologicals.
- Never draw a specimen through a pipette by mouth. This technique is not permitted in the laboratory.
- Always wear gloves.
- Sterilize specimens and any other contaminated materials and/or dispose of them through incineration.
- Wash hands thoroughly before and after every procedure.

Extreme caution and good common sense are essential at all times when working in the laboratory. Regulations and precautions must be followed consistently.

The biohazard symbol (Fig. 2–4) indicates that the material within the container may contain **infectious organisms.** This symbol is placed on all containers that may contain certain disease-producing organisms, such as HBV and HIV. It serves to alert personnel to

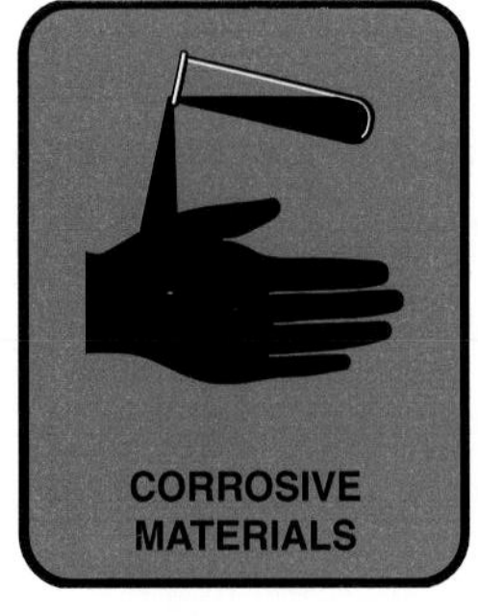

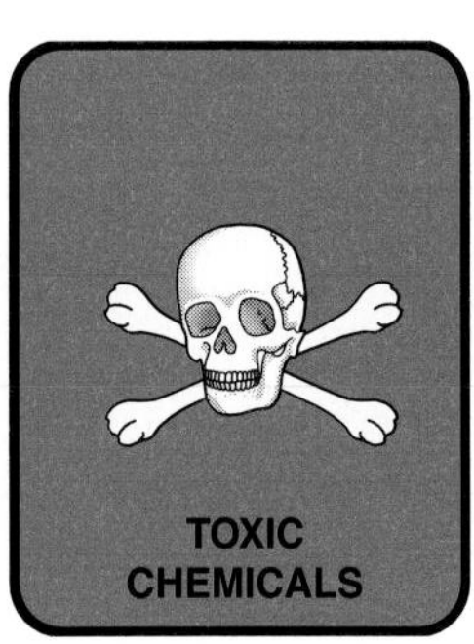

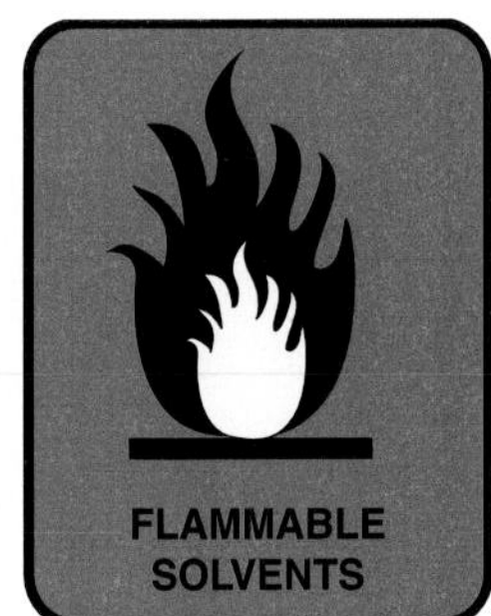

Figure 2–2. *Warning labels identify specific substances.*

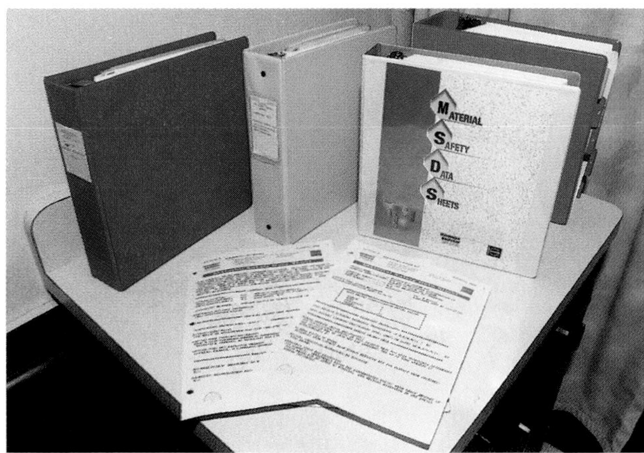

Figure 2–3. *Laboratory MSDS notebook.*

take additional precaution when handling and/or transporting the container. When the biohazard symbol appears on a container, the waste within the container must be incinerated or autoclaved before it is discarded.

Laboratory Safety

Rules

Safety begins with each member of the laboratory staff. Many of the dangers associated with the laboratory can be eliminated, or the risk of danger greatly reduced, if all laboratory employees are personally committed to safety.

GUIDELINES

Mandatory Safety Precepts

- Do not eat, drink, or smoke in the laboratory area.
- Never use a biohazard refrigerator for food or beverage storage.
- Wear a laboratory coat or apron in the laboratory area; remove it when leaving the laboratory area.
- Do not wear jewelry (although a plain wedding band is acceptable).
- Keep hair off your shoulders or contained within a laboratory cap or bonnet.
- Follow universal precautions at all times.

In addition to the guidelines just listed, emergency telephone numbers should be posted near the telephone, in plain view. Emergency numbers should be checked on a periodic basis to ensure that every number is current.

Emergency numbers to be posted should include emergency 911 or community emergency medical system (EMS), police department, fire department, hospital emergency room, and poison control center.

Equipment

A clinical laboratory poses frequent risks to safety because the specimens often contain pathogenic organisms. Standard safety supplies and equipment should be readily available in the clinical laboratory at all times, and all laboratory personnel should be trained in their use. In addition, depending on the type of laboratory, specialized safety equipment may be needed to protect laboratory personnel.

SUPPLIES AND EQUIPMENT

Safety Supplies and Equipment

- Biohazardous waste containers (Fig. 2–5)
- Body shower and eyewash station (Fig. 2–6)
- Fire blanket
- Fire extinguisher
- First aid equipment and supplies
- Latex gloves
- Safety eyewear (goggles)
- Full face shield
- Barrier gowns
- Sharps container (see Fig. 2–5)

Figure 2–4. *Biohazard symbol.*

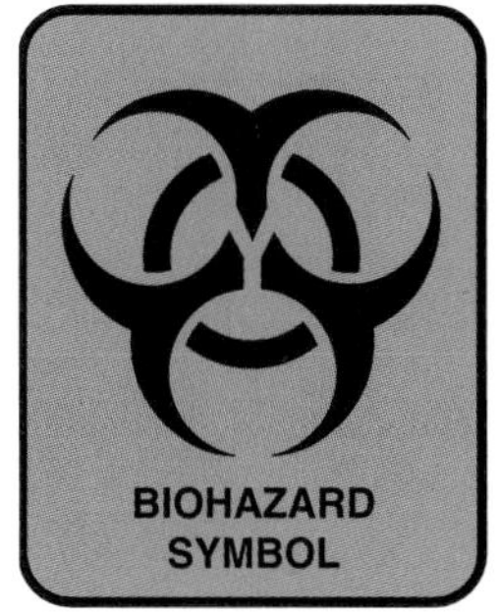

Figure 2–5. *Biohazardous waste and sharps containers.*

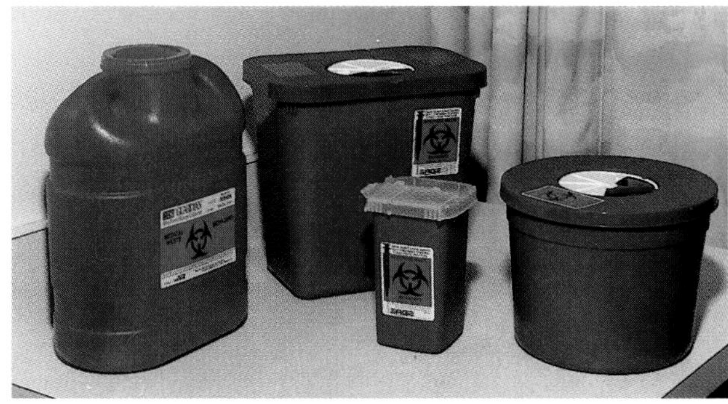

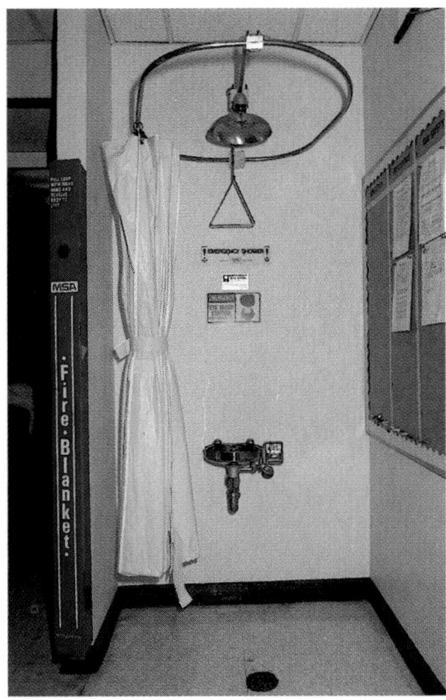

Figure 2–6. *Chemical shower and eyewash station.*

- Ventilated fume hood (Fig. 2–7)
- Biohazardous spill decontamination kits

Personal Safety

The Chain of Infection

The life and growth of pathogens is a cycle, or chain. When you break the chain, you stop the infectious process (Fig. 2–8).

Reservoir Host

Most infections originate with a **reservoir host,** which may be an insect, animal, or human. To survive, **pathogens** must gain access to a host. Once the organism receives nourishment from its host, it can grow and multiply. Pathogens may cause infection in the host, or they may be transmitted from the host to other healthy individuals, who then become reservoir hosts.

Means of Exit

In order for an organism to escape a host and continue to infect others, it must have a **means of exit.** Escape may be through the mouth, nose, eyes, ears, intestines, urinary tract, reproductive tract, or an open wound.

Means of Transmission

After escaping the reservoir host, organisms may spread by either direct or indirect transmission. Direct transmission occurs when another individual comes in direct contact with an infected person or with the discharges of an infected person (e.g., urine, saliva, and **feces**). Indirect transmission occurs when droplets are expelled by a host as a result of coughing or sneezing, when organisms are carried by insects (vectors), when contaminated food or drink is consumed, and when contaminated objects (fomites) are released into the air and taken in by the new host through respiration.

Means of Entry

The organism that has been transmitted–whether directly or indirectly–must find a means of entry into the new host. As with the means of exit, entry is gained through an opening in the body. The same route used to escape the reservoir host can thus be used to enter the new host.

If the host is one that is capable of supporting the growth of the infecting organism, the organism will multiply. Factors affecting susceptibility include the location of entry, the number of organisms (sometimes termed the organism's virulence), the living environment of the host, and the health of the new host.

Environmental Requirements

Certain environmental conditions must be present for microorganisms to survive. These conditions relate to nutrition, oxygen, temperature, darkness, moisture, and pH. **Autotrophs** are microbes that use nonliving substances as their source of food, whereas **heterotrophs**

Figure 2–7. *Ventilated fume hood.*

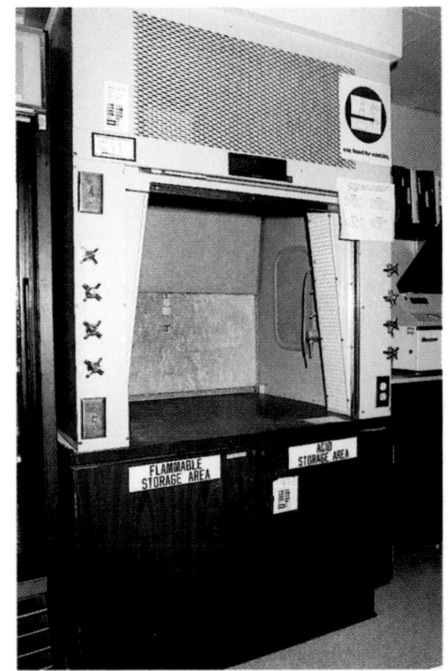

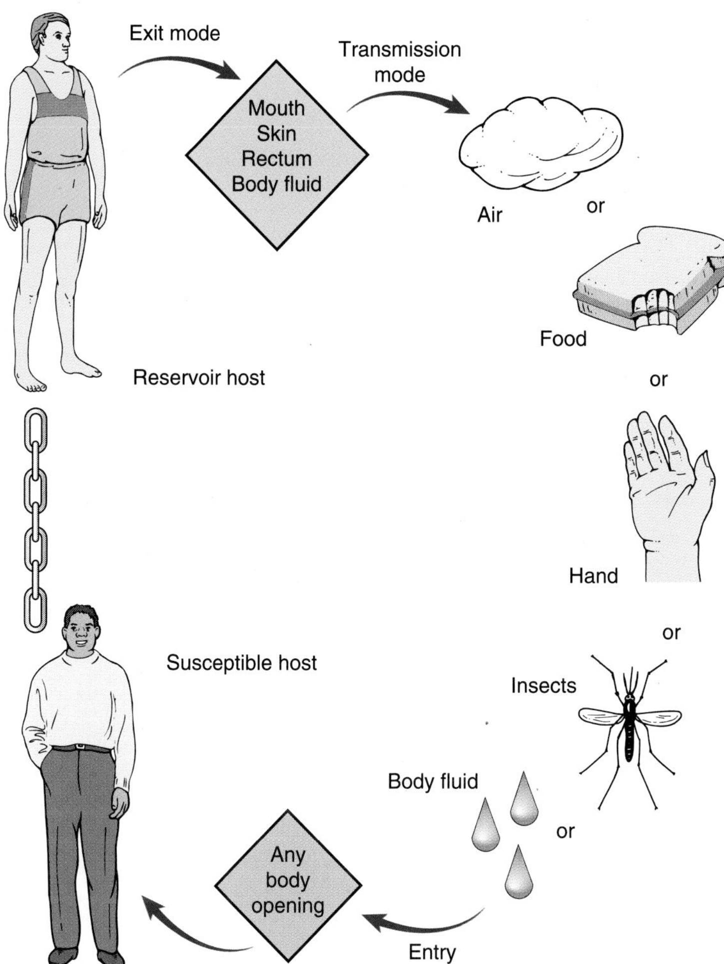

Figure 2–8. *Infectious process. (From Woods, M. A.* The Clinical Medical Assistant. *Philadelphia: W. B. Saunders, 1994, p. 5.)*

are microbes that receive their nourishment from living substances. Organisms that require oxygen to grow are classified as **aerobes;** those that grow best in the absence of oxygen are **anaerobes.** Each microorganism has a temperature at which it grows best, knows as its optimal growth temperature. In humans, this temperature is usually the same as the normal body temperature, or 98.6°F (37°C). Darkness provides an ideal environment for microbe development, as does moisture, which the organism needs for cell metabolism and waste elimination. A neutral pH (neither acid nor alkaline) is preferred by most microbes. If the environment becomes too alkaline or too acidic, the organisms will die. When conditions are right, the organisms reach infectious levels, the susceptible host becomes a reservoir host, and the cycle begins again.

The Inflammatory Response

When pathogenic organisms invade an individual's body, the response is called an inflammation. In order to fight this invasion, the body initiates specific reactions with the aim of destroying the pathogenic organism and its by-products.

1. The blood vessels at the site of injury or invasion dilate, and the number of white blood cells in the area increases, causing *redness.*
2. The white blood cells overpower and consume the pathogenic microorganisms in a process called **phagocytosis.**
3. Fluid in the injured tissues increases, creating edema (*swelling*), which puts pressure on the nerves and causes *pain.*
4. The increased blood supply to the area produces *heat.*

As this reaction proceeds, the cardinal symptoms of disease appear: inflammation, redness, swelling, pain, and heat. If the process is not reversed, it will continue as follows:

5. In a process called **suppuration,** pathogens, tissue cells, and white blood cells will collect in the area, forming a thick white substance known as pus.

6. If the pathogenic invasion is too great for the white blood cells to control, the infection may collect in the body's lymph nodes, where more white cells are present to help fight the battle. This causes swollen glands.
7. If the body is too weak, or the number of pathogens is too great, the infection may spread to the blood. This causes a systemic condition, called **septicemia** or blood poisoning, which ultimately may affect the entire body.
8. Without appropriate medical intervention, death can ensue. Laboratory assays must be done and the proper antibiotics must be administered to help the white blood cells bring the pathogenic invasion under control.

Maintaining an Aseptic Environment

Asepsis means freedom from infection or infectious materials. It can be further defined as the destruction of organisms after they leave the body. When we practice aseptic technique, we are directing our efforts at preventing reinfection or cross-infection. The goal is to isolate microorganisms by following OSHA standards, thereby creating a nonsterile but clean environment.

Handwashing

In a world of dangerous viruses, drug-resistant bacteria, and generally bad germs, the entire medical community has to be continuously reminded to wash their hands. The results of a 1995 study conducted at the State University of New York Health Science Center in Brooklyn revealed that only 14% to 59% of the physicians, 25% to 44% of the nurses, and 23% to 73% of the other health care personnel at that institution washed their hands before caring for patients.

Hands must be washed before and after each patient or activity. When hands are properly washed, infectious organisms are removed, and both the health care worker and the patient are protected. Thus, each laboratory sink should be equipped with a surgical soap dispenser (Fig. 2–9). The sink should also be equipped with a foot pedal for regulating water flow and temperature.

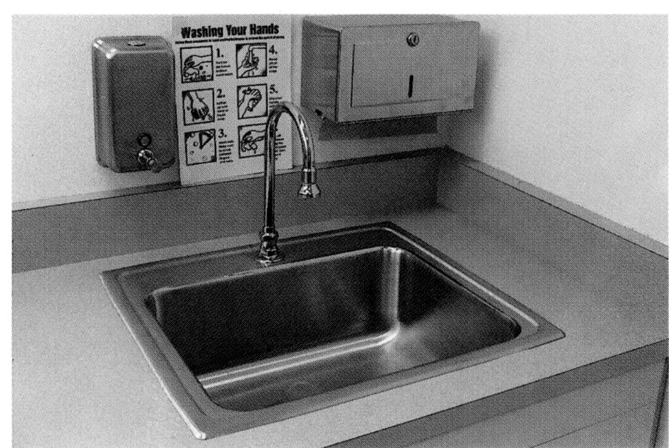

Figure 2–9. *Sink with soap dispenser.*

Proper handwashing depends on two factors: running water and friction. The water temperature should be tepid. Water that is too hot or too cold will chap the skin, and dry, cracked skin can be a source of contamination. Friction means the firm rubbing of all surfaces of the hands. Remember that your fingers have four sides plus fingernails.

GUIDELINES

When Hands Are to Be Washed

- Upon arriving at work each day
- After completing each activity throughout the day, including personal hygiene activities
- Before and after caring for each patient
- Immediately after accidental contact with blood and body fluids, even if gloves have been worn
- Immediately after the completion of any specimen processing
- Before and after eating
- Before and after using the restroom
- Before leaving for the day

PROCEDURE 2–1

Handwashing

Principle

Washing your hands with soap and tepid water and using friction will sanitize your skin before and after performing procedural tasks within the laboratory.

Equipment and Supplies

sink
soap
towels

PROCEDURE 2-1

Handwashing (Continued)

Procedural Steps

1. Remove all jewelry except for your wedding band (no gemstones) and watch.
2. Turn on the water and adjust it to tepid temperature.

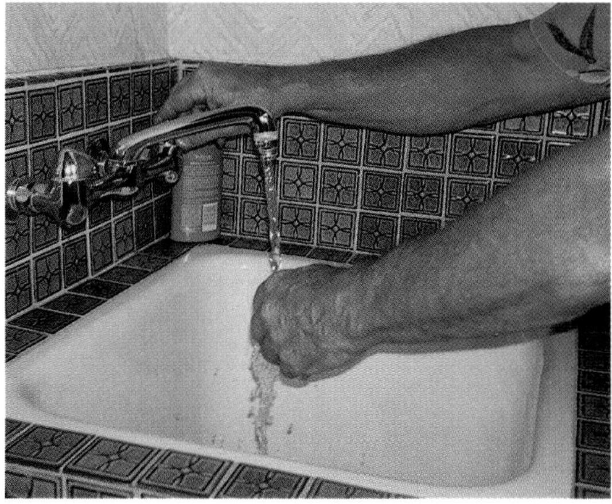

Adjust water to tepid temperature.

3. Wet hands, keeping fingertips lower than your wrists.

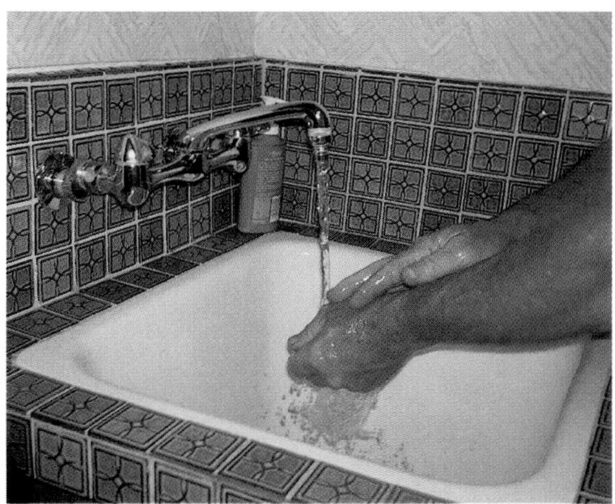

Wet hands, keeping finger tips lower than wrists.

4. Apply soap to both hands.

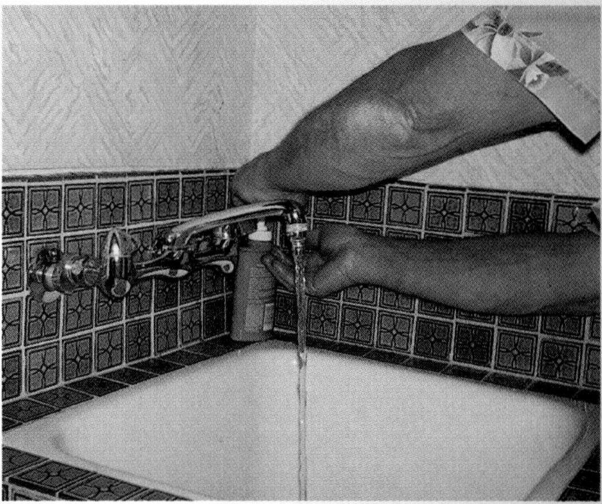

Apply soap to both hands.

5. Completely wash both hands, remembering that there are four sides to every finger.

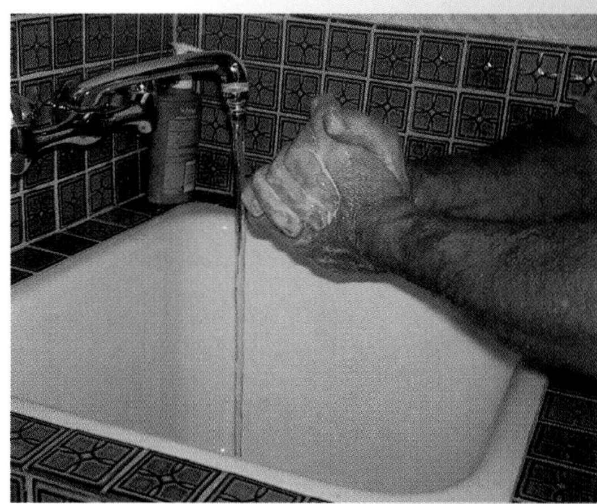

Completely wash both hands.

6. Check under the fingernails for possible debris. Remove any debris that is found.

(continued)

PROCEDURE 2–1

Handwashing (Continued)

7. Rinse your hands, keeping your fingertips below your elbows.

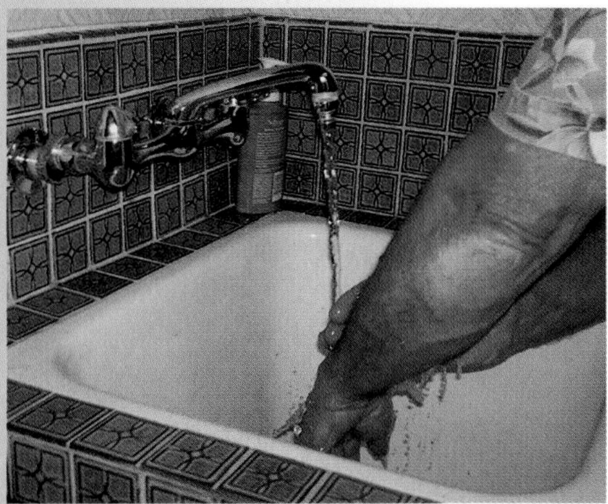

Rinse hands, keeping finger tips below elbows.

8. Dry hands completely.

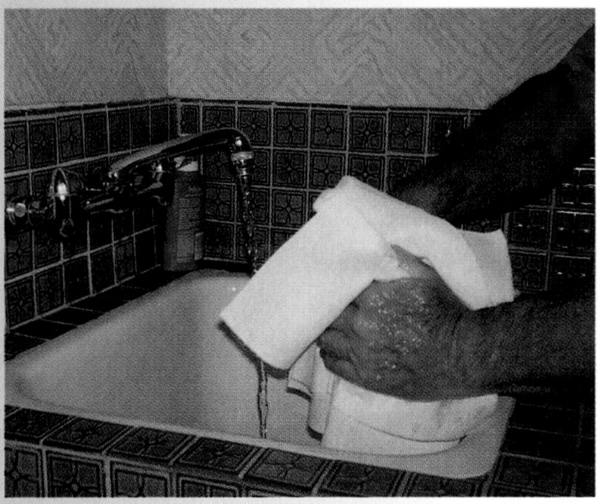

Dry hands completely.

9. Turn off the faucets using your elbow(s), or cover the faucets with a clean paper towel before touching them. DO NOT touch the faucets or the sink with your clean hands.

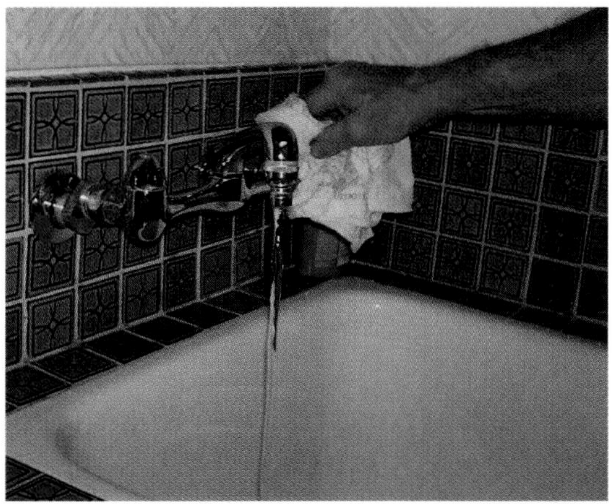

Cover faucets with a towel before turning them off.

Minimizing the Spread of Infection

In the clinical laboratory, the focus of attention is the analysis of body specimens, such as blood, urine, stool, and body exudates. All of these specimens contain pathogenic organisms and serve as a mode of transmission for infection. Everyone who handles and processes specimens must protect themselves against exposure to these pathogenic organisms. To help minimize the spread of infection in the clinical laboratory, all specimens should be handled and processed as if they contained infectious organisms. The exterior surface of specimen containers should always be wiped with a **germicidal agent.** Federal and state guidelines regarding disposal of infectious materials should be closely adhered to, and spills should be cleaned up, using a disinfectant, as soon as they occur.

Hepatitis and Acquired Immunodeficiency Syndrome (AIDS)

Hepatitis and acquired immunodeficiency syndrome **(AIDS)** represent constant threats to the health and safety of laboratory personnel. Both of these potentially deadly diseases are transmitted as a result of exposure to blood and body fluids from an infected individual. The infectious process is similar for both of these diseases.

Hepatitis

To date, scientists have been able to identify at least five types of hepatitis viruses.

Hepatitis A

Hepatitis A (HAV) previously called infectious hepatitis, is caused by type A virus. It is usually spread by the fecal-oral route as a result of improper personal hygiene methods or consumption of contaminated foods, such as shellfish. It is a very common form of viral hepatitis; indeed, approximately 143,000 cases were reported in the United States in 1994.

Hepatitis B

Hepatitis B **(HBV),** previously referred to as serum hepatitis, is caused by type B virus and is acquired **parenterally,** through contact with blood (transfusions, hypodermic needles, dental and surgical instruments) and body fluids (tears, saliva, semen). People who collect and process blood are considered to be at high risk for contracting HBV. Although most infected individuals recover, 10% of the population with HBV become chronic carriers.

Hepatitis C

Hepatitis C is caused by type C virus and is also known as hepatitis non-A, non-B/C virus. It affects approximately 170,000 Americans each year, and is the least known of the hepatitis viruses. Hepatitis C poses a serious health threat, as it often causes debilitating symptoms. In its chronic form, it can lead to severe, sometimes fatal, liver diseases, such as cirrhosis and cancer. Intravenous drug users are at highest risk for becoming infected with the virus, but health care personnel who come in frequent contact with blood and blood products are also at increased risk.

Hepatitis D

Hepatitis D, known variously as the delta virus or the delta agent, is not a complete virus in and of itself. Rather, it infects and causes illness only in persons who are already infected with HBV. When it does become active in the presence of HBV, it is extremely pathogenic.

Hepatitis E

Hepatitis E is also known as enteric (gastrointestinal) non-A, non-B hepatitis. This virus is usually acquired by consuming contaminated food or water. It is not known whether hepatitis E virus is present in the United States.

AIDS

AIDS is not a disease that can be casually contracted. Routine encounters with patients in the laboratory are not sources of **HIV** transmission. Comparing all the sexually transmitted diseases that are known to us, HIV is the most difficult to contract. Although the chances of contracting HIV are low, the serious nature of the infection and the probability of developing AIDS from the infection make it imperative that the laboratory assistant use precautionary procedures. AIDS is caused by a retrovirus known as HIV. Because many HIV carriers are **asymptomatic** and may not be aware that they have the virus, procedures to minimize the risk of exposure to blood and body fluids should be taken with all patients at all times. The current guidelines for diagnosing AIDS are based on the following criteria: (1) the presence of AIDS-related disorders, and (2) the T-cell count of an HIV-infected individual. The normal range for the T-cell count is 800 to 1600/cm of blood. The diagnosis of AIDS is applied to individuals with a T-cell count of 200/cm or less.

Compliance Guidelines

In January 1996 the CDC and the Hospital Infection Control Practices Advisory Committee (HICPAC) issued a new set of mandatory guidelines for isolation precautions. These guidelines are divided into two groups. *Standard Precautions* are a combination of the previous universal precautions, which dealt with reducing the risk of transmission of blood-borne pathogens, and body substance isolation precautions, which dealt with the risk of potential transmission of other body fluids. *Transmission-based precautions* are designed to be initiated in conjunction with the Standard Precautions if the patient is known to be or is suspected of being infected with a contagious pathogen that is transmissable by direct-contact, airborne, or droplet routes. The recommendations for preventing the transmission of HBV and HIV emphasize that Standard precautions be consistently used for all patients in all situations. These standards are divided into categories that must be followed by any employee with occupational exposure, regardless of the place of employment.

Parenteral Exposure

Parenteral exposure refers to the puncturing of the skin or mucous membranes such as occurs with needle sticks, bites, cuts, abrasions, or wounds.

Blood-borne Pathogens

Any exposure to a pathogenic microorganism, such as those that are present in human blood, may result in disease. Examples include HBV and HIV.

Infectious Materials

Many body fluids have the potential for being infectious, including semen and vaginal secretions, saliva, and cerebrospinal, synovial, pleural, pericardial, and amniotic fluids. In addition to these fluids, any fluid that cannot be identified or that contains visible blood should be considered to be hazardous. Unfixed human tissue, tissue cultures, and cells are among the materials included in the OSHA pathogenic standards.

This simple strategy is based on consistent compliance with the recommended procedures for handling body substances of *all* patients. Implementation of this system eliminates the need for warnings. No additional precautions are necessary, even if the patient is infectious. These standards are designed to reduce the risk of cross-infection of any infective agent in any substance in any patient.

Standard Implementation

The OSHA standards require that every laboratory, regardless of its size, have a written plan that includes specific health and safety measures that are taken to minimize the risk of exposure. These measures must be followed closely. This plan must be made available for review by all laboratory employees and must be updated annually.

Control areas that the plan must cover include engineering controls, personal protection, work practice controls, housekeeping controls, and hepatitis immunization.

Engineering Controls

Engineering controls are used to eliminate health hazards from the workplace. These controls must be properly maintained as required to ensure safety for all laboratory personnel. Examples include the availability and use of biosafety cabinets and autoclaves.

Personal Protection Controls

Gloves

Gloves should be changed after contact with each patient and after handling specimens.

GUIDELINES

When to Wear Gloves

- When touching a patient's blood and body fluids, mucous membranes, or skin that is not intact
- When handling items and surfaces contaminated with blood and body fluids
- While performing venipuncture or other vascular interventions
- When handling and processing all specimens of blood and body fluids
- While cleaning and decontaminating spills of blood or other body fluids
- When disposing of bulk blood and supplies used in body fluid procedures

Gowns or Aprons

Gowns or aprons should be changed when soiled or wet and after cleaning body fluid spills.

GUIDELINES

When to Wear Cover Gowns or Disposable Plastic Aprons

- If it is probable that your clothing will be soiled with body substances
- When procedures are likely to generate splashes of blood or other body fluids
- When cleaning and decontaminating spills of blood or other body fluids

Masks and Eye Protection

Regular prescription glasses are not considered protective eyewear. Always change or clean protective wear if soiled or wet.

GUIDELINES

When to Use Masks and Protective Eyewear

- When performing procedures that are likely to generate droplets of blood or body fluids
- When performing laboratory procedures that have a high potential for generating droplets (e.g., blending, ultrasonic procedures, centrifugation, and vigorous mixing)

Work Practice Controls

Needles and Sharp Instruments

Special care must be taken to prevent injuries caused by use, cleaning, or disposal of needles and sharp instruments.

GUIDELINES

Precautions to Observe When Handling Needles and Sharp Instruments

- Do not recap needles.
- Do not bend or break needles attached to syringes.
- Do not remove needles from syringes.
- Immediately after use, dispose of syringes, needles, and scalpels in puncture-resistant containers. The container must be located as close as possible to the area where the procedure was done.
- If a needle cap must be replaced during work with specimens, recap with only one hand. Place the cap on a clean surface and insert the needle into it using the scoop method. Complete this technique with extreme caution (Fig. 2–10).

Laboratory Specimens

All blood and other body fluids from every patient should be considered infective.

GUIDELINES

Proper Method for Handling Specimens

- If a specimen must be sent to another laboratory for testing, place it in a well-constructed container with a secure lid. Then place this in a second container, such as an impervious bag, for transport.
- Use biologic safety cabinets if procedures generate droplets or spattering.
- Immediately decontaminate work surfaces with a disinfectant (e.g., a 1:10 dilution of 5.25% sodium hypochlorite [household chlorine bleach and water] or with a manufactured, OSHA-approved preparation for spill cleanup) after accidental spills of blood or body fluids and at the end of each procedure.
- Decontaminate any equipment that has been contaminated with blood or body fluid before attempting repair in the laboratory or before transport to the manufacturer.

Housekeeping Controls

Blood or Other Body Fluid Spills

GUIDELINES

Steps for Cleaning Up All Spills Involving Blood or Body Fluids

- Use proper barrier protection.
- First, clean and decontaminate all equipment

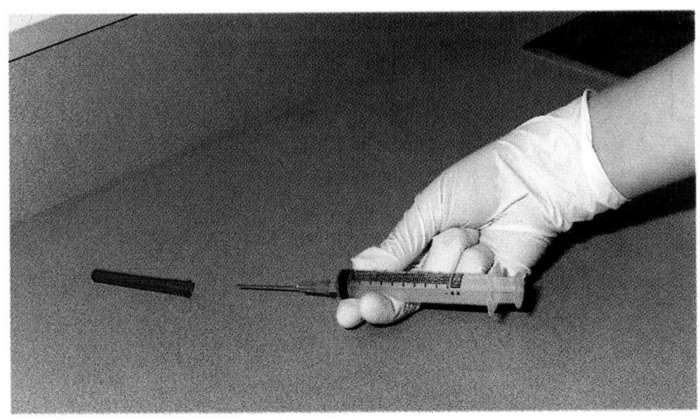

A

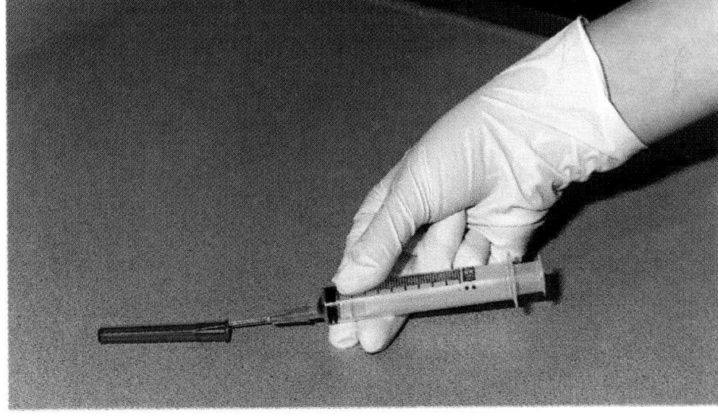

B

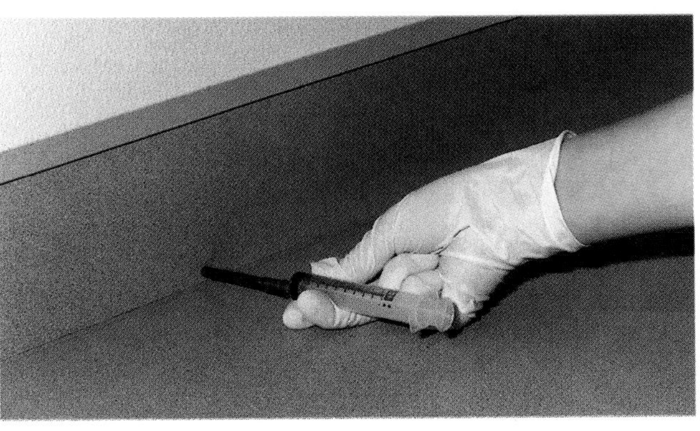

C

Figure 2–10. *Needle recapping procedure.* A, *Align the needle with the protective shield.* B, *Insert the needle into the shield.* C, *Secure the shield over the needle by pushing against a hard surface.*

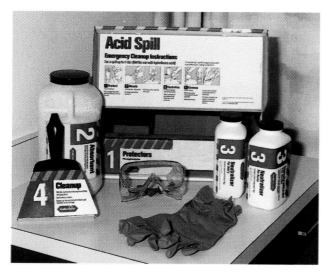

Figure 2–11. *Commercial spill cleanup kit. The kit shown is an acid-spill cleanup kit.*

and work surfaces with an appropriate commercial disinfectant (Fig. 2–11).

- Then place the spilled and the cleaning material immediately into an impervious bag at the spill site.
- Decontaminate the area with chemical germicides that are approved for use as hospital disinfectants. Household bleach solution may be used.
- If the spill is extensive, the contaminated area should be flooded with a liquid germicide and then cleaned and decontaminated with fresh germicidal chemical.
- Dispose of all materials, including gloves, apron, and mask, in a second impervious bag.
- Clean eyewear and wash hands thoroughly.

Infective Waste

Every laboratory should have written policies for the removal of infective materials from the facility. Listed below are precautions to follow, however, the written policies of your laboratory always take precedent.

GUIDELINES

Proper Methods for Removal of Infective Waste

- Decontaminate materials before placing in bags for disposal.
- Autoclave infective waste before disposal in a sanitary landfill or by incineration.

Figure 2–12. *Refusal document.*

Hepatitis B Vaccination Refusal

I have been advised by ______________________ that, due to my occupational exposure to blood or other possible infectious materials, I may be at risk of acquiring the HBV (hepatitis B virus). The risks and consequences involved have been fully explained to me; nonetheless, I refuse to consent to the proposed vaccination.

I hereby release ______________________ and its employees and volunteers from any liability for any ill effects that I may suffer from failure to receive the designated vaccination.

I understand that if, in the future I continue to have occupational exposure to blood or other infectious materials, I can receive the vaccination series, upon request, at no charge to me.

I confirm that I have read and fully understand the above and that all of the blank spaces have been completed prior to my signing.

____
Employee Name (printed)

______________________ ____________
Employee Signature Date

______________________ ____________
Witness Signature Date

____

The form must be signed and placed in the employee's personnel folder.

- Carefully pour bulk blood and body fluids down a drain connected to a sanitary sewer.
- Collect biohazardous waste in impermeable *red polypropylene bags or polypropylene bags that have been clearly marked with a biohazardous waste symbol* and seal tightly.
- Dispose of waste through heat treatment, incineration, steam sterilization, chemical treatment, or other equivalent methods that render the waste inactive.

Hepatitis B Immunization

OSHA standards require physicians to offer the hepatitis B vaccination series free of charge to all medical office personnel who may have occupational exposure. It is a three-dose series that is believed to give immunity to the virus. The immunization must be offered within the first 10 days of employment in an occupational risk area. Laboratory personnel who do not want to be vaccinated must sign a waiver form documenting refusal, which is to be filed in the employee's OSHA record (Fig. 2–12).

Summary

One cannot anticipate or prevent every health and safety risk. However, the risks are greatly reduced when everyone who works in a laboratory setting is conscious of safety in the workplace and diligently follows the established safety guidelines. Use good common sense. If you are in doubt about the safety of a procedure, ask your supervisor. If you are aware of a potential safety problem, report it to the person in charge. Remember, your welfare, the welfare of your co-workers, and the welfare of the patients you serve depends on your commitment to safety.

Chapter Review

True or False

Circle T or F to indicate the correct answers to the following:

T F 1. Universal Precautions were established to protect employers from lawsuits.

T F 2. All blood and certain other body fluids should be treated as if known to be infected with HIV or HBV.

T F 3. When the skin or eyes come in contact with any chemicals, you should immediately wipe them with a clean towel.

T F 4. A type of biological hazard is mouth pipetting.

T F 5. It is acceptable to store your lunch in a biohazard refrigerator as long as it is kept in an airtight container.

T F 6. Two ways an organism can escape its host are via the mouth and eyes.

Fill in the Blanks

Complete the following statements:

7. The environmental requirements needed to keep a microorganism alive are ____________ , ____________ , ____________ , ____________ , ____________ , and ____________ .
8. ____________ use nonliving substances as a source of food.
9. The medical term for blood poisoning is ____________ .
10. Proper handwashing depends on ____________ and ____________ .

Multiple Choice

Circle the letter that represents the single best answer:

11. The type of hepatitis that is of the greatest concern in the laboratory is:
    a. Hepatitis A
    b. Hepatitis B
    c. Hepatitis C
    d. Hepatitis D
    e. Hepatitis E
12. Parenteral exposure refers to:
    a. Puncturing of the skin or mucous membranes
    b. Hereditary diseases
    c. Broken bones
    d. Parent and/or family contacts
    e. Child abuse

Vocabulary

authorized person: an individual authorized under state law to order tests or receive test results, or both

automated testing: laboratory testing in which a series of steps are performed by a preprogrammed analyzer

calibration: the testing and adjustment of test systems to provide a known relationship between the measurement response and the substance value measured by the test

calibration verification: the assaying of calibration materials to confirm that the calibration has remained stable throughout the laboratory's reportable range for patient test results

manual testing: a method for obtaining laboratory test results that involves performing a series of steps by hand or by personal physical means

quality assurance: a set of policies and procedures that are followed to ensure that every test performed is valid

quality control: the process by which final results are validated and variations are quantified

reference value: the range of test values expected for a designated population of individuals (e.g., 95% of individuals presumed to be healthy)

reportable range: the range of test values over which the relationship between the testing instrument, kit, or system's measurement response has been shown to be valid

Chapter Objectives

After reading this chapter, you should be able to:

1. Define quality control and list related policies and procedures.
2. Explain the purpose of the Clinical Laboratory Improvement Amendment (CLIA 1988).
3. List the objectives of quality control.
4. Define JCAHO and describe its purpose.
5. What quality assurance (QA) tools are found in a quality care facility?
6. List the components for implementing a QA program.
7. Outline the areas of preparation for a physician's office laboratory (POL) inspection.

Chapter 3
Quality Assurance/Quality Control

Clinical laboratory personnel performed quality work and provided quality results long before the terms **quality assurance** and **quality control** became popular. Quality assurance (QA) refers to a set of policies and procedures that are followed to ensure that every test performed is valid. These policies assure the patient that the results of the tests performed are accurate and can safely be used to guide treatment. Quality control (QC) is the process by which final results are validated and variations are quantified. The principles of quality are rooted in both fact and perception. Doing the right thing, the right way, the first time, and on time are all aspects of quality. These aspects of quality, when applied to the health care setting, are often driven by outside agencies, whether government-sponsored (e.g., the Food and Drug Administration [FDA]) or voluntary (e.g., accrediting agencies, such as the Joint Commission on the Accreditation of Health Care Organizations [JCAHO]).

Clinical Laboratory Improvement Act (CLIA 1988)

In 1988, with the passage of the Clinical Laboratory Improvement Act (CLIA), clinical laboratories were required to participate in a recognized proficiency testing program for laboratory tests performed (Fig. 3–1).

Programs Recognized for Laboratory Proficiency Testing

- American Association of Bioanalysts (AAB Proficiency Testing Service)
- American Academy of Family Physicians (AAFP): AAFP-PT
- American Society of Internal Medicine (ASIM): Medical Laboratory Evaluation (MLE)
- College of American Pathologists (CAP): External Comparative Evaluation for Laboratories (EXCEL)

HIGHLIGHTS OF CLIA 1988

Purpose of CLIA 1988

In 1988, Congress passed the Clinical Laboratory Improvement Amendments (CLIA 1988) to improve the quality of laboratory testing in the United States. CLIA 1988 consists of federal regulations governing all facilities that perform laboratory tests for health assessment or for the diagnosis, prevention, or treatment of disease. CLIA 1988 includes facilities not previously covered under federal legislation, such as physician's office laboratories (POLs) and nursing homes. The regulations for implementing CLIA, developed by the Department of Health and Human Services (DHHS), consist of four separate sets of rules: laboratory standards, application and user fees, enforcement procedures, and approval of accreditation programs.

Categories of Laboratory Testing

The CLIA regulations establish three categories of laboratory testing based on the complexity of the testing methods:

Low-Complexity Tests: Low-complexity tests are simple procedures, including those that patients can perform at home. Laboratories that perform only low-complexity tests must apply for a certificate of waiver, which exempts them from many of the CLIA oversight requirements. Laboratories with certificates of waiver are still expected to adhere to good laboratory practices, which include following the manufacturer's recommended instructions for each product or testing kit. There are only nine waived laboratory tests:

- Dipstick or tablet reagent urinalysis (nonautomated) for bilirubin, glucose, hemoglobin, ketones, leukocytes, nitrite, pH, protein, specific gravity, and urobilinogen
- Fecal occult blood tests
- Ovulation testing, using visual color comparisons
- Urine pregnancy tests, using visual color comparisons
- Erythrocyte sedimentation rate, nonautomated
- Hemoglobin by copper sulfate method, nonautomated
- Spun microhematocrit
- Blood glucose determination with devices approved by the FDA for home use

Moderate-Complexity Tests: Moderate-complexity tests account for 75 percent of the estimated 10,000 laboratory tests performed in the United States. Examples of moderate-complexity tests performed in the medical office include throat cultures, white blood counts, rapid strep tests, cholesterol, HDL and triglyceride testing with an automated analyzer, Gram staining, urine cultures, pinworm preps, and microscopic analysis of urine sediment.

High-Complexity Tests: High-complexity tests include all procedures related to cytogenetics, histopathology, histocompatibility, and cytology (includes PAP testing). These tests are not usually performed in medical offices; most of these tests are done in laboratories already subject to federal regulation.

Requirements for Moderate- and High-Complexity Testing

Laboratories performing moderate- or high-complexity tests, or both, must meet the CLIA regulations and are subject to unannounced inspections every 2 years by the Department of Health and Human Services. The major components of the CLIA 1988 regulations relating to laboratory standards are listed here:

Patient Test Management: A system must be established to maintain the optimal integrity and identification of patient specimens throughout the testing process and to ensure accurate reporting of results.

Quality Control: To ensure accurate and reliable test results, each laboratory must establish and follow written quality control procedures that monitor and evaluate the quality of each testing process. These include developing a laboratory procedure manual, following the manufacturer's instructions for each product; performing and documenting calibration procedures at least every 6 months and two levels of controls daily; performing and documenting actions taken when problems or errors are identified; and documenting all quality control activities.

Quality Assurance: Each laboratory must establish and follow written policies and procedures to monitor the overall quality of the total testing process.

Proficiency Testing (PT): Proficiency testing is a form of external quality control in which laboratory specimens are prepared by an approved proficiency testing agency. Three times a year, the physician's laboratory must test a shipment of these unknown specimens using the same procedure as for testing a patient's specimen. The results are then forwarded to the proficiency testing agency for evaluation.

Personnel Requirements: The CLIA regulations specify qualifications and responsibilities for personnel for laboratory directors, technical consultants, clinical consultants, and testing personnel. The regulations list specific education and training qualifications for the various positions and also define the responsibilities for the persons who fill these positions. Personnel requirements are most stringent for high-complexity testing.

Figure 3–1. *Highlights of CLIA 1988. (From Bonewit-West, K.* Clinical Procedures for Medical Assistants. *Philadelphia: W. B. Saunders, 1994, p. 294.)*

The health care reforms of 1994 have given rise to numerous discussions within the American Medical Association (AMA), as well as other physicians' groups. The physicians' groups have suggested several proposals that would greatly change the current regulations. The most prevalent reason cited for these changes and discussions is the tremendous number of laboratory functions that now involve totally **automated testing.** Because a machine performs and reads the results of a given test, the physicians believe it is both unnecessary and expensive to require "expert" readings. There is broad-based support for exempting physician's office laboratories (POLs) from proficiency testing requirements.

Although numerous concessions have already been made to ease the regulations for POLs, the AMA is still pushing for complete repeal of CLIA 1988 for their constituents.

In April of 1995, the goal of relaxing the regulatory burdens imposed by CLIA 1988 received a boost with the introduction of remedial legislation entitled "Clinical Laboratory Improvement Act of 1995." The aim of this two-page bill is simply to exempt POLs from the regulations, except for POLs that perform Papanicolaou (PAP) smear testing. It is believed that this bill would increase physicians' level of efficiency and reduce test costs to patients by eliminating the burdensome paperwork and costs associated with compliance.

A major streamlining of the CLIA 1988 regulations may be in the offing as part of a regulatory reform drive. At present, the Centers for Disease Control (CDC) are discussing how to reduce the scope of the CLIA regulations as part of this process.

CLIA Certification Levels for Clinical Laboratories

In 1994, the CLIA established three levels of certification for POLs: low complexity (waiver), moderate complexity, and high complexity. Laboratories may be certified according to the complexity of the tests performed. Thus, a laboratory that is certified as a waiver-level laboratory is authorized to perform only the nine tests identified in the waiver list.

TEST

Nine Low-Complexity Tests (Waiver)

- Dipstick or tablet reagent urinalysis (nonautomated) for bilirubin, hemoglobin, leukocytes, protein, specific gravity, glucose, ketones, nitrite, pH, and urobilinogen
- Fecal occult blood
- Ovulation testing, using visual color comparisons for detection of human luteinizing hormone
- Urine pregnancy tests, using color comparisons
- Erythrocyte sedimentation rate (nonautomated)
- Hemoglobin by copper sulfate method (nonautomated)
- Blood glucose determinations, using monitoring devices approved by the FDA for home use
- Spun microhematocrit
- Hemoglobin determinations (automated), using devices that provide direct measurement and readout

When a laboratory is certified for moderate-complexity testing, it may perform all of the waiver tests plus all of the moderate-level tests. There are 7500 tests included in the list of moderate-complexity tests.

TEST

Examples of Moderate-Complexity Tests

- Automated chemistry
- Automated blood gases
- Automated hematology
- Manual differential counts
- Microscopic urinalysis
- Slide and tube agglutination tests
- Direct antigen tests
- Urine culture and colony counts (kits only)
- Throat culture screening

Laboratories that are classified as high-complexity laboratory facilities may perform all levels of testing. These are usually large hospital laboratories or reference laboratories that are staffed with a full complement of laboratory personnel. There are 2500 tests designated as high-complexity tests.

TEST

Examples of High-Complexity Tests

- All cytologic, cytogenic, histopathologic, and histocompatibility tests
- Chemistries (nonautomated)
- Flame photometry
- Radioimmunoassay
- Bone marrow examination
- Hematology procedures (manual)
- Differential count (manual)
- Isolation and identification of bacteriological cultures

Quality Control (QC)

The primary objective of a laboratory QC program is to ensure the accuracy of test results while detecting and eliminating error. QC is simply the application of methods and means to ensure that test results are reliable and valid, and that errors that may interfere with obtaining accurate test results are detected and eliminated. One method by which this is accomplished is through **calibration verification.** QC is a major part of the routine in most clinical laboratories, and is an ongoing process. Mandated by law, QC programs monitor all phases of laboratory activity, from specimen collection through processing, testing, and reporting results. QC programs monitor supplies, reagents, machinery, personnel, and actual test performance. Equipment performance and maintenance are also monitored. Specially prepared QC samples are tested along with samples from patients. The results of testing performed on the QC samples must be within a pre-established range before patient results can be reported. The QC samples, called controls, are usually supplied with prepackaged kits intended for use in the small laboratory. The controls should be analyzed at specified intervals. For example, the positive and negative controls supplied with pregnancy test kits should be tested along with each patient specimen. Urinalysis dipsticks (used for chemical examination of urine) should be checked daily and each time a new container is opened. Controls for automated chemistry analyses should be monitored at specified intervals during the day. Consistent results of controls ensure constant conditions throughout the testing sequence.

Quality Assurance (QA)

Physicians routinely use clinical laboratory test results for diagnosing and treating their patients. Thus, every step in the formulation of these results must be of superior quality. Clinical laboratories are responsible for the methodology that assures reliable, accurate test results. QA is a comprehensive set of policies and procedures developed to ensure the quality of laboratory testing. It includes quality control, personnel orientation, laboratory documentation, knowledge of laboratory instrumentation, and enrollment in a proficiency testing program. QA focuses on establishing a series of operating policies to produce reliable laboratory results. These policies benefit the patient by providing quality care.

These policies also benefit the physician by reducing liability for inaccurate reporting of test results. In order for a physician to use a laboratory test in establishing a diagnosis, the results must be compared with **reference values.** These values are established for the population in the laboratory's geographic area. Reference values or ranges are often regional, and may differ in other parts of a country or in different countries. Age, sex, and physical conditions may also affect the reference values. Determining the reference values for a patient in your population is an important part of QA.

The QA system enables the laboratory to assess, verify, and document the quality of the test results. These policies provide guidelines for the performance of laboratory duties and make it possible to detect small but significant changes from the usual performance level before erroneous patient test results are reported.

Laboratory Testing Facilities

The number of laboratory tests performed and the site where these tests are conducted depend largely on the nature of the patient's disease or condition and the physician's speciality. For example, an internist would be likely to perform blood chemistry testing in the office, whereas a pediatrician would probably not perform such tests at all.

Physician's Office Laboratories

The medical facility may contain its own laboratory in which simple screening tests and/or automated tests are performed, such as urinalysis and hematocrit and hemoglobin determinations, and where blood samples are drawn for specific analyses to be done in a commercial laboratory. In a POL, you will be required to be proficient in all areas of testing.

It is the physician's responsibility to utilize laboratory test results for both diagnosis and treatment of the patient. It is the responsibility of the POL worker to be certain that all test results are accurate as reported. Most physicians utilize both types of facilities to fulfill their diagnostic needs.

Commercial Laboratories

Commercial laboratories must meet the CLIA regulations based on the three categories of testing complexity. They are subject to unannounced inspections every 2 years by the Department of Health and Human Services. Because of these regulations, commercial testing laboratories provide office laboratories with a laboratory directory to be used as a source of reference for proper methods of specimen collection and handling (Table 3–1).

Table 3–1
Sample Page from a Laboratory Directory

Laboratory Test	***Test #***	***Draw/Requirement***
Cryofibrinogen	1050	1 SST 2 ml serum. *Do not refrigerate or freeze.*
Cryoglobulins (Qual.)	1055	1 SST 2 ml serum. *Do not refrigerate or freeze.*
Cryptococcal antigen, serum or CSF	7605	1 SST or CSF 1 ml serum. Separate from cells, freeze in plastic tube; and/or 1 ml frozen CSF.
Cryptococcus antibody (N1 #3121)	5208	1 SST 1 ml serum
Cryptococcus antigen (N1 #3122)	5206	1 SST or CSF 1 ml serum. Separate from cells, freeze in plastic tube; and/or 1 ml frozen CSF.
Cryptosporidium/giardia (DFA)	8713	Stool sample Submit stool in plastic screw-cap container. Hold sample at room temperature.
Crystals, body fluid	200	Body fluid 2 ml of body fluid in plastic tube. Separate from cells; freeze in plastic tube.
Crystal stone analysis (N1 #2016)	5427	Stone Place stone in plastic tube for transport to lab.
Culture and sensitivity (includes organism I.D.)		Performed per organism when indicated
Culture, AFB	8919	Sample varies Sample in sterile glass container. Hold sample at room temperature. Note source and patient's date of birth.
Culture, bacterial routine	5654	Swab tube or fluid in sterile container Place swab or fluid from appropriate source in transport container. Hold sample at room temperature. Do not refrigerate. Note source on requisition.
Culture, blood	8901	Blood culture bottle Submit bottle after adding the quantity of blood indicated on label. Prepare skin with iodine, no alcohol. Hold sample at room temperature. Incubate at 37°C if possible.
Culture, campylobacter	8750	Stool sample or rectal swab Submit stool in plastic screw-cap container. Hold sample at room temperature. *Do not refrigerate.*

JCAHO's 10 Steps to a Quality Assurance Plan

1. Assign responsibility.
2. Delineate scope of care.
3. Identify important aspects of care.
4. Identify indicators related to these aspects of care.
5. Establish thresholds for evaluation.
6. Gather and organize data.
7. Evaluate care when thresholds are reached.
8. Take corrective action.
9. Assess the effectiveness of the actions; document improvement.
10. Communicate relevant information.

Quality Assurance Programs

QA programs have become part of the laboratory accreditation standards established by the College of American Pathologists. The JCAHO has been instrumental in providing direction to facilities wishing to implement QA programs, and laboratories that implement QA programs are awarded a certificate of registration. Certified facilities are those judged to provide quality care that is effective, acceptable to the patient, accessible, efficient/appropriate, and continuous/consistent. JCAHO has outlined 10 steps involved in designing and implementing a QA program.

JCAHO also believes that the health care staff should be involved in the entire QA process, from design to evaluation. The program can be designed to focus attention on the important aspects of care that are high-risk, high-cost, or problematic.

A well-designed QA program enables laboratory staff to identify problem areas that require corrective measures, as well as areas that are already cost-effective and of high quality.

The laboratory that performs the tests is responsible for preparing the procedure manuals. This information must be provided to every laboratory employee. Adherence to these procedures will reflect accurately a given patient's condition and lead to a positive patient outcome.

Program Implementation

In order for a laboratory to design a QA program, it is necessary to first identify all the elements relevant to a given area. These elements include skills needs, technique, QC, supplies, and perceptions of customer approval. Recognizing which of these elements involve high volume, high risk, or high cost, and which are problematic will provide additional direction in plan design and development. Indicators can then be identified and thresholds established.

Having decided which of these key indicators should be monitored, data can be gathered and ana-

Guidelines for Facility QA Documentation for Quality Care

- Information important to decision making is communicated (usually by memorandums, newsletters, staff meetings, or logbooks).
- Orientation and training are well structured and contain checklists pertaining to the important aspects of the job.
- Continuing education is strongly encouraged and provided.
- Performance is monitored by supervisory personnel, compared with standards, and an annual appraisal is conducted.
- Standard operating procedure manuals are up to date.
- A personnel file exists for every employee.
- Proficiency/competency tests are distributed to the staff on an established methodical basis.
- Participation in scheduled QC and QA activities is included in job descriptions.
- Equipment and instrumentation are calibrated, maintained, and serviced according to an established schedule.
- Computer systems are validated before use and monitored thereafter.
- The workplace and immediate environment are safe.
- There are leaders who actively seek suggestions.
- Documentation of adherence to all of these guidelines is routinely and precisely done.

lyzed at a frequency suitable to the department. Employees are involved in data gathering; supervisory personnel usually summarize and analyze these data, proposing a course of corrective action when necessary.

Whenever an incident occurs that may affect patient perception or specimen quality, it should be reported to the appropriate laboratory supervisor. This information may help the laboratory diagnose problem areas, and the effectiveness of a particular course of action can then be evaluated.

Preparation for Inspection of a POL

The CLIA 1988-mandated inspection begins approximately 1 year prior to the date of the inspection. The *1990 Guide to OSHA Requirements for Hospital, Independent, and Physician Office Laboratories* provides an overview of the areas to be assessed and the steps that must be completed in preparation for the inspection. Remember that the OSHA inspection is usually unannounced.

Area 1

Make a complete laboratory inventory that includes an evaluation of all test procedures and the instruments that support the tests. Once this is completed, request a meeting with the laboratory director to identify the deficiencies that need to be corrected and/or eliminated. Attention should be given to out-of-date, costly, and seldom-used tests. **Remember that all tests must be within the certification level of the POL.**

Area 2

Follow the CLIA and OSHA guidelines to ensure that an adequate QA program exists for all tests, that a safety program is being used, and that there is a laboratory manual containing written documentation for all tests performed.

Area 3

Register the POL with the Health Care and Finance Administration (HCFA). (Request HCFA form 109.)

Area 4

Design a documentation system that includes all steps taken in laboratory testing. These might include, for example, the physician's order, specimen collection, testing procedure, QC measures, instrument and reagent maintenance, and reporting of test results. **Remember that proof is in the written word, NOT the verbal word.**

Area 5

Organize a precise QC program that includes every test performed in your laboratory. The key components should include recording test controls daily, performing statistical analyses monthly, and maintaining a diary of documented problems and the means by which they were resolved.

Area 6

Once all the procedures are running smoothly and procedure documentation is in order, apply for certification.

During this preparation for inspection, you may find that you need further help and guidance. CLIA and OSHA provide laboratory consultation to help you in completing this monumental task. Listed in the 1990 guide are numbers that you can call for assistance in your area. Do not be afraid to use them.

PROCEDURE 3–1

Designing a Quality Assurance Plan

Principle

As health care workers, we must all be concerned with the reliability of our procedures and the responsibility we have to the patients and physicians we serve. As you complete this procedure, never lose sight of this concept.

Procedural Steps

1. Design a model laboratory. List the testing areas, staffing, and possible responsibilities for each staff member. Brainstorm together to develop ideas and suggestions.
2. Design a flow chart. The chart should include

(continued)

PROCEDURE 3–1

Designing a Quality Assurance Plan (Continued)

specimen collection and should chart the path the specimen will follow for test completion and physician notification.

3. Decide on the length of time you think it will take to complete this process. How many tests will you be able to perform in each area over the course of an 8-hour day?
4. Look at ways and means for quality improvement.
5. Decide on the best method for ensuring a reliable quality control process.
6. Outline the guidelines that you feel must be established and followed in order to institute a proper quality assurance program.
7. During class, defend your model and its feasibility.

Summary

Each employee's involvement in the entire process is fundamental to a successful QA plan. Monitoring and evaluating quality is a time-consuming process. It is vitally important that the following QC guidelines be applied consistently:

- Routinely check laboratory equipment for precision accuracy using standards and controls.
- Discard all outdated collection equipment and reagents.
- Follow collecting and testing procedures as written.
- Perform duplicate testing to ensure accuracy of results.
- Perform equipment maintenance at regularly scheduled intervals and as needed.

The regulations established by OSHA and CLIA are sometimes time-consuming to follow, and it may be a task that no one in the laboratory wants to do. However, adherence to these guidelines is mandatory, and benefits, such as positive outcomes, satisfied patients, improved teamwork, and increased profitability, are worth the investment and are important to the laboratory's survival.

Chapter Review

True or False

Circle T or F to indicate the correct answers to the following:

T F 1. Quality control is the process that validates final results and quantifies variations.

T F 2. CLIA 1988 requires all laboratories to participate in proficiency testing.

T F 3. Quality control in the laboratory is designed to ensure the accuracy of most test results and provide tests with a margin of error.

T F 4. Quality assurance benefits the patient by providing rules for quality of care.

Fill in the Blanks

Complete the following statements:

5. Steps you can take when designing and implementing a QA program include ______________ and ______________.
6. The two outside agencies that oversee quality control in the laboratory are ______________ and ______________.
7. The objectives of quality control in the laboratory are to ensure the accuracy of test results while ______________ and ______________ error.
8. The three levels of certification for POLs are ______________, ______________, and ______________.

Multiple Choice

Circle the letter that represents the single best answer:

9. A laboratory that is certified as a waiver-level laboratory can perform all of the following EXCEPT:
   a. Hemoglobin
   b. Differential counts

c. Specific gravity
d. Bilirubin
e. Glucose tolerances

10. The JCAHO's steps to a QA plan include:
    a. Assigning responsibility
    b. Gathering data
    c. Taking corrective action
    d. a and c
    e. a, b, and c

Vocabulary

bacteria: unicellular microorganisms that do not have membrane-enclosed nuclei

Chlamydia: a genus of microorganisms that live as intracellular parasites and that are pathogenic in humans

differential white cell count: a count based on observation of the different kinds of white cells and reported as percentages of the total number of white cells examined. (Usually, 100 cells are examined to determine the percentage of each type.)

eukaryotic: pertaining to organisms with a true nucleus, such as fungi, protozoa, and most algae

fungi: microorganisms that live on decaying organic material

immunology: the study of the reaction of tissues of the immune system of the body to antigenic stimulation

legionella: a small, rod-shaped bacterium that is the causative agent in legionnaires' disease

microbe: a microscopic organism

morphology: the study of the physical shape and size of a specimen

prokaryotic: pertaining to organisms without a true (membrane-bound) nucleus, such as bacteria and viruses

reticulocyte: a nonnucleated immature red blood cell

sediment: a deposit of relatively insoluble material that settles to the bottom of a container of liquid

viruses: an infective agent smaller than bacteria

Chapter Objectives

After reading this chapter, you should be able to:

1. List the characteristics of low-power, high-power, and oil immersion microscopy.
2. Determine when you would need to use high-power microscopy.
3. Name two types of observations that are best accomplished using oil immersion microscopy.
4. Identify the purpose of darkfield microscopy.
5. Locate the area of the laboratory where you would expect to use fluorescence microscopy.
6. Identify the need for phase-contrast microscopy.
7. Compare analyses using the electron microscope and the brightfield microscope.

Chapter 4
The Microscope

Every medical laboratory is equipped with a microscope. This indispensable instrument is used to view objects too small to be seen with the naked eye (Fig. 4–1). The microscope is used to evaluate stained blood smears, urine sediment, and microbacterial smears of the throat, vagina, and semen, as well as to determine blood cell counts.

Microscopes may be monocular, dual, binocular, or triocular. A monocular microscope has one eyepiece for viewing, whereas the binocular microscope has two eyepieces and the triocular microscope has three. The eyepiece, or ocular, is located at the top of the microscope and contains a lens that magnifies what is being seen. The ocular is attached to a barrel or tube that is connected to the microscope arm. Under the arm is the revolving nosepiece, to which are attached the DIN objectives. Most microscopes have three or four objectives, and each has a different magnifying power. The shortest objective, which has the lowest power, is marked 10× or 16 mm. Low power is used for initial focusing and to scan urine **sediment** and blood smears; it may then be used to focus on an area of particular interest. Greater detail is observed with the next longest objective (high power), which is marked 40× or 4 mm. High magnifying power is used to study cells and sediment in greater detail and for manually counting red blood cells. The longest objective (oil immersion), which is marked 100× or 1.8 mm, allows for the finest focusing on an object and is used to view microorganisms, to view a **Gram-stained** specimen, and to obtain **differential white cell counts** and **reticulocyte** counts. If there is a fourth objective, it is labeled 4× and is used in a manner similar to the 10× objective, but with only half the magnification.

When adjusting the objective to a new power, the nosepiece should be rotated using its grip, **NOT THE OBJECTIVES.** Otherwise, the objective may be loosened and seriously damaged by incorrect rotation (Fig. 4–2).

The arm of the microscope connects the objectives and oculars to the base, which supports the microscope and contains the light source. The condenser is mounted under the stage of the microscope and can be low-

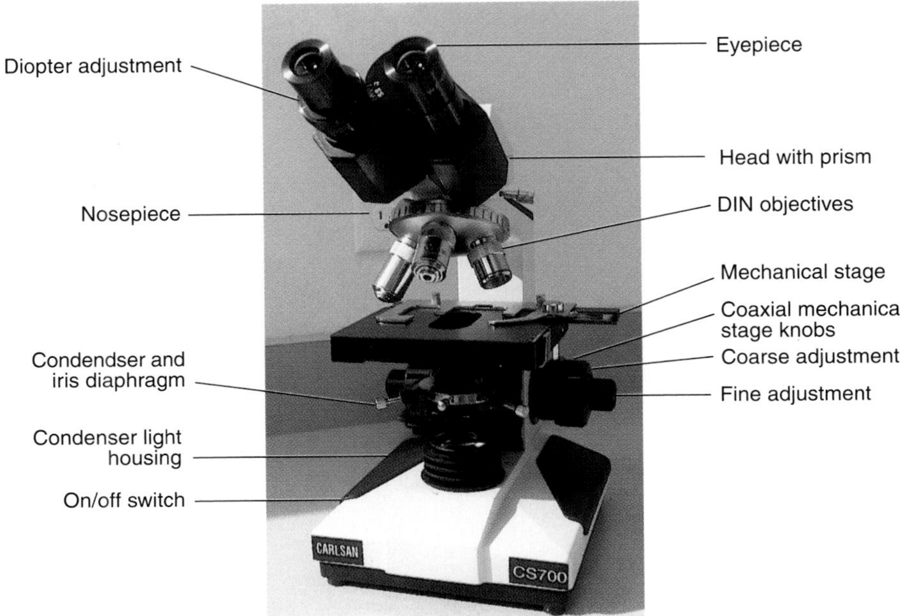

Figure 4–1. *Parts of microscope. (From Woods, M. A.* The Clinical Medical Assistant. *Philadelphia: W. B. Saunders, 1994, p. 184.)*

ered so that each field of view is filled with light rays. The iris diaphragm controls the quantity and quality of light reaching the objective by adjusting the iris leaves under the condenser. Just above the base are the focusing knobs. The coarse adjustment is used only with low power; the fine adjustment is used with both high-power and oil immersion microscopy. The stage of the microscope holds the slide to be viewed.

PROCEDURE 4–1

Identifying the Parts of the Microscope

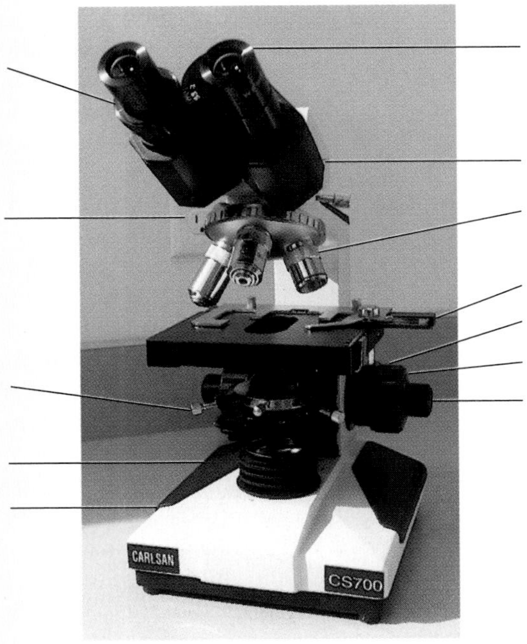

PROCEDURE 4–1

Identifying the Parts of the Microscope (Continued)

Principle

To work in the laboratory, you must be able to successfully identify all the parts of the light microscope.

Procedural Steps

1. Label the parts of the microscope.

A ______________ D ______________

B ______________ E ______________

C ______________ F ______________

G ______________ J ______________

H ______________ K ______________

I ______________ L ______________

2. Explain the correct procedure for turning the light on and off.

____

____

____

Types of Microscopes

Brightfield Microscope

A single magnifying glass usually magnifies the image of an object by 3 to 20 times the object's actual size. The common laboratory microscope today is a compound brightfield microscope with two lenses and a visible light source that passes through the specimen and lenses to the observer's eye, hence the term "brightfield." The eyepiece contains the ocular lens and the second lens is in the objective, near the object to be viewed.

The two-lens system can magnify 40 to 1200 times. The total magnification of a microscope is determined by multiplying the magnifying power of the ocular lens (usually 10×) by the magnifying power of the objective lens (10×, 40×, or 100×). Thus, with the low-power objective, the total magnification is 10 multiplied by 10, or 100×. This level of magnification is used for observing the **morphology** of microorganisms. When a polarized filter is used with the brightfield microscope, it is possible to examine crystals in synovial fluid (Fig. 4–3*A*). With a high-power lens, the total magnification would be 400×. This level of magnification is often used to

Figure 4–2. *Rotating the nosepiece.* A, *Incorrect method.* B, *Correct method.*

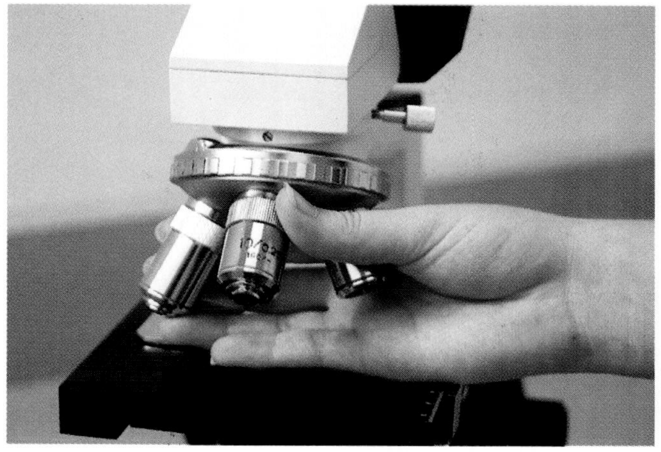

A

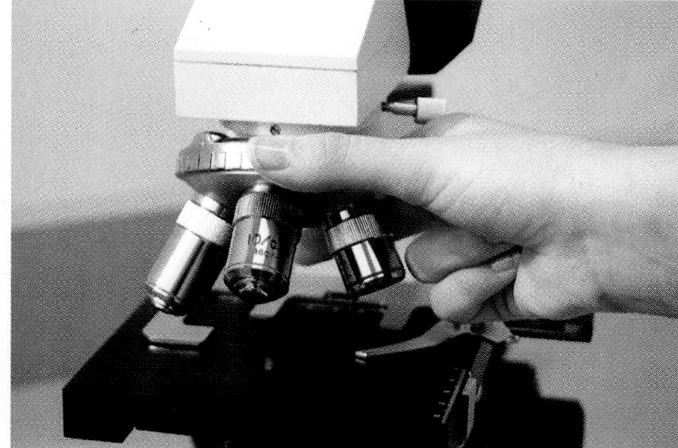

B

view urinary sediment, wet mounts for parasites, and potassium hydroxide preparations for **fungi.** With the oil immersion objective, the total magnification would be 10 times 100, or 1000×; this magnification is used for observing bacteria, for differential white blood cell counts, and red blood cell morphology.

Generally, the higher the magnification, the more light that is needed. When using the oil immersion objective, a drop of immersion oil is used between the slide and the objective lens. This oil reduces the scattering of light, thereby allowing clearer observation of the specimen. The condenser under the stage focuses light on the specimen, and by adjusting the amount of light, the specimen can be brought into focus.

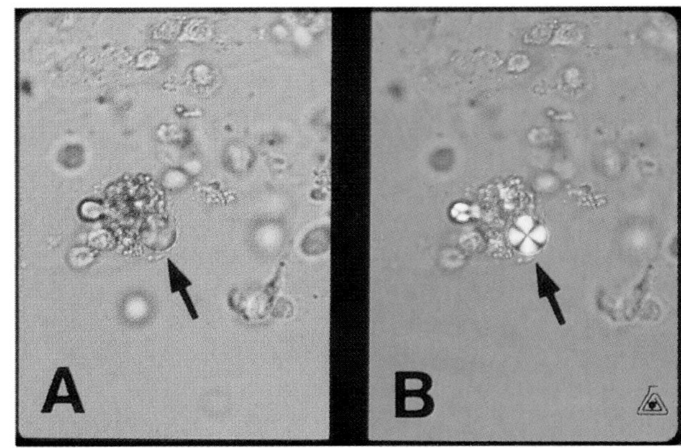

Figure 4–3. *Comparison of brightfield and polarized light.*

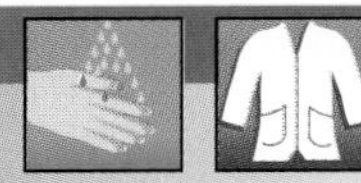

PROCEDURE 4–2

Focusing the Microscope

Principle

Understanding the use of the microscope by focusing a prepared slide under all power magnifications and oil emersion.

Equipment and Supplies

microscope
lens paper
lens cleaner
immersion oil
slides containing specimens
microscope dust cover

Procedural Steps

1. Wash your hands.
2. Gather all of the material needed.
3. Remove the dust cover from the microscope and clean the lenses with lens tissue and lens cleaner.
4. Plug in the microscope and turn on the light switch.
5. Place the slide specimen on the stage and secure it.
6. Turn the revolving nosepiece to low power.
7. Carefully raise the stage while observing the specimen with the naked eye.
8. While looking through the oculars, use the course adjustment knob to focus the specimen and scan the field.
9. Switch to fine adjustment, and focus the specimen in detail.
10. Adjust the amount of light by closing the iris diaphragm and lowering the condenser.
11. Turn the revolving nosepiece to high power and repeat steps 8 through 10.
12. Lower the stage.
13. Place a small drop of oil on the slide.
14. Carefully swing the oil immersion objective into place.
15. Adjust the focus with the fine-adjustment knob.
16. Increase the light by opening the iris diaphragm and raising the condenser.
17. Identify the specimen.
18. Return to low power.
19. Lower the stage.
20. Center the stage.
21. Remove the slide.
22. Switch off the light and unplug the microscope.
23. Clean the lenses with lens tissue, and remove oil with lens cleaner.
24. Wipe the microscope with a cloth.
25. Cover the microscope with the dust cover.
26. Clean the work area.
27. Wash your hands.

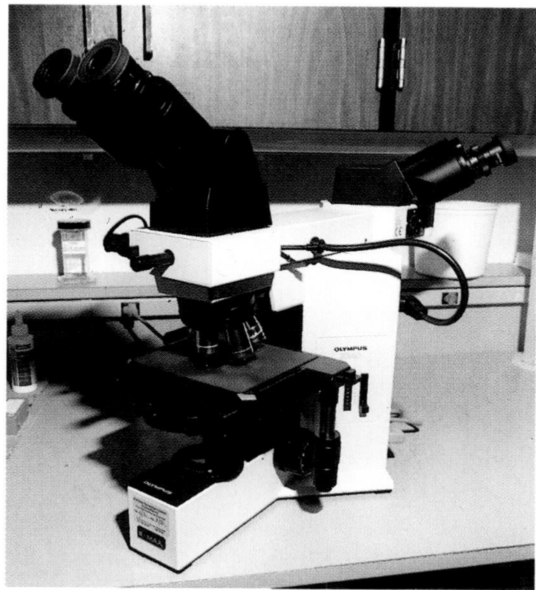

Figure 4–4. *Darkfield microscope.*

Darkfield Microscope

In darkfield microscopy, the light is directed toward the specimen from the side so that the only light to reach the objective is reflected from the **bacteria** or object to be studied. By using this technique, the **microbe** appears as a bright object on a dark background (see Fig. 4–3). A standard laboratory microscope can be used for darkfield microscopy by closing the condenser that shapes the cone of light entering the objective. A large laboratory may be equipped with a specially designed darkfield microscope (Fig. 4–4). This microscopic technique is frequently used to study very small bacteria, such as the spirochete *Treponema pallidum,* which causes syphilis.

Phase-Contrast Microscope

The phase-contrast microscope is of great value as it allows the laboratory worker to observe living microbes without staining. Because the light refracted by living organisms is different from the light refracted from the surrounding medium, the organisms can be seen more easily (Fig. 4–5). Using phase-contrast technique, one can observe dense structures in living **prokaryotic** and **eukaryotic** microorganisms. This technique is also used for identification of urinary sediment and for unstained platelet counts.

Fluorescence Microscope

The microscope used for fluorescence microscopy has an ultraviolet (UV) light source that illuminates the object but does not pass into the objective of the microscope. When UV light strikes certain dyes and pigments, they emit a certain type of light; for example, different types of chlorophyll emit green, yellow, or orange light that can be seen in the microscope against a dark background. The UV light microscope is often used in **immunology** laboratories to show antibodies stained with a fluorescent dye as they combine with specific antigens on bacteria (Fig. 4–6). Its primary use is to detect organisms in cells, tissue, and clinical specimens. Thus, this microscope is used for antinuclear antibody analysis, for detection of tubercle bacillus, and in mycobacterial identification (e.g., **legionella** and **chlamydia.** The fluorescent antibody technique is frequently used as a diagnostic test in bacteriology. Special training in specimen preparation and microscope operation is required.

Electron Microscope

The electron microscope uses an electron beam instead of visible light, and magnets instead of lenses, to focus the beam. A dry specimen is mounted in wax or plastic and the electrons pass through it. The image is then viewed on a fluorescent screen. The picture is usually

Figure 4–5. *Phase-contrast microscope.*

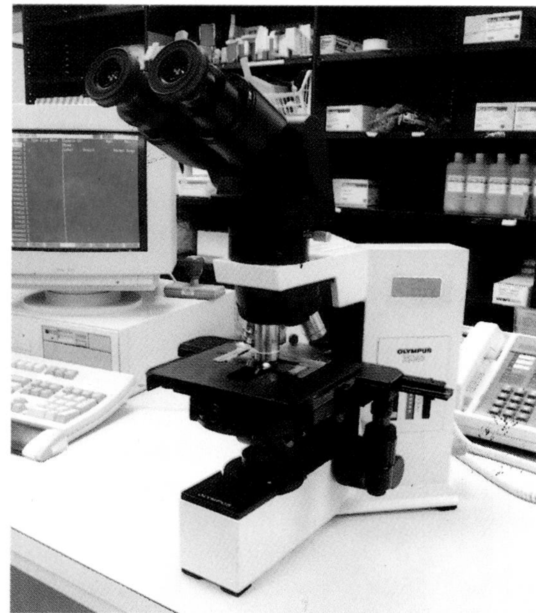

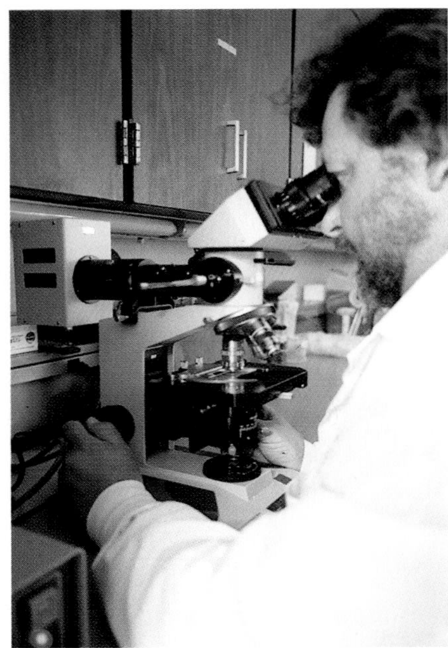

Figure 4–6. *Fluorescence microscopy.*

photographed and enlarged to magnify the object several hundred times, much greater magnification than is possible with any standard ocular microscope. Through this technique, very tiny microbes and **viruses** may be observed. By using thin sections of cells mounted in plastic, the internal structure of cells can be studied by this technique. A recent modification of this microscope resulted in the development of the scanning electron microscope, which is very useful for observing cell surfaces, and mitochondria, and for three-dimensional imagery (Fig. 4–7).

Electron microscopy is a highly specialized field that requires specialized training. The microscope is an extremely expensive piece of equipment and, in most situations, specimens that are to be examined by electron microscopy are sent to a specialized location, which may be some distance from the laboratory where the specimen was obtained. This technique's major application is in the field of research; however, it has been instrumental in diagnosing Reye's syndrome and various genetic/hereditary disorders.

Care of the Microscope

Microscopes are very precise and expensive instruments that require special care in handling and storage. The amount of routine maintenance depends on the amount of daily use.

The objectives and eyepieces are two of the most important parts of the instrument. They should be carefully cleaned, especially the oil immersion objective (100×). If dirt or smudges are found on the optical surface, it should be cleaned carefully with lens paper moistened in a lens-cleaning solution. Xylene and related chemicals are not recommended for routine cleaning because these chemicals can break down the lens-mounting cements. However, some slide preparations may require xylene to remove certain types of smudges from the lens.

If a film or smudge remains, use a clean, double-end cotton swab to clean the surface. Moisten the swab

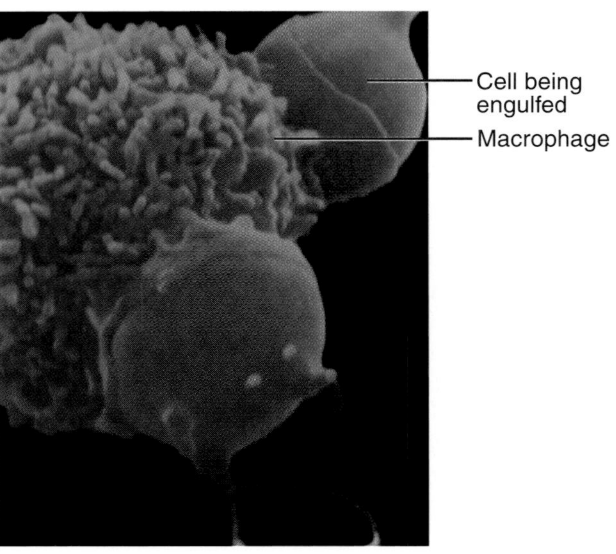

Figure 4–7. *Color-enhanced electron microscopy.*

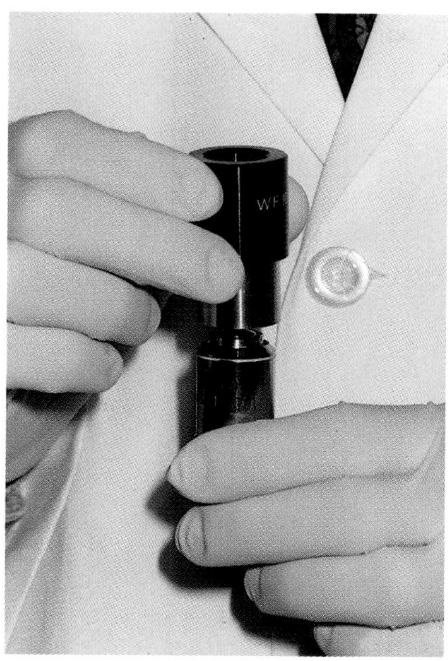

Figure 4–8. *Using the eyepiece to examine an objective.*

in a lens cleaner and, beginning in the middle of the lens, clean the lens using a clockwise, circular motion as you move to the outer edge of the lens. Using the dry end of the cotton swab, work in a counterclockwise direction to the edge of the lens. Do not apply heavy force or use a scrubbing action.

The 100× oil lens should be cleaned immediately after use to prevent a film buildup on its surface. Oil, makeup, dust, and eye secretions all can obstruct vision through the lens, and may cause transmission of infection. If clarity is a problem, the objective may be removed and the eyepiece used as a magnifying glass for examining the bottom element of the objective (Fig. 4–8). Finally, the body of the microscope should be dusted with a soft cloth.

As the microscope is a precision optical instrument, it should be used, maintained, and stored carefully (Table 4–1). Maintenance of this instrument is the same as for other precision instruments. When not in use, it should always be covered with a plastic dust cover and placed in a ventilated, dry, and clean place where no acids, alkalis, or salts are stored.

Table 4–1
Microscope Troubleshooting

Problem	***Possible Causes***	***Remedies***
OBJECTIVES		
Not parfocaled between objectives	Objectives are not screwed in tightly	Tighten the objectives
Objective lens touches the specimen when changing objective.	The slide with the specimen is facing down, not up	Place the specimen or coverslip in the up position
	Coverslip is too thick	Replace the coverslip with a #1 type
Blue colors look green; red colors look pink	A film over the end of the objective	Use a cotton swab to clean the objective
100× objective is focusing some distance from the coverslip	Oil and/or moisture has leaked into the objective tube	Objective will have to be cleaned and resealed or replaced
ELECTRICAL		
Light flickers, changing intensity	Building voltage or room voltage fluctuates	Use a voltage control unit
	Loose connection	Secure both electrical connections
	Bulb is about to burn out	Replace bulb
	Bulb is not the recommended 6-volt, 20-watt, pin bulb	Replace with correct bulb
		NOTE: SURGE PROTECTORS ARE HIGHLY RECOMMENDED
No light	Fuse burned out, wrong fuse	Replace with a new fuse
	Bulb burned out	Replace with a new bulb
	Switch or intensity control is not on	Turn on switch, then increase intensity control
Bulb or fuse burns out too frequently	Wrong bulb or fuse	Replace one or both

(continued)

Table 4–1
Microscope Troubleshooting *(Continued)*

Problem	***Possible Causes***	***Remedies***
VIEWING AREA		
Field of view is shaded on one side	Nosepiece is not clicked in place	Click nosepiece into place
	Condenser is not correctly mounted	Remove and reinsert the condenser
	Head is not centered	Tighten the screw holding the head in place
The image is not sharp	Dirt on the objective, condenser, or eyepiece	Clean optic surfaces carefully
	Dirty specimen	Clean top and bottom of slide
	[100× R oil lens]	Clean and replace immersion oil
	Immersion oil may have bubbles	
	Light is too bright	Reduce the amount of light
	Position of condenser	Raise or lower condenser
	Objective not clicked into position	Click objective into place
FOCUSING	Clean eyepieces and objectives are required	See section on eyepieces and objectives
Specimen is not coming into focus	Slide with specimen is upside down	Turn slide over
	Coverslip is too thick	Need #1 coverslip for oil lens

Microscopes should be placed in a permanent location in the laboratory, on a sturdy table in an area where they are not likely to be bumped. If a microscope must be moved, it should be carried securely, with one hand supporting the base and the other holding the microscope arm. When storing the microscope, it should be left with the low-power objective in the lowest position.

Summary

This chapter described why the microscope is an important instrument in the laboratory, how to use it, and how to care for it. In the physician's office laboratory, it is an important device used to detect microscopic structures that cannot be seen with the naked eye. As vital a device as the microscope is, it is only as efficient as the person using it. Mastering the use of this instrument takes time and practice. Once this is accomplished, the tasks that can be accomplished with the microscope are myriad.

Chapter Review

True or False

Circle T or F to indicate the correct answers to the following:

T F 1. A microscope may have two or three eyepieces.

T F 2. To observe microbes under the microscope, the 10× objective is used for greatest detail.

T F 3. The higher the magnification, the less light needed.

T F 4. Oil increases the scattering of light and allows clearer observation of the specimen.

Fill in the Blanks

Complete the following statements:

5. When using darkfield microscopy, the object will appear ______________ and the background will be ______________ .

6. Fluorescent microscopy is used for the identification of mycobacteria, such as ______________ and ______________ .

7. The electron microscope uses ______________ and ______________ instead of lights and lenses to visualize an object.

8. The electron microscope has been instrumental in diagnosing ______________ ______________ .

Multiple Choice

Circle the letter that represents the single best answer:

9. Two parts of the microscope that are important for visualization are:
   a. Arm and base
   b. Lenses and light source
   c. Objectives and eyepieces
   d. Objectives and lenses
   e. Stage and condenser

10. When cleaning the optical surface of the objective, you should use:
    a. Alcohol
    b. Distilled water
    c. Soap and tap water
    d. Lens cleaner
    e. Immersion oil

Vocabulary

ocular micrometer: a small ruler on a glass disk used in measuring microorganisms under the microscope

protozoa: single-celled microorganisms; the lowest class of life

Chapter Objectives

After reading this chapter, you should be able to:

1. List the basic units of the metric system.
2. Identify the two types of SI units used in the clinical laboratory.
3. Name the base units frequently used in the laboratory.
4. List the commonly used metric abbreviations.
5. Compare and contrast the English system and the metric system of measurement.
6. Demonstrate efficiency in conversion of metric units.
7. Use English/household and metric conversions with confidency.
8. Convert Celsius to Fahrenheit temperatures with ease.
9. Prepare solutions to exact specifications.

Chapter 5
Understanding Laboratory Measurements

The International Standard of Measurement is the metric system. Metric system measures pertain chiefly to length, weight, volume, and temperature. This system was first proposed by a group of European scientists at the close of the 17th century. They presented a concise system of weights and measures that effectively replaced the incompatible systems being used and that was quickly adopted by all European countries. It then was accepted as the International System.

Basic Units of the System

Meter

The *meter* is the basic unit of *length*. A meter is 39.37 inches long. A decimeter would be 3.94 inches long. A centimeter would be about 0.39 inches long, and a millimeter would be about 0.04 inches in length. One thousand meters would equal 1 km. Meters are often used in laboratory reports, charts, and other data requiring linear measurements. For instance, a laboratory procedure might require you to "connect flasks using 0.3 meters of rubber tubing;" this would mean that you must use 12 inches of tubing.

Liter

The *liter* is the basic unit of *capacity* or *volume*. This measure tells us how much space an item occupies. The standard unit for capacity in the International System is expressed in terms of multiples or decimal fractions of the cubic meter. In the laboratory, this unit is too large for everyday use; thus the cubic decimeter is used. The *liter* is accepted as a general designation for 1 cubic decimeter. The liter is used most frequently in the United States by the beverage industry. We are all familiar with the 2-liter soft drink container. A liter is slightly more than 1 qt and is equal to 1000 mL, or the capacity occupied by 2.2 lb of distilled water at 39.2°C.

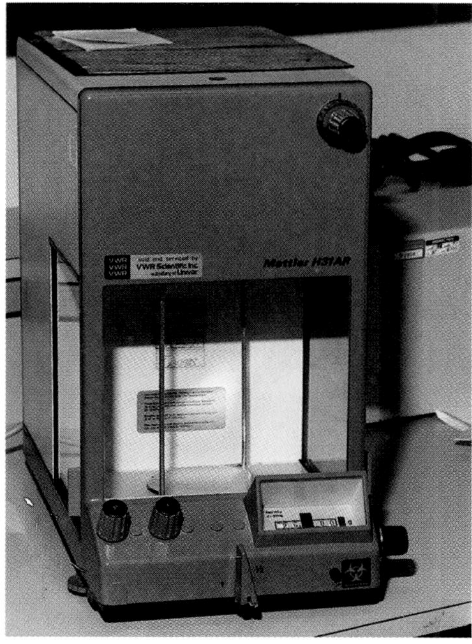

Figure 5–1. *An analytical balance is used to measure very small amounts (micrograms) of laboratory chemicals.*

Gram

The *gram* is the basic unit of *weight* or mass. A measure of weight tells how heavy an item is. One thousand cubic centimeters, the equivalent of 1 cubic decimeter, have the capacity of 1 L and weigh 1000 gm or 1 kg (Fig. 5–1). The *kilogram* is the standard unit of weight and is equivalent to approximately 2.2 lb in the English system of measurement. In the clinical laboratory, the gram (0.001 kg) is used more frequently than is the kilogram. A gram is the weight of 1 cubic centimeter of distilled water at a temperature of 39.2°C.

Table 5–1
International Base Units

SI Base Unit	***Symbol***	***Quantity Expressed***
Ampere	A	Electricity
Candela	cd	Light intensity
Kelvin	K	Temperature
Kilogram	kg	Weight
Meter	m	Distance
Mole	mol	Quantity
Second	s	Time

For practical purposes, the milliliter is considered to be equivalent to a cubic centimeter. Both terms belong to the terminology of the metric system, but *milliliter* is the accurate and preferred term for liquid measurements.

International System

The International System of units (*SI units*) includes two types of units important in clinical laboratories. These are the **base units** and **derived units.** The International Bureau of Weights and Measurements is responsible for maintaining the standards upon which this system of measurement is based. For reference purposes, the instruments used to establish the measurements are still maintained at Sevres, France, and Washington, D.C.

Base Units

The base units are among the most frequently used in the clinical laboratory (Table 5–1).

Table 5–2
Metric Abbreviations

Metric Unit	***Abbreviation***	***Meter***	***Liter***	***Gram***
meter	M (m)			
liter	L (l)			
gram	g or gm			
kilo	k	km	kL	kg
hecto	h	hm	hL	hg
deca	da	dam	daL	dag
deci	d	dm	mL	dg
centi	c	cm	cL	cg
milli	m	mm	mL	mg
micro	μ	μm	μL	μg
nano	n	nm	nL	ng

Table 5–3
Commonly Used Metric Prefixes

kilo = 1000.00	(one thousand)
deci = 0.1	(one-tenth)
centi = 0.01	(one-hundredth)
milli = 0.001	(one-thousandth)
micro = 0.000,001	(one millionth)
nano = 0.000,000,001	(one billionth)

SI-Derived Units

The derived units include measures of area, volume, speed, acceleration, mass density, concentration of a substance, specific volume, and luminescence. These quantities are usually the square or cubic powers of the base unit.

Metric Measurement

Because the metric system is based on 10 and multiples of 10, 100, 1000, etc, the measurements can be expressed in decimals, and decimals can be used in the calculations. Fractions should be changed to their decimal equivalents when working with the metric system.

To express one unit of measure in terms of the next **smaller** unit, **multiply** by 1000. Therefore, 2 gm equals 2000 mg and 0.5 gm equals 500 mg.

To express one unit of measure in terms of the next **larger** unit, **divide** by 1000. Therefore, 2 mg equals 0.002 gm and 50 mg equals 0.05 gm.

Multiples of the metric unit are preceded by prefixes derived from Greek and Latin. The most frequently used prefixes in the clinical laboratory are: kilo (k), milli (m), deci (d), centi (c), micro (μ), and nano (n). Metric abbreviations are listed in Table 5–2.

Prefixes demonstrate the definite relationships to the measure, as shown in Table 5–3.

PROCEDURE 5–1

Obtaining Metric Measurements

Principle

Practice using metric measurements will help to familiarize you in measurement values.

Equipment and Supplies

metric scale
metric ruler
metric tape measure
Celsius thermometer
microscope
laboratory stool
gram scale
distilled water
deionized water

Procedural Steps

1. Obtain the following self measurements:
   Weight: ____________ kg
   Height: ____________ cm
   Temperature: ____________ °C
   Shoe size: ____________ cm
   Waist: ____________ cm
2. Record the weight of the following using a gram scale:
   8 oz of tap water: ____________ gm
   1 L of distilled water: ____________ gm
   500 mL of deionized water: ____________ gm
3. Record the following measurements:
   Area of the microscope base: ____________ cm
   Circumference of a laboratory stool:
   ____________ m
   Length of the blackboard: ____________ km
4. Make a 10% bleach solution from an 80% bleach solution. Show the correct formula and your calculations.

Micro Measurement

Several common metric units are used to describe the size of microorganisms. The meter, which remains the basic unit, is equivalent to approximately 39 inches. It can be divided into 10 decimeters or 100 cm or 1000 mm or 1 million μm or 1 billion nm, etc.

Red blood cells are about 100 μm in diameter. Bacteria vary in width and length from about 0.20 to 10 μm, and viruses range in size from about 0.02 to 0.35 μm. Some very large **protozoa** reach a length of 2000 μm, or 2 mm.

The sizes of microorganisms are calculated by using a microscope stage measuring device, called a *stage micrometer,* to determine the distance between the marks on another measuring device known as the **ocular micrometer,** which is placed in the eyepiece of the microscope. The ocular micrometer is then used to measure the length and width of the microbe on the specimen slide.

Each type of microscope has its limits of visibility. The light microscope can be used for observation of cells larger than 0.2000 μm, whereas the electron microscope can identify objects as small as 0.5000 nm in diameter.

Conversion of Units

In the United States, the household system of measurement is still used. Often, it may be necessary to convert a metric measurement into a household measurement to enable the patient to understand the testing results or the quantity of the specimen needed. The mathematical computations for such conversions are listed in Table 5–4.

Table 5–4
Conversion of Metric Units to English Units

Metric Unit	*Multiplier*	*Household Unit*
LENGTH		
1 kilometer	0.6	Miles
1 meter	3.3	Feet
1 meter	39.37	Inches
1 decimeter	4.0	Inches
1 centimeter	0.4	Inches
1 millimeter	0.04	Inches
WEIGHT		
1 kilogram	2.2	Pounds
1 gram	0.0022	Pounds
VOLUME		
1 liter	1.06	Quarts
1 milliliter	0.03	Fluid ounces

Temperature Conversion

The Fahrenheit and Celsius scales differ (Fig. 5–2). Observation and comparison of the two scales will show the freezing point and boiling point of each. According to the Fahrenheit scale, the freezing point of water is 32 degrees, and the boiling point of water is 212 degrees. Using the Celsius scale, the freezing point is 0 degrees and the boiling point is 100 degrees.

Five degrees on the Celsius scale equals nine degrees on the Fahrenheit scale. Therefore, the fractions 5/9 and 9/5 are used to convert temperatures from one scale to the other. These fractions indicate the ratio between the two scales.

Originally, the term **centigrade** was used instead of Celsius. However, **Celsius** is the correct metric term. Thermometers and other scientific devices that reflect the different scales use the International System of measurement.

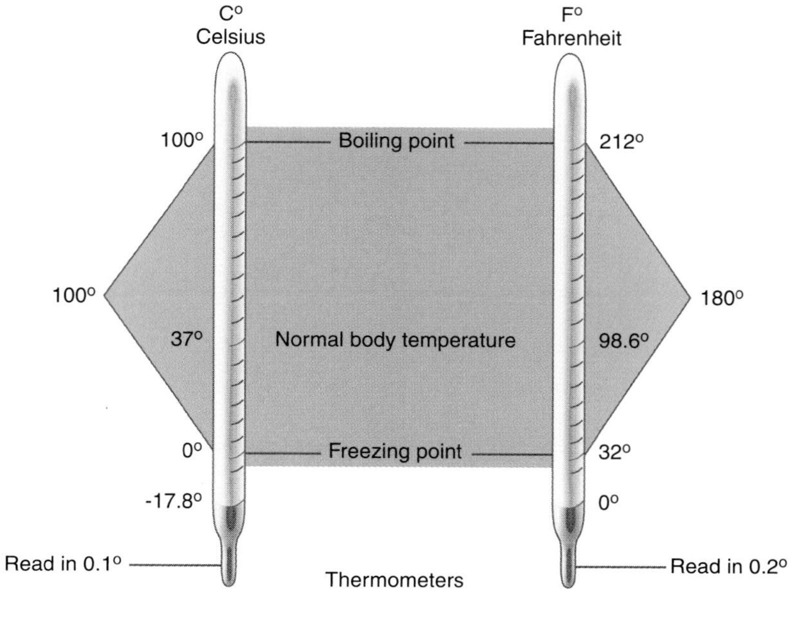

Figure 5–2. *Comparison of Fahrenheit and Celsius temperature scales.*

Conversion Formula

Fahrenheit to Celsius

To convert Fahrenheit to Celsius temperature:

Subtract 32° from the Fahrenheit temperature.
Multiply the result by 5/9.

The formula for this conversion is written as follows:

C = (F − 32) × 5/9

Example: Convert 105°F to Celsius.

C = (F − 32) × 5/9
C = (105 − 32) × 5/9
105 − 32 = 73
73 × 5/9 = 40.6
C = 40.6°

Celsius to Fahrenheit

To convert from Celsius to Fahrenheit temperature:

Multiply the Celsius temperature by 9/5.
Add 32°.

The formula for this conversion is written as follows:

F = 9/5 C + 32

Example: Convert 25°C to Fahrenheit.

F = 9/5 × C + 32
= (9/5 × 25) + 32
= 45 + 32
= 77°

Note: The information in Table 5–5 is provided for reference and comparison.

Table 5–5
Fahrenheit/Celsius Conversion Chart

°F	°C	°F	°C	°F	°C	°F	°C	°F	°C	°F	°C
96	35.6	118	47.8	140	60	162	72.2	184	84.4	206.6	97
96.8	36	118.4	48	141	60.6	163	72.8	185	85	207	97.2
97	36.1	119	48.3	141.8	61	163.4	73	186	85.6	208	97.8
98	36.7	120	48.9	142	61.1	164	73.3	186.8	86	208.4	98
98.6	37	120.2	49	143	61.7	165	73.9	187	86.1	209	98.3
99	37.2	121	49.4	143.6	62	165.2	74	188	86.7	210	98.9
100	37.8	122	50	144	62.2	166	74.4	188.6	87	210.2	99
100.4	38	123	50.6	145	62.8	167	75	189	87.2	211	99.4
101	38.3	123.8	51	145.4	63	168	75.6	190	87.8	212	100
102	38.9	124	51.1	146	63.3	168.8	76	190.4	88	213	100.6
102.2	39	125	51.7	147	63.9	169	76.1	191	88.3	213.8	101
103	39.4	125.6	52	147.2	64	170	76.7	192	88.9	214	101.1
104	40	126	52.2	148	64.4	170.6	77	192.2	89	215	101.7
105	40.6	127	52.8	149	65	171	77.2	193	89.4	215.6	102
105.8	41	127.4	53	150	65.6	172	77.8	194	90	216	102.2
106	41.1	128	53.3	150.8	66	172.4	78	195	90.6	217	102.8
107	41.7	129	53.9	151	66.1	173	78.3	195.8	91	217.4	103
107.6	42	129.2	54	152	66.7	174	78.9	196	91.1	218	103.3
108	42.2	130	54.4	152.6	67	174.2	79	197	91.7	219	103.9
109	42.8	131	55	153	67.2	175	79.4	197.6	92	219.2	104
109.4	43	132	55.6	154	67.8	176	80	198	92.2	220	104.4
110	43.3	132.8	56	154.4	68	177	80.6	199	92.8	221	105
111	43.9	133	56.1	155	68.3	177.8	81	199.4	93	225	107.2
111.2	44	134	56.7	156	68.9	178	81.1	200	93.3	230	110
112	44.4	134.6	57	156.2	69	179	81.7	201	93.9	235	112.8
113	45	135	57.2	157	69.4	179.6	82	201.2	94	239	115
114	45.6	136	57.8	158	70	180	82.2	202	94.4	240	115.6
114.8	46	136.4	58	159	70.6	181	82.8	203	95	245	118.3
115	46.1	137	58.3	159.8	71	181.4	83	204	95.6	248	120
116	46.7	138	58.9	160	71.1	182	83.3	204.8	96	250	121.1
116.6	47	138.2	59	161	71.7	183	83.9	205	96.1	255	123.9
117	47.2	139	59.4	161.6	72	183.2	84	206	96.7	257	125

Solutions and Dilutions

Frequently, it is necessary to make dilutions in the laboratory. For example, blood, serum, or plasma are diluted to produce color reactions that can be used in determining test results. When blood cell counts are done manually, it is necessary to make a dilution before these cells can be counted under the microscope.

Today, most solutions are commercially prepared and come to the laboratory in a ready-to-use package. You have already read that a 10% bleach solution is the solution of choice in cleaning areas where there is the possibility of body fluid contamination. There is always a time that you will need to prepare a solution of a certain strength from a given solution of another strength. Whenever solution preparation is required, accuracy is essential. When preparing a solution, it must be accomplished to exact specifications.

Understanding the Terminology

To understand the principle formulas in preparing solutions, one must first know the terms that are used to describe the process and the result.

When a weaker solution is made from a stronger given solution, the process is called a **dilution.** A dilution requires two solutions: a *concentrate* solution, which is the stronger substance, and a *diluent,* which is the substance that will be used to reduce the strength of the concentrate. When we combine the correct amount of concentrate with the correct amount of diluent, we will obtain the needed dilution.

Solutions are made by mixing a solute and a solvent. This procedure starts with a *solute,* which is usually a powdered substance that is to be dissolved. The *solvent* is the liquid in which the solute is dissolved. When these two are combined in correct proportions, the end product is called a *solution*. The total amount of the newly formed solution is called the *total volume.*

Preparing Solutions and Dilutions

Whenever a dilution is to be prepared, the formula is as follows:

$$\frac{\text{desired strength}}{\text{available strength}} = \frac{X\text{ (amount needed)}}{\text{amount available}}$$

Problem: Make a 10% bleach cleaning solution from 50% stock. The desired strength is 10%, the amount needed is X L, the available strength is 50%, and the amount available is 10 L.

$$\frac{0.1}{0.5} \times \frac{X}{10} = 0.1X = 5$$

$$X = \frac{5}{0.1}$$

$$X = 50\text{ L}$$

Thus, one would add 40 L of diluent to the concentrate (10 L), to yield a new concentration of 10%.

To make a solution, follow the directions on the solute.

Example:

"Mix contents with 10 mL of normal saline. This will make a 30% solution."

Use a flask that will accurately measure the solute, which in this case, is 10 mL of normal saline. Pour it into the bottle containing the powder and mix. This is now a 30% solution, and the total amount in the bottle is the total volume.

Summary

In countries around the world, the metric system is used for all household measurements. However, in the United States, both the household and English systems of measurement are used. In scientific fields, the metric system and the International System are used for measurement because measurements must be exacting. Without consistent units of measurement, reference values and ranges would have no standards, and they would serve no useful purpose for analysis. The laboratory worker needs to know these systems and the conversion formulas in order to understand and accurately record laboratory results, as well as to assist patients in understanding the specimen requirements and the testing results. Within the clinical laboratory, reports for urinalysis, blood chemistries, hematology, and serology use these units of measurement for reference values and reference ranges.

Chapter Review

True or False

Circle T or F to indicate the correct answers to the following:

T F 1. The International Standard of Measurement is the meter system.

T F 2. A millimeter is larger than a centimeter.

T F 3. A liter is the basic unit of length.

T F 4. A gram is the basic unit of weight.

Fill in the Blanks

Complete the following statements:

5. The two SI units that are important in clinical laboratories

   are ______________ and ______________ .

6. 2000 mg = ______________ gm.

7. Some microorganisms can be calculated by using a

   ______________ ______________ .

8. 1 kg = ______________ gm.

9. 5 mg = ______________ mL.

Multiple Choice

Circle the letter that represents the single best answer:

10. The boiling point in Fahrenheit is:
    a. 212°
    b. 200°
    c. 112°
    d. 100°
    e. 32°

11. The freezing point in Celsius is:
    a. 0°
    b. 5°
    c. 10°
    d. 32°
    e. 100°

12. If your temperature is 105°F, what would it be in Celsius?
    a. 35°
    b. 37°
    c. 39.8°
    d. 40.5°
    e. 41.2°

Unit II
Urinalysis

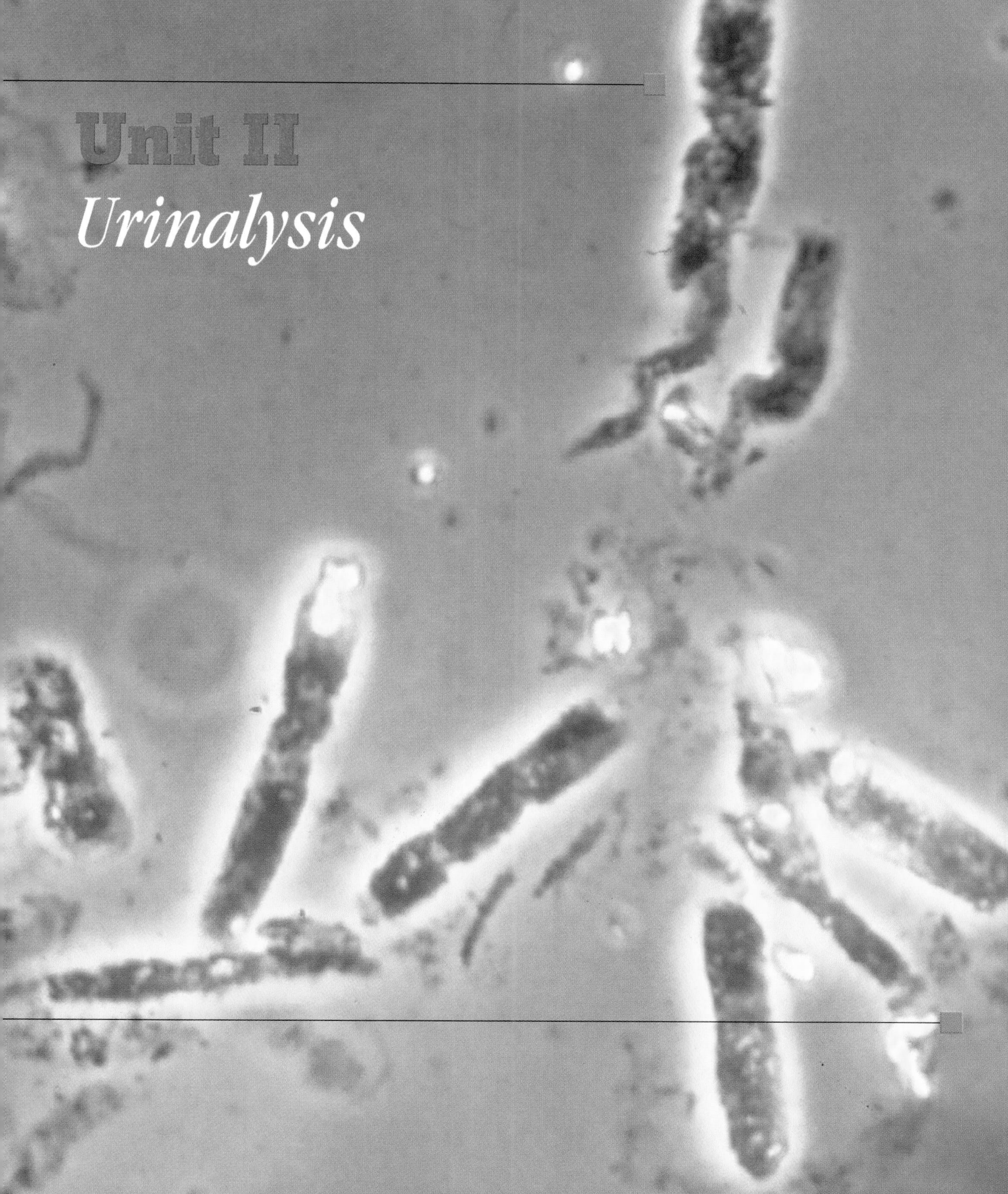

Vocabulary

Bowman's capsule: a cup-shaped membrane surrounding the glomerulus
catheterization: the insertion of a small tube into the bladder through the urethra for the purpose of removing urine
cortex: the outer layer of an organ
glomerulus: a mass of capillaries surrounded by Bowman's capsule
hilum: a notch in the medial border of the kidney
medulla: the inside portion of an organ
micturition: urination
nephron: the basic unit of the kidney
renal corpuscles: bodies forming the beginnings of nephrons and consisting of a glomerulus and Bowman's capsule
renal pelvis: a funnel-shaped basin located at the distal end of the tubules that drain urine from the kidney into the ureter
retroperitoneal: lying behind the peritoneum
tubule: small canal forming the last part of the nephron that the glomerular filtration passes through before entering the renal pelvis
urinary meatus: external opening of the urethra
urination: the discharge or passage of urine out of the body via the urinary meatus
voiding: the process of urinating

Chapter Objectives

After reading this chapter, you should be able to:

1. Name the scientist who perfected the first stable liquid test for the presence of sugar.
2. Identify the anatomic components of the urinary system.
3. Identify the structures of the urinary system and describe the function of each part.
4. List the reasons why quality assurance is important.
5. Explain the responsibility of the laboratory worker in relation to specimen identification.
6. Identify factors that determine how a specimen is handled.
7. List the importance of using controls.
8. List procedures that should be included in a procedure manual.
9. List factors included in responsible instrument maintenance and reagent handling.
10. Explain the importance of urinalysis in the care of patients.
11. List the basic methodologies employed in urinalysis.

Chapter 6
Introduction to the Urinary System and Urinalysis

For centuries, abnormalities in urine have been known to indicate disease. Medical history books contain a wealth of information about the study of urine. One of the earliest recorded urine tests involved pouring urine on the ground to see if it would attract insects. When insects were attracted to it, this was thought to indicate "honey urine," which was noted to be excreted by people with boils. Another early test involved tasting urine for sweetness. These simple tests were the forerunners of modern tests used to detect sugar and to diagnose diabetes.

In 1000 A.D., Ismail of Jurjani, a Persian physician, described seven different observations to be made of urine: quantity, consistency, color, odor, transparency, sediment, and froth. These observations prompted the "Pisse Prophets" of the middle ages to claim to be able to diagnose disease and foretell the future of a person by looking into their urine.

Subsequently, there were really no great urologic advances until the 20th century, when urinalysis became a practical laboratory procedure. The first stable, practical, liquid test for the presence of sugar in urine was perfected by Stanley Benedict. His research paper, published in the *Journal of the American Medical Association* in 1911 when he was a 17-year-old medical student, demonstrated the use of Benedict's solution of alkaline copper sulfate. Shortly after this paper was published, Victor Myers, Ph.D., was appointed head of the first clinical laboratory in the United States at the New York Postgraduate Hospital. He thus became the first practitioner of clinical chemistry, which included urinalysis.

Anatomy of the Urinary System

The urinary tract normally consists of two kidneys, two ureters, one bladder, and one urethra, as depicted in Figure 6–1. A basic understanding of kidney structure and urine formation is important to an understanding of urinalysis and its interpretation.

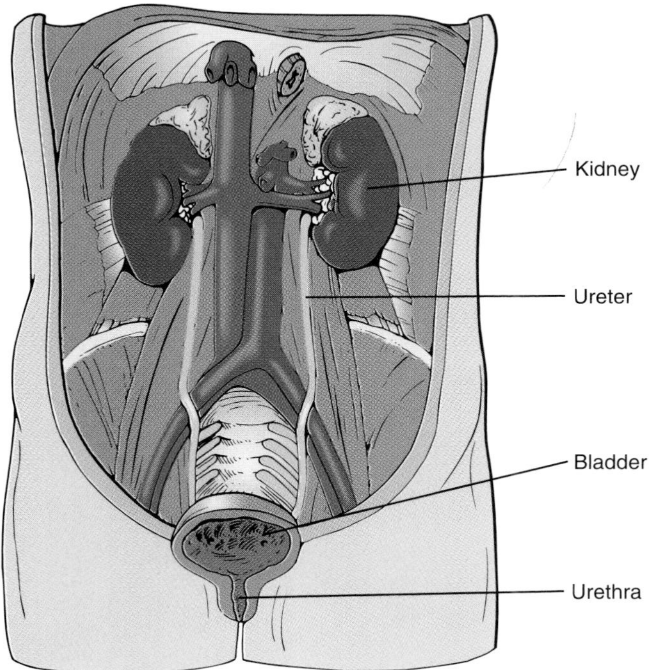

Figure 6–1. *Anatomy of the urinary system.*

Kidneys

The kidneys are dark red, bean-shaped organs measuring approximately 10 to 12 cm in length and 5 to 6 cm in width, having a thickness of 2.5 cm. Each kidney weighs about 8 oz. The kidneys are situated behind the abdominal cavity membrane, and thus have a **retroperitoneal** location. They lie, one on each side of the spinal column, just above the waistline, against the muscles of the back. Each kidney is surrounded by three capsules: the true capsule, a capsule of perirenal fat, and the renal fascia. The true capsule is a smooth, fibrous connective membrane that is loosely adherent to the surface of the kidney. The perirenal fat capsule is the adipose capsule that embeds each kidney in fatty tissue. The renal fascia is a sheath of fibrous tissue that helps to anchor the kidney to the surrounding structures, thereby helping to maintain its normal position. Each kidney consists of an outer region (**cortex**) and an inner region (**medulla**). There is a notch in the medial border (the **hilum**) through which blood, lymph vessels, and nerves pass (Fig. 6–2). About 25% of the total cardiac output enters the kidneys. This means that approximately 1200 mL of blood passes through the renal arteries every minute.

Nephrons

Microscopic examination of the kidney shows about 1 million filtering units, called **nephrons,** which are the structural and functional units of the organ. Each nephron consists of a **renal corpuscle** and a **glomerulus,** comprising a filtering system, and **Bowman's capsule.** Extending from each Bowman's capsule is the proximal convoluted **tubule,** the loop of Henle, and the distal convoluted portion through which the filtered fluid passes before emptying into the collecting tubule. Various changes occur as this fluid moves through the tubules. The cell lining of the tubule reabsorbs certain components of the fluid, whereas other particles are secreted into the lumen for eventual excretion. Generally, almost all of the water that passes through the glomeruli is reabsorbed by the tubules (Fig. 6–3). Located at the distal end of the tubules is the renal pelvis, which transports the urine from the kidney into the ureters.

Ureters

The urine passes through the ureter in peristaltic waves, traveling from the kidney to the urinary bladder. The ureters are muscular tubes, about 10 to 12 inches long, that are lined with mucous membrane.

Urinary Bladder

The urinary bladder is a hollow, muscular sac that acts as a holding reservoir for urine until it is ready to be

Figure 6–2. *Major parts of the kidney.*

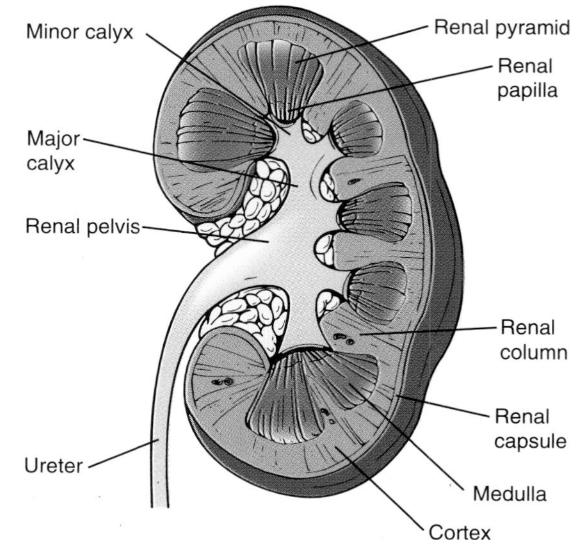

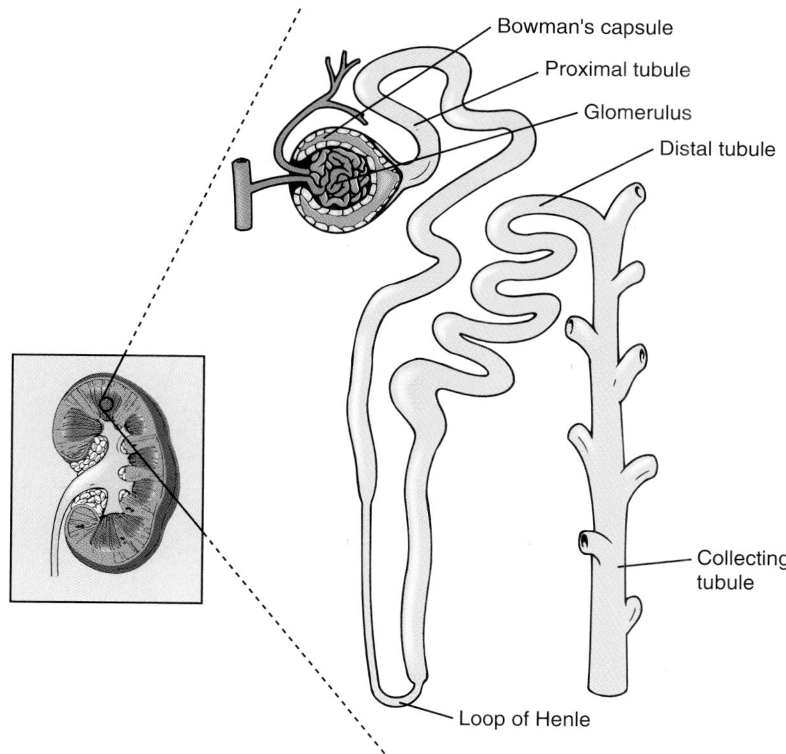

Figure 6–3. *Nephron unit.*

expelled from the body. Urine passes from the body in response to both voluntary and involuntary nervous stimuli.

Urethra

The urethra is a membranous tube through which urine is discharged from the urinary bladder. This tube is approximately 4 cm long in the female and 19 to 20 cm long in the male. The external opening of the urethra is called the **urinary meatus.** Evacuation of urine is variously referred to as **urination, voiding,** or **micturition.**

Urine Formation

The kidney is a highly discriminating organ that maintains the internal environment by selectively excreting or retaining various substances in response to specific body needs. Blood enters the glomerulus of each nephron through the afferent arteriole and flows into the glomerular capillaries.

The walls of the glomerulus capillaries are highly permeable to water and various dissolved substances from blood plasma. These substances filter through the capillary walls and pass into the tubule, where reabsorption of some substances, secretion of others, and the concentration of urine occur.

Certain components, such as glucose, water, and amino acids, are partially or completely reabsorbed by the capillaries surrounding the proximal tubules. In the distal tubule, additional water is absorbed, and potassium and hydrogen are secreted. The urine is concentrated in the loop of Henle and the collecting tubules (Fig. 6–4). The average daily output of urine ranges from 1000 to 2500 mL, depending on the individual's state of hydration. The average adult feels the need to urinate when the bladder contains approximately 300 to 400 mL of urine. Tissue hydration correlates directly to fluid intake and output and fluid loss and retention.

Urinalysis

Urinalysis (UA) is a laboratory procedure that has two purposes, one of which is to detect body disturbances, such as endocrine or metabolic abnormalities. Its second purpose is to detect intrinsic conditions that may adversely affect the kidneys and urinary tract. The com-

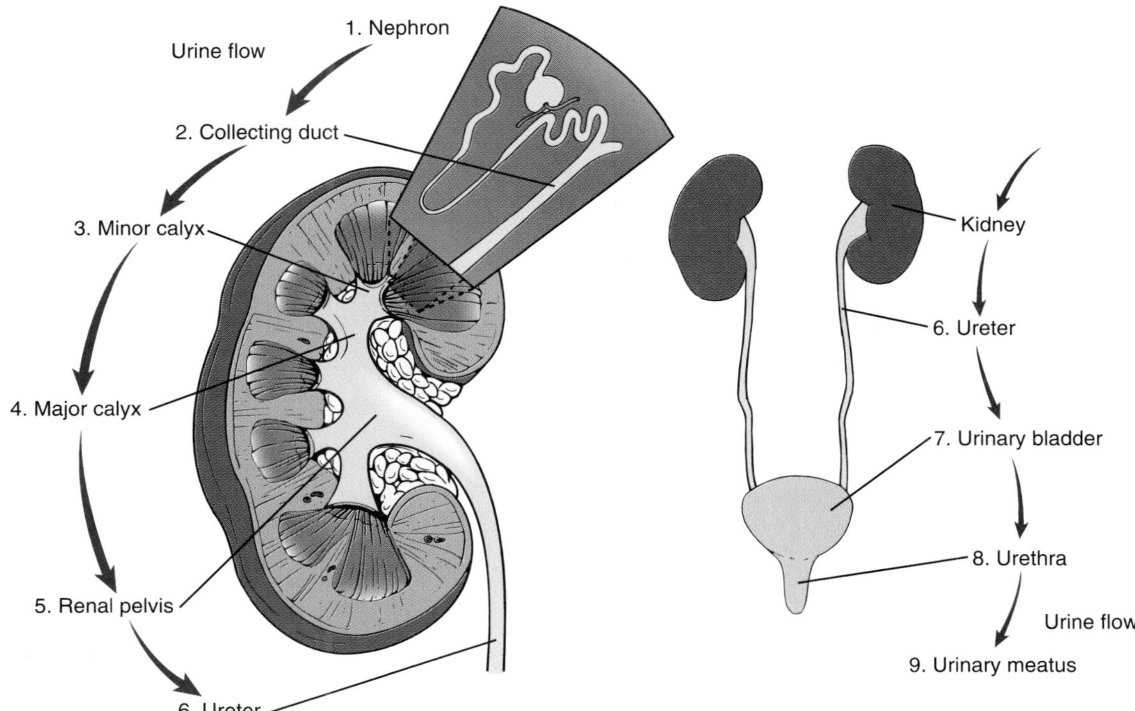

Figure 6–4. *Formation of urine.*

position of urine gives the physician valuable clues as to the well-being of the urinary system and other body systems. A routine UA is an examination of urine to determine the presence of abnormal elements, which may indicate various pathologic conditions.

GUIDELINES

Basic Procedural Steps

- Inspect physical characteristics.
- Analyze urine components through chemical measurements.
- Perform a microscopic examination.

Quality Assurance and Controls

Quality assurance is an important part of urine testing. However, the extreme precision and accuracy required for hematology and chemical assays are not required for routine urinalysis.

ANALYZE

Important Aspects of Quality Assurance in Performing Urinalysis

- Specimen identification
- Specimen handling
- Daily use of controls
- Written procedures
- Instrument maintenance
- Reagent handling
- Record keeping

Specimen Identification

The most frequently encountered laboratory errors involve testing the wrong specimen, or recording the results of a test on the record of the wrong patient. For this reason, it is vitally important that a system for identification of the urine specimen–from the time the urine is voided throughout all testing procedures be established and strictly followed.

GUIDELINES

Identification Procedural Steps

- Identify the patient.
- Record the time the specimen was voided.
- Indicate the time the specimen was centrifuged.
- Note the final testing time.
- Chart the results.

Specimen Handling

Proper procedures for specimen handling should be established so that urine testing is done within 1 hour; otherwise, the specimen should be refrigerated. In either case, the time of collection should be written on the label of the container. Test results may be altered if the urine is left standing at room temperature for an extended period of time. Urine should always be collected in a clean, dry container. A disposable container is highly recommended. Urine specimens may be handled differently depending on the assay to be performed. For example, if tests for urine bilirubin and urobilinogen levels are requested as part of a liver work-up, the specimen should be hand-carried to the laboratory immediately after voiding, as these urine constituents are extremely labile (unstable). They are easily destroyed at room temperature, and may also be affected by laboratory light. In contrast, glucose and ketones are relatively stable in urine unless there are large numbers of organisms in the specimen that metabolize these urine constituents. The best way to temporarily store urine specimens for testing of these constituents is refrigeration. When a bacteriologic culture of urine is to be done, the specimen is usually collected by sterile **catheterization.**

Daily Use of Controls

The use of controls is an important tool to help improve laboratory performance, and to help assure both laboratory staff and patients that the results reported are of the highest quality. Use of control specimens also helps to increase the self-confidence of the personnel performing the testing.

Results obtained on known controls help to assure laboratory personnel that they are performing a test properly, and that the reagents being used have been adequately protected from heat and moisture. A reasonable expectation of results should be established by each laboratory. A commonly suggested control for urinalysis maintains that the test should be considered acceptable if a positive or negative result is obtained on the specimen 95% of the time. Positive specimens used as controls should not be borderline or trace-level–positive. Control values should be posted for easy detection of any trend toward an out-of-control situation, as well as to publicize good, stable, quality controls.

There must also be a written procedure of the steps to follow when a urine test is determined to be "out-of-control." The first step may be simply to repeat the test, after which a decision can be made as to whether or not to do additional testing. **Whatever the corrective procedure established, it must be clearly presented and precisely followed by everyone, with proper records kept. This is mandatory for passing laboratory inspection.**

Written Procedures

Every laboratory must keep an up-to-date manual of laboratory procedures. Every urinalysis procedure used should be included in this manual and should be updated on a regular basis. This manual should also include procedures for microscopic examination of urine sediment, for confirmatory procedures, and for special urine tests.

Instrument Maintenance and Reagent Handling

Keeping reagent strips in a dry, cool place may seem to be a standard, accepted laboratory procedure, but such simple procedures are an important part of quality control. A system for proper handling and storage of reagents needs to be established and closely followed. This should include removing only the necessary number of strips at a time and making certain that the cap is tightly replaced after each use.

It is helpful to maintain a log of instruments and supplies that must be checked daily, weekly, monthly, or at other designated intervals. One person should be responsible for keeping this log, and should see to it that the equipment is maintained as specified by the manufacturer.

Quality assurance should be a simple, set routine that, when maintained, brings satisfaction and confidence to all staff members.

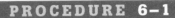

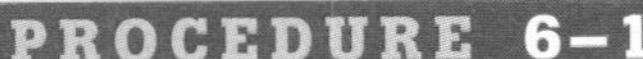

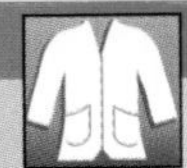

PROCEDURE 6–1

Conducting an Expiration Date Audit

Principle

All testing chemicals and reagents expiration dates must be periodically audited to ensure the validity of testing.

Equipment and Supplies

supply cabinet in which all urinary testing reagents are stored
pencil and paper

Procedural Steps

1. List all of the chemical reagents found in the supply cabinet.
2. Check the expiration date on each bottle.
3. Remove any bottle that has expired.
4. Rearrange stock bottles so that the bottles with the oldest expiration dates are used first. Place those with the newest expiration dates toward the back of the row.
5. List the expired supplies and notify the laboratory supervisor of your findings.
6. Discard the expired reagents according to instructions or accepted laboratory protocols.

Summary

When urinalysis is performed correctly, it can provide valuable information for confirming a diagnosis or ruling out a specific disease. Indeed, in many instances, a chemical change in a patient's urine is the first indication of illness or disease.

Chapter Review

True or False

Circle T or F to indicate the correct answers to the following:

T F 1. The first test to detect sugar was performed by Ismail Jurjani.

T F 2. The kidneys lie within the peritoneal cavity.

T F 3. Perirenal fat is the adipose capsule that embeds the kidney.

T F 4. The average daily output of urine for adults is 300 to 400 mL.

Fill in the Blanks

Complete the following statements:

5. The outer region of the kidney is called the _____________, whereas the inner region is called the _____________.
6. The filtering unit of the kidney is called the _____________.
7. Urine passes through the _____________ on its course from the kidney to the bladder.
8. The female urethra is _____________ cm in length, whereas the male urethra is _____________ cm long.

Multiple Choice

Circle the letter that represents the single best answer:

9. The important aspects of quality assurance as it relates to urinalysis are:
   a. Specimen collection
   b. Specimen identification
   c. Record keeping
   d. Patient preparation
   e. All of the above
10. One of the most frequently encountered laboratory errors relating to specimen identification is:
    a. Obtaining the specimen from the wrong patient
    b. Accidentally spilling the specimen
    c. Recording results on the wrong patient record
    d. Doing the wrong test on the specimen
    e. Failing to report test results to the physician

Anatomy

Label the following parts of the urinary system:

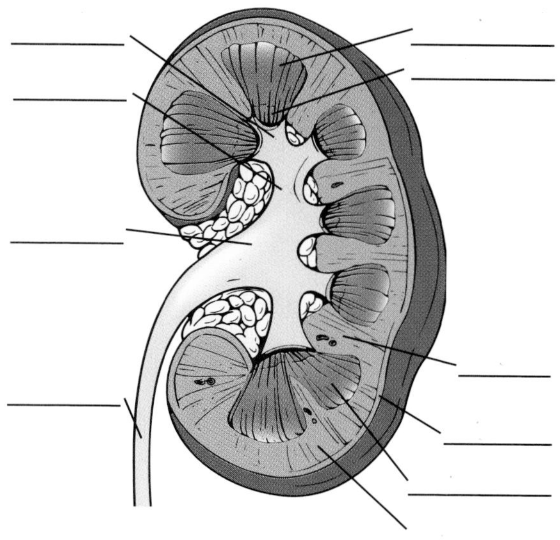

Vocabulary

analyte: a substance or material being chemically analyzed
aseptic: free of infection and/or infectious materials
glans: the cone-shaped enlargement at the end of the penis which, in the uncircumcised male, is covered by the foreskin
labia majora: the two folds of adipose tissue extending from the mons pubis to the perineum in females
labia minora: the two thin folds of epithelial tissue that are situated between the labia majora and the opening of the vagina
sterile: free of all forms of microbial life
urethra: the canal connecting the urinary bladder to the exterior of the body through which urine and sperm (in males) are discharged
urinary meatus: external opening of the urethra
void: urinate

Chapter Objectives

After reading this chapter, you should be able to:

1. Identify the preferred specimen collection method for routine urinalysis.
2. Instruct a female patient on the proper method for obtaining a clean-catch urine specimen.
3. Instruct a male patient on the proper method for obtaining a clean-catch urine sample.
4. State how a timed urine specimen is collected.
5. List tests that may require a 24-hour urine specimen.
6. Explain how a 24-hour urine specimen is collected.
7. State the reasons for adding a preservative to a urine specimen.
8. List the responsibilities of the laboratory worker when a patient presents a urine specimen for processing.
9. Spell and define the words listed in the vocabulary.

Chapter 7
Collecting the Urine Specimen

Whether a specimen is a secretion, excretion, or body material obtained at biopsy, the validity of the results depends on proper specimen collection. Examination of a urine specimen can yield results that will assist in the diagnosis and treatment of the patient. Although medical assistants often collect a variety of specimens for testing outside the physician's office, this chapter focuses on the urine tests that are usually performed within the medical office/clinic.

The manner in which the specimen is collected depends on the test to be performed. The health care worker must adhere to proper urine collection techniques and must be certain to obtain the proper specimen as ordered by the physician. Some specimen collections are complicated and require specially trained personnel and extensive patient preparation. In the medical office, the collection, processing, and/or transport of most specimens can be accomplished without complication. Patient education is the responsibility of the medical assistant, and collecting a urine specimen requires clear and concise instructions.

General Instructions for Urine Collection

Urine specimens may be collected in the medical office or at home. In either situation, it is important to follow appropriate procedures for specimen collection and processing.

GUIDELINES

Instructions for Urine Collection

- Carefully label all specimens. Do not apply the label to the container lid, but place the label on the container itself. Use an indelible marker or make sure that the label will adhere to the container at refrigerated temperatures. On the label, record the patient's name, the date and time of collection, and the type of specimen. Add the physician's name if the specimen is to be sent to a central laboratory facility (Fig. 7–1).

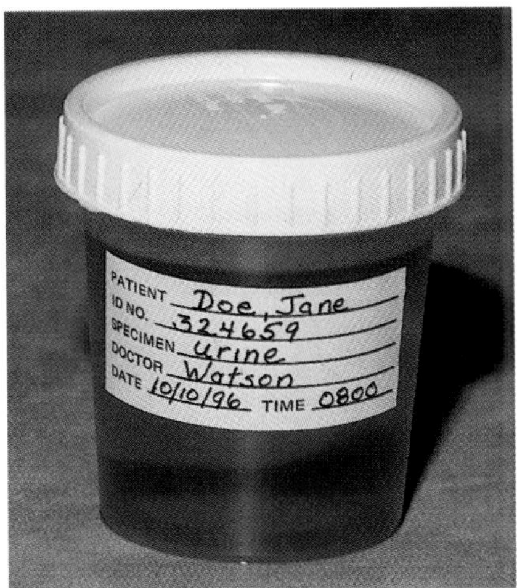

Figure 7–1. *Properly labeled specimen container.*

- Provide a precleaned or sterile disposable container made of plastic or plastic-coated paper (Fig. 7–2). The collection container should have a capacity of 50 to 100 mL and an opening that is 2 inches in diameter. If the specimen is to be obtained from a pediatric patient, the container may be slightly smaller. If the specimen is to be transported, be sure it has a screw-type lid.
- If a bacterial culture is ordered, make sure a sterile container is available. If this is the case, the specimen may have to be obtained through catheterization.
- Advise female patients, with the consent of the physician, that the collection of a urine specimen should be avoided, if possible, during their menstrual period and for several days before and after, as the specimen may be contaminated with blood.
- If the **analyte** is unstable or if the testing is delayed, you may add preservatives to the specimen. Check your laboratory's procedure manual or the procedural manual provided by the referral laboratory to determine the proper preservative for each test. Remember that the preservative must not interfere with the test procedures or results. Always note on the

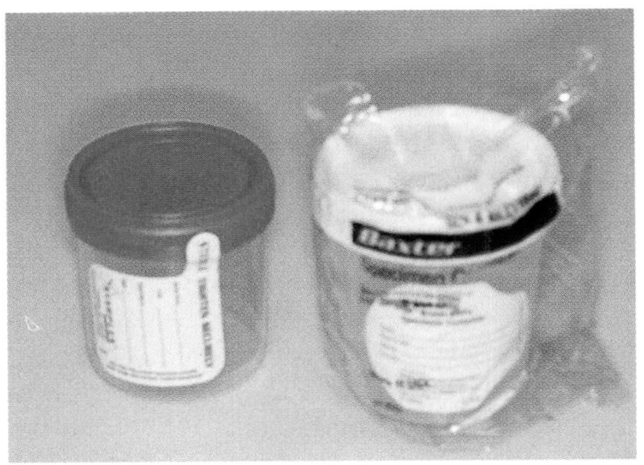

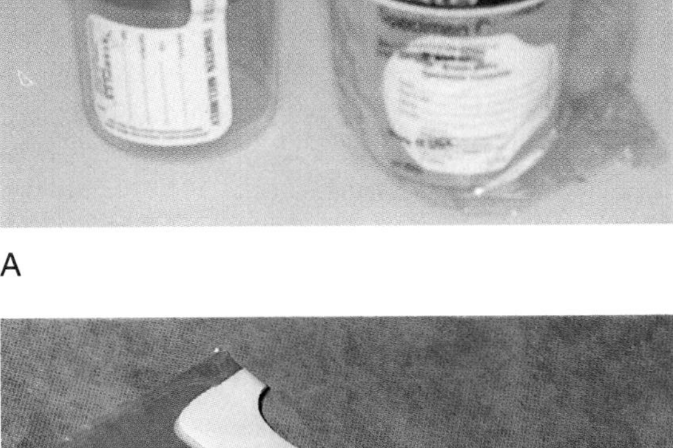

A

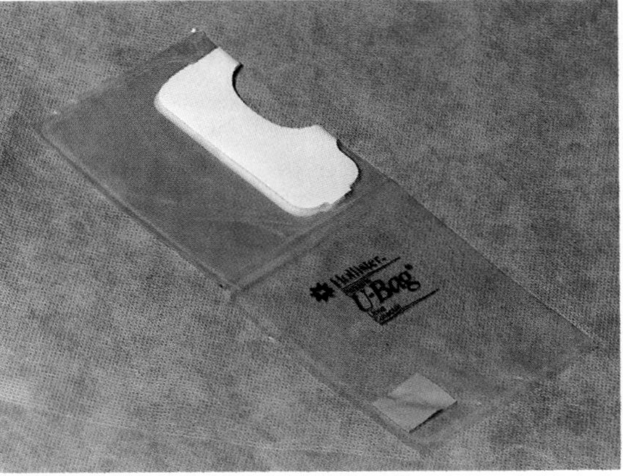

B

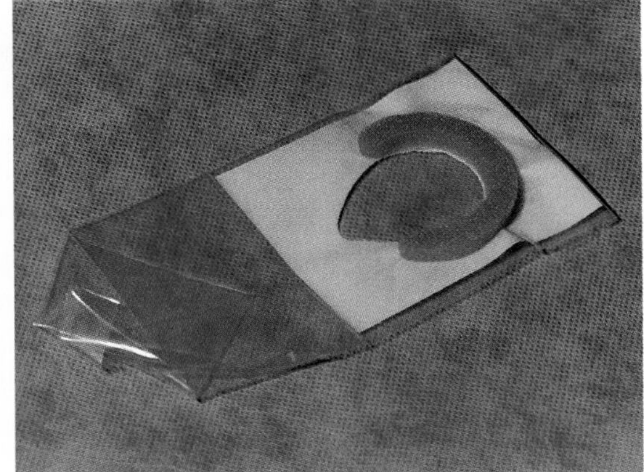

C

Figure 7–2. A, *Adult urine specimen container.* B *and* C, *Pediatric urine specimen containers.*

specimen the type and amount of preservative added.

Types of Specimen Collection

First Morning Sample

A first morning urine sample is the type of specimen most commonly used for routine urinalysis. Because the concentration of urine varies throughout the day, it is usually easiest to identify abnormalities in a relatively concentrated specimen. The first morning specimen may also be called an early morning specimen, as it represents the urine formed over approximately an 8-hour period.

Because it is impractical to collect a first morning specimen in the medical office, the patient must be instructed in the proper collection technique for a clean-catch or mid-stream urine sample. The specimen can then be collected at home and brought to the office. Be certain that the patient knows to refrigerate the specimen until it is transported to the office. (Alternatively, the patient may be instructed to add a preservative to the container.) The laboratory should supply the container (Fig. 7–3), and any preservative to be added, as a container from home may not be properly washed and rinsed prior to use.

When the specimen is delivered to the office or laboratory, the medical assistant should check it for proper labeling and perform the required test(s) immediately. If that is not possible, the specimen may be refrigerated until testing can be done.

Mid-Stream Specimen

A mid-stream urine specimen is one that is collected not at the beginning or end of voiding, but in the middle of urination. The patient is instructed to **void** the first one third of the urine into the toilet. At that point, the patient stops the urine flow, places the specimen container into position, and voids the next one third of the urine into the container. Once the specimen is collected, the patient can then finish emptying the bladder into the toilet. The specimen volume should be at least 25 mL of urine. A mid-stream specimen is thought to be more representative of the contents of the bladder because it is free from the contaminants that may have been in the **urethra** or the **urinary meatus.**

Clean-Catch Specimen

Most laboratories prefer a clean-catch, mid-stream specimen for testing, as it provides the clearest, most accurate results. If the urine specimen is to be tested for bacteria or antibiotic sensitivity and a catheterized specimen is not required, a clean-catch sample will be needed. Collecting this sample requires special cleaning of the external genitalia. Because most patients are not familiar with **aseptic** technique, they must be carefully instructed on the procedure. In the case of a disabled or elderly individual, assistance may be needed in obtaining the specimen.

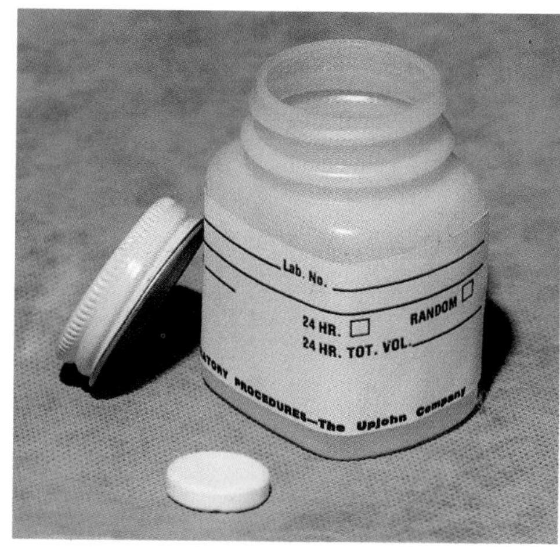

Figure 7–3. *First morning specimen container and preservative.*

Most laboratories and medical offices use a commercial kit that contains all the supplies needed for a clean-catch specimen. This kit contains premoistened towelettes, a **sterile** specimen container, and illustrated instructions (Fig. 7–4).

The female patient should be instructed to first wash her hands before beginning the procedure. Then, she should position herself on the toilet seat with legs spread apart as widely as possible. She then spreads open the **labia majora** using a towelette. Using a clean towelette, she then cleans the **labia minora** on

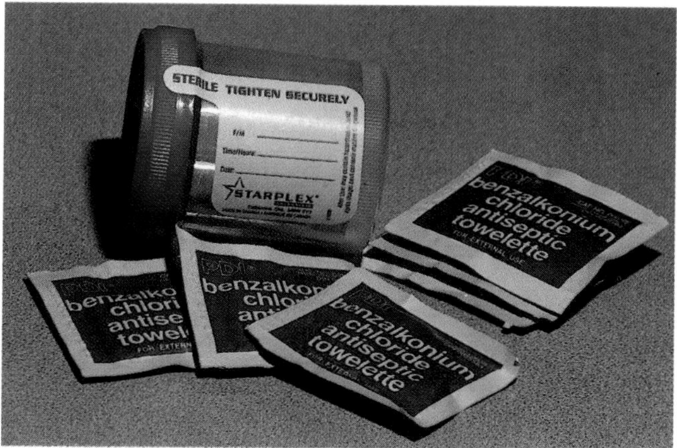

Figure 7–4. *A commercial clean-catch urine collection kit, including a sterile container and antiseptic towelettes.*

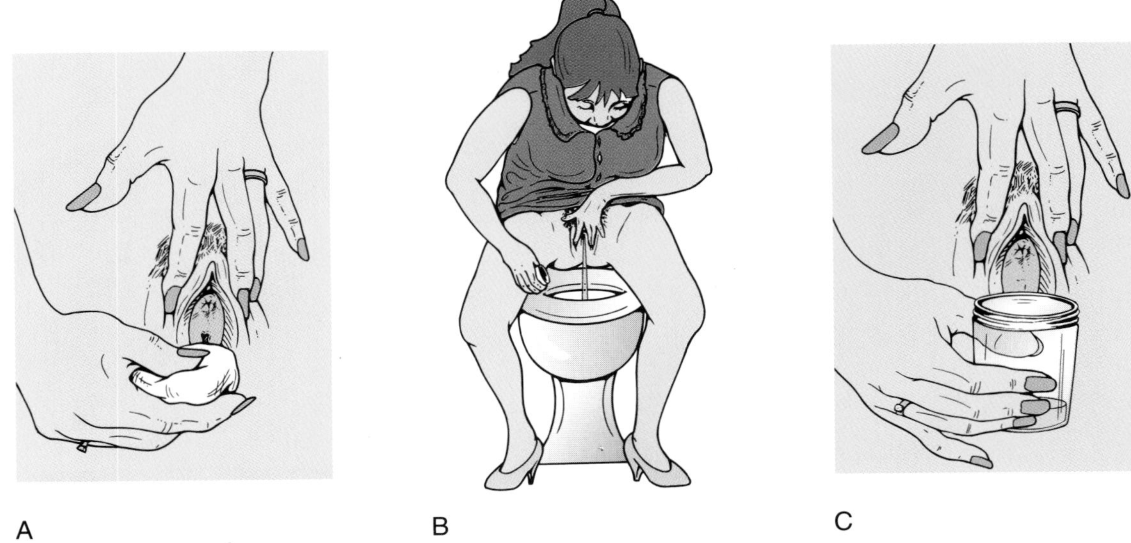

Figure 7–5. *Procedure for obtaining a clean-catch urine specimen in females.*

one side of the urinary meatus with a single stroke, wiping from front to back. She then repeats this procedure, using another towelette, on the opposite side of the meatus. Finally, with a third towelette, she cleans the urinary opening with the same front-to-back motion. After completing this cleaning procedure, she keeps the labia spread while collecting a urine sample using the same procedure as for mid-stream collection (Fig. 7–5).

The male patient should be instructed to retract the foreskin (if not circumcised) using a towelette. Using a clean towelette, he then cleanses the urethral opening with a single stroke directed from the tip of the penis toward the ring of the **glans.** Without touching the cleansed area, he then collects a urine sample according to the procedure for mid-stream collection.

Once the specimen has been collected, the container should be closed immediately. Advise the patient to avoid touching the inside of either the container or the lid (Fig. 7–6).

When the patient delivers the specimen to you, put on gloves before handling the specimen container. Next, wipe the outside of the container with a disinfectant and dry with a clean paper towel. Apply a label that contains all of the needed information. Put the specimen in the designated location and check the restroom and work area to be sure it is clean and ready for the next patient. Remove the gloves and wash your hands.

If the specimen is to be sent to another laboratory for testing, it should be sealed in a plastic bag to ensure safe handling, in case the original container leaks.

Figure 7–6. *Procedure for obtaining a clean-catch urine specimen in males.*

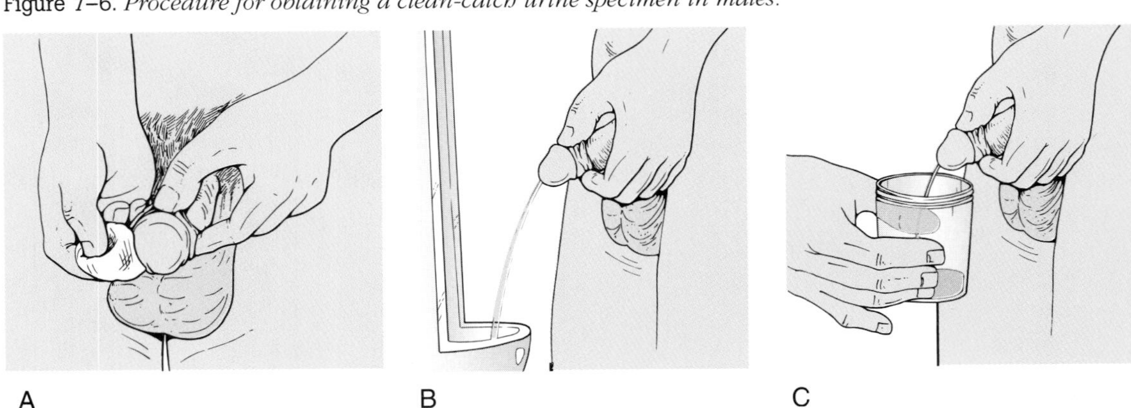

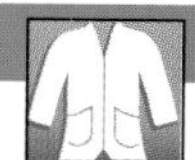

PROCEDURE 7–1

Obtaining a Clean-Catch, Mid-Stream Urine Specimen

Principle

Patient education to ensure proper collection of the sample is vital to the validity of the test results.

Equipment and Supplies

sterile urine specimen container
premoistened towelettes

Procedural Steps

1. Label the specimen container.
2. Read the directions for obtaining the specimen.
3. Go to the restroom and obtain the specimen, carefully following all directions.
4. Place the specimen in the "to be tested" area of the laboratory.
5. To check the accuracy of the collection procedure, your specimen can be cultured. If contaminants appear on the culture media, you failed to follow the instructions and will need to repeat the procedure.

Timed Specimen

A timed urine sample is one that is collected at a specific time or at specific intervals. This type of urinalysis is usually part of a series of tests being done to assess metabolic activity or excretory function. A glucose tolerance test is an example of a type of metabolic testing that requires timed urine samples. After the first blood sample and urine sample have been obtained to establish the basal glucose level, the patient is given a specified amount of glucose to drink. At periodic intervals after glucose ingestion, a blood sample and urine sample are collected to determine the glucose level. The urine samples in this procedure are timed samples because they must be collected at the same time that the blood is drawn.

It is extremely important that you have the proper reagents and containers on hand before beginning any timed test. All specimens must be fully labeled and the collection time MUST appear on the label. After obtaining and labeling the sample, refrigerate it immediately or send it to the referral laboratory according to established protocols.

24-Hour Urine Collection (Addis Test)

Because the concentration of urine changes over a 24-hour period, a single urine sample may not yield results that are representative of the patient's true clinical picture. The Addis test requires pooling of urine over a 3-, 6-, 12-, or 24-hour period. The method of collection is the same for all time periods; only the length of time that the sample is collected varies. The primary purpose of this test is to determine the quantity of an analyte in the specimen.

Because the urine will not be tested until the completion of the designated collection time, it is necessary to add a preservative and to refrigerate the urine to avoid decomposition. Consult the procedural manual for the proper preservative, as it must be one that does not interfere with the analyte.

The normal volume of urine produced every 24 hours varies. Infants and children produce smaller volumes than adults (Table 7–1).

Time is an important parameter in the Addis test. Most patients find it easiest to begin this test upon arising; however, the test may be begun at any time. The first morning voiding is not collected for testing.

Table 7–1
Normal 24-Hour Urine Volumes

Age of Patient	*Urine Volume (mL/24 hr)*
Neonate	20–350
Child (1–9 years)	300–600
Adolescent (10–16 years)	600–1500
Adult	600–2000

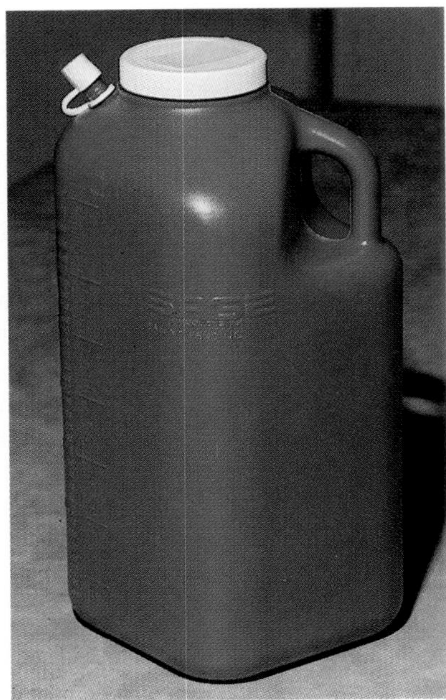

Figure 7–7. *A 24-hour urine specimen container.*

Rather, it is discarded, and the patient notes the time of this voiding. The test thus begins with an empty bladder. The patient then collects all urine voided for the next 24 hours. Individual specimens are collected in a small container and then poured into a large 24-hour container. This collection process continues for the full timed period. At the end of the timed schedule, the patient empties the bladder to collect a final specimen, which is then added to the 24-hour container (Fig. 7–7).

When the patient delivers the container to the office/clinic, the medical assistant will prepare the specimen for transport to the referral laboratory. Be sure that the specimen is thoroughly mixed and the quantity is measured and recorded. After the specimen has been logged, prepare a representative sample from the specimen and send it to the referral laboratory. It is important always to follow the recommended procedure for transport.

Summary

The collection of a urine specimen becomes a routine function in the medical setting. However, to the patient, it seldom is viewed as routine. The culture, language, and educational level of the patient play important roles in how the patient handles this procedure. It is the responsibility of the medical assistant to recognize the patient's needs for help and understanding. Do not assume that, because this procedure seems simple to you, it will also appear simple to the patient. Be sure the patient knows how to collect the specimen and the amount that is needed, and reassure the patient that you are there to assist and that they need not feel embarrassed to ask for clarification or help. Getting it right the first time will save you time and will build the patient's confidence.

Chapter Review

True or False

Circle T or F to indicate the correct answers to the following:

T F 1. The manner in which the urine specimen is collected depends on the nature of the test.

T F 2. It is very important to label the lid of the specimen container.

T F 3. Always be certain to add a preservative to every urine specimen.

T F 4. The first morning specimen is collected 2 hours after the patient awakens in the morning.

Fill in the Blanks

Complete the following statements:

5. A mid-stream specimen is one in which the ______________ portion of the urination is collected.
6. A ______________ - ______________ urine specimen is the most desirable.
7. It is extremely important to have ______________, ______________, and ______________ on hand before beginning a timed test.
8. A 24-hour urine specimen should be placed in the refrigerator to avoid ______________.

Multiple Choice

Circle the letter that represents the single best answer:

9. The normal 24-hour urine volume for an adolescent is:
   a. 100–250 mL
   b. 400–500 mL
   c. 300–600 mL

d. 600–1500 mL
e. 800–2000 mL

10. When labeling a urine specimen, include all of the following EXCEPT:
    a. Name of the patient
    b. Date
    c. Time collected
    d. Date of birth
    e. Physician's name

Vocabulary

albumin: a water-soluble, heat-coagulable protein
bacteriuria: the presence of bacteria in urine
bilirubin: the orange-yellow pigment of bile formed by the breakdown of hemoglobin
crenation: the formation of notches or leaf-like edges in red blood cells, as well as a shriveled surface
glycosuria: the presence of glucose (sugar) in the urine
hematuria: the presence of red blood cells in urine
hemoglobinuria: the presence of hemoglobin in urine
hyposthenuria: the production of urine with low specific gravity
isosthenuria: the production of urine with consistently low specific gravity, regardless of fluid intake
ketonuria: the presence of ketone (acetone) in the urine
lipiduria: the presence of fat in the urine
nephrotic: pertaining to the nephron, which is the fundamental unit of the kidney
polyuria: the excretion of urinary volume exceeding 2000 mL in 24 hours
proteinuria: the presence of an excess of serum proteins in the urine, usually albumin
sediment: the solid (bottom) portion of a centrifuged urine specimen
solute: the substance dissolved in a solution
specific gravity: a measure that reflects the ratio of waste products to fluid in the urine
supernatant: the liquid portion of a centrifuged urine specimen
turbid: clouded or obscured, as occurs with solids that are in suspension in a solution
urea: a systemic osmotic diuretic found in urine
urobilinogen: the presence of bilirubin in the urine
urochrome: the color spectrum of urine

Chapter Objectives

After reading this chapter, you should be able to:

1. Spell and define the vocabulary words.
2. List the three parts of a urinalysis.
3. Explain why the color of urine varies.
4. Identify what causes urine to become turbid.
5. Explain how you would obtain the specific gravity of urine.
6. Identify three reasons why urine may become foul-smelling.
7. List tests that are included in the chemical analysis of urine.
8. Identify the possible causes of the following: glycosuria, proteinuria, ketonuria, hematuria, and urobilinogen.
9. List the microscopic constituents of urine sediment.
10. Explain the need for test confirmation, as well as how it is accomplished.

Chapter 8
Performing Routine Urinalysis

Even in ancient times, health care practitioners recognized the value of the examination of urine. Modern health care practitioners find a routine urinalysis no less valuable than did their predecessors. Because of its ease of collection and the valuable information it can provide, a routine examination of a patient's urine is one of the most commonly ordered clinical laboratory tests. Examination of urine is useful in screening patients for diseases directly related to the kidney or urinary tract, as well as for the diagnosis and treatment of many other diseases.

Like all specimens submitted for laboratory examination, urine that is obtained for routine urinalysis should not be tested until it has been found acceptable for examination.

GUIDELINES

Criteria for Urine Testing

- Identify the patient.
- Label the specimen container.
- Collect the specimen.
- Process the specimen according to laboratory guidelines.

The urinalysis involves the physical, chemical, and microscopic examination of urine (Fig. 8–1).

Physical Examination of Urine

For purposes of urinalysis, the physical examination of urine consists of an evaluation of the urine's color, appearance, specific gravity, and odor.

Color

The normal color of urine is a result of the pigment **urochrome.** The color of normal urine may vary from straw yellow or pale yellow to dark yellow or amber, and may change according to level of hydration, medications,

		LAB
	SER	0496046
Spec. Type: URINE-cathed	Collected: 10/18/96 1515	[2442426]
Result name	Result	Reference Range
Color:	YELLOW	
Character:	CLEAR	Clear
Specific Gravity:	1.030	1.001-1.035
pH:	5.5	4.6-8.0
Protein UA (mg/dL):	NEG	NEG
Glucose (mg/dL):	NEG	NEG
Ketone (mg/dL):	NEG	NEG
Bilirubin (mg/dL):	NEG	NEG
Blood/UA (mg/dL):	NEG	NEG
Nitrite (mg/dL):	NEG	NEG
Urobilinogen (Ehrlich Units):	1	0.1-1.0
Leukocyte:	NEG	NEG
RBC (/HPF):	1	< 3
ASAP	URINALYSIS	
Ord Phys: Dr. HALLS		PRINTED: 05:03 P 1

		LAB
	SER	0496046
Spec. Type: URINE-cathed	Collected: 10/18/96 1515	[2442426]
Result name	Result	Reference Range
Squamous Epithelial (/HPF):	<1	
Amorphous Crystals:	FEW	
Mucus:	OCC	

Figure 8–1. *Laboratory urinalysis form.*

and disease process (Fig. 8–2). **When preparing a female patient for urinalysis, always inquire if she is having her menses at this time, as this must be noted on the laboratory request form.**

Abnormal Urine Colors

Red Urine

The most frequently observed color abnormality is red or red-brown. When the urine appears to be a cloudy pink, red, or red-brown, it may indicate **hematuria,** which is the presence of red blood cells in the urine. **Hemoglobinuria,** the presence of hemoglobin in the urine, results in a clear pink, red, or red-brown color. The presence of *porphyrins,* a group of pigments associated with the production of hemoglobin, is usually responsible for a red or a purple color. The presence of blood in urine with an acid pH may result in a dark brown or even black color. The presence of red blood cells or hemoglobin in the urine is easily confirmed during chemical and microscopic examination.

Yellow-Brown or Green-Brown Urine

Yellow-brown urine that produces a yellow foam when shaken may indicate the presence of **bilirubin** and other bile pigments. Normal, concentrated urine may be dark yellow in color, but will produce a white foam when shaken.

Figure 8–2. *Different colors of normal urine.*

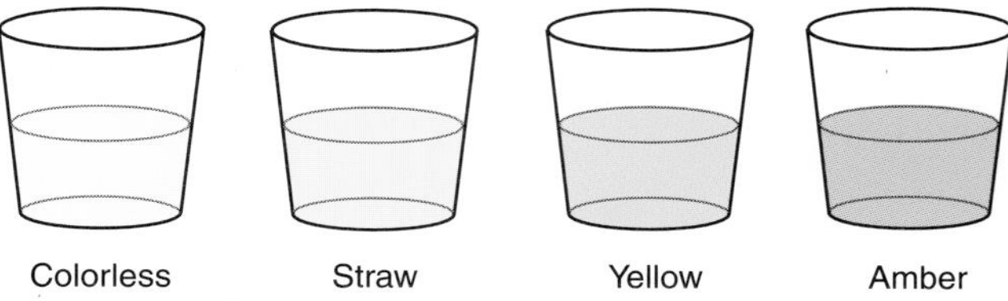

Green-brown urine may be seen in patients with severe obstructive jaundice. Numerous medications and food dyes may also change the color of urine.

Appearance or Character of Urine

Freshly voided normal urine is usually clear. However, cloudy or **turbid** urine may not necessarily be abnormal. Amorphous phosphates in alkaline or basic urine, or urates in acid urine, may cause turbidity. Amorphous phosphates form a white precipitate, which dissolves with the addition of acetic acid. Amorphous urates, leukocytes, or white blood cells may also cause white turbidity. The presence of leukocytes can be confirmed by microscopic examination. Turbidity may also result from the presence of microscopic organisms, such as bacteria, yeast, or parasites, which can result in a hazy appearance. A microscopic examination can confirm or negate the presence of microorganisms. Turbidity or haziness may also result from increased amounts of mucus in the urinary tract. Contamination of the urine with menstrual discharge, feces, or talcum powder has a similar effect (Fig. 8–3).

Lipiduria, the presence of fat globules in urine, can cause haziness or turbidity in the urine of patients with **nephrotic** syndrome or major skeletal trauma. Alternatively, it may simply be attributable to ingesting too much fatty food.

Specific Gravity

The **specific gravity** of urine is the ratio of the weight of a given volume of urine to the weight of the same volume of distilled water at a constant temperature. Specific gravity is the most convenient way of measuring the kidneys' ability to concentrate and dilute. An abnormality in the ability of the kidney to concentrate or dilute urine is an indication of renal disease or hormonal deficiency.

Figure 8–3. *Turbid (contaminated) urine.*

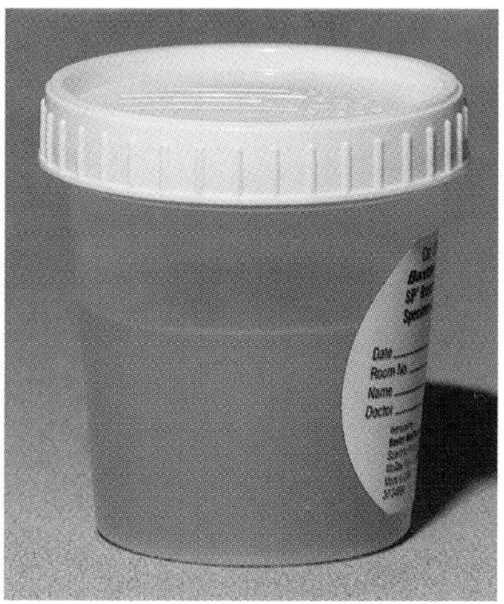

During a 24-hour period, normal adults with normal diets and normal fluid intake produce urine with a specific gravity of between 1.015 and 1.025. The normal range of urine specific gravity for a random collection is 1.005 to 1.030.

Low specific gravity, or **hyposthenuria,** may indicate a concentration problem. Hyposthenuria may occur in patients with *diabetes mellitus* and *diabetes insipidus, glomerulonephritis,* or *pyelonephritis,* to name a few of the more common, related diseases.

High specific gravity, termed hypersthenuria, can result from dehydration, **proteinuria, glycosuria,** adrenal insufficiency, nephrotic disease, and congestive heart failure. It may also be the result of excessive loss of water secondary to sweating, fever, vomiting, and diarrhea. Fixed urine specific gravity, **isosthenuria,** correlates with a specific gravity in the range of 1.010, which varies little from specimen to specimen. Isosthenuria indicates severe renal damage affecting both the concentrating and diluting functions of the kidney.

Methods of Measurement

Urine specific gravity is commonly measured by hydrometer, refractometer, and reagent strip (Fig. 8–4).

Hydrometer

A urinometer is a hydrometer that has been calibrated to measure the specific gravity of urine at room temperature. Measurement of urine specific gravity using a urinometer is based on the principle of buoyancy. The higher the urine specific gravity, the more dense the urine, and thus, the higher the urinometer will float. This method of measurement has been discontinued in many offices.

The urine specimen should be allowed to reach room temperature before using the urinometer. To ensure accuracy, the urinometer should be checked using distilled water, which has a specific gravity of 1.000. The urinometer should also be checked against solutions with known specific gravity to further ensure the accuracy of the urinometer readings. The hydrometer method is the least accurate method of determining urine specific gravity, and is not widely used today.

Refractometer

A refractometer, or Total Solids (TS) meter, is an instrument specifically designed for measuring the total solids of a solution. A refractometer measures the refractive index of a solution. The refractive index is the ratio of the velocity of light in air to the velocity of light in the solution. Most refractometers used to measure

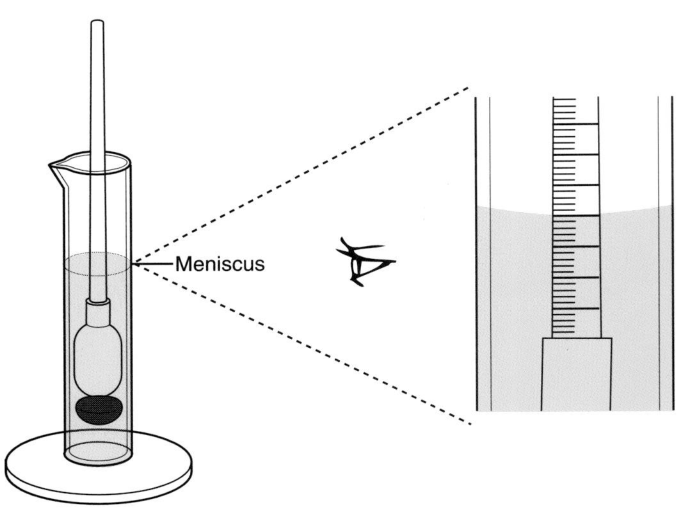

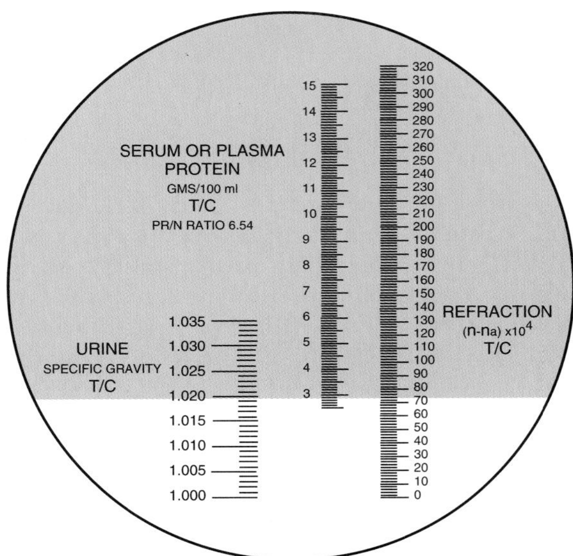

A

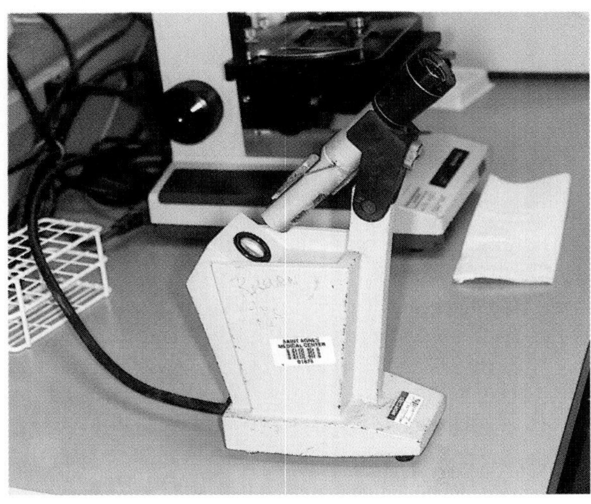

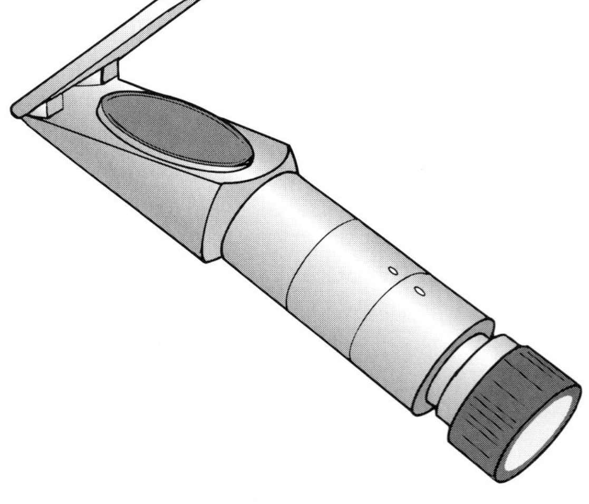

B

Figure 8–4. A, *Refractometer.* B, *Hydrometer.*

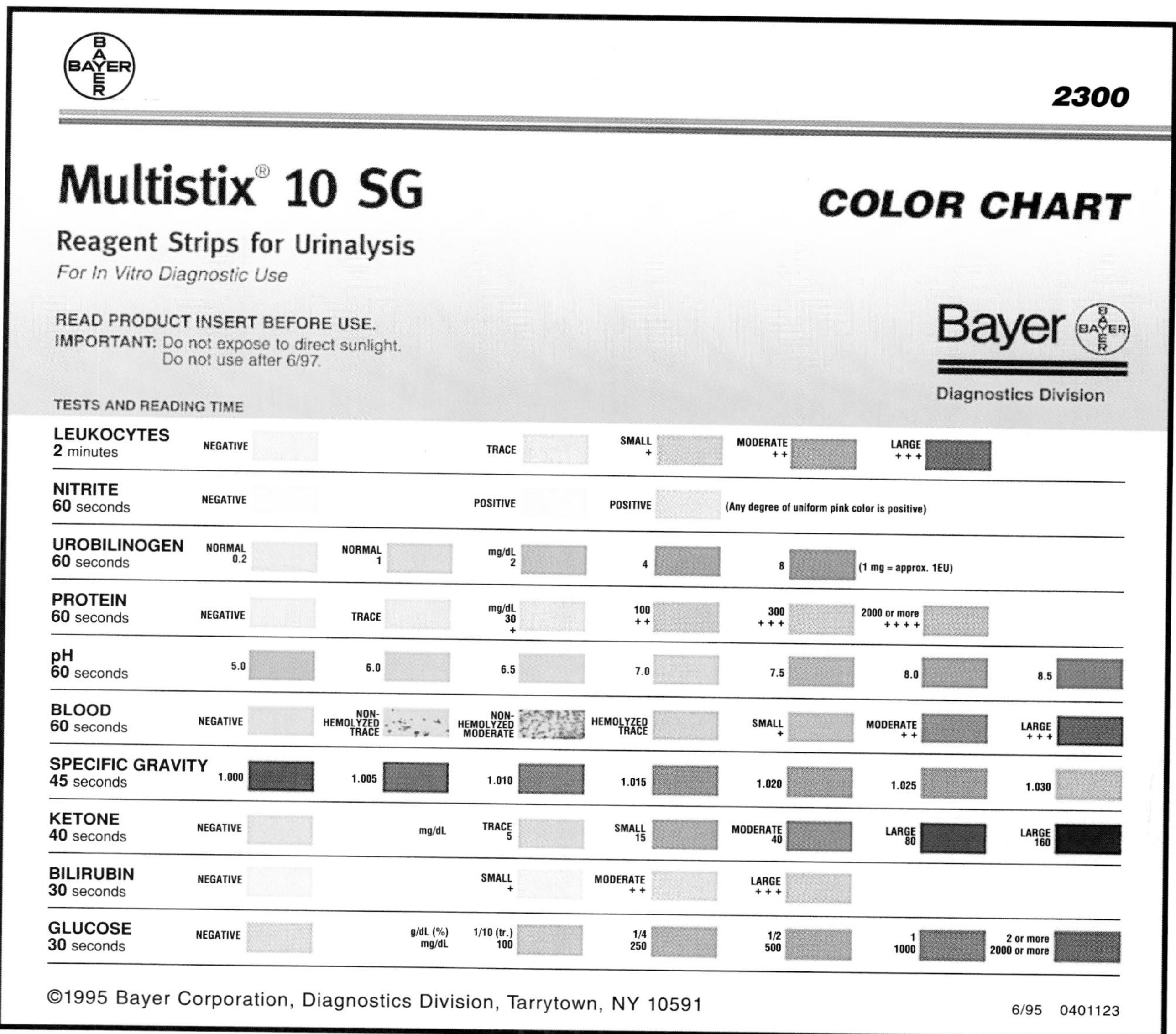

Figure 8–5. *Ames color table for reagent testing. (Courtesy of Diagnostic Division, Bayer Corporation)*

urine specific gravity have been calibrated in terms of specific gravity, refractive index, and total solids. The refractometer should also be calibrated daily to ensure the greatest accuracy possible. A refractometer is preferable to the urinometer in that it only requires one drop of well-mixed urine and has greater accuracy.

Reagent Strip

The newest and most common method of determining specific gravity is the colorimetric reagent strip method. The reagent strip method is a convenient method for estimating specific gravity on the basis of a color reaction. The reagent strip pad changes color according to the concentration of ions in the urine specimen. The resultant color is then compared to a chart to determine the specific gravity (Fig. 8–5).

Osmolality

Urine osmolality, like urine specific gravity, is a measure of the total **solute** concentration in urine. However, urine osmolality is not affected by the density solute, such as glucose and protein. Therefore, osmolality is a better indicator of the ability of the kidneys to concentrate and dilute. Osmolality is not a part of the routine urinalysis. A freezing point depression method is the most frequently used test protocol. Normal urine osmolality in an adult is 500 to 850 mOsm/kg of water.

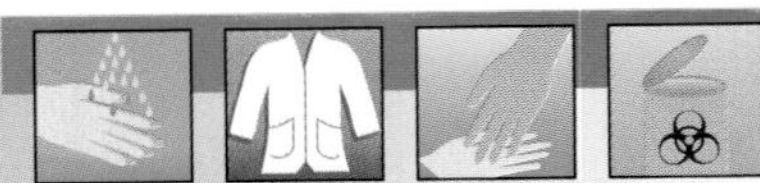

PROCEDURE 8–1

Measurement of Specific Gravity Using a Hydrometer

Principle

Examine and record the specific gravity of urine.

Equipment and Supplies

hydrometer (urinometer)
urine cylinder
filter paper

Procedural Steps

1. Wash hands with disinfectant and put on gloves.
2. Assemble equipment and supplies.
3. Check the calibration of the hydrometer by reading the specific gravity of distilled water. The specific gravity of distilled water should be 1.000.

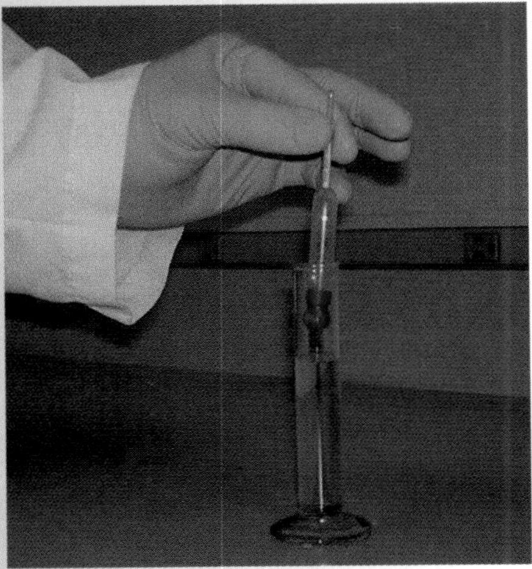

Checking specific gravity of distilled water

4. Obtain a fresh urine specimen.
5. Fill a clean cylinder three-fourths full of well-mixed, freshly voided urine.

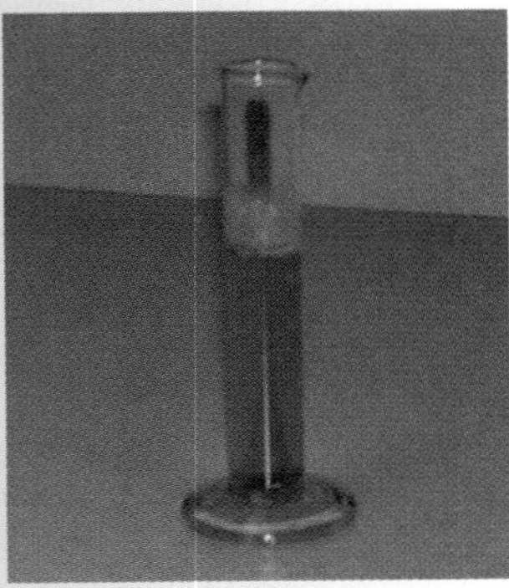

Filling cylinder three-fourths full of well-mixed urine

6. Remove any foam using filter paper.

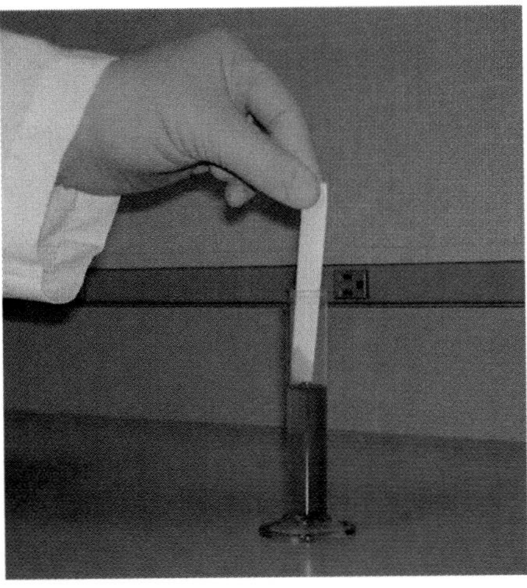

Removing foam with filter

7. Gently insert the hydrometer into the urine using a gentle spinning motion.

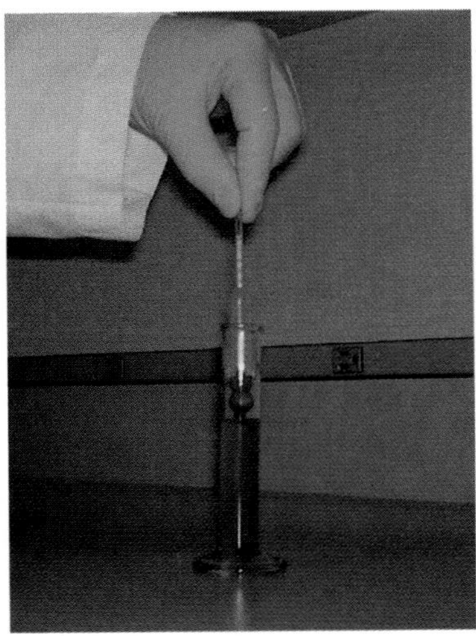

Inserting hydrometer with a gentle spinning motion

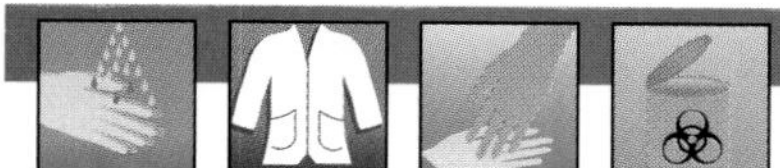

PROCEDURE 8–1

Measurement of Specific Gravity Using a Hydrometer (Continued)

8. The specific gravity is determined by reading the level of the meniscus on the scale of the hydrometer at eye level.

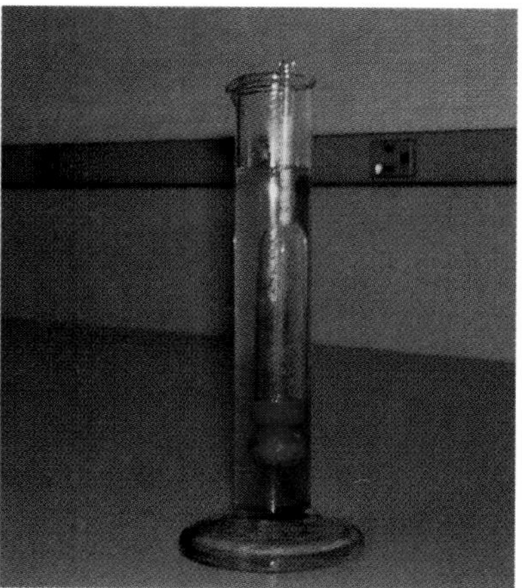

Reading urine-specific gravity with a hydrometer

9. After consulting with the physician or laboratory technologist, discard the urine sample according to laboratory policy.
10. Record your findings on the proper forms.
11. Disinfect the equipment and work area.
12. Remove gloves and wash your hands.

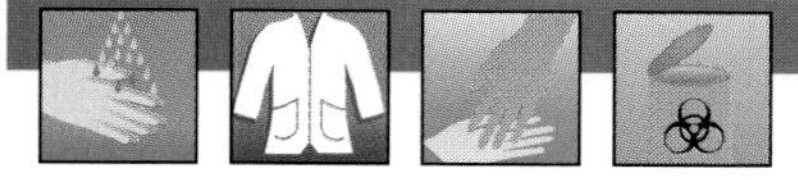

PROCEDURE 8–2

Measurement of Specific Gravity Using a Refractometer

Principle

Measure the refractive index of the urine.

Equipment and Supplies

urinary refractometer
filter paper

Procedural Steps

1. Wash hands and put on gloves.
2. Assemble equipment and supplies.
3. Check the calibration of the refractometer by reading the specific gravity of distilled water. The specific gravity of distilled water should be 1.000.
4. Collect a well-mixed, fresh urine specimen in a clean, dry container.
5. Place one drop of well-mixed urine on the prism of the calibrated refractometer.
6. Determine the specific gravity by reading the level on the scale.
7. After consulting with the physician or laboratory technologist, discard the urine sample according to laboratory policy.
8. Record your test results on the proper form(s).
9. Clean and disinfect all equipment and the work area.
10. Clean the refractometer prism and dry it with lint-free tissue.
11. Remove and discard gloves.
12. Wash hands.

Odor

Normal, freshly voided urine has a faint, not offensive, aromatic odor. Odor can be important in determining whether a urine specimen collected for urinalysis is acceptable. Urine that has been standing for a period of time after collection may develop an ammonia odor that results from the breakdown of urea by a bacteria in the urine.

Urine that has a foul smell may indicate a urinary tract infection. Urine from patients with diabetes mellitus may have a fruity odor owing to the presence of ketone in the urine.

Diet can affect the odor of urine as well. Asparagus and garlic are foods that can produce an abnormal urine odor. Abnormal urine odors are also often associated with amino acid disorders. These observations of abnormal odor should be noted on the laboratory slip.

Urine Volume

The normal volume of urine produced by an adult in a 24-hour period is 600 to 2000 mL. **Polyuria** is a 24-hour urine output that exceeds 2000 mL. In normal patients, the predominant factor affecting urine output is water intake. Urinary output is measured by doing a 24-hour urine collection (see Chapter 7).

Chemical Examination of Urine

The chemical phase of the urinalysis includes qualitative and quantitative testing.

Qualitative tests usually involve comparisons with a color chart, with the results being recorded in terms of trace, +1, +2, +3, or +4. Sometimes, it is only necessary to record the results as negative or positive. These types of readings are quick and easy to perform in the medical office and are useful for screening purposes.

Quantitative urine tests usually involve the use of more complex equipment and testing procedures. Frequently, these tests are performed in a larger laboratory, as they are time consuming and the equipment required is prohibitively expensive for a medical office laboratory. These tests indicate the exact amount of a chemical substance that is present, and the results are reported in measurable units (e.g., grams per liter).

TEST

Tests Performed in the Chemical Examination of Urine

- pH
- Glucose
- Ketone
- Protein
- Blood
- Bilirubin
- Urobilinogen
- Nitrite
- Leukocyte esterase

The configuration of all of these chemical tests available on reagent strips and the number of tests per strip depends upon the type of reagent strip used. In the physician's office laboratory (POL), chemical examination of urine is usually accomplished using a reagent strip. Confirmatory tests and other procedures may be required for special circumstances or different conditions. For example, screening tests for reducing substances are often included in the routine urinalysis of the urine specimen of a child.

Reagent strips should be stored and handled carefully to ensure the best possible test results. Strips should be stored in the container supplied by the manufacturer. They should be kept in a cool, dry place, not refrigerated. Always check the expiration date on the container before using the reagent strips. Whenever a new lot number is received, the manufacturer's instructions should be reviewed for any changes in test protocol.

The best results are obtained when the urine is tested as soon as possible after collection. Urine that cannot be tested within 1 hour of collection should be refrigerated. Refrigerated specimens are acceptable for testing for up to 8 hours after collection. The best results are obtained when the urine is allowed to return to room temperature before testing. The reagent strip should be quickly dipped in a fresh, well mixed, unspun urine sample. The strip should remain in the urine for 1 second or less. Any excess urine is then removed by gently tapping the suspended strip. The strip is then read, following the exact timing requirements for each chemical test while holding the reagent strip close to the color chart for comparison. Great care should be taken in reading the strip to avoid inconsistencies in reporting results. A good light source should always be available to ensure the most accurate reading possible. When manually comparing the strip to the color chart, take care **NOT** to get urine on the color chart. Reagent strips are most commonly read manually, but instruments that detect color changes electronically are available. When possible, the use of an instrument for reading reagent strips is preferable because it eliminates inconsistencies in interpretation.

In many large POLs and in all hospital laboratories, automated strip readers are used. This helps to lower the rate of erroneous readings that occur when the strips are not read at the correct times or when urine runs between the test squares and falsifies the readings (Fig. 8–6).

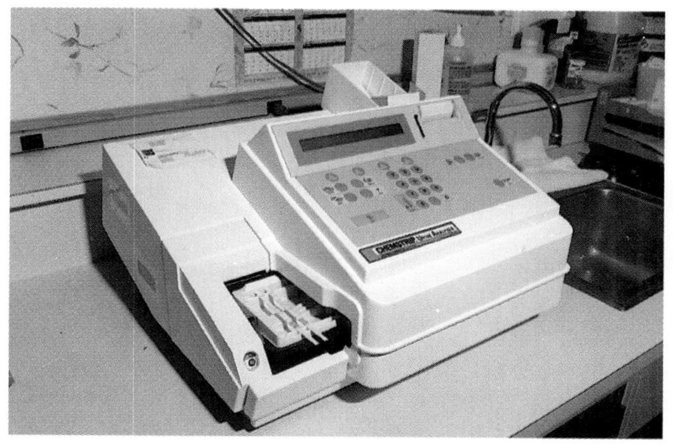

A

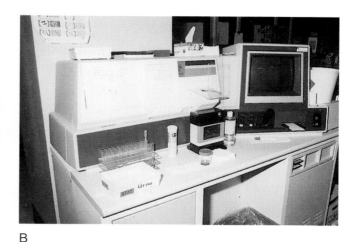

B

Figure 8–6. *Automated strip readers.*

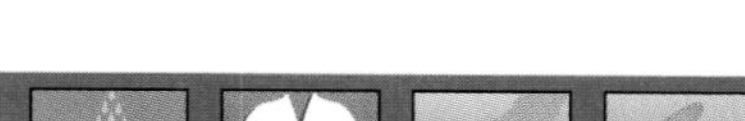

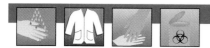

PROCEDURE 8–3

Chemical Examination of Urine Using Reagent Strips

Principle

Test and report the chemical analysis of urine.

Equipment and Supplies

reagent strips
color comparison chart

Procedural Steps

1. Wash hands and put on gloves.
2. Assemble equipment and supplies.
3. Collect a well-mixed, fresh urine specimen in a clean, dry container.
4. Remove one (1) reagent strip from the bottle and replace the cap.
5. Fully immerse the reagent pad area of the strip in the urine sample.
6. Quickly remove the excess urine from the strip.

   Remember to keep the strip horizontal to prevent mixing of chemicals from adjoining reagent pads.
7. Compare the reagent pad areas to the corresponding areas on the bottle or the color chart provided. Carefully match the appropriate reagent pad, but avoid contaminating the color chart with the inoculated reagent strip.
8. Follow the timing requirements for each test as specified on the bottle or color chart. Proper timing is critical for accurate results.
9. Record the results on the proper laboratory form(s).
10. After consulting with the physician or laboratory technologist, discard the used reagent strip and urine sample according to laboratory policy.
11. Remove and discard gloves.
12. Wash hands.

Routine Urine Chemistry Tests

Urinary pH

The *pH,* or the percentage of hydrogen ion concentration of a solution, is a reflection of the acidity or alkalinity of that solution. A pH of 7.0 is considered to be neutral. The pH of distilled water is 7.0. A pH of 0 to 7.0 is considered to be acidic, whereas a pH of 7 to 14 is considered to be alkaline or basic.

The body's acid–base balance is regulated by the lungs and the kidneys. Volatile substances that affect acid–base balance are removed from the body by the lungs during expiration. Nonvolatile substances that affect the body's acid–base balance are excreted by the kidneys.

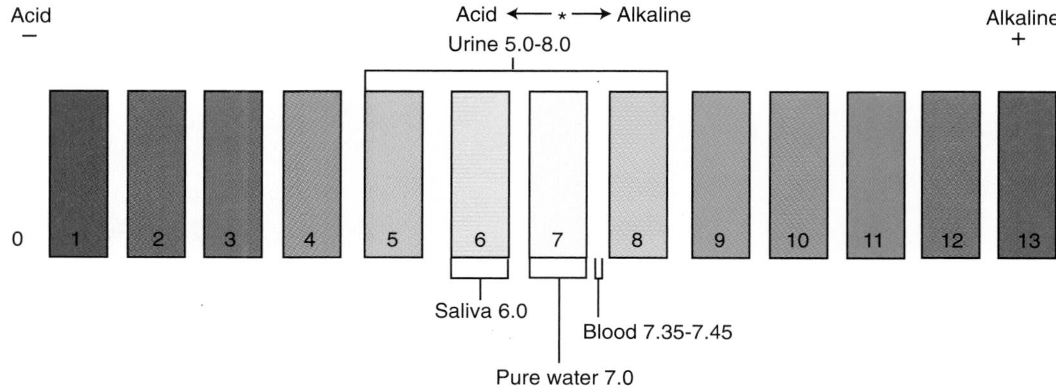

Figure 8–7. *pH scale.*

Diet, medication, and disease may affect body pH level. A diet that is high in protein will create an acidic urine. An alkaline urine can be the result of a diet high in vegetables and citrus fruits. The pH of urine may be regulated by medication to prevent the production of kidney stones, to fight bacterial infections, and to increase the excretion rate of a specific substance. Diseases, such as respiratory acidosis and metabolic acidosis, urinary tract infections, starvation, and diarrhea, can cause the pH to fluctuate.

A normal, freshly voided urine will usually have a pH of 4.5 to 8.0. Within this range, the urine pH of most healthy patients is around 6.0.

An accurate measurement of urinary pH requires a freshly voided urine specimen. Unless refrigerated, urine become alkaline upon standing owing to the loss of carbon dioxide and the conversion of urea into ammonia by bacteria. The pH portion of the reagent strip uses the indicators methyl red and bromthymol blue. These indicators show a color range that changes from orange to green to blue as the pH becomes more basic (Fig. 8–7).

When a precise measurement of urinary pH is desired, pH can be measured by use of a pH meter. A pH meter is an instrument that uses a glass electrode and provides a direct readout of pH (see Fig. 8–6).

Urinary Glucose

Glucose is the sugar typically found in urine. Other sugars, such as lactose, fructose, galactose, and pentose, may be detected in urine under specific circumstances. Glucose is present in urine when the blood glucose level exceeds the renal threshold. Glycosuria is the presence of glucose in urine.

Patients with diabetes mellitus have glycosuria, along with polyuria and thirst. The reagent strip tests for glucose rely on enzymatic tests that are specific for glucose. A common reagent strip urinary glucose enzymatic method uses glucose oxidase. The glucose oxidase reacts specifically with glucose. Sugars, such as lactose, fructose, and others, are not detected by the glucose oxidase method. A copper reduction test is a commonly used confirmatory and screening test for glucose and other reducing substances in urine. Copper reduction tests are used in pediatric patients to detect increased levels of glucose that may not be detected by the specific enzymatic test found on most reagent strips (Fig. 8–8).

Figure 8–8. *Pediatric copper reduction testing.*

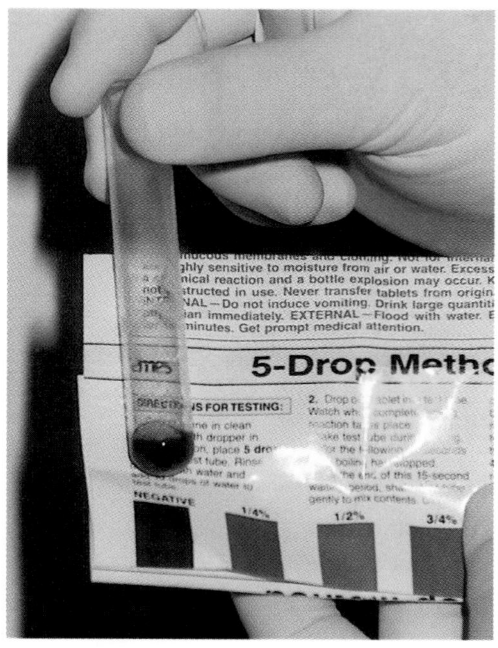

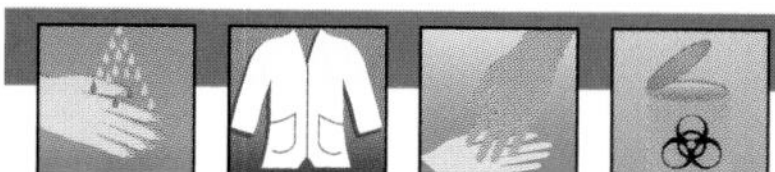

PROCEDURE 8–4

Performing a Clinitest for Reducing Substances

Principle

Perform confirmatory testing for glucose in the urine using Clinitest.

Equipment and Supplies

urinary test tube
medicine dropper
distilled water
Clinitest tablet
color comparison chart
watch with second hand

Procedural Steps

Carefully follow the manufacturer's instructions.

1. Collect a well-mixed, fresh urine specimen in a clean, dry container.
2. Place 5 drops of urine in a test tube. Add 10 drops of distilled water to the same test tube.
3. Drop one (1) Clinitest tablet into the test tube once the latter has been placed in a rack. (Remember that the tube will become too hot to hold.) Observe the test tube while a complete boiling reaction takes place.
4. Fifteen (15) seconds after the end of the boiling reaction, shake the test tube gently to mix the contents.
5. Compare the color of the liquid in the test tube to the color chart.
6. Record the results properly.
7. After consulting with the physician or laboratory technologist, discard the urine sample according to laboratory policy.

Caution: Clinitest contains sodium hydroxide, which is caustic and can cause severe burns. Therefore, the instructions on the package should be followed carefully.

Urinary Ketones

Ketonuria is a term that indicates the presence of ketone in the urine as a result of incomplete fat metabolism. Ketonuria may occur as a result of vomiting, diarrhea, starvation, and diabetes mellitus, among other conditions. Ketonuria in patients with insulin-dependent diabetes is important because it indicates that a change in insulin dosage or other treatment may be warranted.

The reagent strip test for ketone is based on a nitro-oxide reaction. Ketone, in the form of acetone and acetoacetic acid, reacts to create a violet color. The reagent strip pad changes color from beige (negative) to violet (positive).

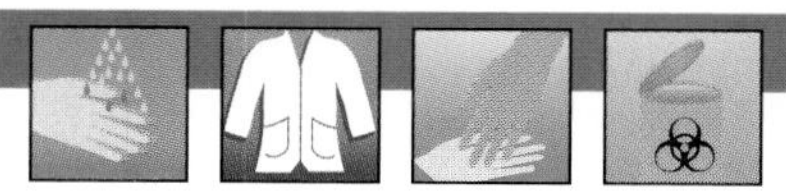

PROCEDURE 8–5

Performing an Acetest for Ketones

Principle

Perform confirmatory testing for ketones in the urine using Acetest tablets.

Equipment and Supplies

Acetest tablet
color comparison chart
medicine dropper
watch with a second hand
white paper or filter paper

(continued)

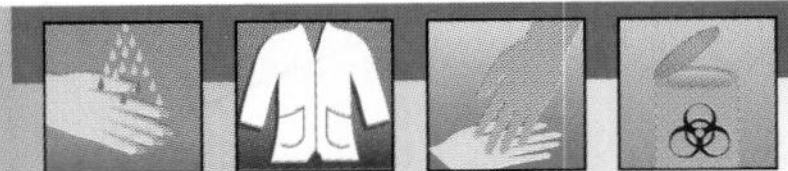

PROCEDURE 8–5

Performing an Acetest for Ketones (Continued)

Procedural Steps

Carefully follow the instructions provided by the manufacturer.

1. Wash hands and put on gloves.
2. Assemble equipment and supplies.
3. Place an Acetest reagent tablet on a piece of white paper or filter paper.
4. Place 1 drop of fresh, well-mixed urine on the tablet. (Serum, plasma, or whole blood may also be tested using the Acetest tablet.)
5. After 30 seconds, compare the color of the tablet to the color chart provided with the Acetest kit.
6. Record the results, either positive or negative, on the proper laboratory form(s).
7. After consulting with the physician or laboratory technologist, discard test materials according to laboratory policy.
8. Disinfect the equipment and work area.
9. Return all equipment to its storage area.
10. Remove gloves and wash hands.

Urinary Proteins

In normal patients, there is only a scant amount of protein in the urine. Urinary proteins consist mainly of **albumin** and globulin. These urinary proteins are derived from plasma and the urinary tract.

Proteinuria is an increase in urinary protein. Proteinuria can occur after strenuous exercise or dehydration, and it may also be an indicator of extrarenal disease or a significant sign of renal disease. The detection of urinary protein by the reagent strip method, coupled with a microscopic examination of the urinary sediment, is important in diagnosing renal disorders.

Because of the importance of a positive result on a reagent strip protein test, all positive strips should be confirmed by a second method. A commonly used confirmatory test is the sulfosalicylic acid precipitation test. Urinary protein precipitates in the presence of sulfosalicylic acid, and the turbidity caused by the precipitation can be graded from negative to +4.

Certain diseases are characterized by the presence of a particular type of protein. Bence Jones proteinuria is associated with multiple myeloma. Albumin may be associated with strenuous exercise, pregnancy, infections, and glomerulonephritis. Globulins are associated with glomerulonephritis and renal tubular dysfunction. Other proteins, such as hemoglobin, fibrinogen, **urea,** and nucleoproteins are associated with other specific conditions (Table 8–1).

The reagent strip test is based on the ability of proteins to alter the color of some acid–base indicators without altering the pH. The reagent strip method uses the indicator tetra bromphenol blue, buffered at a pH of 3; the color changes from yellow (no protein) to green and then blue with increasing amounts of protein.

Table 8–1
Proteins Found in Urine

Protein	*Associated Cause(s)/Conditions*
Albumin	Strenuous physical exercise Emotional stress Pregnancy Infection Glomerulonephritis Neonates (first week)
Globulins	Glomerulonephritis Renal tubular dysfunction
Hemoglobin	Hematuria Hemoglobinuria
Fibrinogen	Severe renal disease
Nucleoprotein	White blood cells (WBCs) in urine Epithelial cells in urine
Bence Jones	Multiple myeloma Leukemia

Courtesy of Diagnostics Division, Bayer Corporation

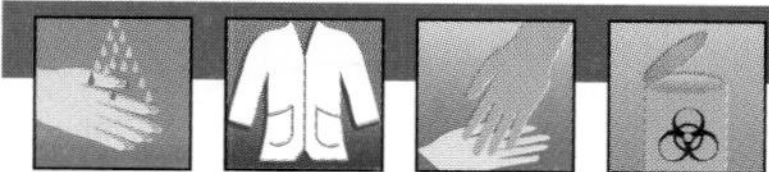

PROCEDURE 8–6

Performing a Sulfosalicyclic Acid Test for Protein

Principle

Perform and report the testing results for the presence of urine protein using SSA precipitation test.

Equipment and Supplies

centrifuged urine
urine measuring device (mL)
urine test tube
3% Sulfosalicylic acid

Procedural Steps

1. Place 3 mL of centrifuged, fresh, well-mixed urine in a test tube.
2. Add 3 mL of 3% sulfosalicylic acid.
3. Mix thoroughly and estimate the amount of turbidity present.
4. Record the results as negative, trace, +1, +2, +3, or +4.
5. After consulting with the physician or laboratory technologist, discard test materials according to laboratory policy.
6. Record the test results on correct laboratory form.
7. Properly clean and store all equipment.
8. Clean equipment and work area.
9. Remove gloves and wash hands.

Urinary Blood

Hematuria is the presence of red blood cells in the urine. Hemoglobinuria is the presence of free hemoglobin in the urine. Blood in the urine may be in the form of intact red blood cells or in the form of free hemoglobin. A "smokey" red urine or cloudy red urine is an indicator of hematuria, whereas a clear pink or clear red urine is an indicator of hemoglobinuria.

Bleeding in the urinary tract may occur with renal disorders, infectious diseases, trauma, or neoplasms, and after excessive exercise. Free hemoglobin may be found in hemolytic diseases, transfusion reactions, and any condition or disease that causes damage to the red blood cells.

The detection of blood in the urine is most commonly done by a reagent strip method. The reagent strip pad is saturated with an indicator that changes from orange (negative) to green and then dark blue with increasing amounts of urinary blood (see Fig. 8–7).

Urinary Bilirubin

Bilirubin is a product of the breakdown of hemoglobin in bone marrow, spleen, and liver. Bilirubin is transmitted in the blood by protein. This unconjugated bilirubin will not pass through the glomerular membrane of the kidney. When bilirubin is conjugated in the liver, it becomes water-soluble and is then able to pass through the glomerular membrane.

Conjugated bilirubin in the urine indicates that there may be obstructive disease. Bilirubin may also appear in the urine of patients with viral hepatitis; therefore, care should be taken in the handling of any urine with a positive bilirubin. The urine of patients with an elevated bilirubin level usually appears dark yellow or amber, with a yellow foam (Fig. 8–9).

The reagent strip method of detecting urinary bilirubin involves the use of diazotized 2, 4-dichloroaniline, which reacts with bilirubin to form a brownish to purplish color.

A positive bilirubin test by the reagent strip method can be confirmed by testing with Ictotest Reagent Tablets.

Figure 8–9. *Amber urine with yellow foam (indicating an elevated bilirubin level).*

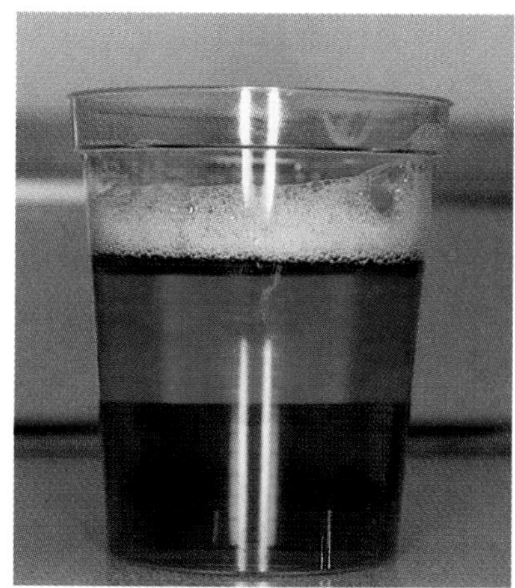

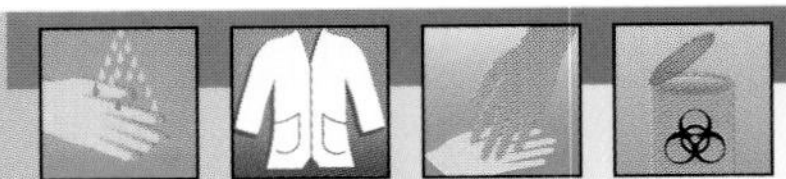

PROCEDURE 8-7

Performing an Ictotest for Bilirubin

Principle

Test and report the chemical results for bilirubin in urine using Ictotest.

Equipment and Supplies

Ictotest
distilled water
watch with a second hand

Procedural Steps

Be sure to follow the manufacturer's directions precisely.

1. Wash hands and put on gloves.
2. Assemble equipment and supplies.
3. Place a square of the absorbent test mat, supplied with the Ictotest, onto a paper towel. Place 10 drops of fresh, well-mixed urine in the center of the test mat.
4. Place one (1) Ictotest reagent tablet onto the center of the moistened mat. **Remember not to handle the tablet with your fingers. Put the tablet in the cover of the bottle and then put it onto the mat or use tweezers to transfer the tablet to the mat. Recap the reagent tablet bottle immediately.**
5. Place 1 drop of distilled water onto the reagent tablet. Wait 5 seconds and then place a second drop of water on the reagent tablet so that water runs off the tablet onto the mat.
6. Observe the colorless to pale blue color of the mat around the tablet after 60 seconds.
7. The presence of a deeper blue color (record bluer color) on the mat indicates that bilirubin is present.
8. Record the results either as positive or negative.
9. After consulting with the physician or laboratory technologist, discard test materials according to laboratory policy.
10. Return all equipment to its proper storage area.
11. Disinfect the testing area.
12. Remove and discard gloves and wash hands.

Urinary Urobilinogen

Bilirubin that finds its way into the intestinal tract via the bile duct from the liver is converted into a group of compounds known as **urobilinogen.** In normal patients, a small amount of urobilinogen may be present. In normal urine, urobilinogen concentration is typically in the range of 0.1 to 1.0 Ehrlich units/dL.

The amount of urobilinogen present in the urine relates to the amount of bilirubin produced. Common reagent strip methods of urobilinogen detection involve the reaction of urinary urobilinogen with para-diethylaminobenzaldehyde, and an acid buffer solution.

Urinary Bacteria

Enteric gram-negative bacteria that are always nitrite positive can convert urinary nitrate to nitrite. A positive nitrite test is an indication that a significant number of bacteria are present in the urine. **Bacteriuria** is the presence of bacteria in the urine.

Urinary Leukocytes

The presence of increased numbers of leukocytes or white blood cells in the urine is an indicator of bacteriuria or urinary tract infection (UTI). Granulocytic leukocytes release esterase when the cells lyse. Testing for leukocyte esterase by the reagent strip method is used in tandem with the microscopic examination of urine sediment for the diagnosis of bacteriuria or UTI.

A positive test by the reagent strip method is indicated by a purple color. The greater the amount of leukocytes/esterase present, the greater the intensity of the purple color.

UTIs are best confirmed by bacterial culture and sensitivity testing. A clean-catch mid-stream urine sample is usually required for any bacterial culture. For this reason, **it is ALWAYS wise to collect a clean-catch urine specimen; do not dispose of the specimen until the physician directs you to do so.**

Microscopic Examination of Urine Sediment

The microscopic examination of urine **sediment** is an important part of the urinalysis. The examination of urine sediment is a significant tool in the diagnosis and interpretation of renal and/or urinary tract disease. Urine sediment consists of cellular elements, casts,

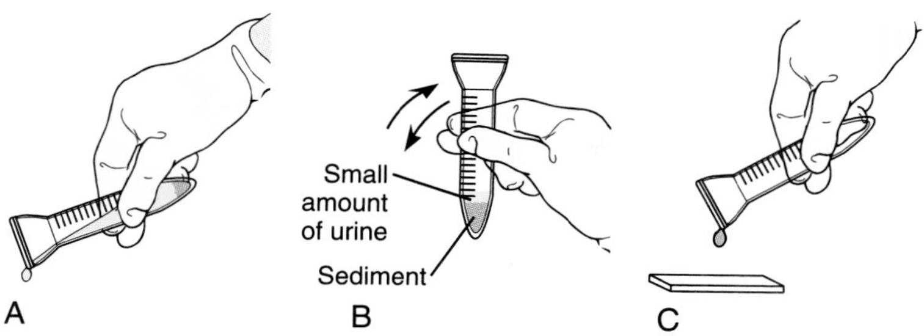

Figure 8–10. *Pouring off supernatant and resuspend sediment.*

crystals, microorganisms, and numerous miscellaneous constituents. The identification and enumeration of the constituents of urine sediment require that only highly skilled and qualified individuals undertake the microscopic examination of urine sediment. It is also important that each of the three aspects of the routine urinalysis be considered together when evaluating urinalysis.

The results of microscopic examination of urinary sediment must always be verified by a second form of testing. This usually is accomplished through the use of a reagent-strip test. For example, if the leukocyte esterase reagent strip tests positive, then microscopic examination would be used to verify the presence of white blood cells. Whenever there is a disagreement among the tests for the same sample, results should be held until the same urine sample can be retested or a new sample can be obtained from the patient and tested to confirm results.

Urine Collection and Processing

A freshly voided (preferably clean-catch) urine specimen is required for urinalysis. The urine sediment must be examined while the urine specimen is fresh. That is, the sediment must be examined within 1 hour of collection if it is unrefrigerated, or within 8 hours of collection if the specimen is to be refrigerated. A midstream urine specimen is appropriate for a urinalysis, but because a bacteriological culture and sensitivity may be required, it is always advisable to obtain a clean-catch collection. The specimen should be handled with care to avoid contamination that could affect the culture and sensitivity results. A first morning specimen, when available, provides the most accurate information relating to urinary sediment.

Urine sediment is obtained by centrifugating a 10- to 12-mL sample of well-mixed, freshly voided urine. After the urine sample has been transferred into a special centrifuge tube, the tube is placed in a centrifuge. A *centrifuge* is an instrument that uses centrifugal force to separate the sediment (solid matter) from the **supernatant** (liquid matter) (Fig. 8–10). This is done by spinning the sample at high speeds (at a predetermined number of revolutions per minute) for an appropriate time. After centrifugation, the supernatant is decanted (poured off) and a small button of sediment is resuspended into the remaining supernatant. The resuspended urinary sediment is then examined under a microscope (see Fig. 8–10).

Microscopic Examination

Typically, urinary sediment is examined unstained, using a brightfield microscope. For improved microscopic detail, the sediment may be stained with a supravital stain. Supravital stains, which are available commercially, are used to stain cells while still living. Sedi-Stain (Clay-Adams) and KOVA Stain (ICL Scientific) are two of the more common commercial stains (Fig. 8–11). The KOVA Stain is a standardized slide

Figure 8–11. *Sedi-Stain and KOVA Stain for microscopic examination of urine sediment.*

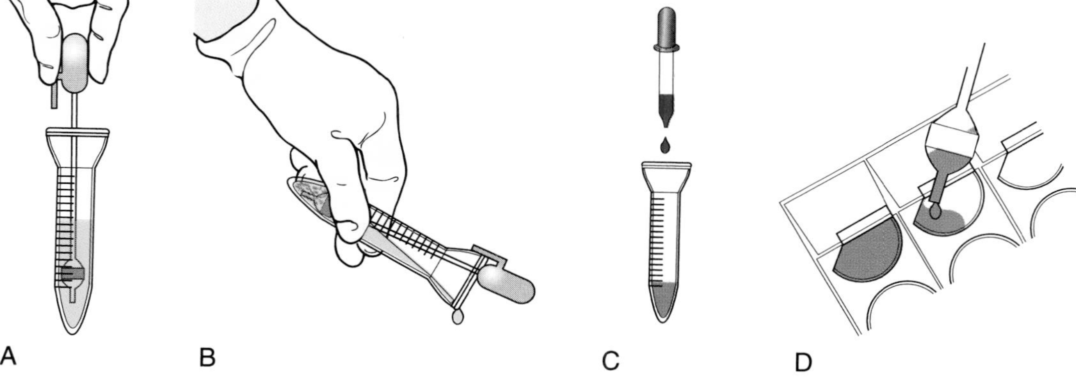

Figure 8–12. *Casts found in urine. (Courtesy of Diagnostics Division, Bayer Corporation)*

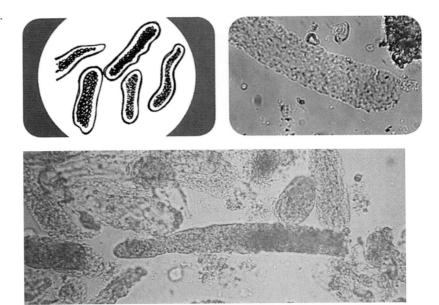

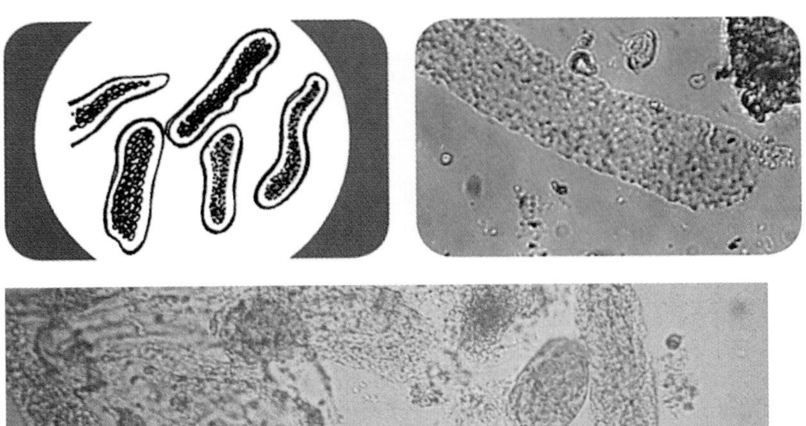

Granular cast

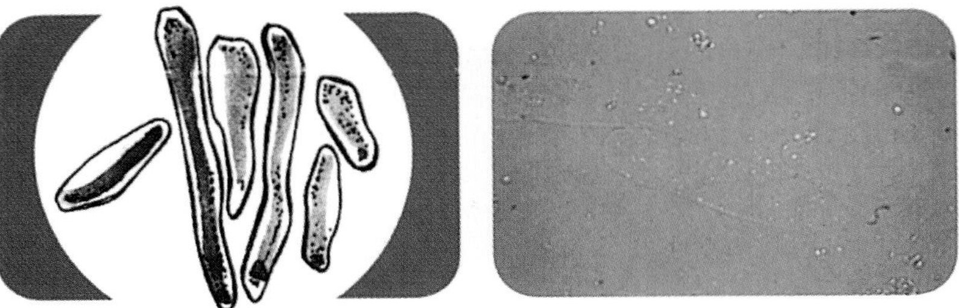

Hyaline cast

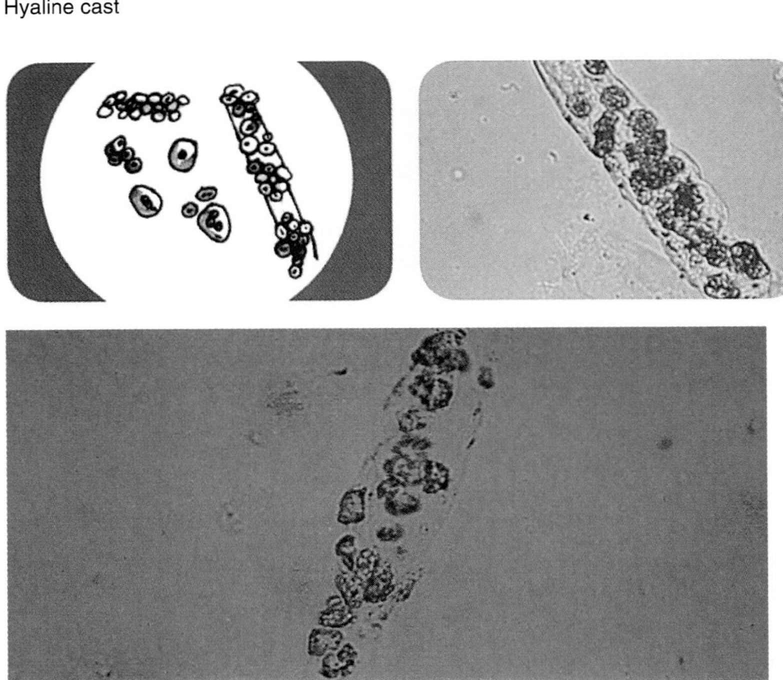

WBC cast

Figure 8–12 *Continued*

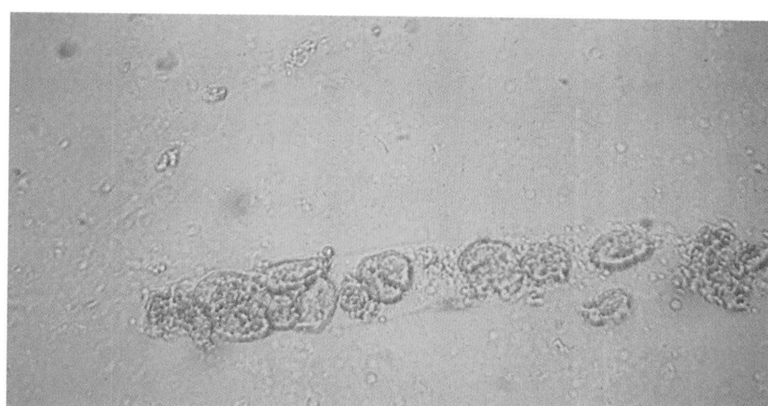

Epithelial cell cast

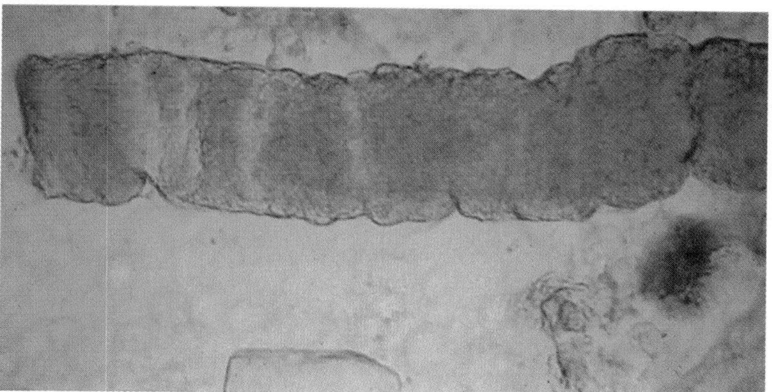

Broad cast (waxy)

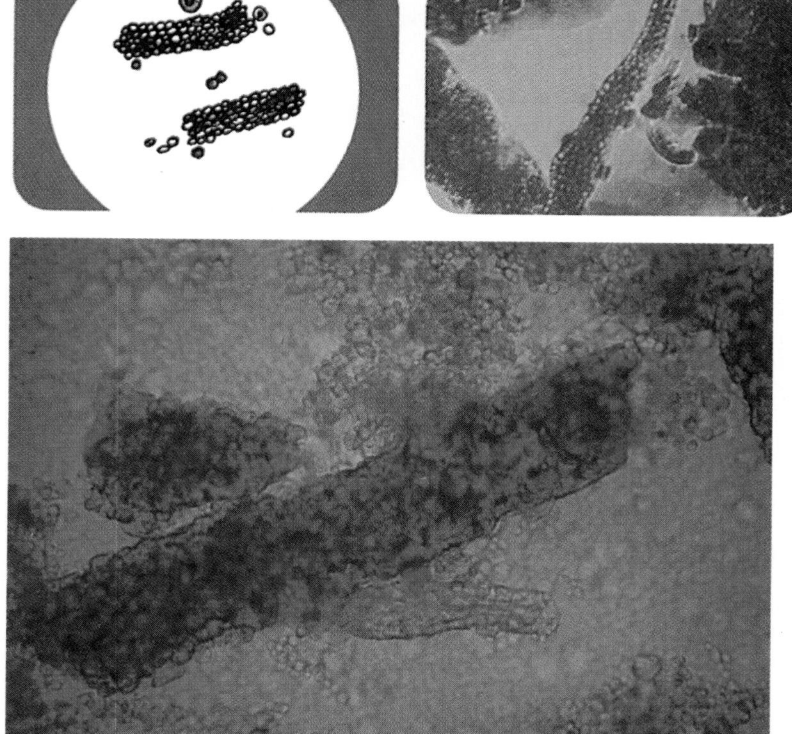

RBC cast

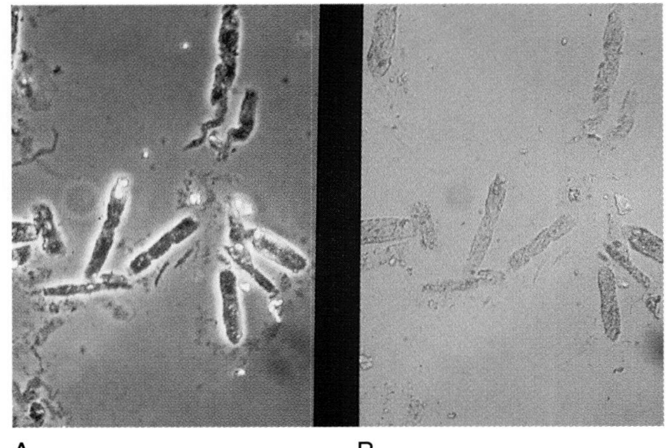

Figure 8–13. *Appearance of casts in urine examined with brightfield* (A) *and phase-contrast* (B) *microscopy.*

procedure that yields more reproducible results than conventional methods.

Improved sediment detail may also be obtained by using different types of microscopy. Polarized microscopy is useful in the identification of crystals. Phase-contrast microscopy improves the visibility of translucent material within the urinary sediment.

Microscopic Constituents in Urine Sediment

Casts

Casts found in urine are formed in the renal tubules when proteins precipitate after accumulation (Fig. 8–12). Protein forms a matrix that can trap granular and/or cellular material. The protein in the cast matrix is called Tamm-Horsfall protein. Casts take on the size and shape of the renal tubules at the site of their formation. Casts are cylindric, and may be short or long and have flat or rounded ends. Casts are classified according to the type of matrix and cellular or granular inclusions. Casts are washed into the urine from the renal tubules and may be associated with renal disease. They are not commonly seen in the urine of healthy people, except after strenuous exercise. Casts will dissolve in the presence of bacteria or in alkaline urine, so it is important that a freshly voided urine be examined promptly. Casts are most readily visible using phase-contrast microscopy (Fig. 8–13).

Figure 8–14. *Hyaline casts.*

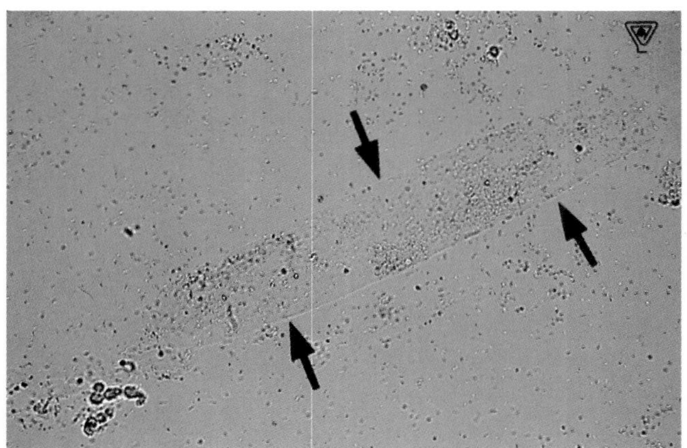

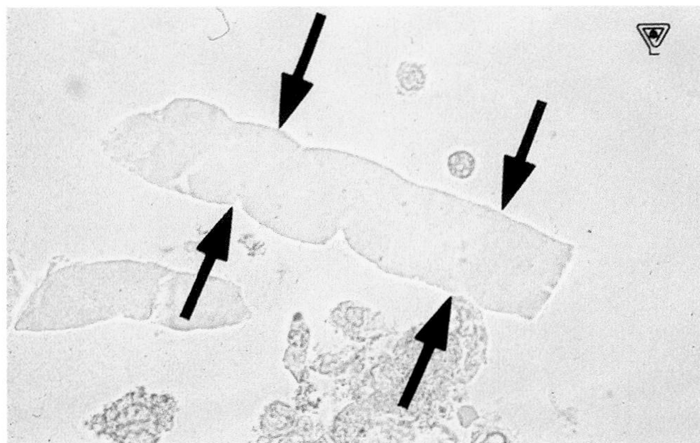

Figure 8–15. *Waxy casts.*

Hyaline Casts

Hyaline casts are usually pale and transparent, and usually have parallel sides. Hyaline casts may be found in persons with renal disease or may appear following strenuous exercise (Fig. 8–14).

Waxy Casts

Waxy casts are refractive, homogeneous casts with flat ends and fractures along the edges. Waxy casts are often seen in patients with chronic renal failure (Fig. 8–15).

Figure 8–16. *Granular casts.*

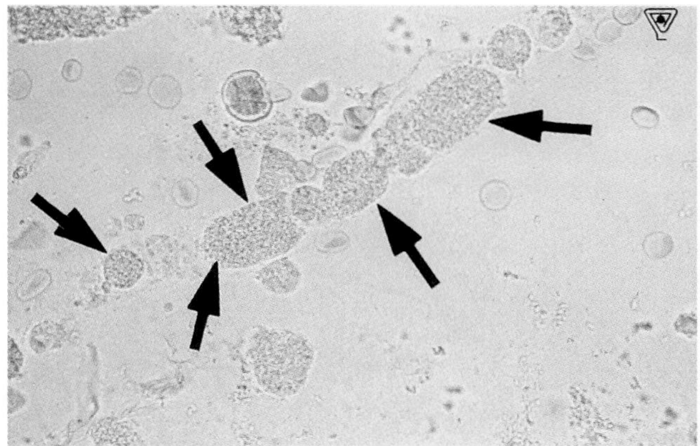

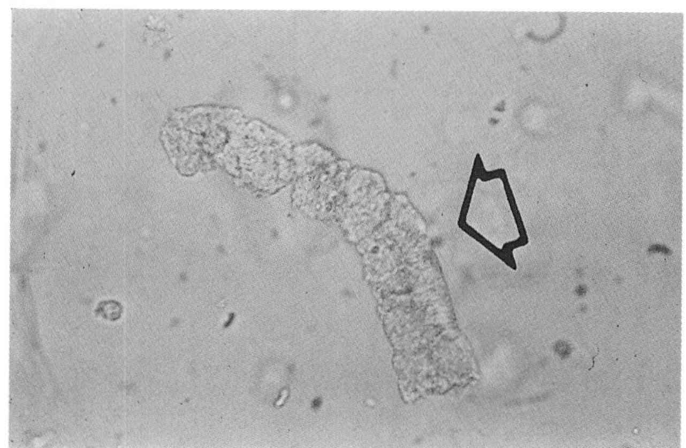

Figure 8–17. *Cellular casts.*

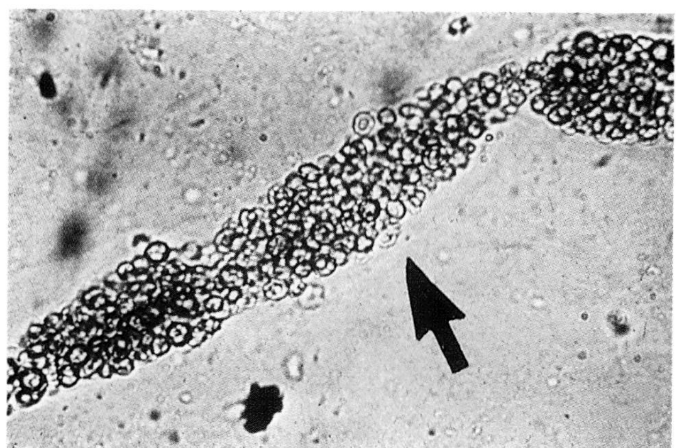

Figure 8–18. *Red blood cell casts.*

Granular Casts

Granular casts are common and may display fine or coarse granulation. Granular casts may be transient when they result from strenuous exercise. Patients with renal disease may also exhibit granular casts (Fig. 8–16).

Cellular Casts

Cellular casts may contain red blood cells, white blood cells, or renal tubular epithelial cells. The presence of red blood cells is significant, and is diagnostic of glomerular damage or disease (Fig. 8–17).

Red Blood Cell or Erythrocyte Casts

Red blood cell, erythrocyte blood cell, white blood cell, or leukocyte casts are most commonly seen in pyelonephritis. Casts containing renal tubular epithelial cells are usually an indication of excessive kidney damage. Common causes are shock, acute tubular necrosis, viral disease, or exposure to drug or heavy metal toxicity. Commonly, more than one cell type may be found in single casts. Casts with more than one cell type are routinely classified as mixed-cell casts (Fig. 8–18).

Miscellaneous Casts and Structures

Casts may also contain fatty material, crystals, hemosiderin granules, hemoglobin, microorganisms, and abnormal cells, such as tumor cells (Fig. 8–19).

Cells

Cells that derive from the lining of the genital urinary tract and the circulating blood are commonly seen in urine sediment.

Red Blood Cells (Erythrocytes). Red blood cells may be found in normal urine in small numbers. The presence of red blood cells in the urine is known as hematuria. Hematuria may be acute or chronic, and may result from an inflammation or injury. Red blood cells may appear in unstained urine as pale, biconcave disks. Red blood cells are smaller than white blood cells and have no nucleus. If the urine sediment is not examined promptly, red blood cells may begin to fade. Red blood cells may undergo **crenation** in hypertonic or concentrated urine. In hypotonic or dilute urine, red cells often swell and burst. Care must be taken not to confuse red blood cells with oil droplets or yeast cells. Red blood cells are destroyed in the presence of acetic acid. Oil droplets vary in size and are refractile, whereas red blood cells are nonrefractive and more uniform in size and shape (Fig. 8–20). Yeast cells in urine sediment often exhibit budding.

Mucous Threads

Mucous threads in urine appear as long, wavy, threadlike structures with pointed ends. In small amounts,

Figure 8–19. *The appearance of cholesterol under polarized light.* A, *Light side—brightfield microscopy.* B, *Deep blue—polarized light.*

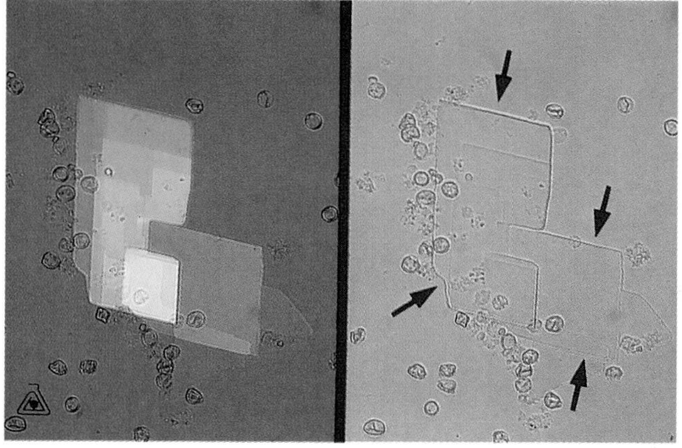

A B

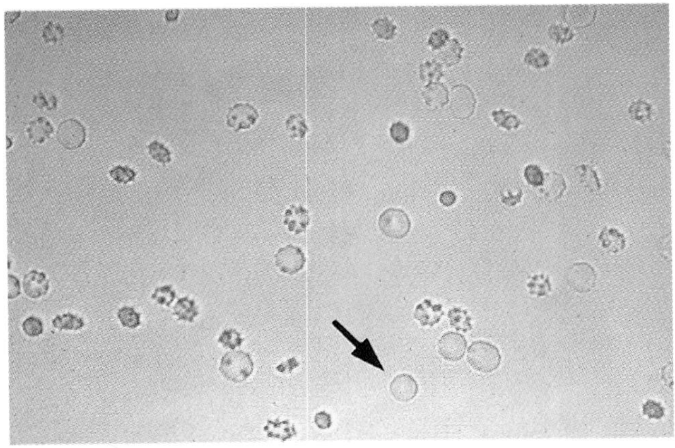

Figure 8–20. *Red blood cells in urine.*

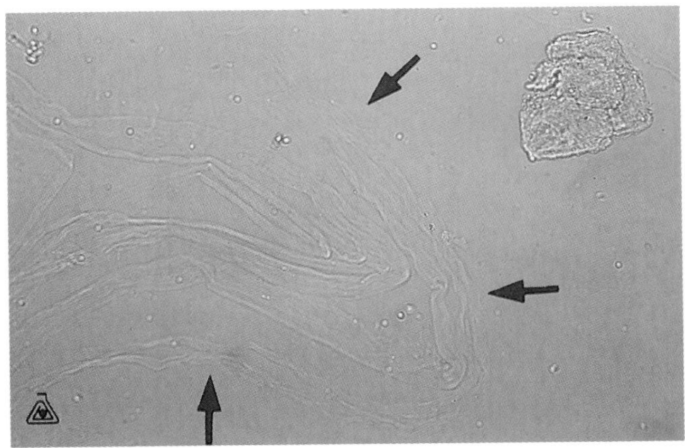

Figure 8–21. *Mucous threads in urine.*

Figure 8–22. *Epithelial cells: renal* (A), *bladder* (B), *and squamous cells* (C).

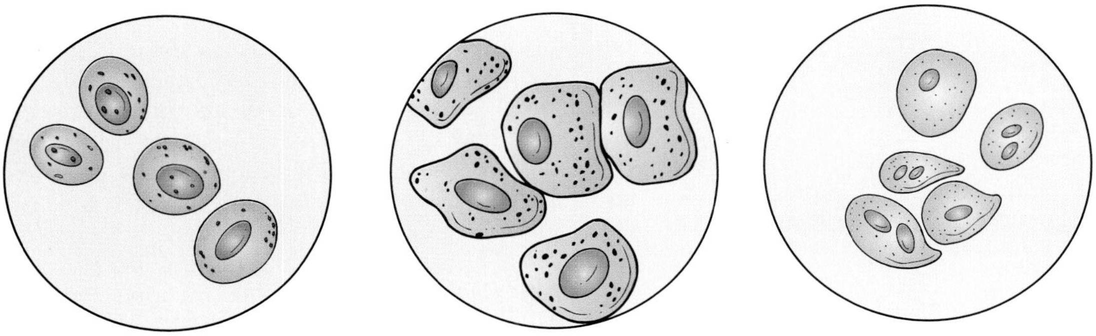

Renal tubular

Renal epithelial

Renal transitional

A

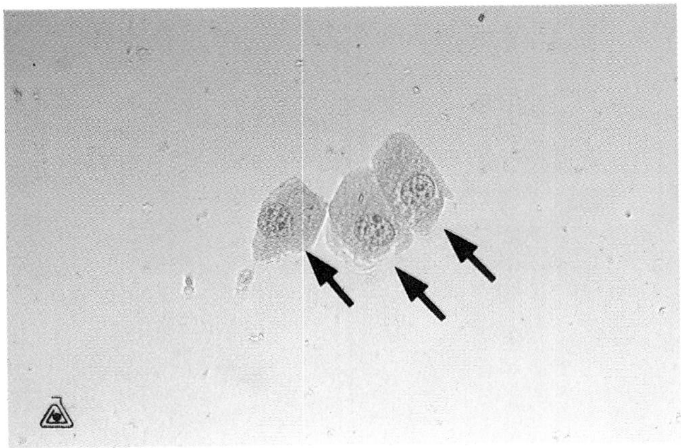

B

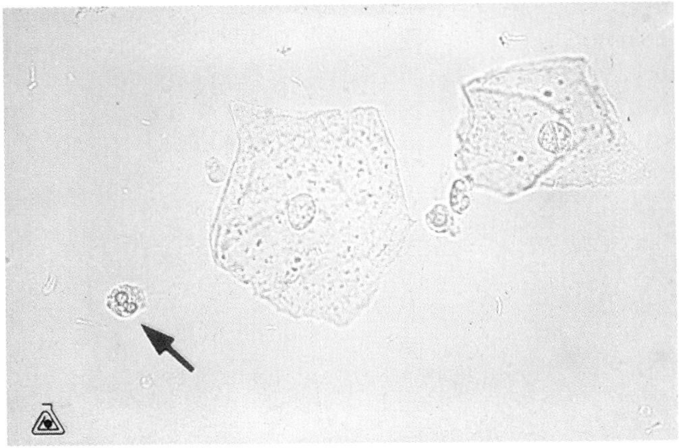

C

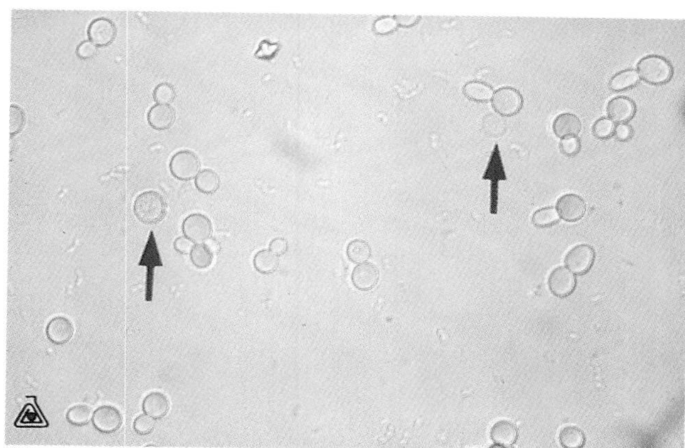

Figure 8–23. *Fungus (yeast) in urine.*

these structures are considered to be normal (Fig. 8–21).

Epithelial Cells

When examining urine sediment, it is normal to see an occasional epithelial cell or even a clump of cells because the renal tubules and their epithelial cell layer are always being replaced. If the renal epithelial cells are shed at an increased rate, however, it is indicative of disease damage to the renal tubular epithelium. These cells appear as round cells that are slightly larger than leukocytes, and they have a large, single nucleus (Fig. 8–22*A*).

Bladder cells are even larger renal epithelial cells, but are smaller than squamous cells (Fig. 8–22*B*).

The squamous cells that are often found in urine originate in the urethra, vulva, or vagina. They are large, flat cells with a single nucleus. Their presence is of little significance unless they appear in "sheetlike" form, in which case one should always note this on the laboratory slip (Fig. 8–22*C*).

Fungus

Yeast is the most common type of fungus found in urine sediment. It is colorless, varies in size, and frequently shows budding. The suspicious colony must be examined carefully, as yeast cells are sometimes confused with red blood cells. Yeast is most frequently seen in urine from female patients (Fig. 8–23).

Parasites

The parasite most frequently seen in urine is *Trichomonas vaginalis*. These are unicellular parasites with anterior flagella which are commonly recognized by their swimming motions. Trichomonas, which is seen most commonly in the urine of female subjects, may resemble flattened, ovoid, epithelial cells (Fig. 8–24).

Crystals

The most important factor in identifying crystals in urine is the pH of the urine. Most crystals are of limited significance, but because there are a few with clinical indications, it is important to be able to recognize and identify urinary sediment crystals. Crystals commonly seen in urine sediment include urates, oxalates, and phosphates (Fig. 8–25).

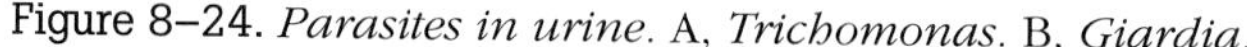

Figure 8–24. *Parasites in urine.* A, *Trichomonas.* B, *Giardia.*

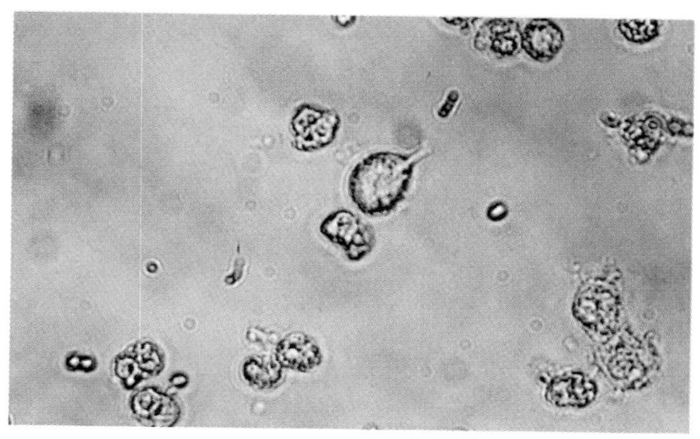

A

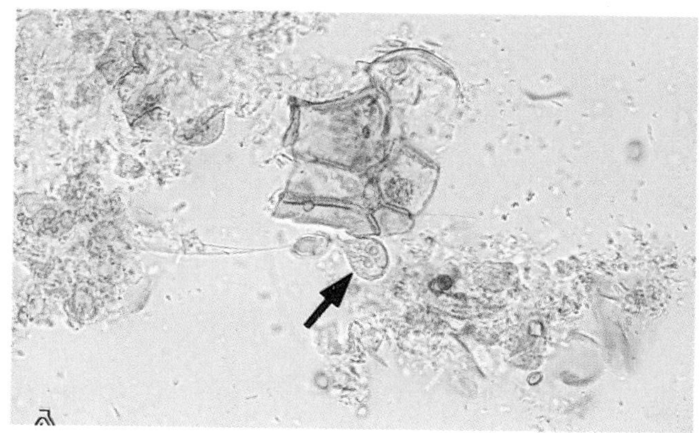

B

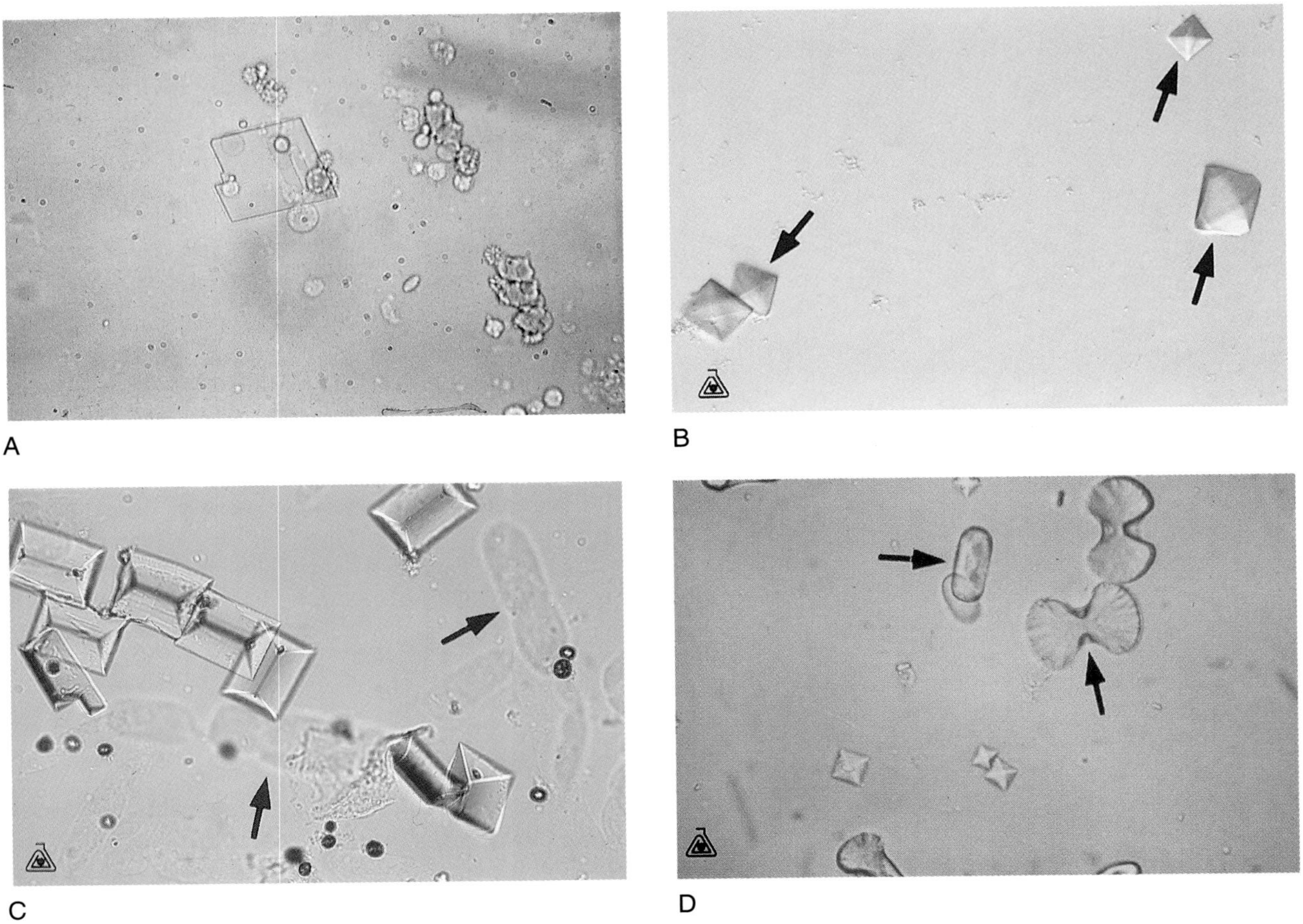

Figure 8–25. *Crystals in urine.* A, *Cholesterol.* B, *Calcium oxalate.* C, *Triple phosphate.* D, *Sulfonamide.*

PROCEDURE 8–8

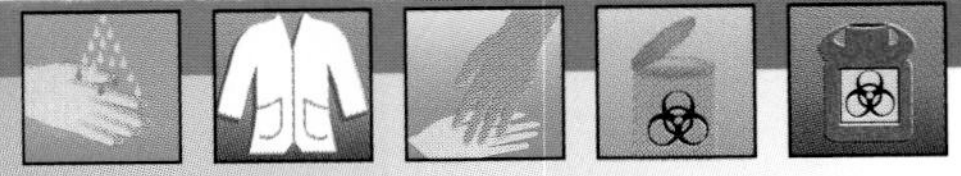

Microscopic Examination of Urine Sediment

Principle

Examine urine microscopically to determine the presence of normal and abnormal elements.

Equipment and Supplies

centrifuge
12 mL of fresh, well-mixed urine
medicine dropper microscope
microscopic slides and coverslips

Procedural Steps

1. Wash hands and put on gloves.
2. Assemble equipment and materials.
3. Obtain 12 mL of fresh, well-mixed, centrifuged urine.
4. Pour off the supernatant.
5. Resuspend the urine sediment.
6. Place 1 drop of the resuspended urine sediment onto a clean glass slide and cover with a coverslip.
7. Place the slide on the microscope stage.

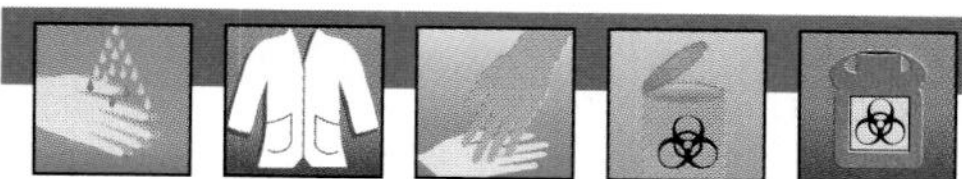

PROCEDURE 8-8

Microscopic Examination of Urine Sediment (Continued)

8. Examine the slide under low and high power, beginning with the low-power objective and ending with the high-power objective.
9. Scan the slide to identify any casts, blood cells, bacteria, yeast, epithelial cells, mucus, or crystals.
10. Record your findings.
11. After consulting with the physician or laboratory technologist, discard test materials according to laboratory policy.
12. Clean and disinfect the equipment and work area.
13. Return all equipment to its proper storage area.
14. Remove gloves and wash hands.

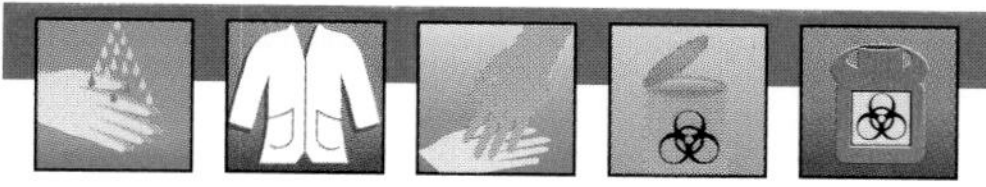

PROCEDURE 8-9

Microscopic Examination of Urine Using the KOVA Method

Principle

Using the KOVA method, complete a microscopic examination and report the normal and abnormal elements found in urine sediment.

Equipment and Supplies

laboratory coat/apron and disposable gloves
centrifuge
microscope
KOVA microscopic slides
KOVA pipette
KOVA KUP
2 KOVA tubes with KAPS
glass-marking pen
KOVA rack
KOVA stain

Procedural Steps

1. Wash hands. Put on laboratory coat/apron and gloves.
2. Collect and assemble equipment and supplies.
3. Label the KOVA tube with necessary patient information.
4. Give the patient the KOVA tube, tube cap, and KOVA collection cup and provide instructions for urine collection.
5. Secure a urine sample from the patient and record patient identification information on the specimen container using a marking pen.
6. Secure the KOVA KAP on the tube and place it in the KOVA rack.
7. Centrifuge the 12 mL of urine at 1500 rpm for 5 minutes.
8. Remove the sample from the centrifuge and insert the KOVA pipette until it sits firmly on the bottom of the tube.
9. Decant 11 mL of urine from the centrifuged tube and place this amount into a second tube.
10. Remove the pipette.
11. Add 1 drop of KOVA stain to the remaining mL of urine sediment.
12. Return the pipette to the KOVA tube.
13. Mix the sediment and stain together.
14. Prepare the KOVA microscopic slide by placing it flat on the workspace, with the covered (half-moon) chambers uppermost.
15. Using the pipette, draw up a small amount of sediment.
16. Place the sediment sample on the open, recessed area of the KOVA slide.
17. Tilt the KOVA slide on its edge to allow the sediment to flow down into the chambers.

(continued)

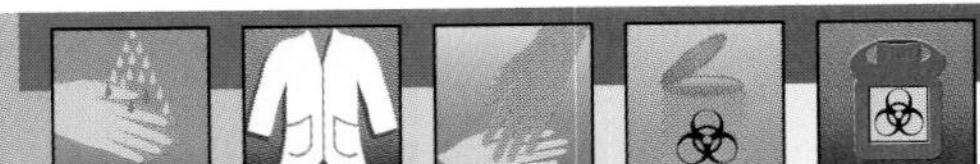

PROCEDURE 8–9

Microscopic Examination of Urine Using the Kova Method (Continued)

18. Let the specimen stand for 60 seconds to allow settling.
19. Place the slide under the microscope objective.
20. Using reduced light and low-power magnification, scan the entire area covered by the coverslip. Identify and record ALL formed elements observed.
21. Note the number of casts in 10 to 15 low-power fields.
22. Set the microscope to high-power magnification, increase the light, and observe 10 to 12 fields.
23. Identify and enumerate the significant formed elements. Note the presence of yeast, bacteria, or sperm.
24. Record your findings on the laboratory slip.
25. After consulting with the physician or laboratory technologist, discard test materials according to laboratory policy.
26. Clean and disinfect the equipment and work area.
27. Return all equipment to its proper storage area.
28. Remove gloves and wash hands.

Summary

Urinalysis is a valuable diagnostic tool because the physical and chemical constituents of normal urine remain constant, so abnormal conditions or diseases may be detected quickly and easily. This is why all tests must be done with accuracy and precision. Despite its great diagnostic value, microscopic examination of urine sediment remains the most imprecise and inaccurate part of the urinalysis. Pathologic findings should always be verified by using two different testing methods. Careless handling of the urine specimen or failure to adhere to the testing procedure may have serious consequences. Remember, the patient and the physician are depending on you for accurate results.

Chapter Review

True or False

Circle T or F to indicate the correct answers to the following:

T F 1. A complete urinalysis includes the physical, chemical, and microscopic examination of a urine specimen.

T F 2. The color of urine depends on what the person drinks.

T F 3. Hematuria means red urine.

T F 4. All urine will produce foam when it is shaken.

Fill in the Blanks

Complete the following statements:

5. Specific gravity is the most convenient way of measuring the kidneys' ability to ____________ and ____________.
6. You can measure specific gravity with a ____________, ____________, or ____________ ____________.
7. Urine osmolality is a measurement of the total ____________ concentration of urine.
8. A urine output of greater than 2000 mL/24 hr is called ____________.

Multiple Choice

Circle the letter that represents the single best answer:

9. The chemical examination of urine includes measurement of:
   a. pH
   b. Blood
   c. Albumin
   d. Nitrites
   e. All of the above

10. An acidic urine specimen would have a pH of:
    a. 8.0
    b. 7.6
    c. 7.3
    d. 7.1
    e. 6.7
11. The sugar that is typically found in urine is:
    a. Galactose
    b. Glucose
    c. Lactose
    d. Fructose
    e. Pentose
12. If a urine specimen is refrigerated, it is acceptable for testing for:
    a. 5 hours
    b. 6 hours
    c. 8 hours
    d. 12 hours
    e. 24 hours

Vocabulary

acidosis: an abnormal increase in the body's hydrogen ion concentration resulting in a blood pH of less than 7.4

agglutination: the clumping together of cells as a result of interaction with specific antibodies called agglutinins

electrolyte: an element or compound which, when dissolved, turns into ions that are able to conduct an electric current

gestation: the period of time between conception and birth

porphyrin: group of nitrogen-containing organic compounds forming in protoplasm

qualitative test: a test that determines the presence or absence of a substance

quantitative test: a test that determines the amount of a substance per unit volume or unit weight

solid-phase: immunoassay separation technique where the antibody is bound to the reaction vessel

syndrome: a group of signs and symptoms resulting from a common cause or appearing in combinations

urethra: a small tube that carries the urine from the urinary bladder to the outside of the body

Chapter Objectives

After reading this chapter, you should be able to:

1. Describe three types of pregnancy tests.
2. Identify three common specialized urine tests.
3. Name two of the most frequently used immunoassay tests.
4. Determine whether the human chorionic gonadotropin (hCG) test is negative or positive.
5. List some of the possible causes for a false-positive hCG test result.
6. Identify five of the common urinary chemical constituents.
7. Compare and contrast the tests associated with increased/decreased chemical levels.
8. List the advantages of urinary drug screening over blood screening.
9. List the laboratory findings you would expect to find associated with urinary calculi.

Chapter 9
Specialized Urine Tests

As you have just learned, urinalysis is a very valuable diagnostic tool. However, the examination of urine may involve more than a routine urinalysis. There are many specialized urine tests that are equally important in diagnosing and managing disease.

Specialized urine testing may involve **qualitative tests,** or screening tests. Alternatively, **quantitative tests,** or definitive tests, may be indicated.

In this chapter, some of the more common specialized urine tests are discussed, such as urine pregnancy testing, urine osmolality, and testing for specific urinary constituents, such as sodium, potassium, and creatinine.

Urinary Pregnancy Testing

Probably the most common specialized urine test is the pregnancy test. Human chorionic gonadotropin (hCG), also known as uterine chorionic gonadotropin (UCG), is produced in the placenta and is detectable in the blood and urine early in the **gestation** period. hCG is not normally found in the urine of young, healthy, nonpregnant women. Because of hCG's early appearance during gestation, increased levels of hCG are a natural marker for pregnancy.

Testing Methods

Immunoassay Tests

hCG can be measured in the urine using a number of testing methods. Qualitative, or screening, procedures are most commonly used for this purpose. **Agglutination** inhibition immunoassay and enzyme immunoassay tests are the two most popular tests. These types of immunoassay are easy to perform and inexpensive, and produce reliable results within minutes. When more definitive, or quantitative, results are required, radioimmunoassays are often used. The disadvantage of radioimmunoassay is that it requires the use of a radioisotope and special instrumentation. Its chief ad-

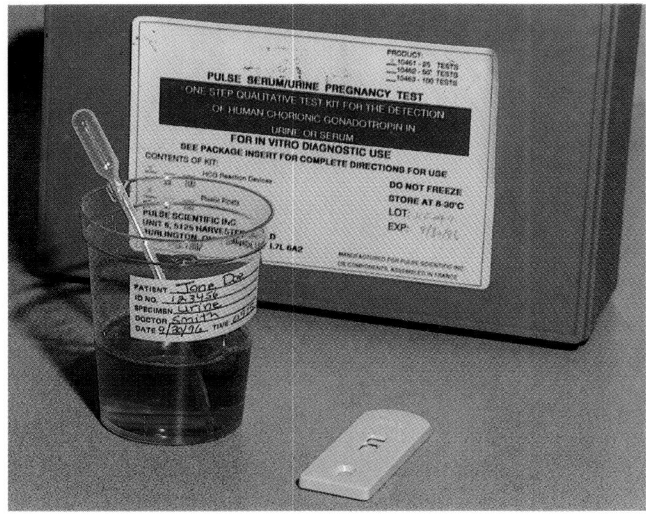

A

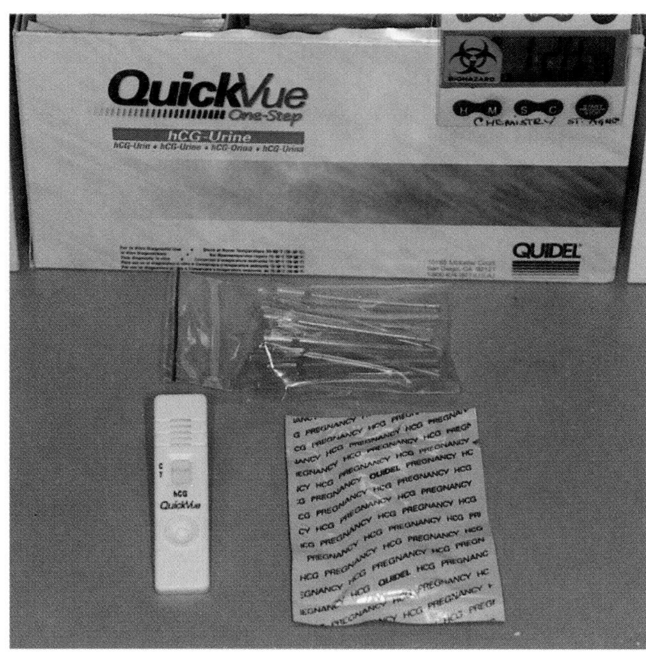

B

Figure 9–1. A, *Pulse serum/urine pregnancy test.* B, *Quick Vue pregnancy kit (hCG urine).*

vantage is increased sensitivity. **Solid-phase** immunoassays include the Tandem ICON II hCG, ICON II hCG, QTest Pregnancy, and Kodak Sure Cell hCG-Urine Test Kit. These tests have the ease and rapidity of qualitative tests but have a sensitivity approaching that of radioimmunoassays without the requirement of special instrumentation or radioisotopes (Fig. 9–1).

Agglutination Tests

Slide Agglutination Test

The slide agglutination test is commonly used in the physician's office, as it only takes 2 minutes to complete. Positive test results are based upon the inhibition of latex particle agglutination. The absence of agglutination on the slide test, termed *agglutination inhibition,* indicates a positive reaction for pregnancy. However, if agglutination occurs on the slide, the test results are reported as negative (Fig. 9–2). When hCG coats with latex, agglutination occurs, which can be seen and read as a negative reaction by the medical assistant. Without the latex, agglutination would not be visible when the hCG antigen and antibody combine.

Test Tube Agglutination Test

The test tube agglutination test involves the interaction of a patient's hCG with hCG antiserum, which produces an antigen-antibody reaction. It is the most sensitive of the pregnancy agglutination tests, and takes 2 hours to complete.

The test begins exactly like the slide agglutination test. Thus, if the patient's urine contains hCG, it will react with the hCG antiserum, creating an antigen-antibody reaction. However, in the test tube test, red blood cells (RBCs) coated with hCG are added to the test tube. If an antigen-antibody reaction has already occurred, no available hCG antiserum is left in the specimen to react with the hCG. Thus, the RBCs settle in a sharp, precise ring on the bottom of the tube, yielding a positive test result. When the urine specimen does not contain hCG, the available hCG antiserum combines with the antigen-bound RBCs, and a small round film of agglutination settles at the bottom of the tube, yielding a negative test result.

Test Results

A positive test result normally indicates pregnancy. However, false-negative results and false-positive results are always possible. False-negative tests commonly occur when urine is diluted, or when it is too early in the pregnancy for detectable levels of hCG to be present. Detectable levels of hCG vary depending upon the testing method and the manufacturer of the urine pregnancy test kit. False-positive test results are usually associated with drug interference, hematuria, or proteinuria, among other reasons. Before performing the urine pregnancy test, the procedure and literature provided in each test kit should be reviewed thoroughly and understood. Always use positive and negative controls and test urine specimens immediately, unless the urine sample is refrigerated. Although it is acceptable for urine specimens to be collected at any time, **hCG is most concentrated in the first urine of the morning.**

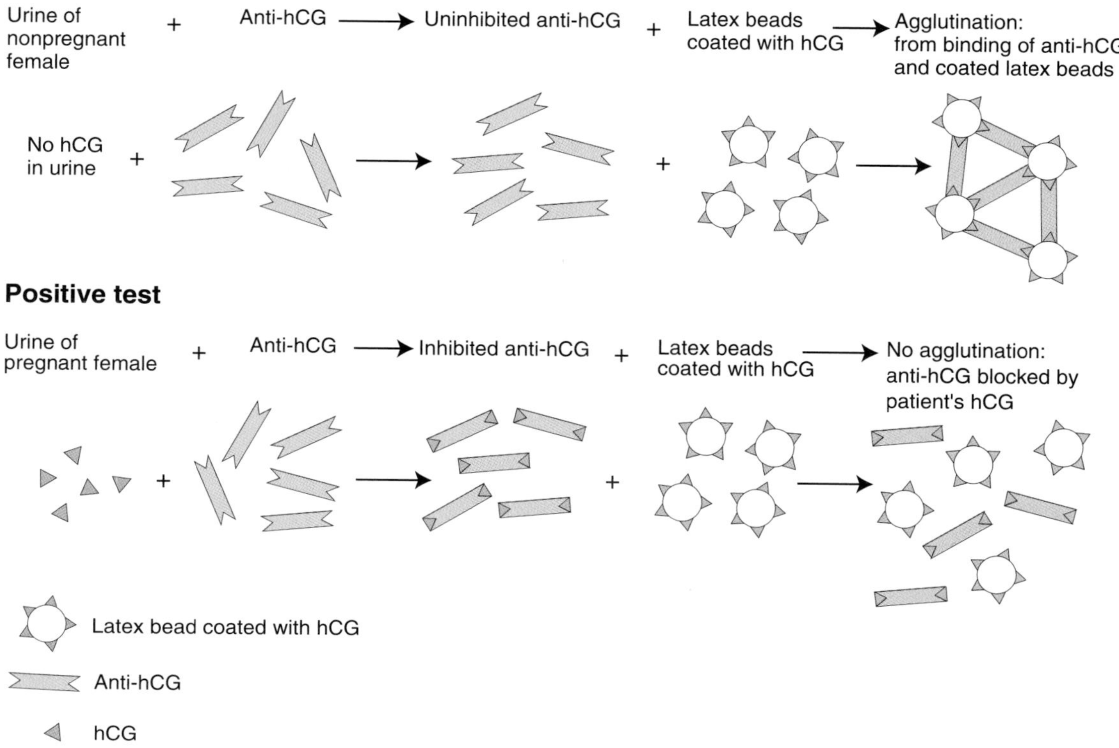

Figure 9–2. *Process of hCG agglutination inhibition.*

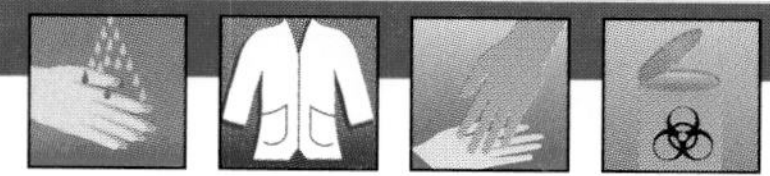

PROCEDURE 9–1

Performing a Pregnancy Detection Test

Principle

Perform and report results of pregnancy testing of urine using the Wampole method.

Equipment and Supplies

urine specimen
clean test slide
reagents
Wampole One Step hCG
disposable mixing sticks
eye droppers

Procedural Steps

1. Wash and dry hands. Put on gloves.
2. Assemble and prepare all testing equipment.
3. Obtain a urine specimen (minimum of 0.250 mL) in a clean container.
4. Label the handle of the absorbent device or the conjugate tube with the patient's name and control number.
5. Remove and discard the stopper from the conjugate tube.

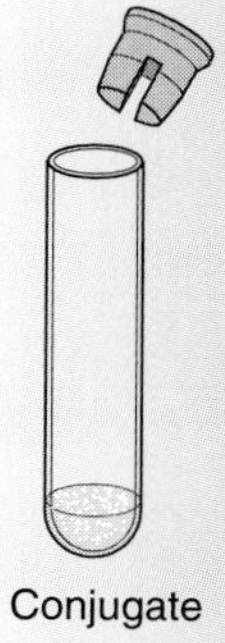

(continued)

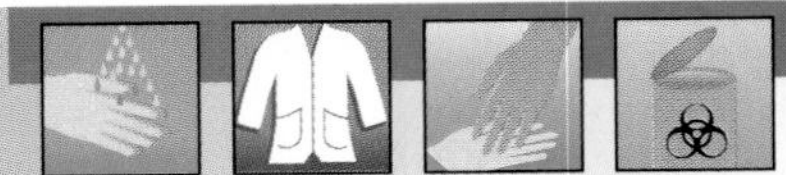

PROCEDURE 9–1

Performing a Pregnancy Detection Test (Continued)

6. Using a disposable specimen dispenser, draw the urine specimen to the 0.250-mL calibration line and expel the specimen into the conjugate tube.

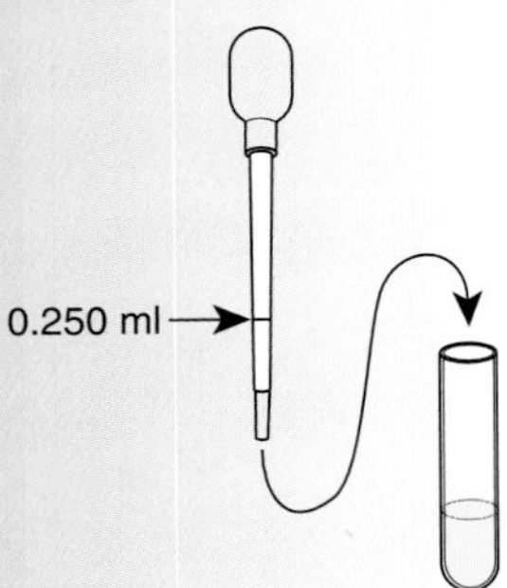

7. Mix the urine in the tube briefly, using a side-to-side motion, to reconstitute the conjugate. Do not turn the tube upside down. A vortexed specimen is neither required nor recommended. The mixture will appear cloudy.

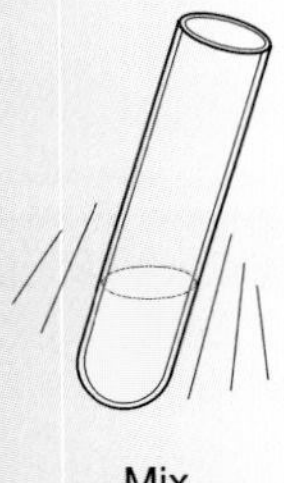

Mix

8. Place the conjugate tube into the work station.
9. Place the labeled device into the conjugate tube.

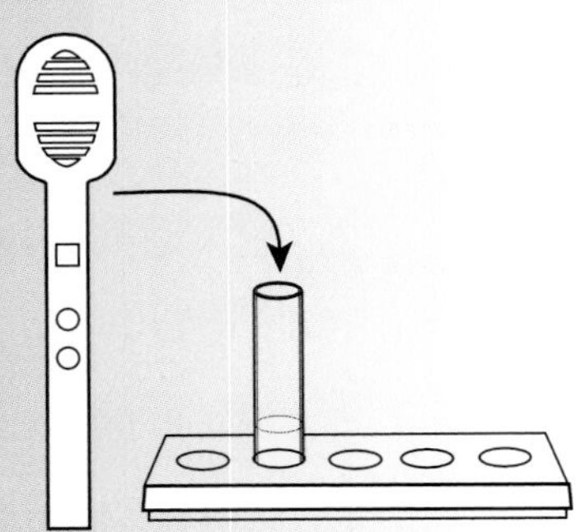

10. Read the reactions after 5 minutes. The absorbent device MUST be left in the conjugate tube when reading results.
11. To read the results, compare the color development in the three reaction zones. If the pink-rose color in the sample reaction is darker than the negative control zone, the test result is positive. If the pink-rose zone in the sample reaction zone is equal to the color in the negative control zone, the test result is negative.

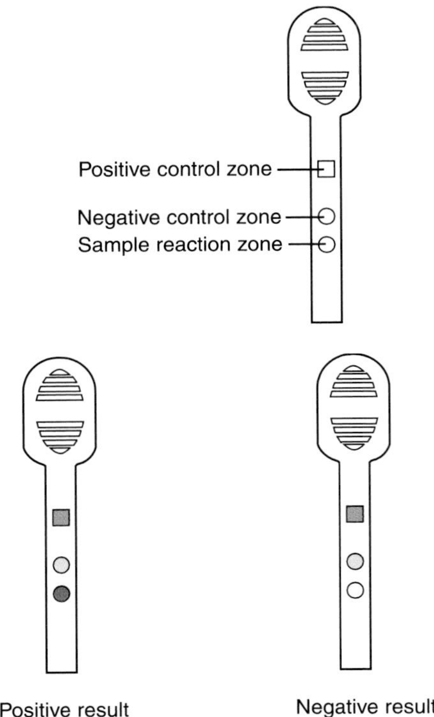

12. Record the test results.
13. Once test results have been verified, discard the specimens according to laboratory policy.
14. Dispose of all used testing equipment in proper biohazard waste containers. Clean the area.
15. Remove and discard gloves and wash hands.

Figures reprinted with permission from Kinn, Woods, Derge. *The Medical Assistant: Administrative and Clinical,* 7th ed. Philadelphia: W. B. Saunders, 1993.

Testing for Common Urinary Chemical Constituents

The measurement of urinary sodium, potassium, and chloride levels is an important tool for determining a patient's **electrolyte** balance. Urinary measurements of sodium, potassium, and chloride are quantitative, and are usually based on the amount excreted in the urine within a 24-hour period. Sometimes, urinary specimens are collected over a shorter interval, as with a 2-hour or a 12-hour urinary sodium test. However, the preferred testing method involves 24-hour collection.

Sodium, potassium, and chloride measurements are valuable for monitoring and diagnosing problems of electrolyte balance, water balance, acid–base balance, and renal or adrenal disturbances.

Sodium

The primary regulator of the body's ability to excrete or retain water and to maintain the proper acid–base balance is sodium. Sodium is the predominant basic substance in the blood. Because of its ability to bind with chloride and bicarbonate, sodium helps regulate the body's acid–base balance and also helps to maintain the normal balance of electrolytes in intracellular and extracellular fluids. Increased levels of sodium may be caused by dehydration, starvation, chronic renal failure, or diabetic **acidosis.** Decreased levels of sodium are associated with congestive heart failure, diarrhea, acute renal failure and malabsorption **syndrome.**

Potassium

Potassium functions as part of the buffer system of the body. Along with sodium (sodium-potassium pump), potassium helps to maintain the normal electrolyte balance in the intracellular and extracellular fluids. Sodium and potassium are also important in the function of muscles, nerves, and heart.

Increased levels of potassium may be associated with dehydration, starvation, chronic renal failure, or diabetic acidosis. Decreased levels of potassium may be found in acute renal failure, diarrhea, and malabsorption syndrome.

Chloride

Urine chloride levels are important for diagnosing dehydration and are useful in monitoring patients for whom a reduced-salt diet has been prescribed as well as patients with cardiovascular disease, kidney disease, liver disease, or hypertension. The urine chloride level is increased in association with dehydration and starvation and decreased in patients with congestive heart failure, diarrhea, or malabsorption syndrome.

Protein

A 24-hour urine sample is also useful in the diagnosis of renal disease. The urine of normal, healthy individuals contains little or no protein. The passage of protein from the blood into the urine is blocked by the glomerulus. The presence of large amounts of protein in the urine (*proteinuria*) is usually the result of some type of glomerular damage.

Proteinuria can also occur in association with many nonrenal conditions and diseases. Heart disease, liver disease, fever, and trauma are a few of the nonrenal diseases and conditions that can result in proteinuria.

A 24-hour urine test for protein is helpful in indicating the degree of proteinuria. It is also helpful in determining whether the proteinuria is persistent or intermittent. It is important to remember that the most common cause of errors in quantitative protein examinations is improper collection technique.

Creatinine

Creatinine is a product of muscle energy metabolism. In normal, healthy individuals, creatinine is excreted by the kidneys. The rate at which creatinine is cleared from the blood by the kidneys is an indication of glomerular filtration in the kidneys. A 24-hour creatinine clearance test is usually performed in conjunction with the quantitative measurement of other urinary constituents, such as sodium, potassium, chloride, and protein. In performing a creatinine clearance test, the patient's urinary creatinine and blood creatinine levels are measured. Urinary creatinine is measured in mg/24 hours, whereas blood creatinine clearance is measured in mL/minute.

Urine Osmolality

Urine osmolality and urine specific gravity measurements are indicators of total urinary solute concentration. Specific gravity determination is part of a routine urinalysis. Osmolality is a special urinary test that provides a more exact measurement of urine concentration. Osmolality is not affected by the type of particles in the solute concentration. Particles, such as sugar and protein, affect urine specific gravity more than urine osmolality. Therefore, a urine osmolality test is indicated when a precise measurement of solute concentration is required, usually when evaluating the ability of a patient's kidneys to concentrate and dilute urine.

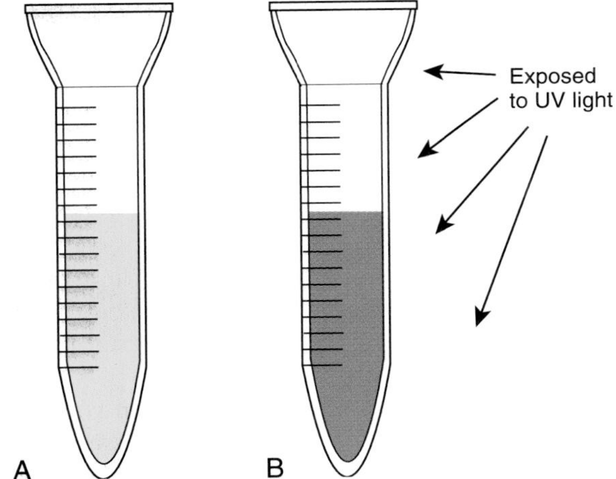

Figure 9–3. *Porphyrins fluorescing.*

Porphyrins

Porphyrins are mainly produced in the liver and bone marrow. Bone marrow porphyrins are important in the synthesis of hemoglobin, and liver porphyrins are important in the synthesis of other hemoproteins, such as myoglobin. Hemoglobin is the main component of the erythrocytes (RBCs). Its main function is to transport oxygen from the lungs to the cells and to remove and transport carbon dioxide from the cells to the lungs for elimination. In normal, healthy individuals only minute amounts of porphyrins are excreted in the urine.

Overproduction of porphyrins results in elevated urinary excretion. Disorders of porphyrin metabolism may be inherited or acquired. The most common inherited porphyrin disorder is acute, intermittent porphyria. Lead poisoning is a common acquired disorder of the porphyrin metabolism.

Porphyrins fluoresce when exposed to black light or ultraviolet light. A common screening test for urine porphyrins involves the exposure of urine to black light or ultraviolet light after urinary porphyrins have been extracted (Fig. 9–3).

Urinary Drug Screening

Blood testing is the best means for determining precise information about drug levels. However, urine is the preferred specimen for *screening* patients for unknown drugs. Although blood and gastric specimens provide valuable information, urine drug screening is commonly used for a number of reasons. Urine specimens are easily obtained, and drug concentrations are typically more elevated in urine than in blood. Indeed, some drugs are not detectable in blood, and urine drug levels may remain elevated even after a drug is no longer detectable in the blood. An exception would be that blood is the preferred specimen when testing a patient's ethyl alcohol levels.

Urine drug screening may be performed for medical reasons or legal reasons. It is often a condition of employment, and is done routinely as part of pre-employment physical examinations. Urine drug screening is also used to detect drug abuse in the workplace. Urine drug screening is common when public safety is a factor, as with employment with a railroad or an airline company. Urine drug screening is also important in differentiating drug-induced diseases from other disease processes (Table 9–1).

Because of the implications of the presence of drugs of abuse, great care should be taken in ensuring that specimens are properly collected, identified, and tested. Confirmation testing is usually required in legal and/or employment situations when positive results are obtained.

Urine specimens for legal or employment drug screening must be collected in such a way as to preserve the chain of custody. This may require that the actual collection of the specimen be witnessed by a trained individual. Check to be certain that the state in which you are employed allows medical assistants to collect specimens for drug testing.

The major disadvantage of urine drug testing is that a positive test result indicates only the presence of a drug in urine and does not provide any information when the drug was taken or if it is still present in the blood. Thus, a positive urine drug test does not tell us whether the person is physically or mentally impaired by the drug. This is one of the primary reasons for the controversy surrounding drug testing in the workplace.

Table 9–1
Drugs Detectable in Urine

Alcohol	Phencyclidine (PCP)
Amphetamines	Lysergic acid diethylamide (LSD)
Barbiturates	Analgesics
Benzodiazepines	Sedatives
Cocaine/"crack"	Major tranquilizers*
Opiates	Stimulants
Marijuana (THC)	Sympathomimetics

From Fischbach, F. *A Manual of Laboratory and Diagnostic Tests,* 5th ed. Philadelphia: Lippincott-Raven Publishers.

*Minor tranquilizers are almost completely metabolized in the gastrointestinal system, and unless there has been an overdose, it is not likely that they will be detected.

Urinary Calculi

Urinary calculi, or kidney stones, are a common finding in patients older than 30 years of age. The calculi are typically formed in the kidneys. Passage of the calculi down the ureter causes severe pain. Small stones may also be passed through the **urethra.** Obstruction, infection, and hematuria are common findings in patients with urinary calculi.

The most commonly found urinary calculi are formed from calcium oxalate. Urinary calculi may also be formed from other substances, such as cystine. Urinary calculi may have a sandy or gravelly appearance, or they may resemble stones.

Urinary calculi are most commonly identified by gross inspection and chemical analysis.

Specialized Urinary Tests for Other Urinary Constituents

Quantitative 24-Hour Urine Collections

Quantitative 24-hour urine collections are also used for determining uric acid, calcium, magnesium, and amylase levels. Levels of other substances, such as 5-hydroxyindoleacetic acid, 17-ketosteroid, 17-hydroxycorticosteroid, and vanillylmandelic acid, are also commonly determined by 24-hour urine specimen testing.

Urine and blood tests are performed in neonates to detect phenylketonuria (PKU). Phenylketonuria is a genetic disease which, if left untreated, leads to mental retardation and brain damage.

Summary

Every year, more than 12 million people in the United States seek medical attention for urinary tract problems. Every one of these individuals will rely on the results of a urinalysis to guide their medical treatment care plan. As the health care worker responsible for obtaining the urine specimen and performing the urinalysis, it is our duty to perform the necessary tests quickly and accurately. Often, we lose sight of the importance of such "routine" tests. Always remember, though, that a health problem is not considered by the patient to be routine, and they are relying on us to do our part to assist them to regain their state of health.

Chapter Review

True or False

Circle T or F to indicate the correct answers to the following:

T F 1. Urine tests may be qualitative or quantitative.

T F 2. hCG is usually found in healthy young females.

T F 3. Immunoassay testing is more definitive than radioimmunoassay testing.

T F 4. Agglutination indicates a positive pregnancy test.

T F 5. In test tube agglutination, a ring of RBCs forms at the bottom of the test tube if the patient is pregnant.

Fill in the Blanks

Complete the following statements:

6. hCG is most concentrated in the ____________ specimen.
7. Measurements of ____________, ____________, and ____________ are important indicators of a patient's electrolyte balance.
8. Sodium binds with ____________ and ____________ to help regulate the body's acid–base balance.
9. Potassium helps maintain the normal electrolyte balance in both ____________ and ____________ fluids.

Multiple Choice

Circle the letter that represents the single best answer:

10. Chloride levels are decreased in:
    a. Heart failure
    b. Diarrhea
    c. Malabsorption syndrome
    d. Dehydration
    e. All of the above
11. Creatinine clearance is measured in:
    a. mg/hour
    b. ms/day
    c. mg/liter
    d. mL/minute
    e. mL/hour
12. A blood specimen is preferred over a urine specimen when testing for the consumption of:
    a. Cocaine
    b. Alcohol
    c. Marijuana
    d. PCP
    e. Opiates

13. Urinary calculi are a common finding in patients older than:
    a. 20 years of age
    b. 30 years of age
    c. 40 years of age
    d. 50 years of age
    e. 60 years of age

14. Quantitative 24-hour urine collections are used to determine levels of:
    a. Uric acid
    b. Calcium
    c. Magnesium
    d. Albumin
    e. All of the above

Unit III

Hematology

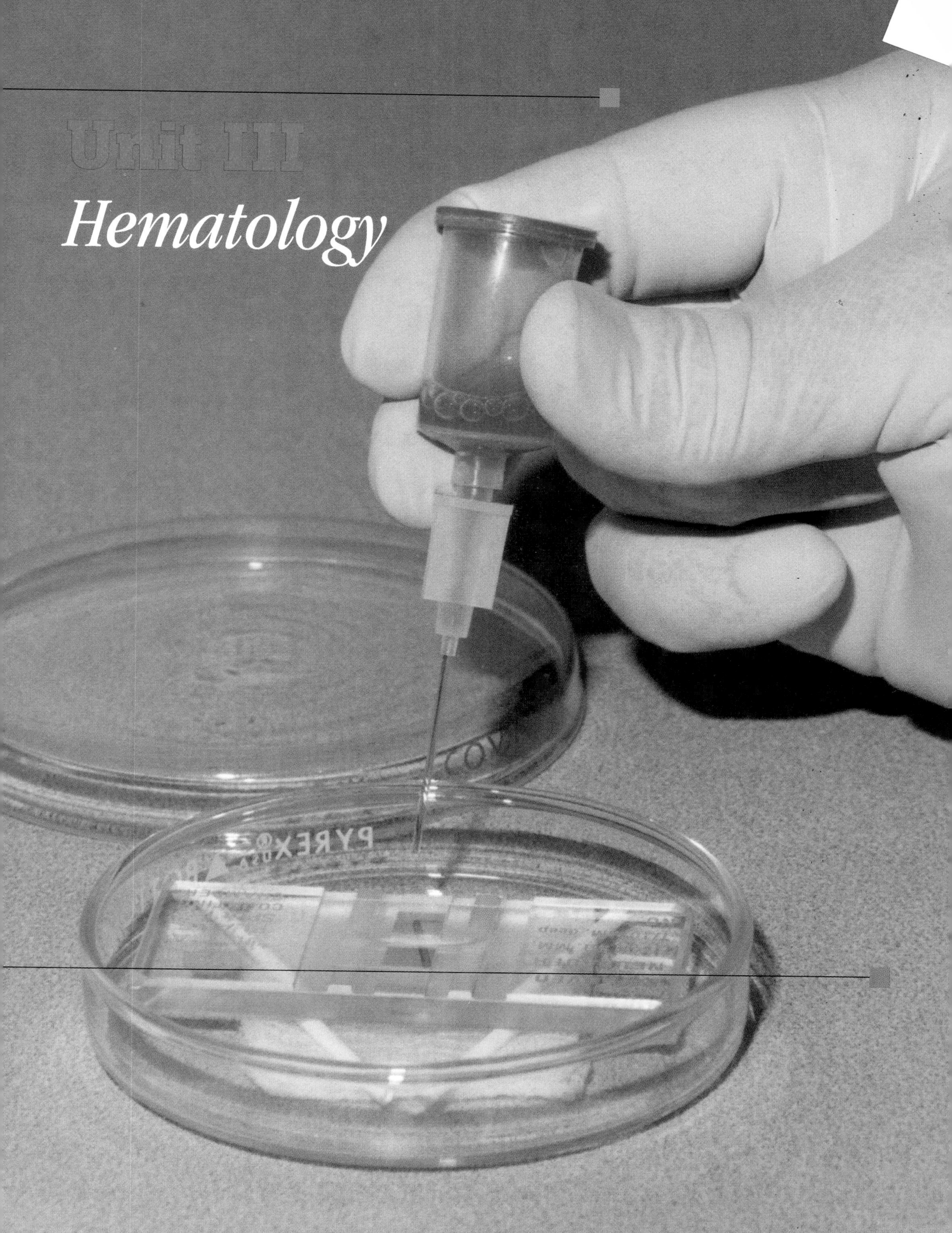

Vocabulary

bone marrow: specialized soft tissue located in the cancellous bone of the epiphyses
centrifuge: a laboratory machine used to separate particles of different densities within a liquid by spinning them at very high speeds
cytoplasmic: pertaining to all of the substances of a cell other than the nucleus
dyscrasia: a morbid condition, usually referring to an imbalance of the components of blood or bone marrow
enzyme: a protein produced by living cells
hormone: a chemical substance secreted by an endocrine gland and carried by the blood to its designated target
phagocyte: a white blood cell that is able to surround, engulf, and ingest microorganisms and debris
polymorphonuclear: having a multilobed nucleus (e.g., the neutrophil)
urea: end product of protein metabolism after ammonia is broken down by the liver

Chapter Objectives

After reading this chapter, you should be able to:

1. Describe the composition and the function of blood in the human body.
2. List the primary responsibilities of the red blood cell.
3. Describe the major role of the white blood cell.
4. Identify the five classifications of white blood cells.
5. Compare and contrast white and red blood cells.
6. Describe the location of the buffy coat and explain what it contains.
7. Discuss the formation and function of the platelet.

Chapter 10
Anatomy and Physiology of the Blood

Hematology is the study of the blood-forming tissues, the blood itself, and the components of blood. Through the centuries, scientists and nonscientists alike have been drawn to the study of the blood. Early medical experimentation with blood involved transfusions using animal blood and blood letting. Myths about blood became the bases for sacrificial religious ceremonies, medical practices, art, literature, and even poetry. Although these ancient beliefs about blood have, for the most part, disappeared, some remain to frustrate modern medical procedures. In certain rural areas, obtaining blood samples is forbidden because it is believed that vital spirits needed to keep the body alive might be removed with the blood. Another primitive belief retained by some is that blood cannot be replaced once it is removed from the body.

The average body holds 2500 to 3000 mL of blood (10 to 12 pints). The heart pumps this blood through the circulatory system more than a thousand times every day. There are more than 70,000 miles of vessels that carry blood throughout the body. The blood contains more than 25 trillion blood cells, and every second of life, the body replaces 8 million old red blood cells (RBCs) with 8 million new RBCs.

Blood Cell Formation

Hematopoiesis (sometimes called *hemopoiesis*) is the production and formation of blood cells. This synthesis occurs in the hematopoietic tissue of the red bone marrow, lymph nodes, spleen, thymus, and gastrointestinal tract.

All blood cells are derived from stem cells in the bone marrow. Stem cells then form blast cells, including erythroblasts, which mature into erythrocytes, and myeloblasts, which mature into granulocytic leukocytes. Agranulocytic leukocytes have their own precursor blast cells. Monocytes are derived from monoblasts and lymphocytes from lymphoblasts. Throm-

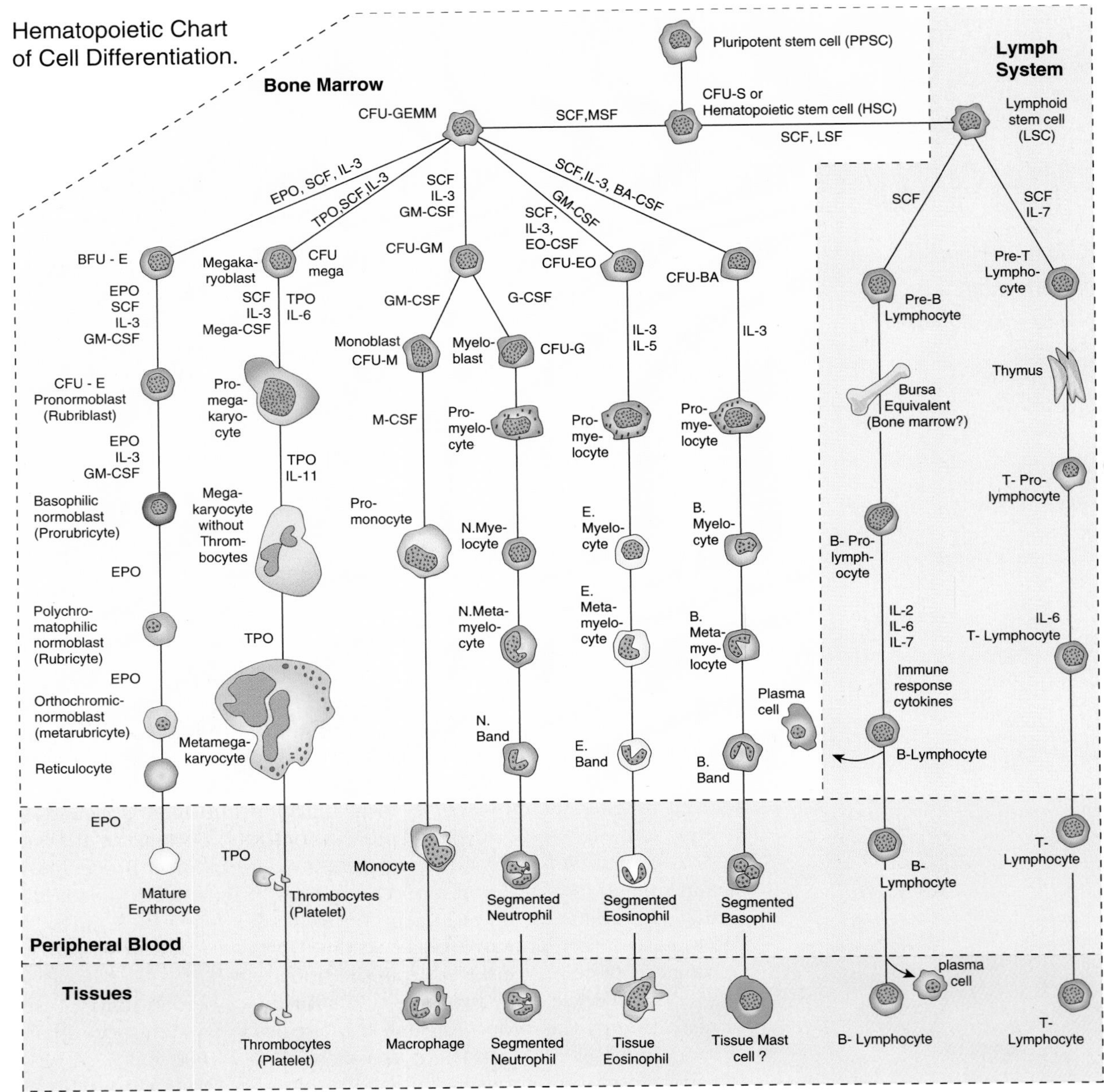

Figure 10–1. *Hematopoiesis chart. (From Stevens, M. L.* Fundamentals of Clinical Hematology. *Philadelphia: W. B. Saunders, 1997, p. 40.)*

bocytes (platelets) are formed from megakaryocytes, which have developed from megakaryoblasts. Blood cell formation is a complex process including many developmental stages (Fig. 10–1).

Impairment in hematopoiesis or unusual destruction of blood cells results in blood **dyscrasia.** Anemia, thrombocytopenia, thrombocytosis, and polycythemia are blood dyscrasias involving erythrocytes and thrombocytes. Leukemia, leukopenia, and lymphoma are dyscrasias involving leukocytes. Bleeding and clotting malfunctions occur as a result of disorders affecting thrombocytes and plasma clotting factors.

PROCEDURE 10–1

Analyzing Major Diseases of the Blood

Principle

By understanding the effect certain diseases have on the blood system, we can be better prepared for the testing procedures that will be needed.

Equipment and Supplies

paper
pencils
reference books on diseases

Procedural Steps

Look up each of the diseases listed on the right to determine what blood cells are altered and why these cells are at the center of focus of laboratory testing procedures.

Allergy
Acquired immunodeficiency syndrome (AIDS)
Hemophilia
Thrombocytopenic purpura
Acute monoblastic leukemia
Aplastic anemia
Polycythemia vera
Thalassemia
Sickle cell anemia
Rouleaux

Blood Function

The blood is propelled through the circulatory system by the pumping action of the heart. The blood is contained in a closed system of vessels, the largest of which is the aorta and the smallest of which are the capillaries, which are only a single cell layer thick. These thin, permeable walls allow certain materials to pass back and forth between the blood and the surrounding tissue.

Besides supplying body cells with the nutrients and oxygen they need, the blood also carries away carbon dioxide and urea, which are the waste by-products of normal cell activity. These wastes would kill the cells if they were allowed to accumulate. Carbon dioxide is carried in the blood to the lungs, where it is released in normal breathing through exhalation. **Urea,** along with other wastes, is carried to the kidneys, where the blood is filtered and the wastes are removed from the body by excretion in the urine. In addition, the blood also distributes **enzymes, hormones,** and other chemicals the body uses for control and regulation.

Blood Composition

Whole blood is composed of cellular or formed elements suspended in a clear liquid portion called *plasma*. Plasma represents about 55% of the blood volume. The remaining 45% of blood consists of the cellular elements, which include erythrocytes, leukocytes, and thrombocytes. Blood is the vital circulating fluid of the body and has, at times, been referred to as the "river of life." It is a transportation system bringing numerous substances of nourishment to all the cells of the body for growth, function, and repair, as well as carrying away waste products for disposal. In addition, blood functions to maintain the body at a uniform temperature; to keep the other body fluids in a state of equilibrium between alkalinity and acidity; and to carry hormones from the various glands to distant tissues where they are needed.

The blood can perform these many functions owing to the complex composition of the blood tissue. A common laboratory procedure is to spin a sample of blood in a **centrifuge** (Fig. 10–2). This causes the blood to separate into three major components. The straw-colored liquid part is called plasma; the narrow, grayish-white part is called the buffy coat; and the more solid red part is the erythrocyte layer. The red cellular part of the blood is made up of erythrocytes and the buffy coat, which is located between the red cells and the plasma and which contains the leukocytes and the platelets. The upper portion of the centrifuge tube contains the pale yellow liquid called plasma (Fig. 10–3).

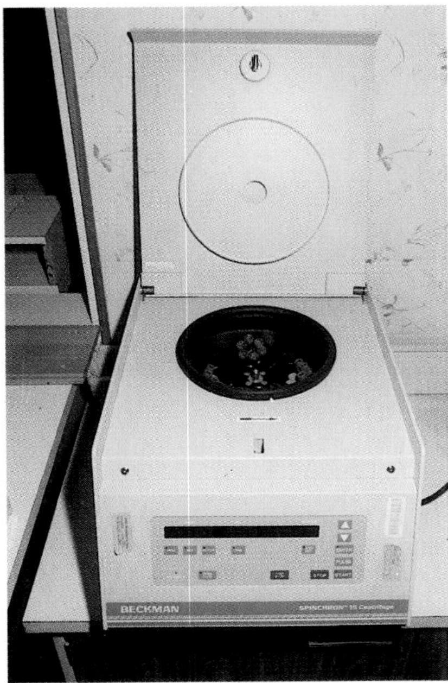

Figure 10–2. *A centrifuge used for processing blood.*

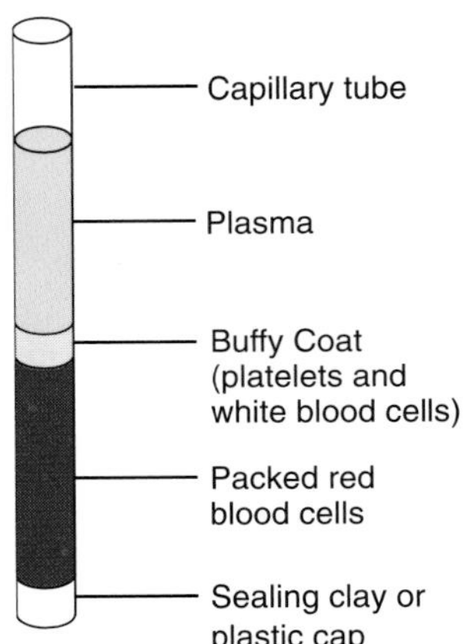

Figure 10–3. *Blood components (hematocrit).*

Plasma

Plasma is a highly complex liquid that is involved in the structure and function of cellular components, the function of thrombocytes (platelets), and the coagulation of blood. Plasma transports the formed cellular components and other noncellular components throughout the body. Some of the noncellular components of the plasma are proteins, carbohydrates, fats, hormones, enzymes, mineral salts, gases, and waste products. Plasma comprises about 90% water, 9% protein, and 1% noncellular components. When the plasma proteins and other components are used up during the clot formation process, the remaining liquid is called *serum*.

Proteins are a significant part of the plasma and play an important role in clotting, blood volume, blood pressure, and molecular transport. These proteins, which are synthesized in the liver, circulate throughout the body. Prothrombin and fibrinogen are important clotting factors; albumin contributes to the maintenance of blood volume and blood pressure; and globulin assists in the transportation of molecules, such as fats.

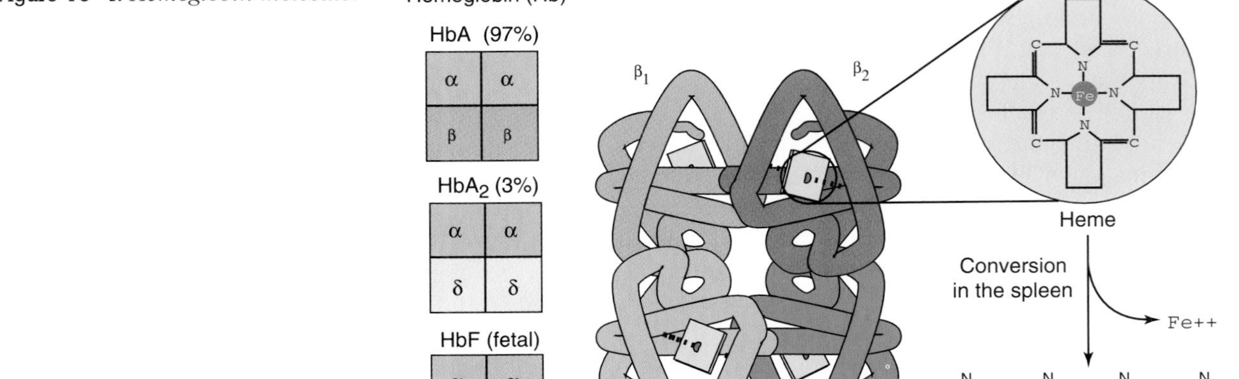

Figure 10–4. *Hemoglobin molecule.*

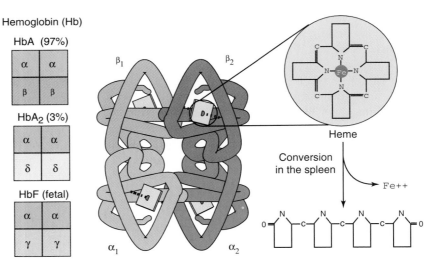

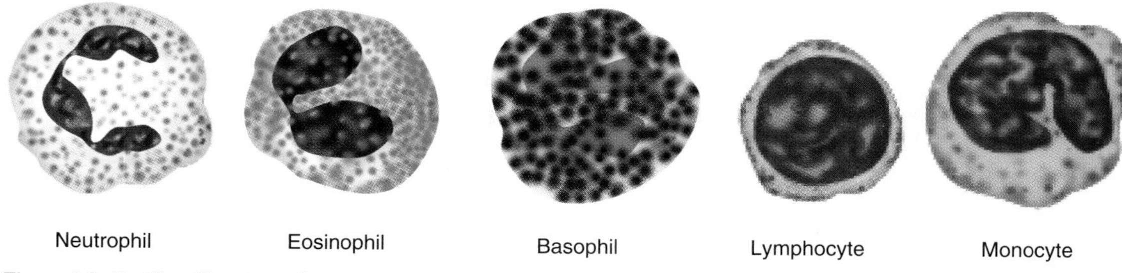

Figure 10–5. *Classification of WBCs.*

Erythrocytes

It is up to the RBCs to distribute oxygen throughout the body. They do this by means of an iron-containing protein in the RBCs called hemoglobin (Fig. 10–4). As the blood circulates through the lungs, oxygen is picked up by the hemoglobin in the RBCs. The combination of oxygen and hemoglobin turns the blood to its familiar red color. This oxygen-rich blood then circulates throughout the body, releasing oxygen to the cells in accordance with the cells' level of activity. The cells generating the most activity get the most oxygen.

The blood returning to the lungs has been depleted of most of the oxygen it was carrying, and so the cells contain carbon dioxide. This is why blood returning to the lungs is a purplish color, whereas blood that is well oxygenated is bright red. The continuous circulation of blood throughout the body is bound to take its toll on individual blood cells. Thus, our bodies continuously manufacture new RBCs in the **bone marrow** to replace the worn-out ones. Assisting the bone marrow in the production and maturation of the blood's cellular components are the spleen and lymphoid organs. The average RBC lives only about 4 months. To keep the number of RBCs at approximately $5{,}000{,}000/mm^3$, the body must produce new ones at the astonishing rate of 2 million cells per second.

Leukocytes

The second cellular component of the blood is the leukocyte (white blood cell [WBC]). There are approximately 10,000 leukocytes per cubic millimeter, or one WBC for every 700 RBCs. The role of the WBC is body defense.

Our body has five different kinds of white cells, each of which performs a different function and protects us in a slightly different way. The three types of granulocytic leukocytes are the basophil, neutrophil, and eosinophil; the two types of agranulocytic leukocytes are the monocyte and lymphocyte (Fig. 10–5).

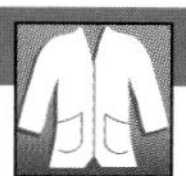

PROCEDURE 10–2

Microscopic Examination of Blood Cells

Principle

To analyze and be able to identify the different cells on a prepared blood slide using a microscope

Equipment and Supplies

microscope
prepared commercial blood cell slide

Procedural Steps

1. Analyze the various cells of the blood under a microscope.

(continued)

PROCEDURE 10–2

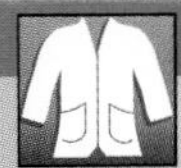

Microscopic Examination of Blood Cells (Continued)

2. Compare the cells you see with the pictures of each in your text; then draw the following:

Lymphocyte **Monocyte** **Basophil**

Eosinophil **Neutrophil** **Erythrocyte**

Granulocytes

Polymorphonuclear leukocytes, also known as granulocytes, are the most numerous among the leukocytes, constituting about 60% of these cells. Basophils contain dark-staining **cytoplasmic** granules that stain with a basic (alkaline) dye. The granules contain heparin, which is an anticlotting substance, and histamine, which is a chemical that is released in allergic responses. Eosinophils contain granules that stain with a red acidic dye called eosin. These granulocytes increase in number during allergic responses and are thought to engulf substances that trigger allergies. Neutrophils contain granules that are neutral; therefore, they do not stain intensely with either dye. Neutrophils are **phagocytes** that accumulate at sites of infection, where they engulf and destroy bacteria and debris. All granulocytes are polymorphonuclear.

Agranulocytes

Agranulocytes are mononuclear leukocytes that do not have dark-staining granules in their cytoplasm. They include both lymphocytes and monocytes.

Lymphocytes arise in the lymph nodes and circulate both in the blood and in the lymphatic system. Lymphocytes play an important role in the immune response that protects the body against infection. They are able to attack foreign matter directly and to make antibodies, which neutralize and destroy antigens.

Monocytes are phagocytic cells that also fight disease. When an infection occurs, they squeeze out between the cells in the capillaries, extending into the tissue to the site of infection. Here, they surround and consume the agents causing the infection, a process called *phagocytosis*.

Figure 10–5 shows the different types of leukocytes, their numbers in the blood, and their function.

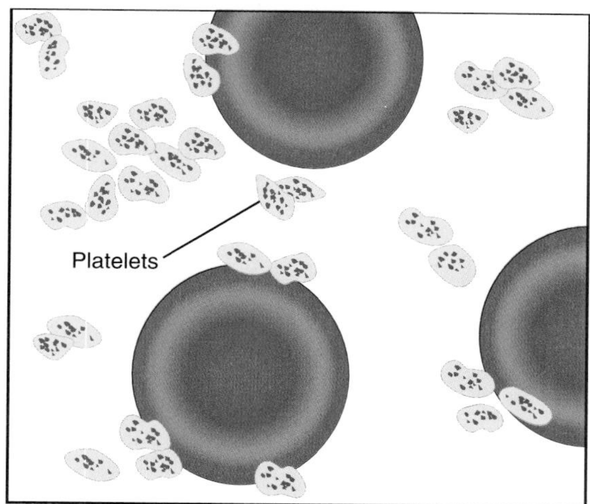

Figure 10–6. *Megakaryocyte with platelets attached.*

Platelets

Platelets, or thrombocytes, are formed in the red bone marrow from giant multinucleated cells called megakaryocytes (Fig. 10–6). Tiny fragments of the megakaryocyte break off from the cell to form platelets. These cells look like cell pieces under the microscope and do not have a nucleus. Their main function is to help in the coagulation of blood. *Coagulation* is the formation of fibrin clots through interaction with platelets to stop bleeding.

Humans cannot survive for long without the continuous flow of blood nourishing the cells and protecting the body from disease. That is why a cut or scratch could be disastrous if it resulted in the loss of too much blood. Fortunately, such disasters rarely occur because of the blood's own mechanism for sealing off broken vessels. Whenever a blood vessel is damaged and bleeding occurs, the complex chemical mechanism of clotting is set into motion. At least 15 different components in blood play a role in this process. First, the platelets stick to the edges of the cut and form a temporary plug that prevents more blood from escaping. As the platelet plug forms, a group of blood proteins, called clotting factors, is activated. One after another, these clotting factors form a net of fibers around and through the platelet plug, sealing and protecting the wound (Fig. 10–7).

The clotting process functions remarkably well in most, but not all, people. *Hemophilia* is one disease in

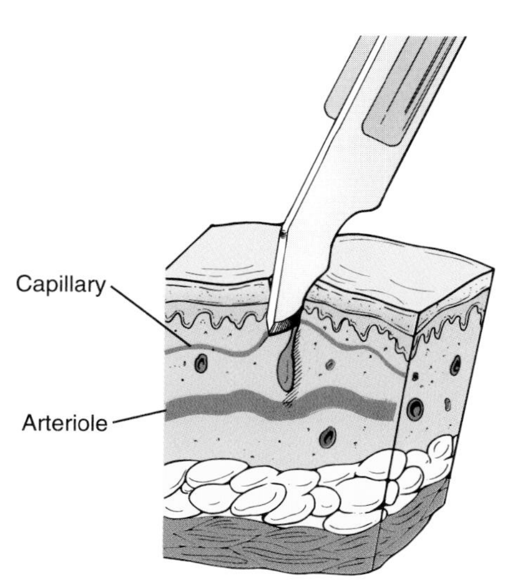

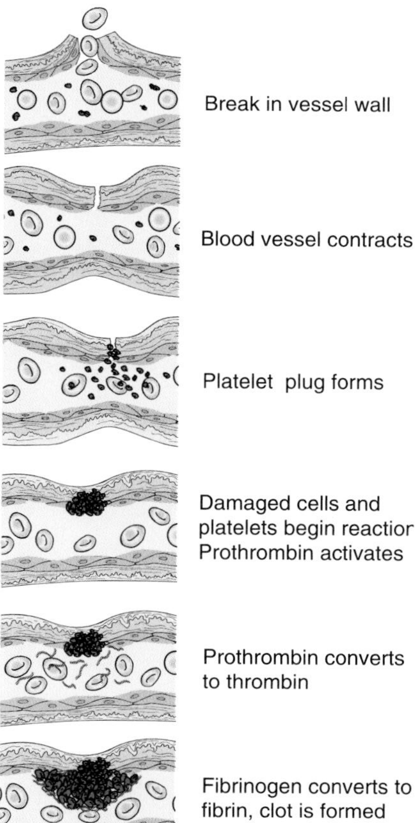

Figure 10–7. *Process of clot formation.*

which the clotting function is impaired. People having this disease can die from fairly minor wounds. To keep this from happening, hemophiliacs must receive regular transfusions of the clotting chemical that is missing from their blood, usually a protein called factor VIII.

Summary

The oxygen/carbon dioxide exchange within our body is only one of the many functions of the blood as it works to maintain stability within the body. Hormones, enzymes, nutrients, wastes, and cellular activity within the blood all have a role in the intricate mechanisms that give and sustain life.

As the blood tissue changes and adapts to the needs of the body as a whole, it reflects the body's overall state of health and stability. Thus, it is easy to understand why physicians and scientists have learned to rely on blood studies to identify illnesses and to evaluate an individual's overall well-being.

CHECK APPENDIX A FOR SPECIMEN REJECTION POLICY AND PROCEDURE.

Chapter Review

True or False

Circle T or F to indicate the correct answers to the following:

T F 1. The average body holds 3000 to 3500 mL of blood.

T F 2. The largest vessel in the body is the aorta.

T F 3. Carbon dioxide and urea are nutrients needed by all cells.

T F 4. Oxygen is released by the lungs upon exhalation.

Fill in the Blanks

Complete the following statements:

5. ______________ makes up 55% of the blood volume, and the remaining 45% is composed of ______________, ______________, and ______________.

6. Platelets are formed in the ______________ ______________.

7. The three major components of blood are ______________, ______________, and ______________.

8. Leukocytes are divided into two classifications: ______________ and ______________.

Multiple Choice

Circle the letter that represents the single best answer:

9. Some noncellular components of plasma are:
   a. Fats and hormones
   b. Hormones and RBCs
   c. RBCs and WBCs
   d. WBCs and serum
   e. All of the above

10. Oxygen is distributed to the cells of the body by:
    a. Platelets
    b. Leukocytes
    c. Erythrocytes
    d. Plasma
    e. Hormones

11. Erythrocytes are formed in the:
    a. Liver
    b. Bone marrow
    c. Kidney
    d. Brain
    e. Blood

12. All of the following are leukocytes EXCEPT:
    a. Platelets
    b. Basophils
    c. Neutrophils
    d. Monocytes
    e. Lymphocytes

13. Hemophiliacs lack clotting factor ______________.
    a. VII
    b. V
    c. VIII
    d. X
    e. XII

14. A WBC that can engulf and digest microorganisms is a:
    a. Monocyte
    b. Eosinophil
    c. Phagocyte
    d. Lymphocyte
    e. Neutrophil

Vocabulary

antecubital: the area in front of and at the bend of the elbow
anticoagulant: an agent that prevents or delays the clotting mechanism of the blood
bifurcation: the point of forking or separating into two branches
cyanotic: pertaining to a bluish discoloration of the skin and mucous membranes
edematous: pertaining to an abnormal collection of interstitial fluid that causes swelling
heparin: a naturally occurring antithrombin factor that prevents intravascular clotting
invasive procedure: a diagnostic or therapeutic technique that requires entering a body cavity
Luer-Lok: the syringe mechanism that securely holds a needle in place
sclerosis: abnormal hardening of tissue
stat: immediately

Chapter Objectives

After reading this chapter, you should be able to:

1. Locate and describe the site generally used for venipuncture.
2. Name the four important steps you must be familiar with when performing venipuncture.
3. List the equipment and the supplies that you will need when drawing blood by the syringe method.
4. List the equipment and supplies you will need for obtaining a blood specimen using a Vacutainer system.
5. Describe the steps to be followed in preparing a patient for venipuncture.
6. Identify the four areas of concern immediately following venipuncture.
7. List the information that must be included on the specimen label.
8. Explain the circumstances for which a butterfly setup would be appropriate for use.
9. Discuss the seven possible blood collection complications, including their cause and effects.
10. Name three possible sites for microcapillary puncture.
11. Explain why venipuncture is an invasive technique.

Chapter 11
Blood Collection Procedures

There is a saying in the medical laboratory that a blood test result can only be as good as the collected specimen. In addition to proper collection technique, it is also very important to select the proper syringe or Vacutainer tube and the appropriate needle.

For many hematologic tests, an adequate blood sample can be obtained by capillary puncture. If a sample of greater volume is required, the blood specimen can be obtained from a vein by venipuncture.

Venipuncture

The most common method of obtaining blood for hematologic testing is venipuncture (phlebotomy). With venipuncture, the blood is taken directly from a superficial vein. The vein is punctured with a needle and the blood is collected in either a syringe or a Vacutainer tube. Although venipuncture is a safe procedure when performed by a trained individual, the procedure must always be performed with care. One must routinely use appropriate barrier precautions when handling blood specimens. Moreover, it is important to preserve the condition of the veins; therefore, practice is required to become skilled and confident in the art of venipuncture.

Generally, veins in the forearm or the **antecubital** area are used as venipuncture sites (Fig. 11–1). The site should be selected carefully after inspecting both arms. The vein most frequently used is the median cephalic vein of the forearm. Alternative sites are indicated if this area is **cyanotic,** scarred, bruised, **edematous,** burned, or otherwise traumatized. Veins on the lower forearm, the back of the hand, or the wrist may also be used. Foot or ankle veins are used only if the patient has good circulation in the legs and permission has been granted by your supervisor or the physician to do so.

Venipuncture involves several important steps with which the laboratory assistant must be thoroughly familiar prior to performing the procedure.

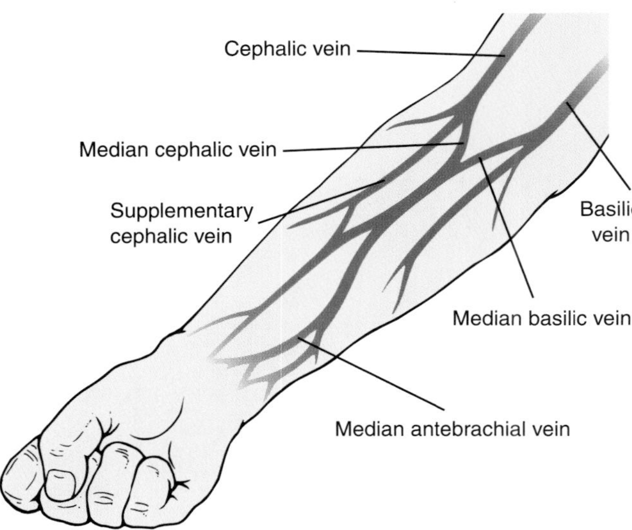

Figure 11–1. *Veins of the arm.*

GUIDELINES

Steps for Performing Venipuncture

- Select the proper method for venipuncture.
- Prepare the patient for the procedure.
- Perform venipuncture and specimen collection.
- Examine/observe the puncture site before releasing the patient.

Selection of Venipuncture Method

Syringe Method of Venipuncture

When veins are very small or fragile, the syringe method of venipuncture may be used.

SUPPLIES AND EQUIPMENT

Equipment Required for the Syringe Method of Blood Collection

- Sterile syringe and hypodermic needle
- Tourniquet and gloves
- 70% Isopropanol (alcohol) prep pads or the preferred antiseptic for the test to be performed (e.g., povidone-iodine for blood cultures and blood alcohol levels)
- Blood collection tube (Fig. 11–2)
- Gauze pads or rayon balls
- Sharps disposal container
- Hypoallergenic tape or bandage
- Permanent marking pen

Most laboratories use disposable needles and syringes and individually packaged alcohol prep pads. The needle and syringe must be assembled carefully to maintain sterility. Do not touch the tip of either the needle or the syringe, and do not uncap the needle until just prior to the actual puncture. For venipuncture, 20- to 22-gauge needles are used. The needle should be visually inspected to ascertain that it is sharp and smooth. The syringe plunger should be checked for free movement and left completely pushed into the barrel so that no air remains in the syringe.

Figure 11–2. *Venipuncture equipment (syringe method).*

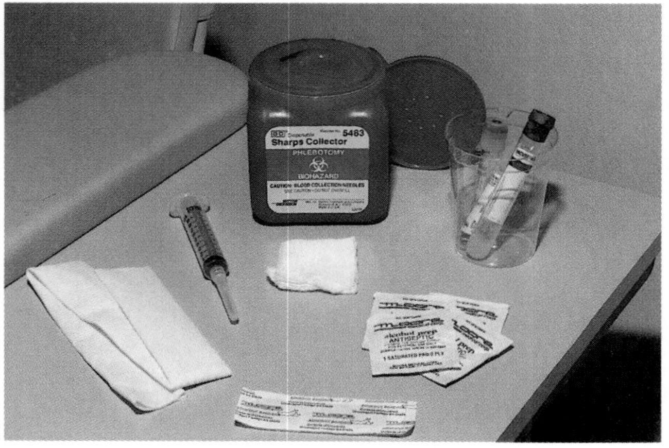

Vacutainer Method of Venipuncture

The Vacutainer system (Becton-Dickenson Company) is the most common collection system in use. It consists of evacuated tubes of various sizes with color-coded tops indicating tube contents; sterile, disposable, double-ended needles of different lengths and gauges for single or multiple draws; and a reusable plastic adapter that holds the needle in place and guides the tube. Both pediatric and adult-size adapters and tubes are available (Fig. 11–3).

If you look at the needle, you will see that it has two sharp ends. The short end is fitted into the adapter, and the long end is used to puncture the vein. After entering the vein, the tube is pushed onto the needle in the adapter, and blood is drawn into the tube

Figure 11–3. *Venipuncture equipment (Vacutainer method).*

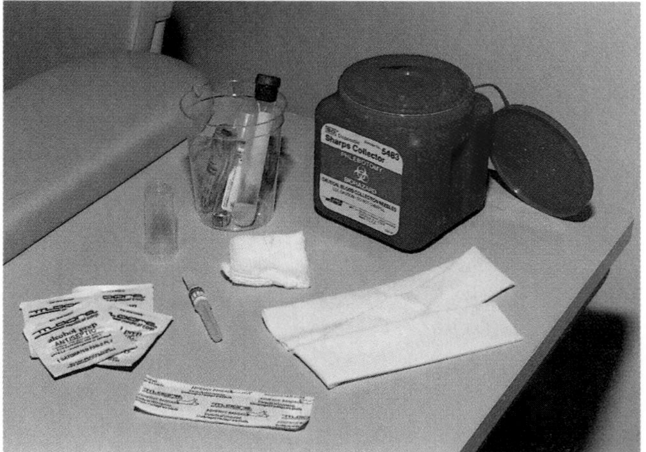

by vacuum. If more than one tube of blood is needed, the full tube can be replaced by another tube without loss of blood.

Several tubes of blood can be collected in a variety of color-coded tubes with a single venipuncture using a multidraw needle. Tubes containing ethylenediaminetetra-acetic acid (EDTA) **anticoagulant** additive are recommended for use when doing hematologic studies. White blood cells and platelets are best preserved by this additive, and improved red blood cell morphology results will be obtained with this type of tube. EDTA has no adverse effects on the blood sample when a sufficient quantity of blood is obtained. However, misleading results and an incorrect diagnosis can occur when too little blood is placed in the tube with the additive.

SUPPLIES AND EQUIPMENT

Equipment Required for the Vacutainer Method of Blood Collection

- Gloves and tourniquet
- Alcohol prep pads or preferred antiseptic for the test to be performed
- Gauze pads or rayon balls
- Needle and evacuated tube holder (assembled, as in Fig. 11–4)

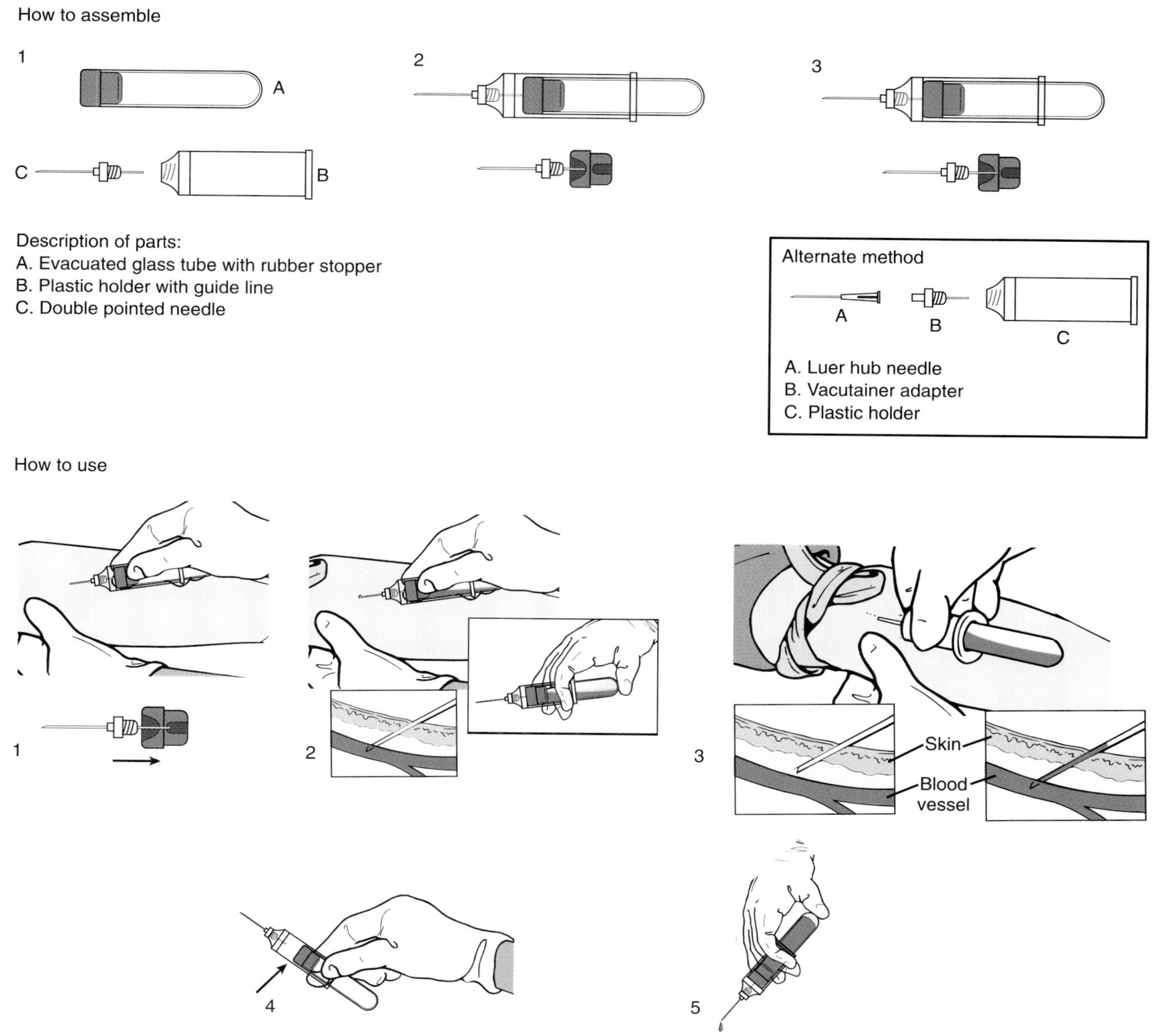

Figure 11–4. *Venipuncture equipment using the Vacutainer method. (Courtesy of Becton Dickinson Company)*

Table 11–1
List of Common Stoppers, Additives, and Laboratory Uses

Vacutainer Colors*	***Color***	***Hemogard Colors***†	***Additive/Additive Function***§	***Laboratory Use***‡,§	***Optimum Volume/Minimum Volume***
Adult Tubes					
Yellow		Yellow	Sodium polyanetholesulfonate (SPS); prevents blood from clotting and stabilizes bacterial growth	Blood or body fluid cultures	5 mL/NA
Red		Red	None	Serum testing; chemistry studies, blood bank, serology	10 mL/NA
Red/gray (marbled)		Gold	None, but contains silica particles to enhance clot formation	Serum testing	10 mL/NA
Light blue		Light blue	Sodium citrate; removes calcium to prevent blood from clotting	Coagulation testing	4.5 mL/4.5 mL
Green		Green	Heparin (sodium/lithium/ammonium); inhibits thrombin formation to prevent clotting	Chemistry testing	10 mL/3.5 mL
Green/gray (marbled)		Light green	Lithium heparin and gel for plasma separation	Plasma determinations in chemistry studies	2 mL/2 mL
Yellow/gray (marbled)		Orange	Thrombin	Stat serum demonstrations in chemistry studies	2 mL/2 mL
Lavender		Lavender	Ethylenediaminetetra-acetic acid (EDTA); removes calcium to prevent blood from clotting	Hematology testing	7 mL/2 mL
Gray		Gray	Potassium oxalate/sodium fluoride; removes calcium to prevent blood from clotting; fluoride inhibits glycolysis	Chemistry testing, especially glucose/alcohol levels	10 mL/10 mL
Royal blue		Royal blue	Sodium heparin (also sodium EDTA); inhibits thrombin formation to prevent clotting	Chemistry trace elements	7 mL
Pediatric Tubes					
Red		Red			2 mL/NA; 3 mL/NA; 4 mL/NA
Lavender		Lavender			2 mL/0.6 mL; 3 mL/0.9 mL; 4 mL/1 mL
Green		Green			2 mL/2 mL
Light blue		Light blue			2.7 mL/2.7 mL

From Rodak, B. F. *Diagnostic Hematology*. Philadelphia: W. B. Saunders, 1995, p. 10.

*Stopper colors are based on Becton-Dickinson Vacutainer tubes.

†Hemogard closures provide a protective plastic cover over the rubber stopper as an additional safety feature.

‡Sterile needles come in a variety of lengths and gauges (bore or opening size). Needles are also made to fit the evacuated tube holder by screwing in or by attaching to the tips of syringes. Most evacuated tube needles have a rubber sleeve to prevent blood from dripping into the holders when tubes are changed; these are called multiple-sample needles. The open end of the needle containing the point has a slanted side (bevel), which must be facing up when the needle is inserted into the vein. Needle positioning is very important in drawing blood. The angle of entry in relation to the skin surface should be 15 degrees. The most common needle size for adult venipuncture is 21 gauge.

§Additives, additive functions, and laboratory uses are the same for both pediatric and adult tubes.

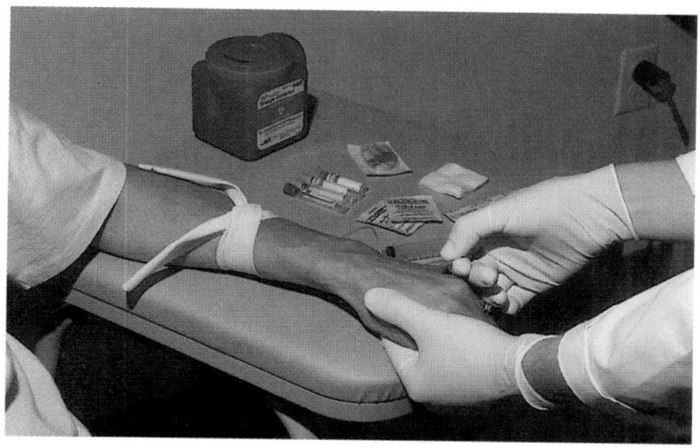
A

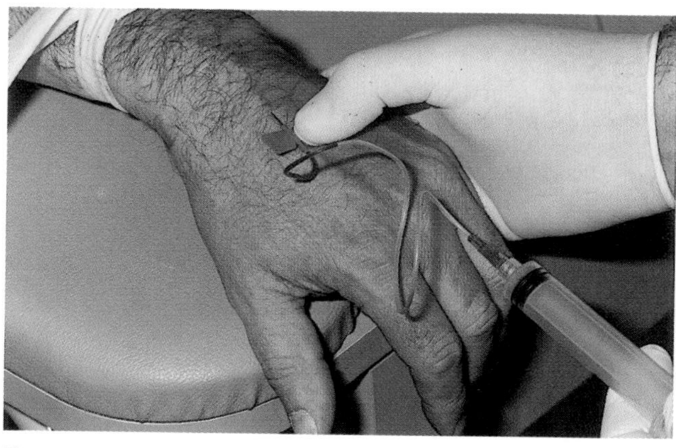
B

Figure 11–5. *Butterfly setup for collecting blood specimens.* A, *The patient's hand is in position for the blood draw.* B, *Drawing blood. Note the position of the hand.*

- Appropriate tubes for the tests to be performed, arranged in the order in which they will be drawn (Table 11–1)
- Needle disposal container
- Hypoallergenic bandage or tape
- Permanent marking pen

The Butterfly Needle Set

A butterfly needle set (Fig. 11–5), sometimes referred to as a winged infusion set, may be the venipuncture method of choice when attempting to draw blood from infants or small children, or from adults with difficult veins, such as those in the hand or wrist.

When using a butterfly set, the butterfly device with a multiple-sample **Luer-Lok** adapter is preferred. The adapter can be attached directly to an evacuated tube holder. A 23-gauge needle is used in the setup, as this size will easily penetrate small veins without rupturing them. Carefully select the small-volume pediatric tubes in which to collect the specimen. Large-volume tubes may create too great a vacuum pressure on the vein and cause it to collapse, or they can cause hemolysis of the specimen. You may need to use the syringe method.

All steps taken to prepare the patient and to ensure a sterile environment when using the Vacutainer or syringe methods of venipuncture are also followed when using a butterfly needle set. Refer to Procedure 11–1 for more detailed information on this method.

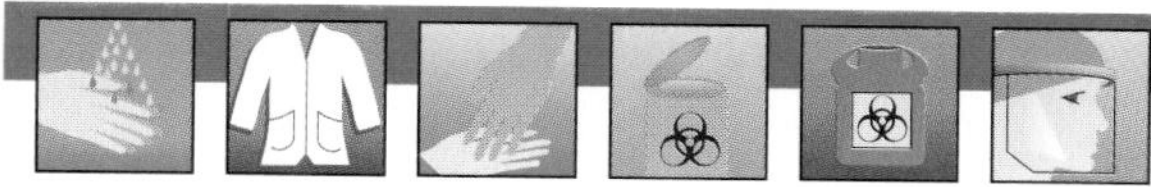

PROCEDURE 11–1

Performing a Butterfly Blood Draw from a Hand Vein

Principle

To obtain a venous blood sample for analysis from a hand vein using a butterfly needle assembly

Equipment and Supplies

tourniquet
alcohol prep pads or other antiseptic pads
gauze pads or rayon balls
butterfly needle set
appropriate pediatric tubes, arrange in order of the samples to be drawn, or a syringe, if necessary
pediatric Vacutainer shell
needle disposal container
nonallergenic bandage
permanent marker pen

(continued)

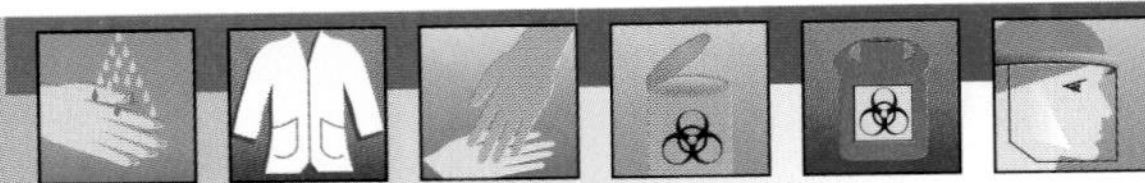

PROCEDURE 11–1

Performing a Butterfly Blood Draw from a Hand Vein (Continued)

Procedural Steps

1. Wash hands, dry them thoroughly, and don glove.
2. Remove the butterfly device from the package. Extend the tubing its full length and stretch it slightly to keep it from recoiling.
3. Attach the butterfly collection device to the evacuated tube holder.
4. Seat the first tube in the holder.
5. Apply a tourniquet to the patient's wrist, proximal to the wrist bone.

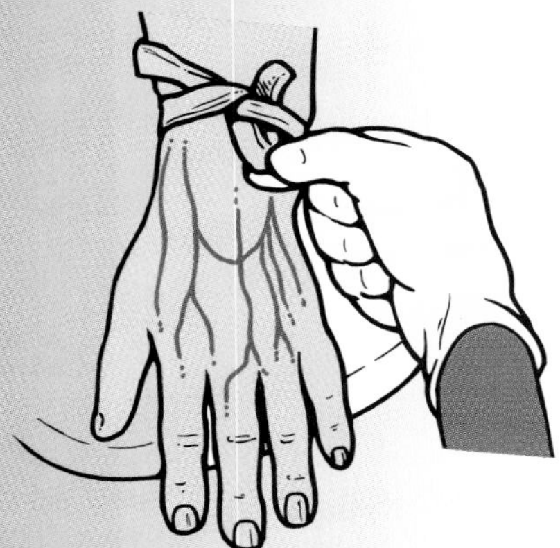

6. Make sure the patient's arm is well supported with a towel or armrest.
7. Hold the patient's hand lightly in your nondominant hand.
8. Select a vein and cleanse the site at the **bifurcation.**
9. Using your thumb, pull the patient's skin taut over the knuckles.
10. Holding the needle bevel-up and aligned with the vein, enter the vein at a 10- to 15-degree angle. When the needle enters the vein, there will be a "flash" of blood in the tubing.

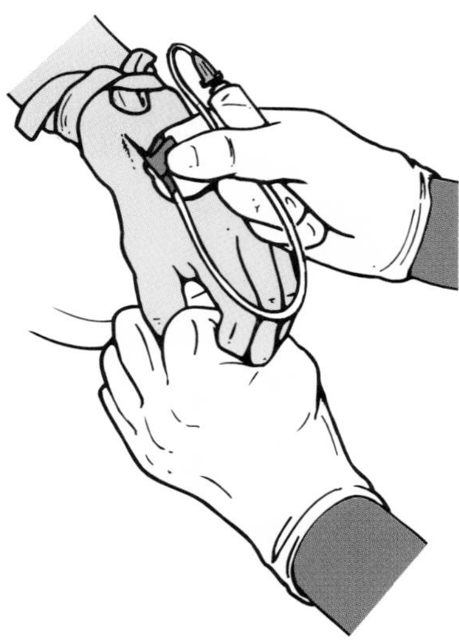

11. "Seat" the needle by threading it up the lumen of the vein slightly so that it will not twist out of the vein if you let go of the needle.
12. Push the blood collecting tube onto the end of the holder or draw blood into the syringe. (Note the position of the hands).

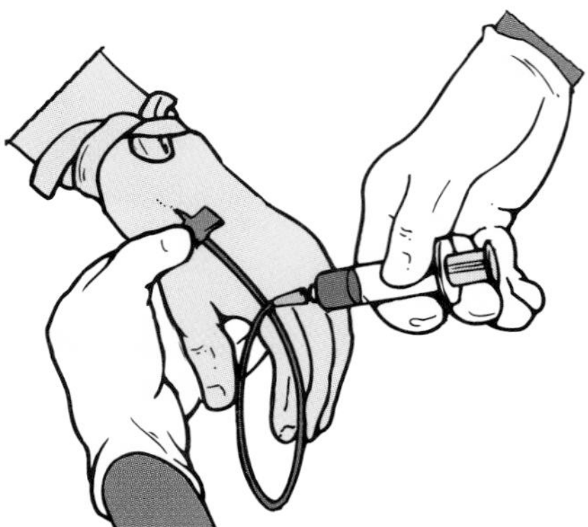

13. Release the tourniquet when blood appears in the tube.
14. Keep the tube and holder in a downward position so that the tube fills from the bottom up.

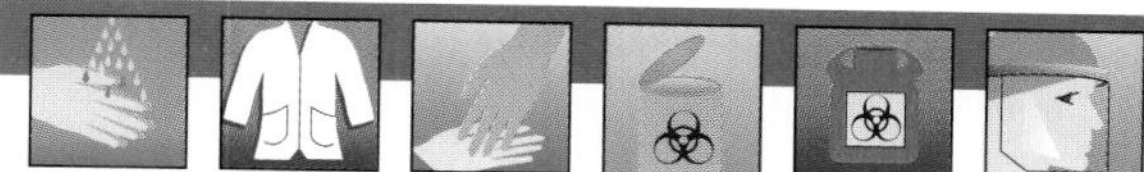

PROCEDURE 11–1

Performing a Butterfly Blood Draw from a Hand Vein (Continued)

15. Place a gauze pad over the puncture site and remove the needle.

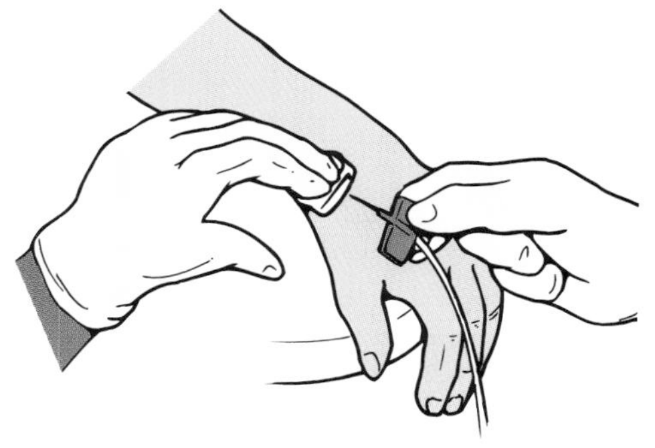

16. Apply slight pressure to the puncture site using the gauze pad.
17. Dispose of used equipment in a sharps container.
18. Check the puncture site and apply a bandage if there is no oozing.
19. Label the blood specimen and place it in the proper collection area.
20. Remove gloves, wash and dry hands thoroughly, and enter the procedure in the laboratory logbook.

Patient Preparation

The most important part of preparing a patient for venipuncture is to correctly identify the patient. After greeting and identifying the patient, a brief explanation of the procedure should be given so as to minimize anxiety. The patient should be seated in a phlebotomy chair (Fig. 11–6). If the patient appears to be apprehensive, it is advisable to ask the patient to lie down for the procedure. Explain to the patient the importance of holding the arm still, and assist the patient by providing adequate support. A child's cooperation can be gained by having him or her take an active part in the procedure, such as holding the gauze pads for you. **NEVER allow the patient to remain standing or to sit on a high stool during the procedure,** for if the patient faints, the risk of injury is greatly increased. Special venipuncture chairs are used in most drawing stations. These chairs have adjustable arm rests and a safety mechanism that prevents the patient from falling should fainting occur.

All necessary supplies should be within easy reach. When using the Vacutainer method, you should have extra tubes available in case you encounter a tube with a bad vacuum. The most common tourniquets used are flat, broad, elastic straps, but Velcro tourniquets are now available which are easy to apply and adjust, and which come in several sizes. The chief disadvantages of the Velcro strap are its cost and the fact that it can be difficult to keep free of blood. Blood pressure cuffs may also be used, especially in geriatric patients whose skin may tear if an elastic tourniquet is used.

Needle disposal units should be readily available. **Remember that used needles may not be recapped.**

Keep your supplies clean and in order. The expiration dates of the evacuated tubes should be checked on a daily basis to be certain that outdated supplies are removed. Commercial venipuncture trays are now available to allow convenient stocking of necessary

Figure 11–6. *Phlebotomy chair.*

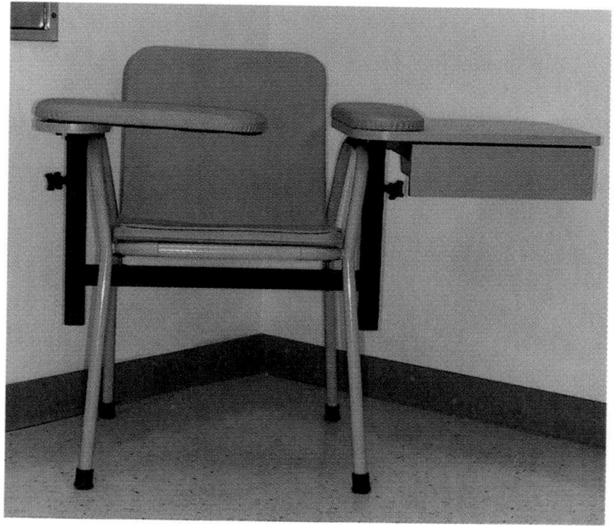

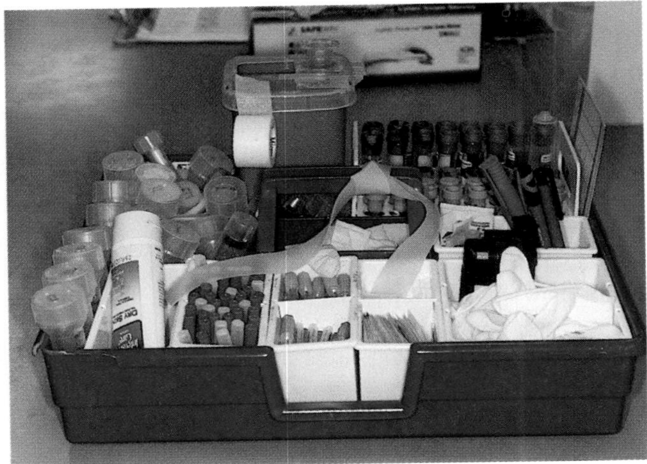

Figure 11–7. *Fully stocked venipuncture tray.*

venipuncture supplies. Figure 11–7 shows a fully stocked venipuncture tray.

Specimen Collection

The patient's arm is fully extended and supported. A tourniquet is applied to the arm, 2 inches above the elbow, to make the veins more prominent by slowing, but not stopping, blood flow (Fig. 11–8*A*). The puncture site is located by gently palpating (pressing on) the veins with your fingertips (Fig. 11–8*B*). This determines the direction of the vein and its approximate size and depth. The area around the puncture site is cleansed, using an outward-moving circular pattern, with the correct antiseptic (Table 11–2). The site is then allowed to air dry or is blotted dry with sterile gauze (Fig. 11–8*C*). **DO NOT FAN OR BLOW DRY the puncture site.**

The syringe or Vacutainer system is held in one hand at a 15- to 30-degree angle to the patient's arm. The needle is positioned bevel-up and pointing in the same direction as the vein. Ask the patient to make a fist, as this tenses the skin, facilitating puncture. The skin and vein are entered with one smooth motion until the needle is in the lumen of the vein (Fig. 11–8*D*). The blood specimen is obtained by gently pulling back on the plunger with the other hand while holding the syringe and needle motionless (Fig. 11–8*E*). When using the Vacutainer method, place two fingers at the end of the holder and, while holding the needle and the adapter motionless, push the tube into the adapter with your thumb. Release the tourniquet as soon as blood begins to fill the tube or to flow into the syringe (Fig. 11-8*F*). When you have obtained the required amount of blood, place a dry, sterile gauze over the puncture site and remove the needle from the vein

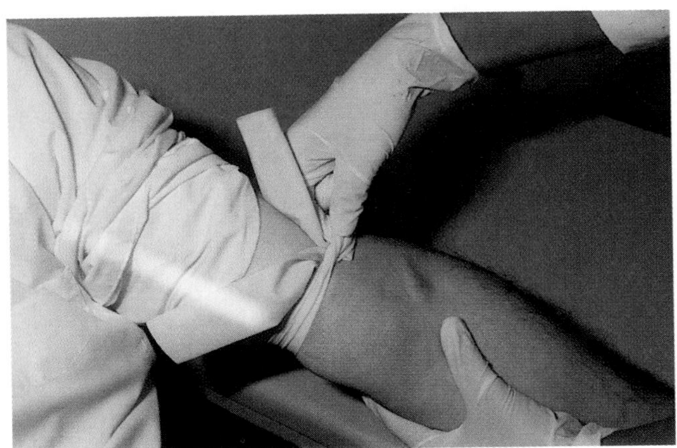

A

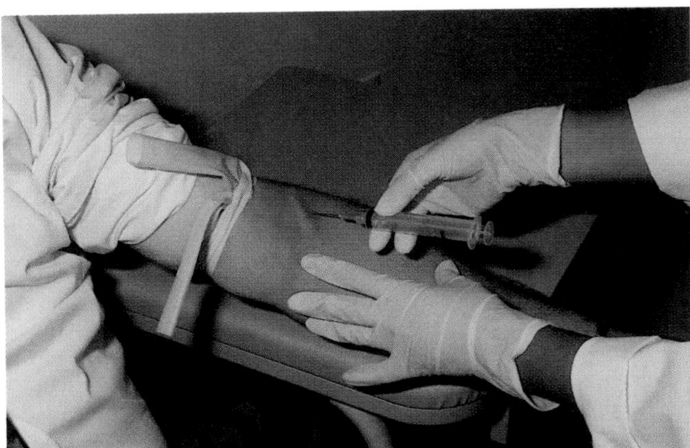

D

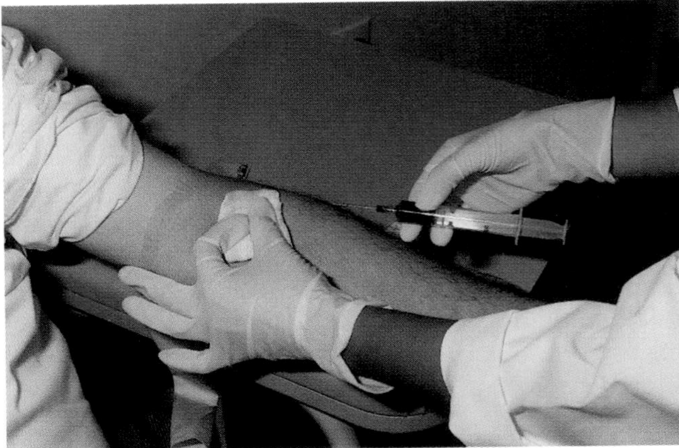

G

Figure 11–8. *Venipuncture—syringe method.* A, *Applying the tourniquet.* B, *Palpating the vein.* C, *Cleansing the site.* D, *Puncturing the vein.* E, *Filling the syringe.* F, *Releasing the tourniquet.* G, *Removing the needle.* H, *Transferring the specimen to the sample tube.* I, *Applying a bandage to the venipuncture site.*

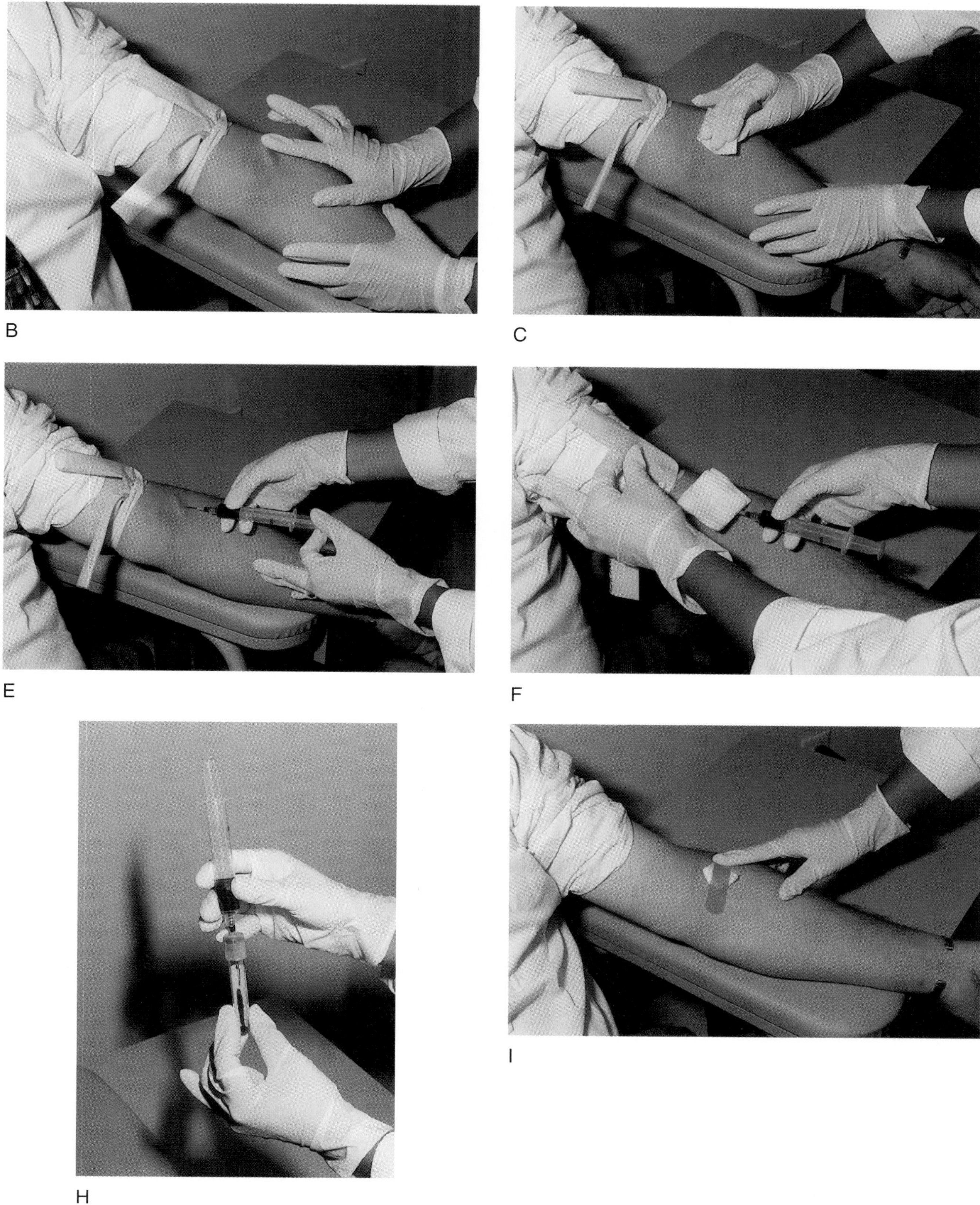

B

C

E

F

H

I

Table 11–2
Antiseptics Used in Puncture Site Preparation

Antiseptic	***Recommended Use***
70% isopropyl alcohol	Most routine blood draws
Povidone-iodine (Betadine)	Arterial blood gas studies and blood culture draws
Benzalkonium chloride (Zephiran)	Draws for blood alcohol levels

(Fig. 11–8*G*). Never apply pressure on the needle site until the needle is completely removed from the vein.

If you have used the syringe method, the blood must be transferred to a tube at this time (Fig. 11–8*H*). Gently insert the needle through the rubber stopper of a vacuum tube using precaution to prevent a needle stick. The vacuum will draw the required amount of blood into the tube. When using tubes that contain additives, gently invert the tube containing the blood 8 to 10 times to mix in the additive.

Postprocedural Concerns

Puncture Site

Apply pressure to the puncture site for a few minutes. You may ask the patient to elevate the arm. To prevent oozing of blood, the patient should not bend the arm.

After 1 or 2 minutes, check the patient's arm to see if bleeding has stopped. If the bleeding has stopped, apply a hypoallergenic bandage over several layers of folded gauze to the puncture site (Fig. 11–8*I*). Advise the patient to remove the bandage in about 30 minutes. Some laboratories prefer not to bandage the puncture site because bandages tend to irritate the skin and leave a sticky film on the skin. Check your procedure manual or consult your supervisor to determine your laboratory's protocol.

Figure 11–9. *Disposing of sharps in a biohazard container.*

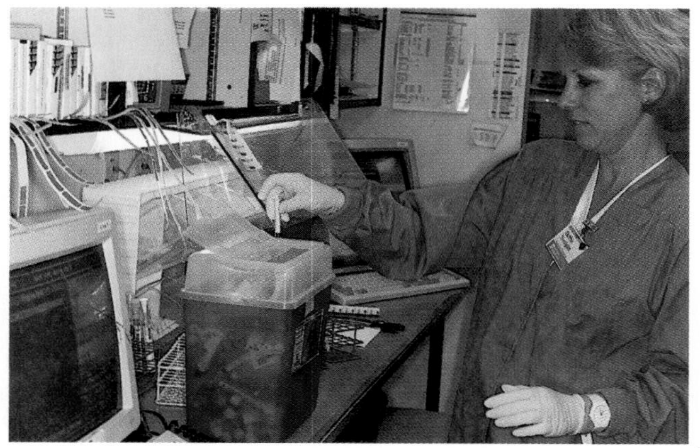

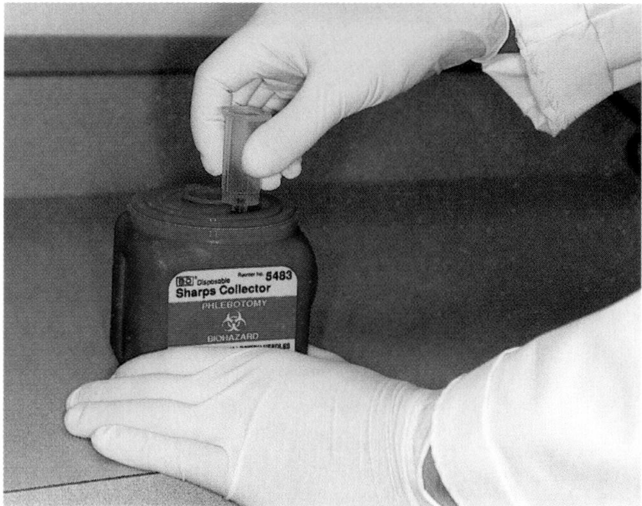

Figure 11–10. *Separating the adapter from the needle using a sharps container.*

Needle Disposal

If the syringe method was used for venipuncture, dispose of the needle and the syringe immediately by placing it in the designated biohazardous waste container (Fig. 11–9). Do not place it on any surface, and do not recap it. If the Vacutainer method was used, place the needle in the proper slot of a biohazard sharps container and turn it counterclockwise until it unscrews from the evacuated tube holder (Fig. 11–10). If the needle refuses to separate from the holder, throw the entire unit away in the biohazard container.

Specimen Handling and Transport

The importance of proper labeling of a blood specimen cannot be overemphasized. You should be familiar with the specimen labeling protocols for your laboratory.

GUIDELINES

Specimen Label Information

- Print the patient's name.
- Fill in the patient's chart number or date of birth.

Figure 11–11. *Properly labeled specimen tube.*

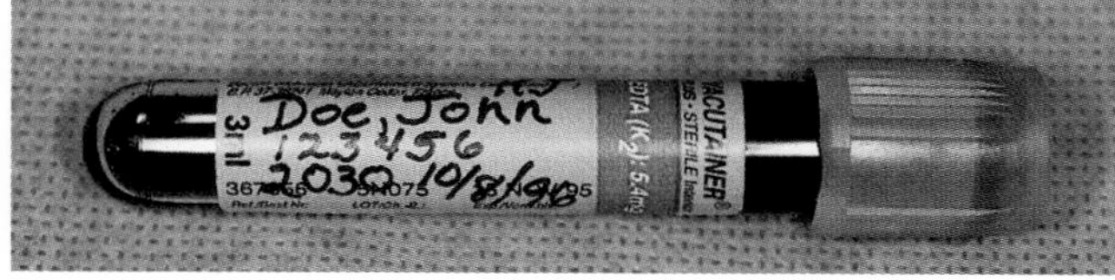

- Record the time of collection.
- Indicate the test(s) ordered.
- Add the date and your initials (Fig. 11–11).

If any specimens require mixing (blue- or purple-stoppered tubes), gently invert the tube several times. You should also be aware of any special transportation requirements. Does the specimen need to be transported on ice? If this is a cold agglutinin test, it will need to be maintained at 37°C. How do you handle a **stat** analysis? Will you need to protect this specimen from the light, as for bilirubin testing?

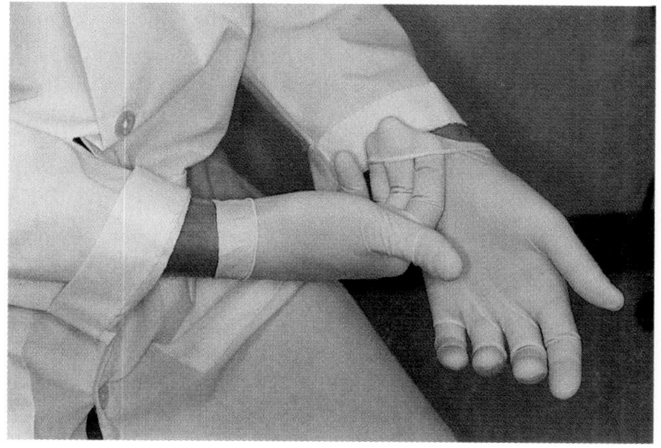

A

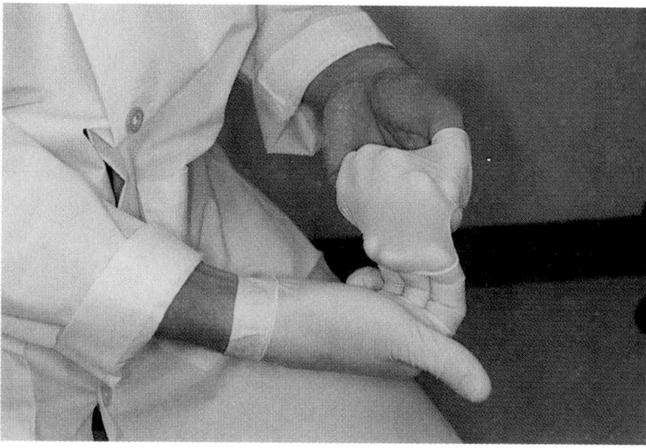

B

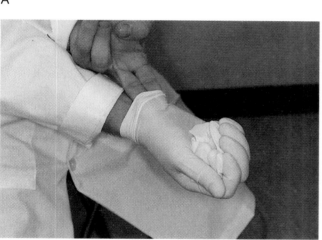

C

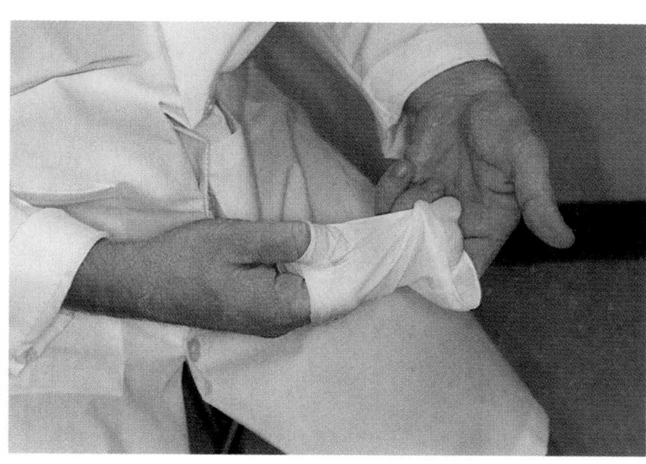

D

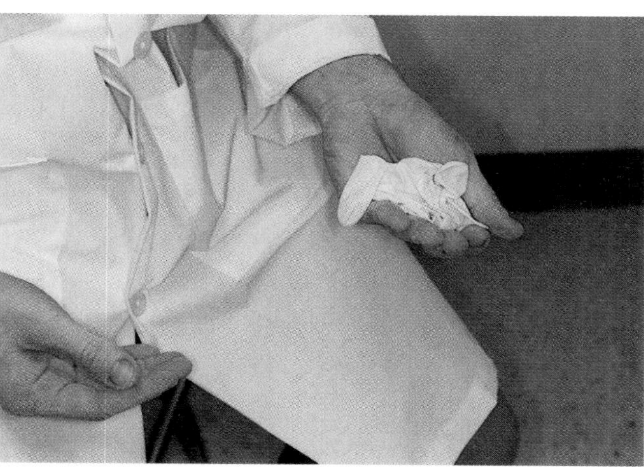

E

Figure 11–12. *Procedure for glove removal.*

Enter the specimen information into the laboratory log book or computer. The collection of laboratory specimens must be documented for verification. Place the specimen and the laboratory request forms in the designated location for prompt processing.

Glove Removal

Remove your gloves by grasping one glove at the wrist and pulling it inside out and off of the hand (Fig. 11–12*A*), ending up with it in the palm of the still-gloved hand. Slip your nongloved fingers under the second glove at the wrist (Fig. 11–12*B*) and pull it off of the hand (Fig. 11–12*C*), ending with one glove inside of the other with the contaminated surfaces to the inside (Fig. 11–12*D*). Avoid "snapping" the gloves as you remove them. Place the gloves in a biohazardous waste container, not the sharps container. Wash your hands and dry them thoroughly.

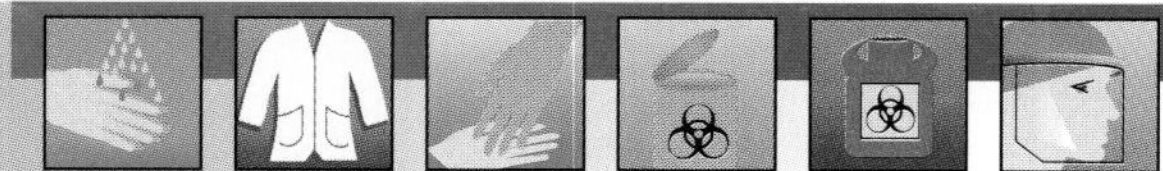

PROCEDURE 11–2

Collecting a Venous Blood Specimen

Principle

To collect a venous blood specimen using the Vacutainer system or syringe method

Equipment and Supplies

needle, syringe, and specimen tubes or a Vacutainer needle (single-draw or multiple-draw, depending on the test[s] ordered)
70% isopropyl alcohol
sterile gauze pads
tourniquet
nonallergenic bandage
permanent marking pen

Procedural Steps

1. Check the requisition form to determine the tests ordered; then gather the necessary supplies.
2. Put on an apron, glasses, and mask.
3. Wash your hands, dry them thoroughly, and put on gloves.
4. Identify the patient and explain the procedure.
5. Offer the patient a comfortable seat and place the patient's arm in a well-supported position, angled slightly downward.
6. Inspect the patient's veins.

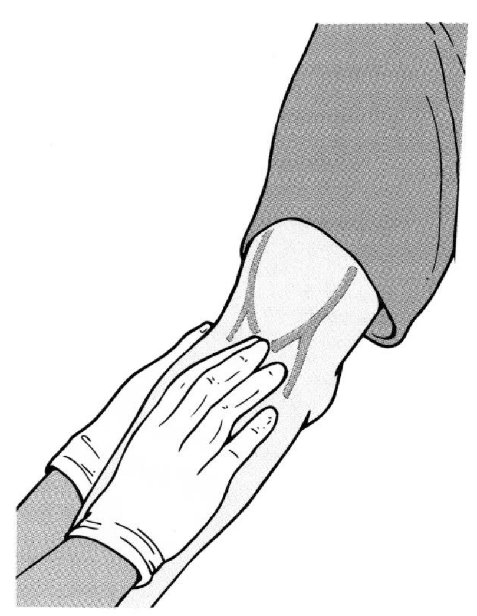

7. Assemble the preferred equipment.

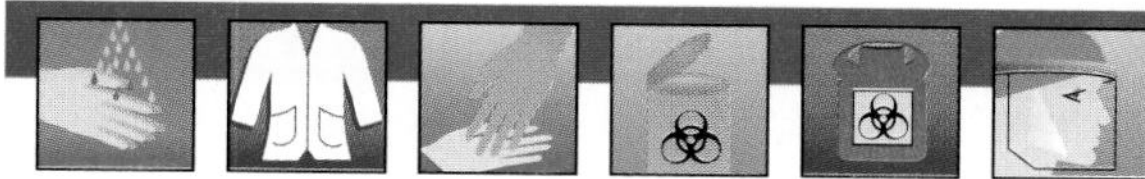

PROCEDURE 11–2

Collecting a Venous Blood Specimen (Continued)

8. Apply a tourniquet around the patient's arm 2 inches above the elbow.

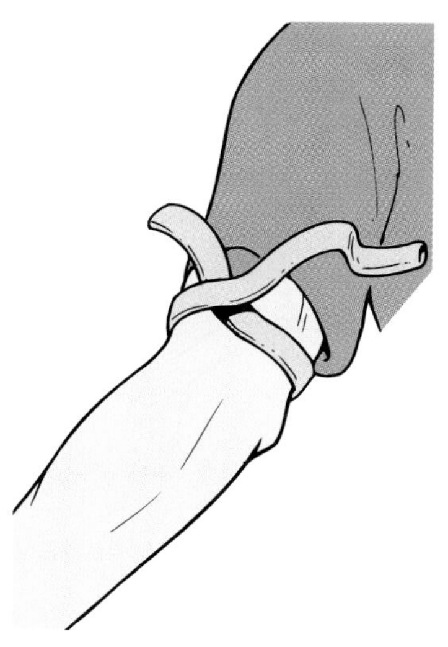

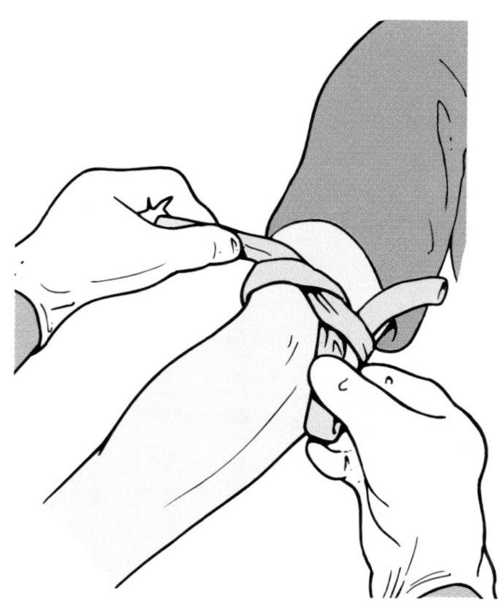

9. Select the venipuncture site by palpating the antecubital site.

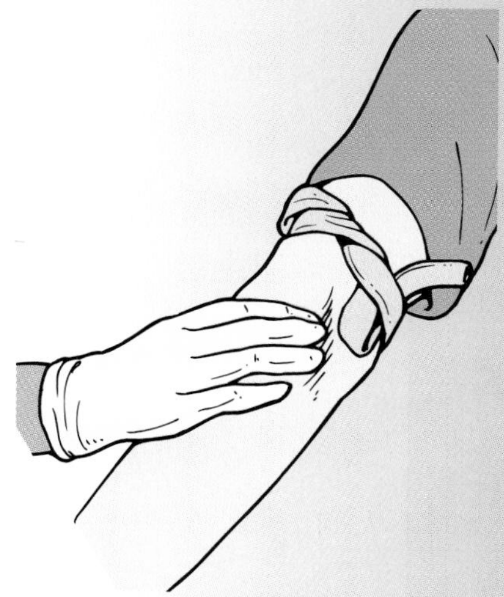

10. Ask the patient to open and close his or her hand several times.
11. Cleanse the site.

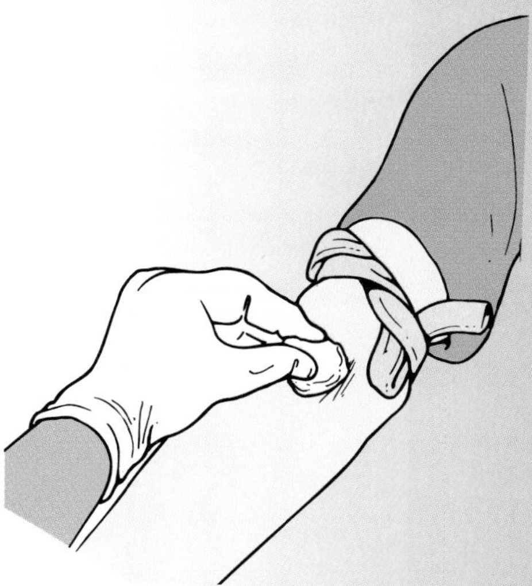

12. Dry the site with sterile gauze.
13. Remove the needle sheath.

(continued)

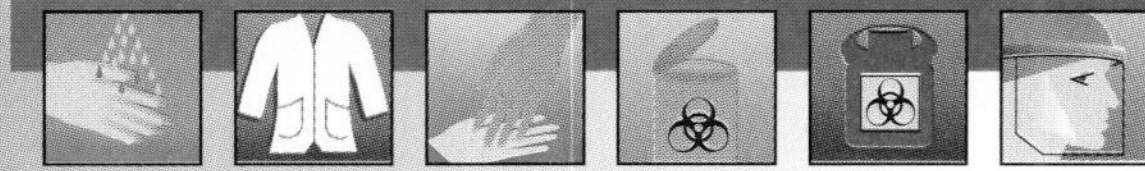

PROCEDURE 11–2

Collecting a Venous Blood Specimen *(Continued)*

14. Hold the syringe or Vacutainer assembly in your dominant hand with your thumb on top and your fingers underneath.
15. Grasp the patient's arm with your nondominant hand and use your thumb and forefinger to draw the skin taut over the site, thereby anchoring the vein.
16. Insert the needle into the vein, bevel-up, at a 15-degree angle.

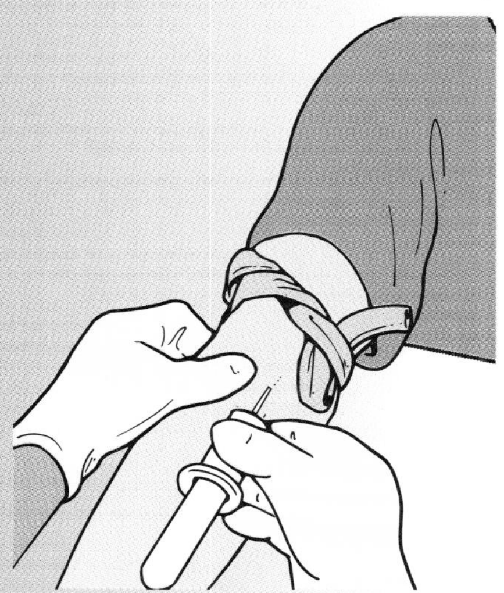

17. Slowly pull back on the syringe with the nondominant hand OR place two fingers on the flanges of the Vacutainer adapter and, with the thumb, push the tube onto the needle in the side of the adapter.

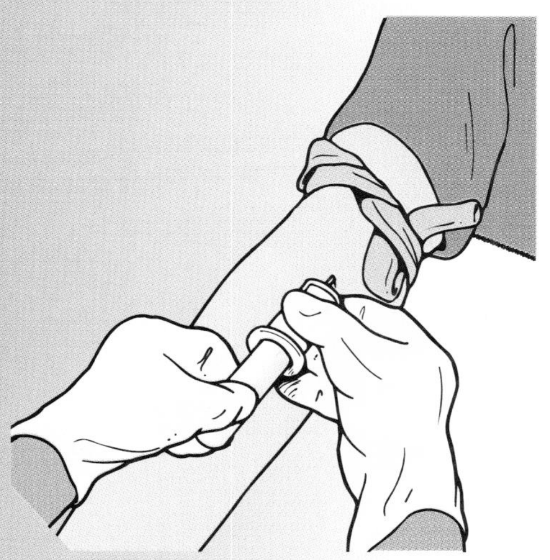

18. Allow the syringe or tube to fill with blood.
19. Release the tourniquet when the venipuncture is complete. **The tourniquet must be released before the needle is removed from the arm.**

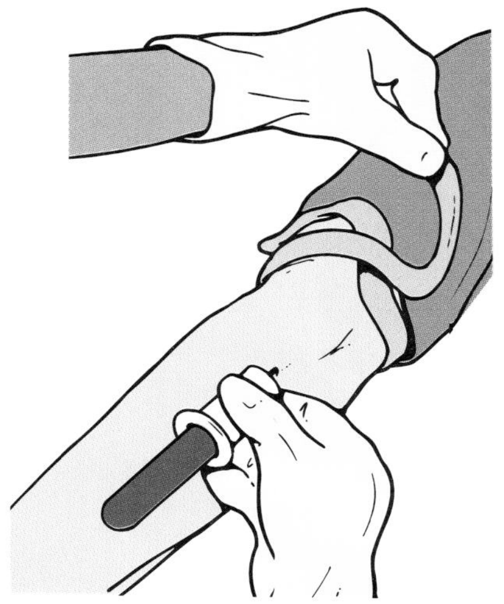

20. Remove the needle and syringe from the vein OR remove the Vacutainer tube from the adapter prior to removing the needle from the vein.
21. Place a sterile gauze square over the puncture site as the needle is withdrawn.

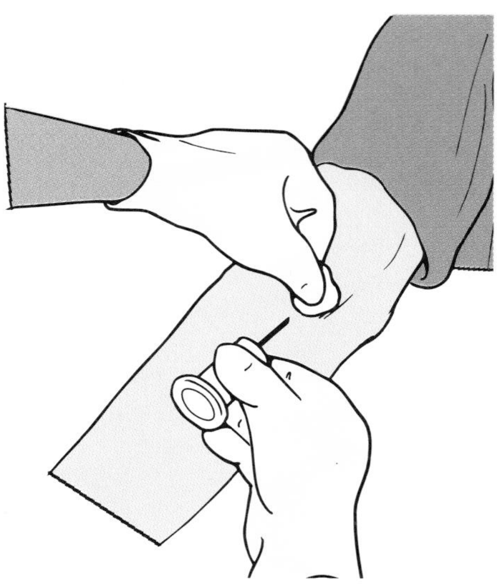

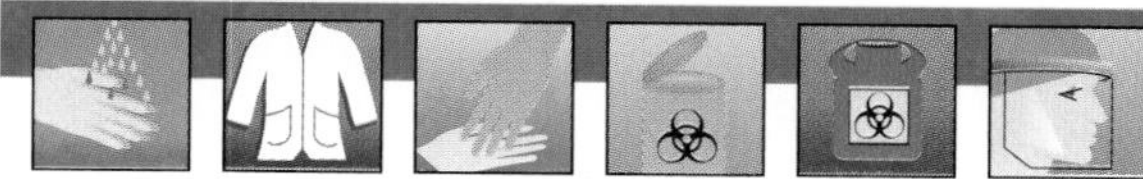

PROCEDURE 11–2

Collecting a Venous Blood Specimen (Continued)

22. Instruct the patient to apply pressure to the puncture site without bending the affected arm.
23. If using a syringe, transfer the blood specimen to the appropriate laboratory tube. Gently invert the tube(s) to mix anticoagulants/preservatives with the blood.
24. Properly dispose of the syringe or Vacutainer needle in a sharps container.

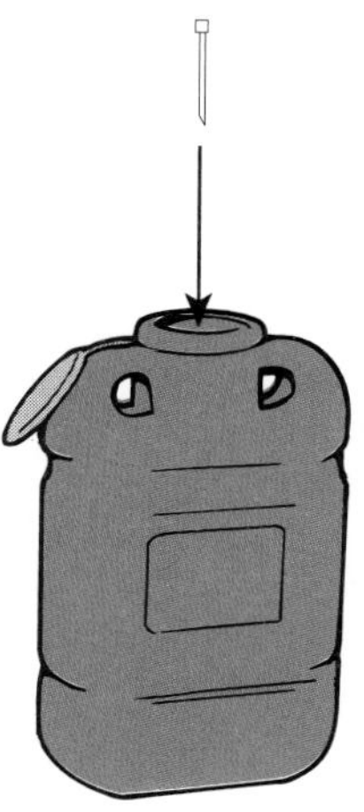

25. Label all tubes with pertinent information.

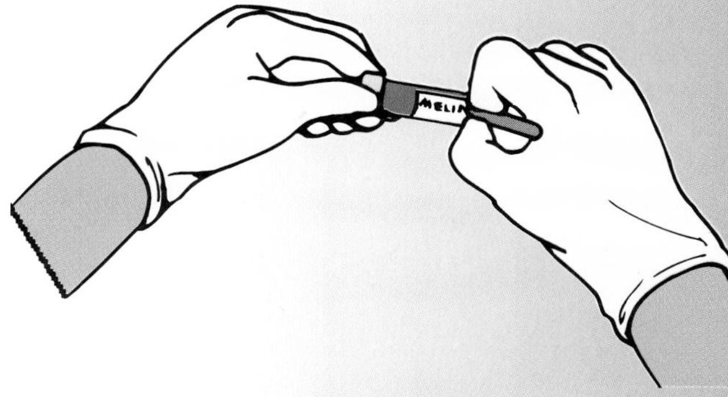

26. Check the puncture site and apply a nonallergenic bandage.
27. Clean the work area according to OSHA standards.
28. Complete the laboratory slips and routing forms if needed. Enter in logbook.
29. Remove gloves and wash your hands.

Potential Complications of Blood Collection

Failure to Obtain Blood

The inability to obtain blood can be caused by a number of factors. Being aware of these factors and how to correct them may determine whether you obtain blood on the first try or whether you will have to repeat the procedure. When you fail to obtain blood, it is important to remain calm so that you can think clearly, systematically determining the cause of the problem. Table 11–3 lists some possible solutions if the problem lies in the positioning of the needle. As a general rule, it is wise to limit yourself to two attempts to obtain blood from any one patient. If you fail on the second try, ask the patient whether he/she would prefer having someone else in the laboratory try or whether he/she would prefer to come back at another time. This will alleviate the apprehension and allow the patient to feel that they are in control of the situation. At one time or another, almost everyone fails to obtain a needed blood sample, so you need not feel inadequate. Very likely, you will be the one who is able to obtain a blood sample from another patient after a coworker has tried unsuccessfully to obtain a specimen.

Syncope (Fainting)

A number of patients become lightheaded or dizzy at the thought or sight of blood. It is important for you to be aware of the patient's condition throughout the procedure. If fainting occurs, terminate the procedure immediately. Be sure that the patient is in a safe position and cannot fall or be otherwise injured. Call for assistance; never attempt to move the patient by yourself. The patient should not be allowed to leave before he/she has recovered fully. Document the event on the laboratory log or, if necessary, complete an incident report.

Table 11-3
Managing Blood Draw Complications

Possible Complication	***Strategies***
Burned area	Must be avoided, as these areas are prone to infection
Convulsions	Stay calm. **Remove the needle;** then, help guide the patient to the floor, protecting him/her from injury. Call for help.
Damaged/scarred veins or infected areas	Look for an alternate site; DO NOT draw blood from scarred or infected areas.
Edema	Avoid the area; look for an alternative site.
Hematoma	Adjust the depth of the needle or remove the needle and apply pressure.
Intravenous (IV) therapy/blood transfusion sites	Blood samples should not be drawn from an arm that is also the site for IV infusion or blood transfusion owing to the dilution factor.
Mastectomy	DO NOT draw blood from the site of the mastectomy, as mastectomy surgery causes lymphostasis, which may produce false results.
Nausea	Place a cold cloth on the patient's forehead, give the patient a basin, in case of vomiting, and instruct them to take deep breaths. Alert the physician.
No blood	Manipulate the needle slightly, or remove the Vacutainer and perform the blood draw again using a syringe or butterfly setup.
Petechiae	Loosen the tourniquet, as this complication usually results from the tourniquet being in place for longer than 2 minutes.
Syncope (fainting)	Position the patient's head between the knees (if in a sitting position). Check and record the patient's pulse, blood pressure, and respiration rate, and continue to observe the patient. **Never leave the patient unattended.**

Hematomas

A hematoma is caused by blood leaking into the tissues; this will cause the area around the puncture site to swell. This can happen when the needle goes completely through the vein, when the bevel opening is only partially into the vein, or when insufficient pressure is applied to the puncture site after the needle has been removed. The result will be a large, painful, bruised area that will last for several days. If a hematoma forms, discontinue the procedure immediately, apply pressure to the area for 3 minutes, and then apply ice to the area. Notify your supervisor. Observe the site to determine if the bleeding has stopped. File an incident report.

Obesity

Large, heavy arms generally have veins that are difficult to visualize and palpate and usually require that the needle be inserted at an angle exceeding 30 degrees (Fig. 11–13). If the vein is missed, you must avoid excessive probing with the needle, as you may cause rupture of red blood cells (RBCs) and release of tissue clotting factors. If you feel uncomfortable about the draw, ask for assistance.

Damaged Veins

Veins that have been damaged by repeated puncture, as may occur with **sclerosis** or inflammation, often are scarred and feel very hard when palpated. As it is difficult to obtain a blood specimen from such veins, you should look for an alternative site from which to obtain the samples needed.

Allergies

Before cleansing the chosen puncture site, determine whether the patient has any possible allergy to the

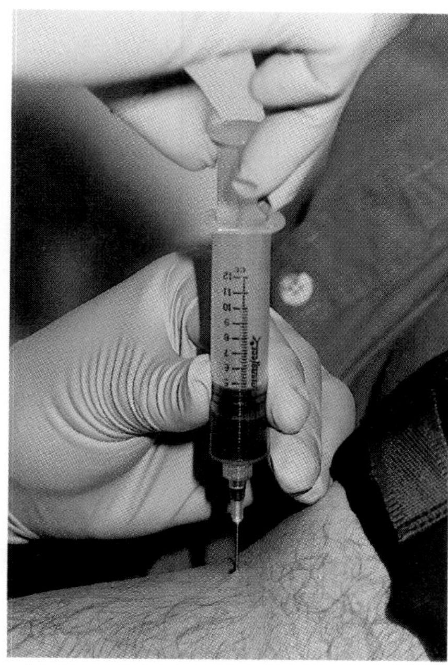

Figure 11–13. *When drawing blood from an obese patient, the angle of needle insertion is usually increased.*

cleansing solution you are about to use, or whether he/she has previously experienced an allergic reaction to certain types of tape or bandage. If so, use an alternative cleansing method and/or bandaging material. Consult the laboratory procedure manual located in the laboratory area for acceptable alternatives.

Burned, Scarred, or Traumatized Areas

Scarred, burned, or noticeably traumatized skin areas are highly sensitive and are susceptible to infections. The veins in a scarred area will be difficult to palpate and may also be damaged. Choose an alternative site for your blood draws.

General Considerations

Besides the complications just discussed, there are four other factors the medical laboratory assistant must consider when preparing to obtain a blood sample:

- The number of times the patient has been "stuck" in one day
- The volume of blood needed in relation to the age of the patient
- The overall health of the patient
- Steps to take if the patient refuses to have blood drawn

These are concerns that should be answered by the physician. It is advisable to have the physician's written protocols available in the laboratory procedure manual.

Microcapillary Blood Collection

Microcapillary blood collections are used primarily in patients without adequate veins for venipuncture or in those with burns, skin irritations, or severe needle apprehension. The capillary puncture is an efficient means of collecting a blood specimen when only a small amount of blood is required.

Patient Preparation

In adults and children, the usual puncture site is the ring finger, but capillary blood can be obtained from the great finger, toe, earlobe, or heel (Fig. 11–14). The puncture is made at the tip and slightly to the side of the finger.

The puncture site is first prepared by gently massaging the finger or placing it in warm water. This will increase blood circulation and allow an adequate flow of blood. The site is then cleansed with an alcohol

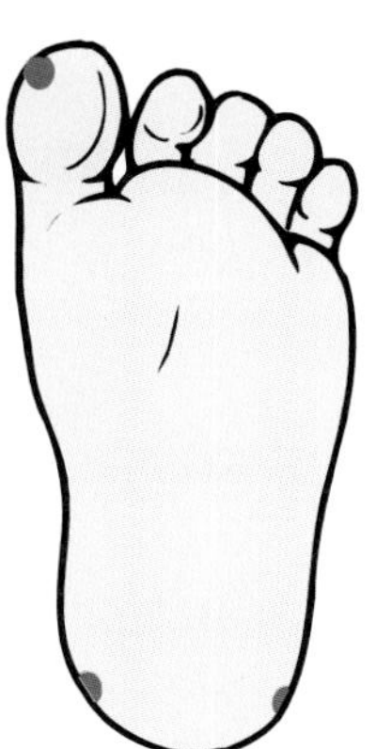

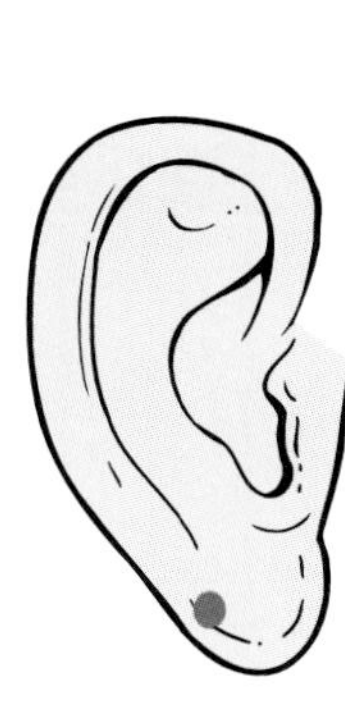

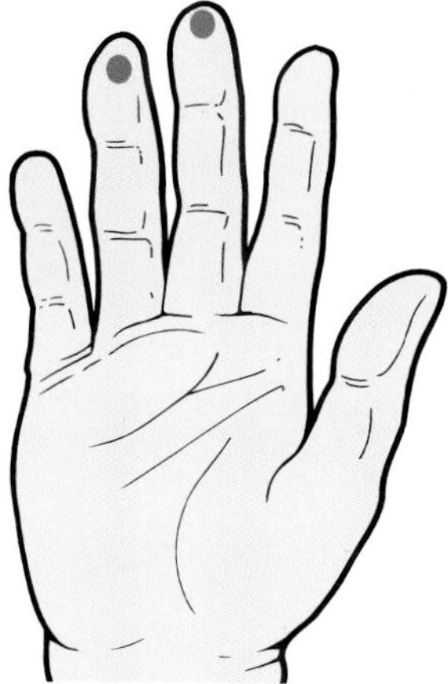

Figure 11–14. *Skin puncture sites for microcapillary blood collection.*

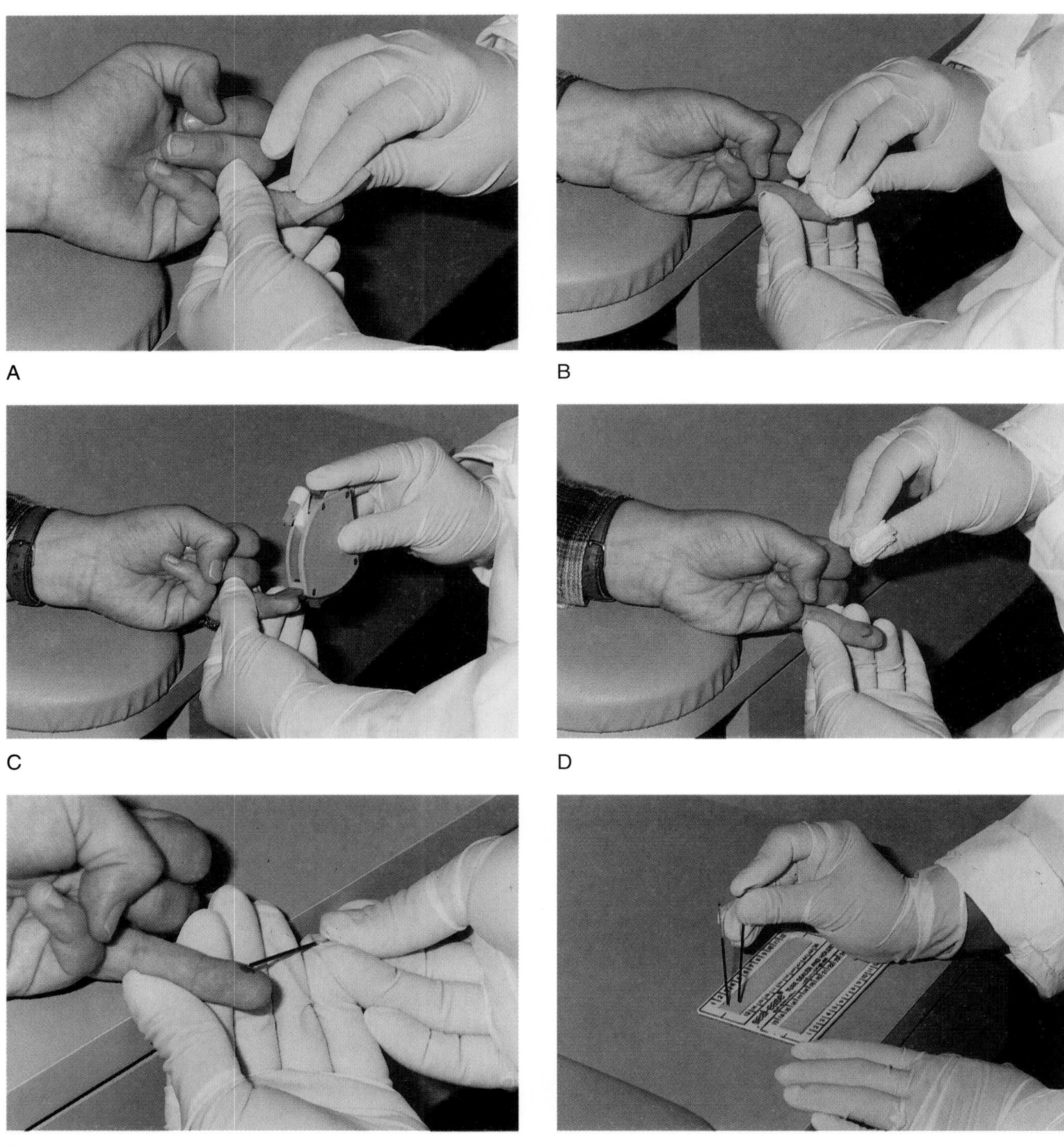

Figure 11–15. *Procedure for capillary blood collection.* A, *Cleansing the site.* B, *Drying the site.* C, *Puncturing the site.* D, *Wiping away the first drop of blood.* E, *Filling the capillary tube.* F, *Placing the capillary tube in sealing clay.*

prep pad or designated antiseptic (Fig. 11–15*A*) moving outward from the puncture site in a circular pattern, and is wiped dry with a gauze pad or rayon ball (Fig. 11–15*B*).

Specimen Collection

The patient's hand is held in a lateral position with the patient's arm supported. Select the appropriate finger and pull the skin near the puncture site taut. A sharp-pointed blade called a lancet is used. Capillary punctures may also be performed using semiautomated devices, such as the *Autolet* (see Fig. 11–15*C*). The puncture is performed in one quick, smooth motion. The lancet should puncture the site to a depth of 3 to 4 mm. The first drop of blood is wiped away (Fig. 11–15*D*) because it contains tissue fluid and would dilute any results. The second and following drops are used. The finger is gently massaged to increase blood flow. Squeezing the finger should be avoided, as this forces tissue fluid to dilute the blood and increases the speed of clotting. Samples must be collected quickly to avoid clotting. For this reason, it is very important for you to assemble all equipment needed before performing the microcapillary puncture.

Blood is collected in glass blood-diluting pipettes, self-filling disposable pipettes, capillary tubes (Fig. 11–15*E*), or on glass slides. Self-filling and self-measuring disposable micropipette systems are also available for counting leukocytes, erythrocytes, and platelets. Once the pipette is filled, the end is placed in sealing clay to prevent blood from escaping (Fig. 11–15*F*). The Unopette system consists of a disposable, self-filling, diluting pipette and a plastic reservoir prefilled with a precise amount of diluting fluid. It is designed to be used for blood cell counts.

A microcollection system can be used for obtaining small amounts of blood (Fig. 11–16). These collection tubes allow for easy measuring, color coding, stoppering, centrifugation, and storage of the blood samples. The collection caps are often shaped like a scoop, which eliminates the need for microcapillary tubes when collecting the blood sample.

Capillary tubes are available with and without the anticoagulant **heparin.** Tubes with a red ring around one end contain heparin, whereas those with a blue ring are nonheparinized; the latter are commonly called "plain" capillary tubes. The microhematocrit specimen can be collected directly from the finger using the heparinized tube.

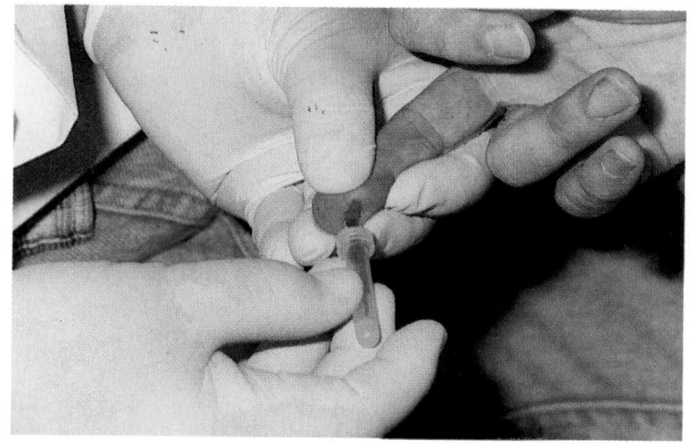

A

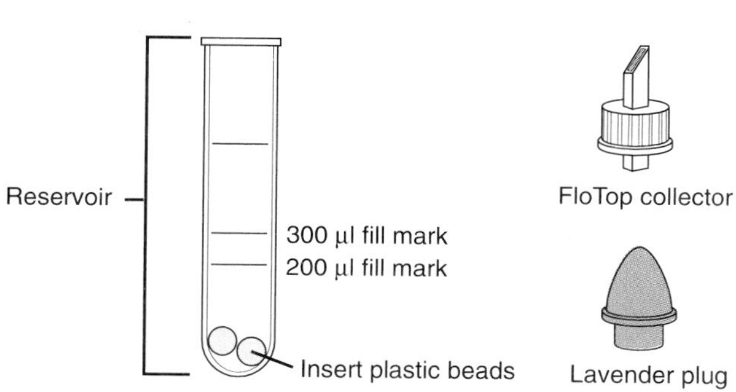

B

Figure 11–16. A, *Obtaining a capillary blood sample using the Microtainer system.* B, *Microtainer system.* (B *Courtesy of Becton Dickinson Company)*

The best specimen for a blood smear is a drop of capillary blood touched directly onto a glass slide and then smeared. The smear is then stained, at which time the morphology of the cellular components can be studied.

Postprocedural Responsibilities

At the completion of the blood collection procedure, you or the patient must maintain pressure on the puncture site until the bleeding has stopped. Special attention should be given any patient who is taking anticoagulant medication. All equipment needs to be cleaned and returned to its storage location, and all used materials, including protective coverings, must be disposed of properly. Remember that the lancet must be placed in a puncture-proof biohazard sharps container. Other materials, such as gauze and gloves, are placed in the biohazardous waste bags or containers. **As with all other procedures involving body fluids, you must wash your hands before caring for the next patient.**

PROCEDURE 11–3

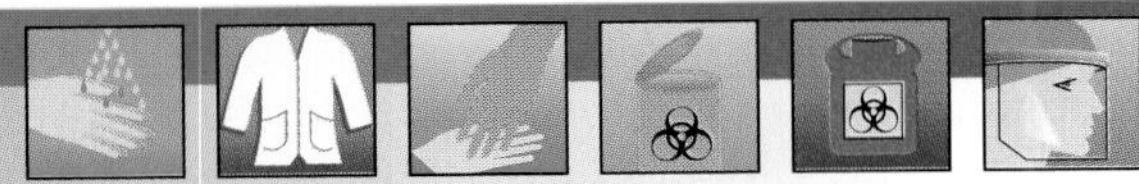

Obtaining Blood by the Microcapillary Method

Principle

To collect an adequate capillary blood sample for testing using a finger puncture and microcapillary collection method

Equipment and Supplies

alcohol prep pad or designated antiseptic prep gauze or rayon balls
manual lancet or Autolet with Autolet platforms
collection devices (glass slides, capillary tubes, Microtainer)
sealing clay or caps for capillary tube
nonallergenic bandage
permanent marking pen

Procedural Steps

1. Wash your hands, dry them thoroughly, and don gloves.
2. Identify the patient and explain the procedure.
3. Assemble all needed equipment.
4. Select the puncture site. Use the patient's nondominant hand if possible.
5. Very gently rub or massage the patient's finger.
6. Cleanse the puncture site and dry it.

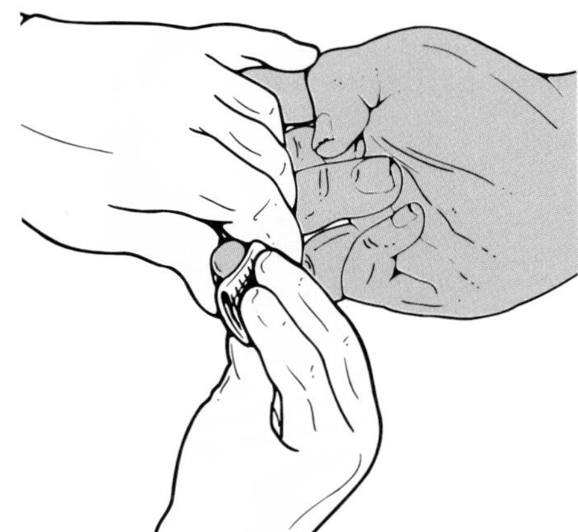

7. Using your nondominant hand, grasp the patient's finger on the sides near the puncture site.

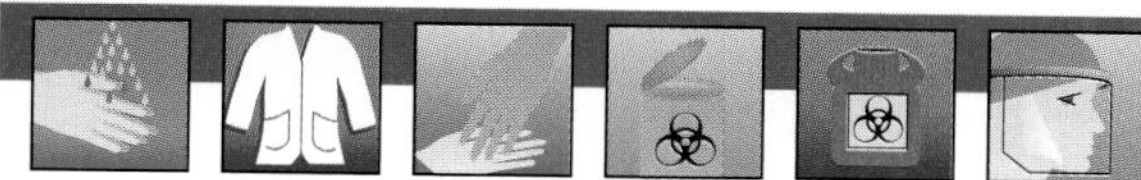

PROCEDURE 11–3

Obtaining Blood by the Microcapillary Method (Continued)

8. Holding the lancet or Autolet at a right angle to the patient's finger, rapidly make a deep puncture on the patient's lateral fingertip.

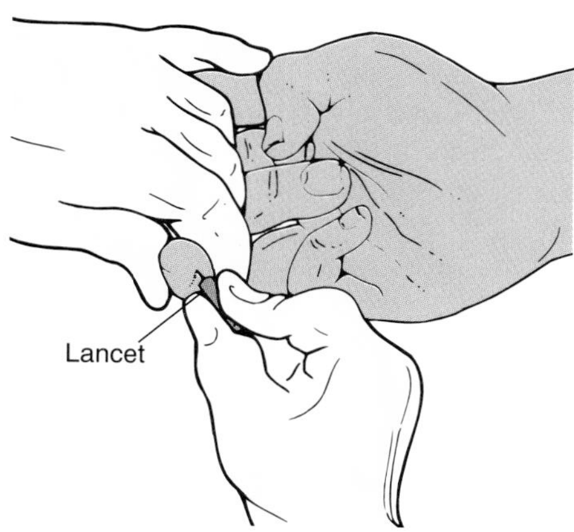

9. Wipe away the first drop of blood.

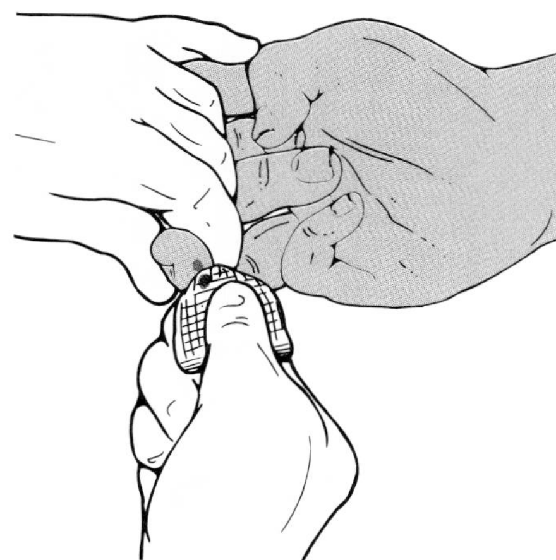

10. Apply gentle pressure to facilitate free flow of blood.

11. Collect blood samples.

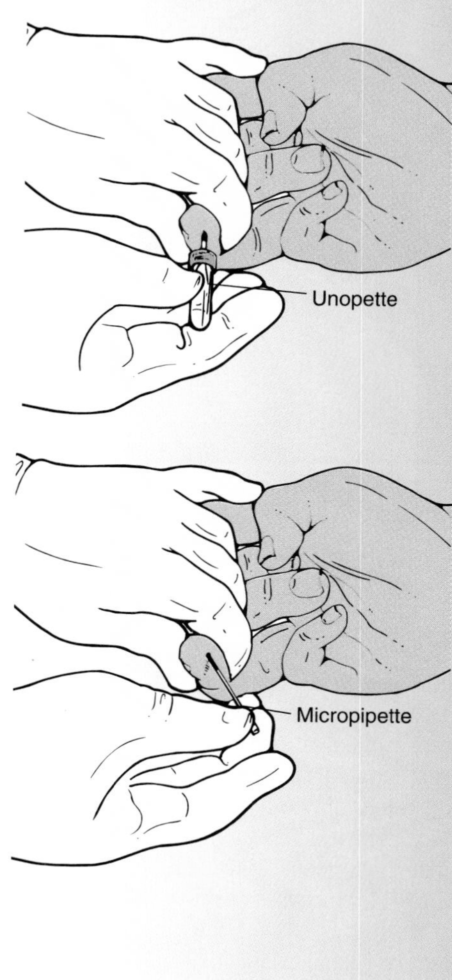

(continued)

PROCEDURE 11-3

Obtaining Blood by the Microcapillary Method (Continued)

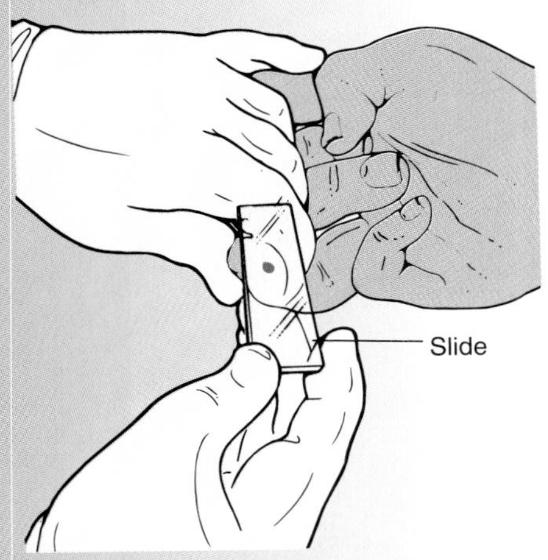

12. Apply pressure to the site until bleeding stops.
13. Label all samples and place them, along with corresponding request forms, in the proper collection location.
14. Check the puncture site for bleeding and apply a bandage if necessary.
15. Properly dispose of all materials used.
16. Clean and return equipment to the storage area.
17. Remove gloves and wash and dry your hands thoroughly.
18. Record the procedure in the laboratory logbook.

Summary

Venipuncture and microcapillary blood collection are **invasive procedures** in which a sterile needle/lancet is inserted into a vein or beneath the skin covering. The procedure is subject to the laws and regulations for surgical procedures because the skin is penetrated and body fluid is removed. When performing venipuncture, these regulations must be enforced, and deviations from them should never be allowed or tolerated. Be sure to follow the procedures established by the laboratory in which you are employed. You must also be familiar with the regulations and standards established by local and state agencies, as well as the Clinical Laboratory Improvement Amendment (CLIA), and the Occupational Safety and Health Administration (OSHA). As a laboratory representative, you share responsibility with every member of the facility for adhering to regulations and protocols.

Chapter Review

True or False

Circle T or F to indicate the correct answers to the following:

T F 1. In a venipuncture blood draw, blood is drawn from a small artery in the arm.

T F 2. Antecubital veins are found on the back of the hand.

T F 3. The most commonly used vein for a blood draw is the median cephalic vein.

T F 4. The Vacutainer system is the collection system of choice in the laboratory.

T F 5. EDTA is a preservative to help the blood clot.

T F 6. When preparing a patient for venipuncture, you should seat him/her on a comfortable stool that is high enough to allow you to perform the procedure without bending over.

Fill in the Blanks

Complete the following statements:

7. When drawing blood, place the tourniquet a distance of ______________ above the elbow.

8. The Vacutainer tube should be held at a ______________ angle to the patient's arm.

9. Always dispose of the needle and syringe in the ______________ waste container.

10. ______________ is a semiautomated device used for capillary puncture.

Multiple Choice

Circle the letter that represents the single best answer:

11. When labeling blood tubes, you should always include:
    a. Patient's name
    b. Date
    c. Time of draw
    d. Your initials
    e. All of the above
12. The butterfly needle set is the needle of choice for:
    a. Adolescents
    b. Fainters
    c. Infants
    d. Differential draws
    e. Most physicians
13. If a hematoma occurs, you should apply pressure for:
    a. 1 minute
    b. 2 minutes
    c. 3 minutes
    d. 5 minutes
    e. 10 minutes
14. Microcapillary collections are primarily used for patients with:
    a. Burns and skin irritations
    b. Severe needle apprehension
    c. Excessively fat arms
    d. Nausea and vomiting
    e. All of the above
15. If you are unable to obtain blood on the first attempt, you should:
    a. Continue trying until you obtain the specimen.
    b. Try a second time and, if still unsuccessful, get help.
    c. Ask the patient for permission to continue trying.
    d. Ask the patient to come back on your day off.
    e. b and c

Vocabulary

chronic: recurring; developing slowly and persisting over a long period of time
EDTA: ethylenediaminetetra-acetic acid; an anticoagulant commonly used in hematologic studies
enumeration: listing or counting
hemolytic: pertaining to the breakdown of red blood cells and the release of hemoglobin
leukopenia: abnormal deficiency in the white blood cell count
morphology: the study of size, shape, and maturity
peripheral: pertaining to an outside surface or the area surrounding a body part
polycythemia vera: a condition of unknown origin that is characterized by a marked increase in total blood volume, RBCs, WBCs, platelets, and hemoglobin
splenectomy: surgical removal of the spleen
thalassemia: an anemia in which different types of hemoglobin are present that are normally found only in the fetus

Chapter Objectives

After reading this chapter, you should be able to:

1. List nine analyses included in a routine complete blood count.
2. Name the anticoagulant of choice for hematologic specimens.
3. Explain the procedure for using a Neubauer hemocytomometer.
4. Identify three important indications of anemia.
5. List the possible causes for an increased or decreased white blood cell count.
6. List the possible causes for an increased or decreased red blood cell count.
7. Discuss the criteria for a properly prepared blood smear.
8. Identify the normal range for each white blood cell type in the differential cell count.
9. Describe hemoglobin and explain its function.
10. Explain the cyanmethemoglobin method of determining hemoglobin.
11. Name three substances that typically interfere with hemoglobin analysis.
12. Explain the purpose of determining the hematocrit.
13. Identify two pathologic conditions that can cause a decrease in the hematocrit and two that can cause an increase.
14. Identify the pathologic condition that will cause an elevated eosinophil count.
15. Identify the blood values that are indicative of the various types of anemia.
16. List the four inflammatory diseases that can cause an abnormal erythrocyte sedimentation.

Chapter 12
Hematologic Testing Procedures

Blood for hematologic testing is either peripheral blood collected by capillary puncture or venous blood collected by venipuncture. Venous samples are preferred. However, capillary specimens are adequate for many tests, particularly those done in a physician's office laboratory (POL) and small laboratories. Venous blood for hematologic analysis is collected in a special tube containing an *anticoagulant.* An anticoagulant is a chemical that interferes with and prevents initiation of the clotting mechanism of the blood. The blood remains whole or liquid even though it may appear to separate. Without an anticoagulant, the body's clotting mechanism will be initiated, and the cellular elements and plasma proteins will be bound up into the clot. As the clot ages, it retracts (shrinks), thereby expressing liquid. This liquid is called *serum.*

The Complete Blood Count

The complete blood count (CBC) is one of the most frequent laboratory tests performed on blood. Despite the dynamic nature of blood, a CBC yields an informative analysis of the cellular components of the blood and is an important tool utilized by physicians to evaluate a patient's health.

TEST

Tests Performed in CBC Analyses

- Red blood cell (RBC) count
- RBC morphology (size and shape)
- RBC indices
- White blood cell (WBC) count
- Differential WBC count
- Platelet count
- Platelet morphology
- Hemoglobin determination
- Hematocrit determination

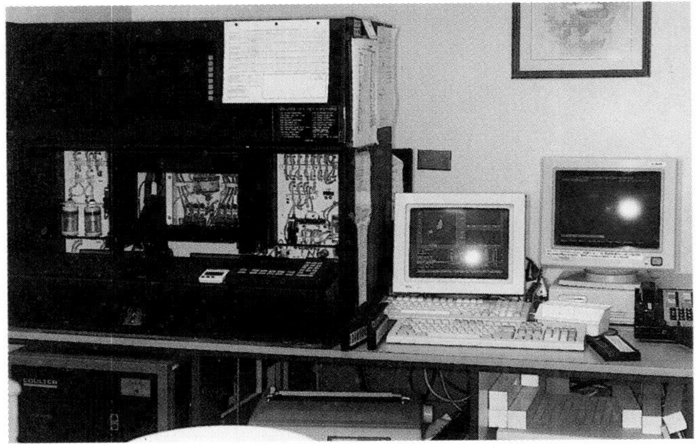
A

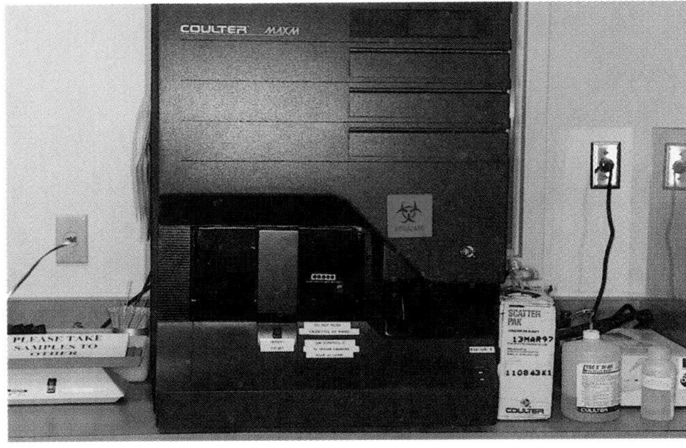

B

Figure 12–1. A, *Large automated cell analyzer.* B, *POL cell analyzer. (Courtesy of Coulter Corporation)*

Blood Cell Counting

An important part of the CBC is the **enumeration** of erythrocytes, leukocytes, and platelets. Enumeration of these blood cells is expressed as a concentration (cells per unit of volume of blood).

Automated Blood Cell Counting

Today, most clinical laboratories use automated methods for blood cell counting. Automated hematologic instruments can perform all of the analyses included in a CBC. These instruments range from very sophisticated, multiple-sample analyzers, which simply require an operator to place a blood sample combined with ethyleneaminetetra-acetic acid **(EDTA)** into the apparatus and start the instrument running (Fig. 12–1*A*), to single-test rudimentary instruments, which require that the operator add diluting and lysing fluids (Fig. 12–1*B*).

When selecting an automated instrument for the POL, several factors are important to consider. Three primary criteria for selection are listed below.

1. The cost of purchasing, operating, and maintaining the device
2. The range of hematologic tests that will be performed routinely in the POL
3. The ease with which the device can be operated

The most common automated methods apply the principle of electrical impedance. Simply stated, this principle involves blood cells passing through an aperture across which an electrical current is flowing. When the cells pass through the current, their electrical resistance changes, which, in turn, creates a voltage pulse. These pulses are then counted (Fig. 12–2).

The electron-optical cell counter counts the blood cells by using light-scattering events. This method incorporates a laser lamp and photomultiplier tube (PMT) sensor. This instrument is seldom used in the POL because it is designed to process large volumes of samples, and it would be prohibitively expensive for the small laboratory.

Fully automated blood cell analyzers perform all three of the following functions:

1. Precise dilution of the blood specimen
2. Sampling of this dilution in a measured volume
3. Blood cell counting within that measured volume

Manual Blood Cell Counting

Noncoagulated blood (using EDTA) is collected by venipuncture. EDTA is the anticoagulant of choice for hematologic analyses. In the past, blood cell dilution for manual blood cell counts was done using reusable glass Sahli or Thoma pipettes. Today, most manual blood cell counts are performed using the Unopette system (Fig. 12–3).

Figure 12–2. *Coulter principle. (Courtesy of Coulter Corporation)*

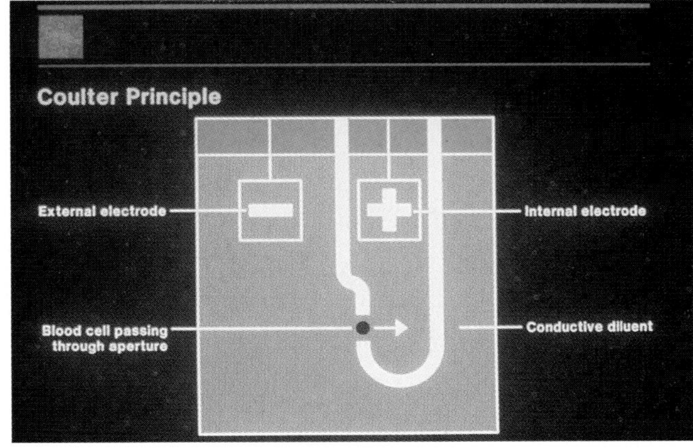

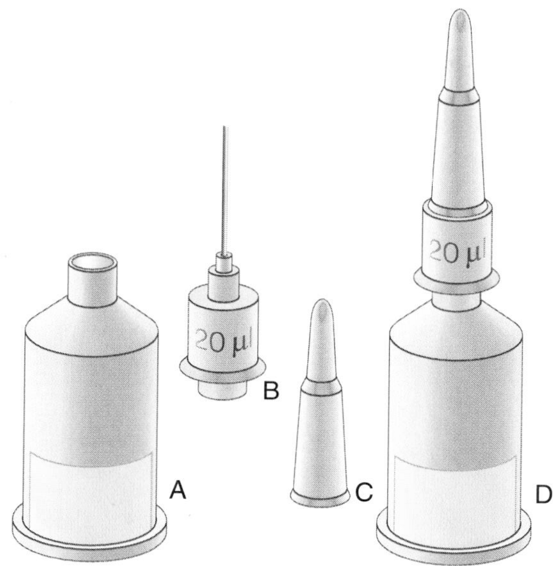

Figure 12–3. *Components of a disposable blood-diluting unit, such as the Unopette system.* A, *A prefilled reservoir, containing premeasured diluting fluid, is sealed with a diaphragm.* B, *A capillary pipette with overflow chamber and capacity marking.* C, *A pipette shield.* D, *Assembled unit.*

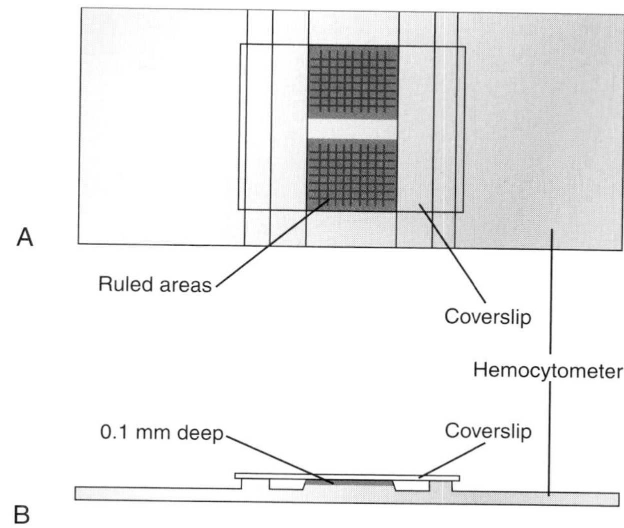

Figure 12–4. *Hemocytometer: top* (A) *and side* (B) *views. The blood sample should fill the shaded areas when the chamber is properly filled. (From Kinn, Woods, Derge.* The Medical Assistant: Administrative and Clinical, *7th ed. Philadelphia: W. B. Saunders, 1993.)*

The Unopette system has the advantages of being accurate, reliable, and disposable. Before attempting a manual blood cell count using the Unopette system, the manufacturer's instructions should be read and followed closely. Unopettes are available for counting RBCs, WBCs, platelets, and eosinophils. The appropriate diluting fluid is premeasured into a reservoir. Accompanying the diluting reservoir is a microcapillary tube that has been calibrated to fill with an appropriate amount of whole blood. A pipette shield is used to puncture the plastic seal of the reservoir, and the blood is transferred from the microcapillary tube to the dilution fluid. The sample is then mixed. The pipette shield also serves as a cap to prevent evaporation. The reservoir with the microcapillary tube attached can then be used to charge the hemocytometer (Fig. 12–4).

The hemocytometer method of manual cell counting may be performed on a capillary sample or an anticoagulated sample. A *hemocytometer* is a uniform, precise, counting chamber consisting of a heavy glass slide with a mirrored and etched counting surface and a special coverslip. Cell counts performed using a hemocytometer are expressed as the number of cells per cubic millimeter. Most clinical laboratories no longer routinely use a hemocytometer except for platelet counts and for confirmation of low leukocyte counts. However, it is still important for those working in clinical laboratories to be familiar with the procedure for using a hemocytometer. When viewed from the top, the hemocytometer has two raised surfaces surrounded by depressions on three sides. Each raised surface is a separate counting area. The counting area of each raised surface is mirrored and etched with lines that define squares of specific dimensions. The Neubauer-type counting chamber is the most commonly used hemocytometer. In this device, each ruled area consists of a square measuring 3 × 3 mm. Each 3 × 3 mm area is divided into nine equal squares, each of which is 1 mm^2. The WBC counting area consists of the four large corner squares. Each WBC counting area is divided into 16 equal squares measuring 0.25 × 0.25 mm (Fig. 12–5).

Figure 12–5. *Arrangement of counting squares.*

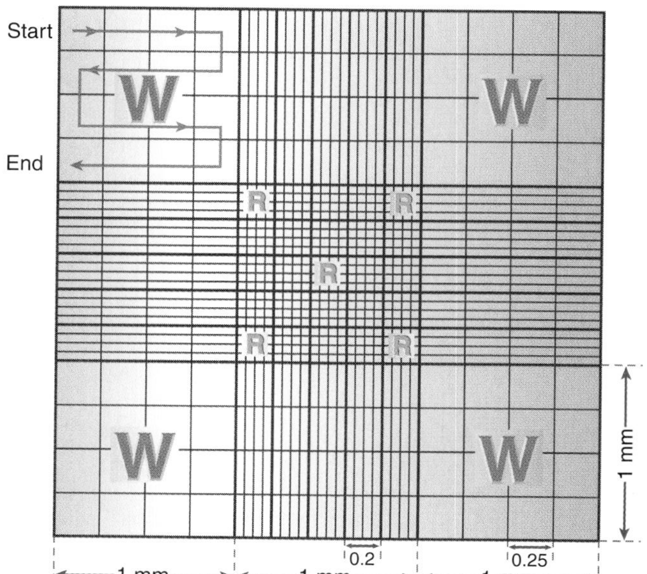

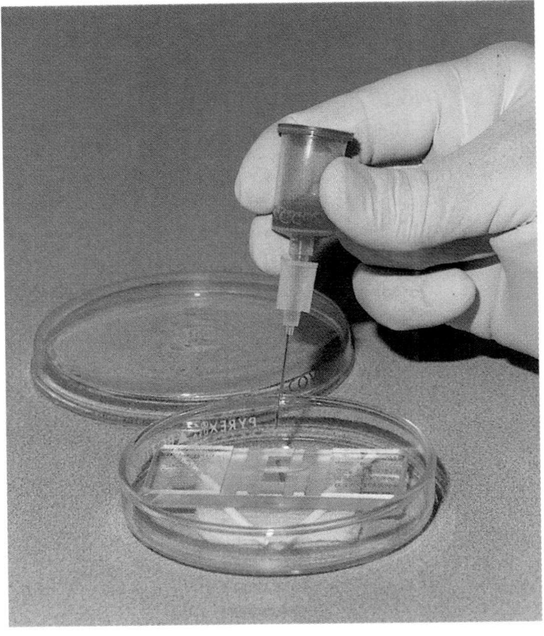

A

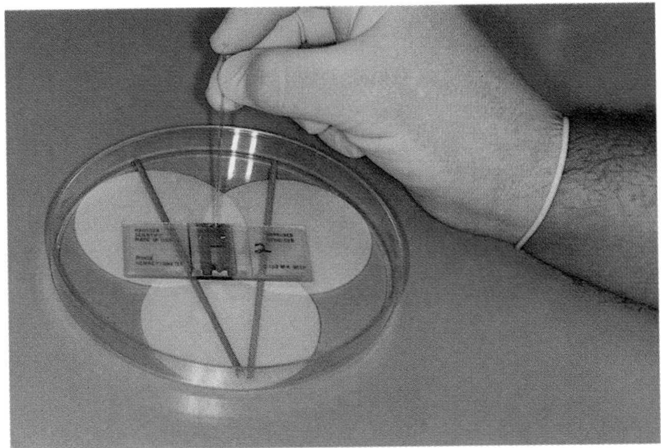

B

Figure 12–6. *Charging a counting chamber using a Unopette system* (A) *and a capillary pipette* (B).

The center square of each counting surface is used to count RBCs. The center square is divided into 25 uniform squares measuring 0.2 × 0.2 mm; each of the smaller squares is further divided into 16 smaller squares. The four corner squares and the center squares are used to count RBCs. To fill or charge the hemocytometer, a special hemocytometer coverslip is positioned over the raised counting surfaces. When the cover is properly positioned, the specimen is added by way of capillary action when the microcapillary pipette is placed at the juncture between the charging well and the coverslip. Both sides of the counting chamber are filled (Fig. 12–6).

After the cells have been allowed to settle for 10 minutes, the hemocytometer is placed on a microscope for counting. The low-power objective (10×) is used for counting WBCs. The high-power objective (40×) is used for counting RBCs. Once the counting area is properly focused, accuracy and reproducibility of cell counts require that the same counting pattern be followed for every blood cell count. A serpentine counting pattern of left-to-right and right-to-left, starting in the upper left corner, is used to ensure that the cells are counted only once. All cells within the squares are counted, including cells touching the top and left boundary lines (Fig. 12–7).

Erythrocytes (RBCs)

Erythrocytes (RBCs) are the most numerous of the blood cells (Fig. 12–8). As discussed in Chapter 10, the primary function of RBCs is to transport oxygen to the tissues and to return from the tissues to the lungs with carbon dioxide to be exhaled. A decrease in the number of circulating RBCs is the primary cause of anemia. The various forms of anemia are characterized by one or more of the following indicators.

ANALYZE

Indicators of Anemia

- Decreased hemoglobin levels
- Decreased RBC production

Figure 12–7. *Neubauer counting chamber.*

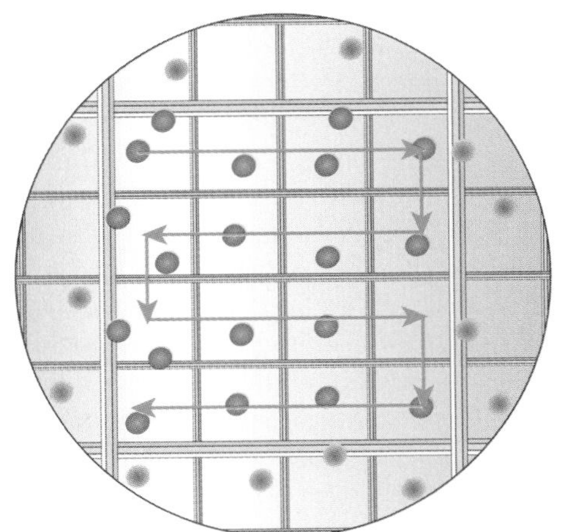

- Increased RBC destruction
- Blood loss

The RBC count, hematocrit value, hemoglobin value, and RBC indices are important indicators of the type and severity of anemia, which is discussed later in this chapter.

A decrease in the number of RBCs may be associated with decreased RBC formation, which can be caused by leukemia, certain **chronic** inflammatory diseases, and nutritional deficiencies. Excessive blood loss secondary to hemorrhage or the destruction of RBCs as a result of a hemolytic condition may also decrease the number of RBCs. A decreased RBC count is termed *erythropenia*. *Erythrocytosis* is an abnormal increase in RBCs. This condition is usually seen in patients with dehydration, severe burns, or **polycythemia vera.** In addition, those who live at high altitudes have an increased RBC count as a means of adapting to the lowered oxygen content of the air.

Normal RBC values range from approximately 4 million cells/mm^3 to 6 million cells/mm^3. Male patients usually have higher RBC counts than do female patients of child-bearing age (Table 12–1). Table 12–2 provides a listing of reference values for the complete blood count.

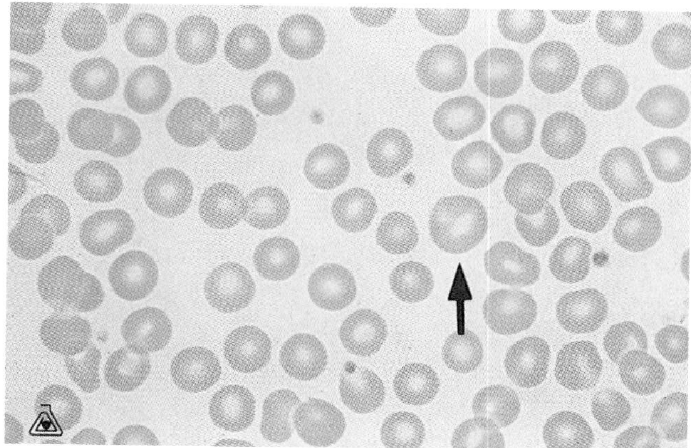

Figure 12–8. *Red blood cells viewed with macrocyte.*

Leukocytes (WBCs)

The leukocyte or WBC count is an enumeration of the total number of leukocytes in the circulating blood. The total leukocyte count makes no distinction between the five normal cell types (Fig. 12–9, *A–E*).

1. Neutrophils
2. Eosinophils
3. Basophils
4. Lymphocytes
5. Monocytes

Leukocytes play an important role in defending the body against infectious agents (bacteria and viruses) and providing immunity. A decrease in the WBC count is known as **leukopenia.** Leukopenia is often associated with viral infections or overexposure to therapeutic agents, such as radiation therapy, drugs, and certain chemicals. An increase in WBC count, termed *leukocytosis,* is most commonly associated with the presence of infectious disease. A dramatic increase in the WBC count may be seen in leukemia. Leukocytosis may also have a physiologic basis (e.g., exercise, stress, pregnancy).

The normal WBC count of a healthy adult ranges from 4500 to 11,000 WBCs/mm^3.

Thrombocytes (Platelets)

Platelets (thrombocytes) (Fig. 12–10) are the smallest of the formed elements in the blood. Platelets are essential to hemostasis, maintaining vascular integrity and blood coagulation. Platelet development occurs primarily in the bone marrow. The formation of the platelet plug is an essential element of hemostasis.

Platelets are the most difficult of the cellular elements of the circulating blood to count because of their small size. Like RBCs, platelets lack a nucleus and are small, irregularly shaped objects. Before the recent advances in automation for blood cell counting, platelet counts were estimated from stained **peripheral** blood

Table 12–1
Comparison of the Number of RBCs, WBCs, and Platelets in Men and Women

	Men	*Women*
RBCs	4.5–6.0 million/mm^3	4.0–5.5 million/mm^3
WBCs	4500–11,000 cells/mm^3	Same as for men
Platelets	150,000–400,000 cells/mm^3	Same as for men

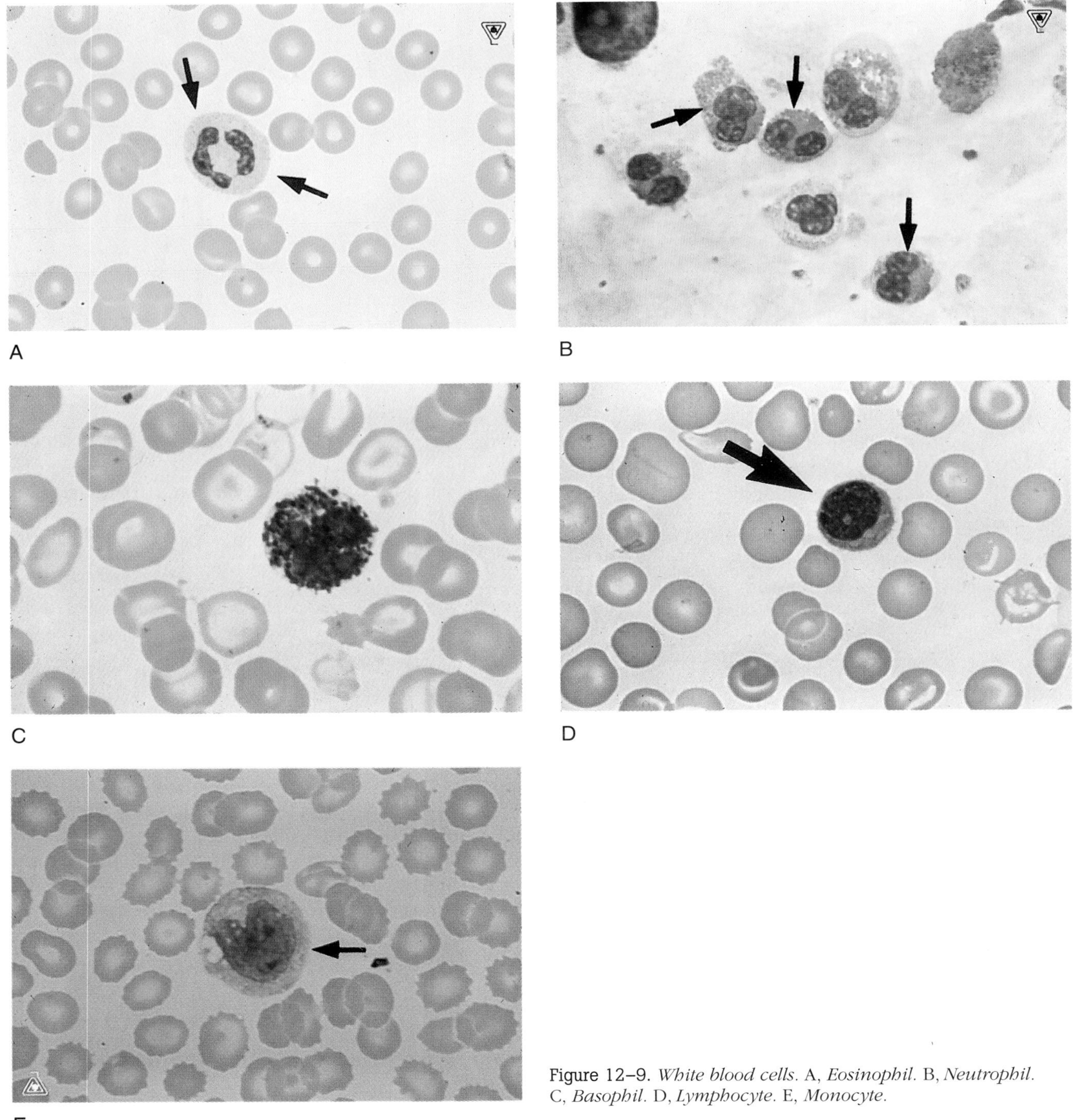

Figure 12–9. *White blood cells.* A, *Eosinophil.* B, *Neutrophil.* C, *Basophil.* D, *Lymphocyte.* E, *Monocyte.*

Table 12–2
Reference Ranges for a Complete Blood Count

Test	*Neonates*	*Infants (6 mo)*	*Children*	*Adults*	
				Men	*Women*
RBCs	4.8–7.1 million/mm³	3.8–5.5 million/mm³	4.5–4.8 million/mm³	4.5–6.0 million/mm³	4.0–5.5 million/mm³
Hematocrit (Hct)	44–64%	30–40%	35–41%	42–52%	36–45%
Hemoglobin (Hgb)	17–21 gm/dL	10–15 gm/dL	11–16 gm/dL	15–18 gm/dL	12–16 gm/dL
RBC Indices					
MCV	96–108 μm			82–98 μm	
MCH	32–34 pg			26–34 pg	
MCHC	31–33 gm/dL			31–37 gm/dL	
WBCs	9000–30,000/mm³	6000–16,000/m³	5000–13,000/mm³	4000–11,000/mm³	
Differential WBC count					
Neutrophils	≥45% by 1 week of age	32%	60% for children 2 yr of age and older	50–65%	
Bands	—	—	—	0–7%	
Eosinophils	—	—	0–3%	1–3%	
Basophils	—	—	1–3%	0–1%	
Monocytes	—	—	4–9%	3–9%	
Lymphocytes	≥41% by 1 week of age	61%	59% for children 2 yr of age or older	25–40%	
Platelets	140,000–300,000/mm³	200,000–473,000 /mm³	150,000–450,000 /mm³	150,000–400,000 /mm³	

smears, and platelet quantity was further evaluated by manual platelet counts.

Thrombocytopenia, which is the term for a decrease in the number of platelets, may be associated with acute leukemia, viral infections, hemorrhage, radiation therapy, and chemotherapy. *Thrombocytosis,* or an increase in the number of platelets, is seen in polycythemia vera, chronic leukemia, and certain anemias, as well as after **splenectomy.** In healthy adults, platelet counts range from 150,000 to 400,00/mm³.

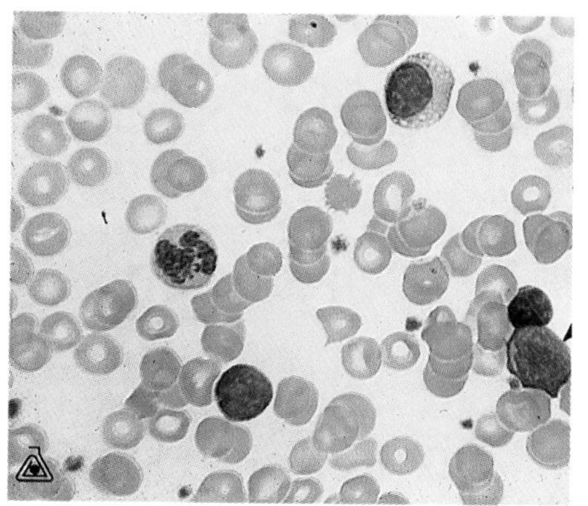

Figure 12–10. *Platelets (thrombocytes).*

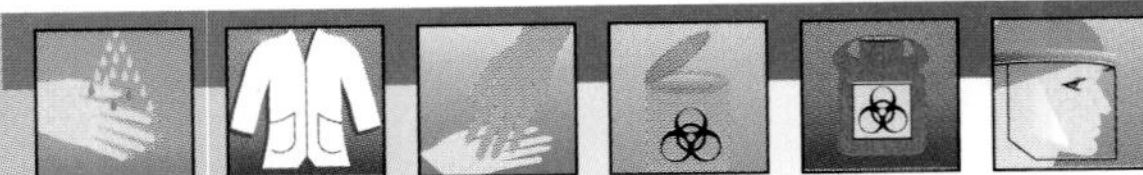

PROCEDURE 12–1

Performing a Blood Cell Count Using the Unopette and Neubauer Ruled Hemocytometer

Principle

To locate the appropriate counting areas for RBC, WBC, and platelet counts, and to determine the count for each cell using the proper technique

Equipment and Supplies

Neubauer ruled hemocytometer
hemocytometer coverslip
lint-free tissues
70% alcohol
appropriate Unopette system (capillary pipette, pipette shield, diluting reservoirs for RBCs and WBCs)
microscope
hand tally counter
filter paper
EDTA-coagulated blood specimen or capillary puncture specimen
gauze pads
test tube
Petri dish with lid

Procedural Steps

1. Wash and dry hands, following OSHA standards. Put on gloves and other protective gear.

Filling a Unopette

2. Remove a Unopette reservoir from the storage container and recap the container tightly. Be sure to use the appropriate reservoir. Use separate reservoirs for RBCs, leukocytes, and platelets.
3. Use the protective shield on the capillary pipette to puncture the diaphragm of the Unopette reservoir. The hole must be large enough to allow the pipette to enter freely.

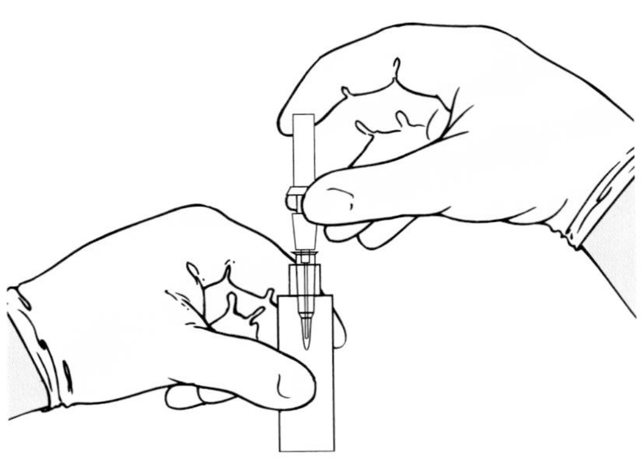

4. Remove the pipette shield.
5. Hold the pipette nearly horizontal.

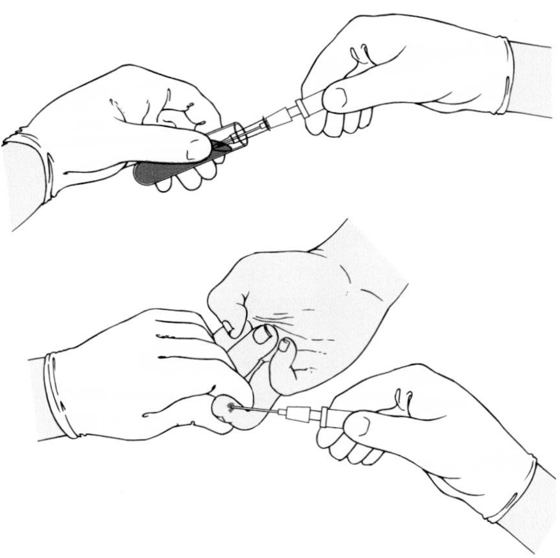

6. Place the tip of the pipette into a well-mixed tube of EDTA-anticoagulated blood, and allow the pipette to fill by capillary action until the blood reaches the end of the pipette. Alternatively, you may perform a finger stick and fill the capillary tube.

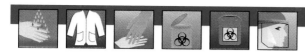

PROCEDURE 12–1

Performing a Blood Cell Count Using the Unopette and Neubauer Ruled Hemocytometer (Continued)

7. Place a finger over the hole in the pipette to prevent the loss of any of the blood sample. Carefully wipe the outside of the pipette with gauze to remove all traces of blood.

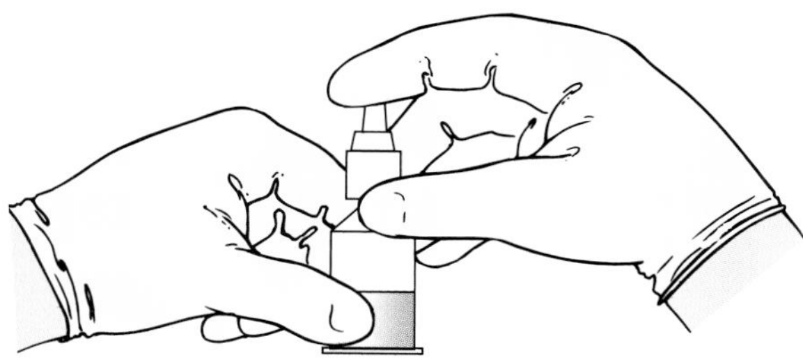

8. Squeeze the reservoir gently with one hand to force out air. Do not expel any liquid. Maintain pressure on the reservoir.
9. While holding the index finger over the hole in the top of the pipette, insert the pipette in the reservoir with a firm, twisting motion.
10. Release the pressure on the reservoir and remove the finger from the top of the pipette. The sample will be drawn into the reservoir. You may place the shield at the open end of the pipette to prevent spilling and possible contamination.
11. Gently (so that the WBCs are not destroyed) squeeze and release the reservoir several times to rinse all blood from the pipette into the reservoir. The reservoir fluid should rise to the overflow chamber but should not be forced out of the top of the pipette.
12. Gently mix the contents in the Unopette by inverting the container or rolling it between the palms of your hands.

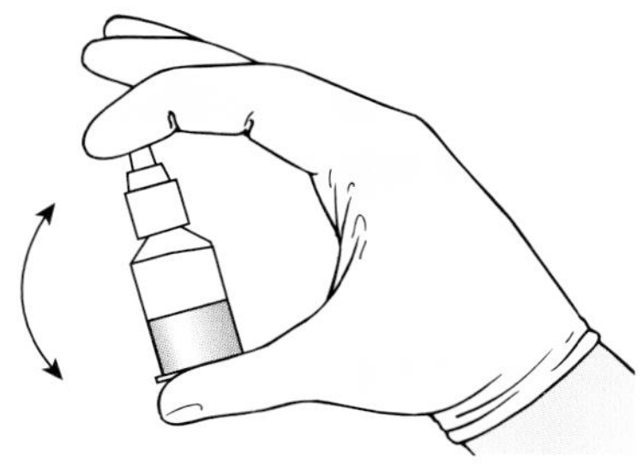

13. Label the Unopette with the appropriate information.

Charging (Filling) a Hemocytometer

14. Convert to dropper assembly by withdrawing the pipette from the reservoir and reseating it securely in reverse position.

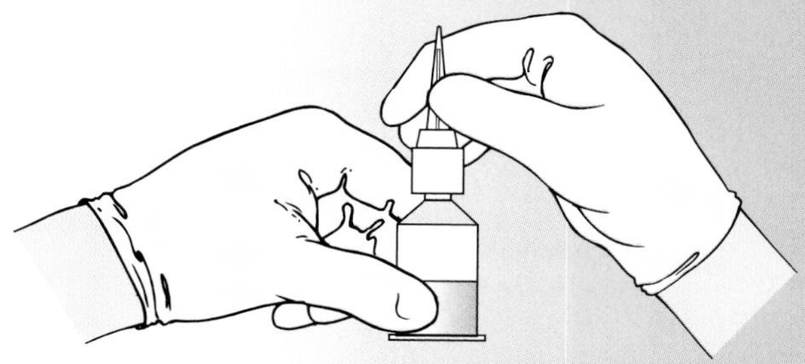

15. To clean the capillary bore, invert the reservoir and gently squeeze the sides, discarding the first three or four drops.

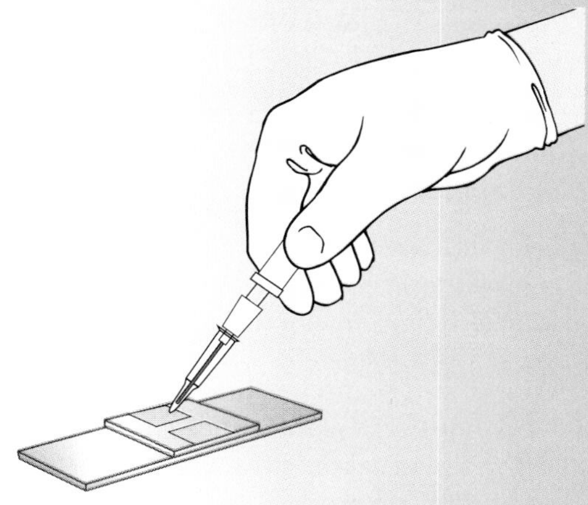

16. For *RBC counts,* proceed as follows:
    a. Touch the tip of the pipette to the edge of the coverslip in the loading area of the chamber.
    b. Controlling the flow, gently fill the chamber in one smooth motion. Fill the chamber slowly and smoothly to avoid introducing air bubbles or overfilling.
    c. Fill both sides of the hemocytometer.

(continued)

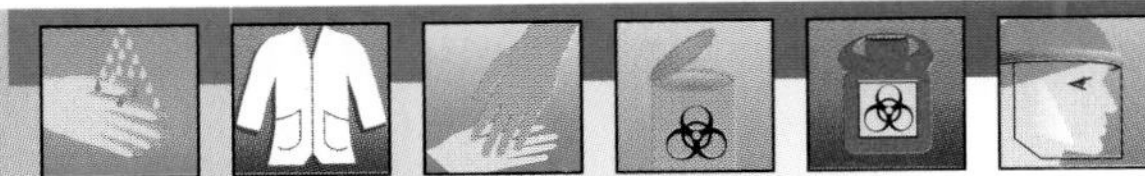

PROCEDURE 12–1

Performing a Blood Cell Count Using the Unopette and Neubauer Ruled Hemocytometer (Continued)

17. For *WBC and platelet counts,* proceed as follows:
    a. Place the hemocytometer on moistened filter paper in a Petri dish. Cover it and allow it to stand 10 minutes to permit the cells to settle. (Moistened filter paper retards evaporation.)

Counting and Calculating Cells

18. *For RBCs,* proceed as follows:
    a. Under magnification 430×, count the erythrocytes in the four corner squares and the one center square within the large center square following the serpentine pattern shown in Fig. 12–5 and described in the next section on WBCs. Between the squares, the number should vary by no more than 20 cells. A greater variation indicates an unevenly filled hemocytometer. If this occurs, recharge the hemocytometer and start again. 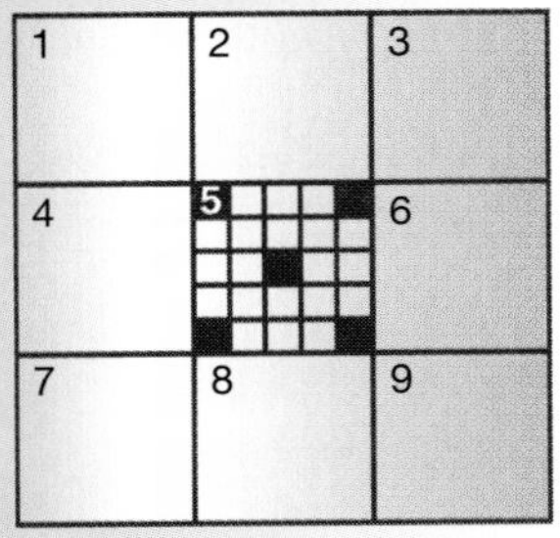
    b. Count the second side of the chamber and then average the two sides.
    c. Multiply by 10,000 the average number of cells counted in the five squares on each side. This is the total RBC count per mm^3.
19. *For WBCs,* proceed as follows:
    a. Under magnification 100×, count the leukocytes in all nine large squares of the counting chamber.
        (1) Use the serpentine counting pattern (see Fig. 12–5), beginning at the top row on the far left.
        (2) Count the top row of leukocytes, moving from left to right. When the end of the top row is reached, drop to the second row and count the second row moving from right to left. Continue in this zig-zag pattern until reaching the small square at the bottom left. 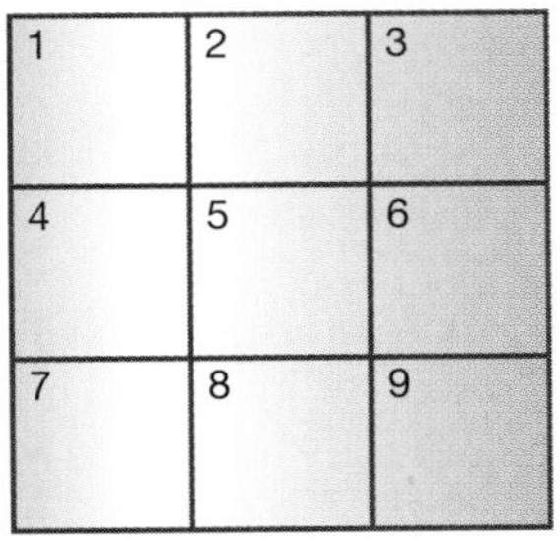
        (3) Count all cells within the boundaries of the square, as well as the cells touching the top and left-hand lines of the square.
        (4) Do not count the cells touching the right-hand or bottom lines of the squares.
        (5) When you have finished counting the cells within a large square, record that number.
        (6) Return the hand tally to zero, move to the next large square, and begin to count again. A properly filled counting chamber will have the cells evenly distributed.
        (7) Count the remaining squares and determine the number of cells in each. The counts from each square should vary by no more than 10 cells. Any variations exceeding that number indicate an unevenly filled hemocytometer. If this occurs, recharge the hemocytometer and recount the cells.
        (8) Count the second side of the chamber in the same manner, then average the counts from both sides.
        (9) Add 10% of the count to the averaged total number of cells counted. (This step simplifies the calculation, which actually entails dividing the number of cells by the number of squares counted and multiplying by 10 to correct for the depth of the chamber.)
        (10) Multiply this figure by 100 to calculate the total leukocyte count per mm^3.
20. Record/report the test performed and the results.
21. Clean the work area. Follow OSHA standards for proper disposal of all used materials.
22. Remove your gloves and wash your hands.

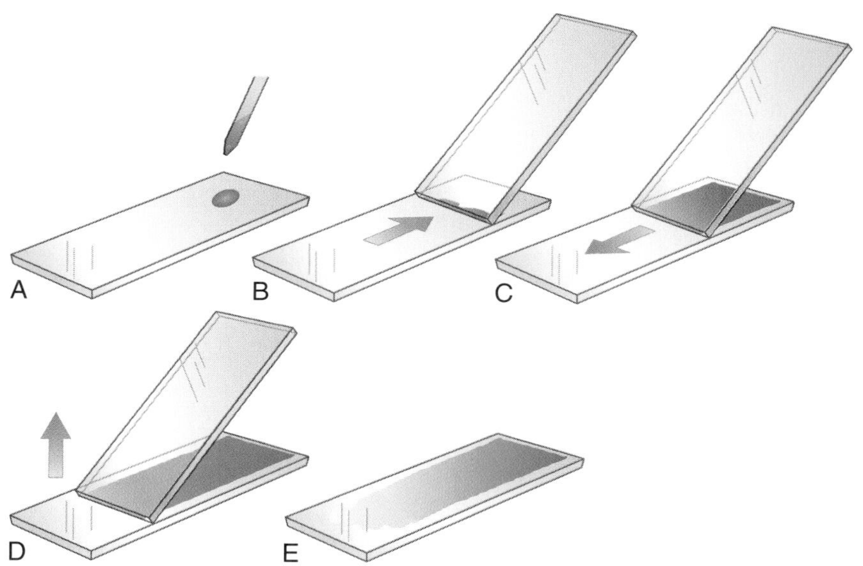

Figure 12–11. *Blood smear slide preparation (feathered edge).*

Differential Cell Count

Preparation of Blood Smears

A blood smear enables you to view and study the cellular **morphology** of leukocytes, erythrocytes, and platelets, including their size, shape, and maturity. A blood smear is prepared by spreading a drop of blood on a clean glass slide. The slide must be free of dust and grease. The best specimen for a blood smear is capillary blood that has not had anticoagulant added to it. However, blood that has been combined with EDTA anticoagulant can be used provided the smear is made within 2 hours of specimen collection.

There are several methods for spreading the drop of blood on the slide to obtain a good smear. The method of choice is to place a small drop of blood ½ inch from the right end of a glass slide. The end of a second glass slide is then placed in front of the drop of blood, at an angle of 30 to 35 degrees, and used as a "spreader." The spreader slide is brought back onto the first slide with a quick but smooth gliding motion. The spreader slide is then pushed to the left with a quick, steady motion, spreading the blood across the slide (Fig. 12–11).

A good smear should cover one half to three quarters of the slide. It should show a gradual transition from a thick coating to a thin end with a feathered edge. It should have a smooth appearance with no ridges, holes, lines, streaks, or clumps. Upon microscopic examination, the cells should be distributed evenly.

After making the smear, allow it to dry by placing it on its narrow end, thick end down, leaning against another surface. Do not blow on the slide to dry it, as this can cause artifacts or distortion of the RBCs due to the moisture in your breath. Once dry, the slide can be labeled over the thick portion of the smear by writing the patient's name in the dried blood film. If slides with frosted ends are used, the information can be written on the frosted end with a pencil or glass marking pen.

Following labeling, the slide is fixed in methanol, which preserves and prevents changes or deterioration of the cellular components. Many of the quick stains available on the market contain fixative in the stain.

Staining of Blood Smears

The stains commonly used for examination of blood cells are called *polychromatic* because they contain dyes that will stain various cell components different colors. These stains usually contain methylene blue, a blue stain, and eosin, a red-orange stain. These stains are attracted to different parts of the cell. Thus, the cells and their structures can be more easily visualized and differentiated. The most commonly used differential blood stain is Wright's stain.

Wright's stain is applied to the slide for approximately 1 to 3 minutes. A buffer is added on top of the stain and is mixed by gently blowing until a green metallic sheen appears. This usually takes 2 to 4 minutes. The slide is then gently rinsed and is allowed to air-dry. A properly stained smear should appear pinkish to the naked eye.

Semi-automated slide stainers are frequently used in large laboratories (Fig. 12–12). These machines are capable of staining a large number of blood smears with consistency and reliability. Small laboratories gen-

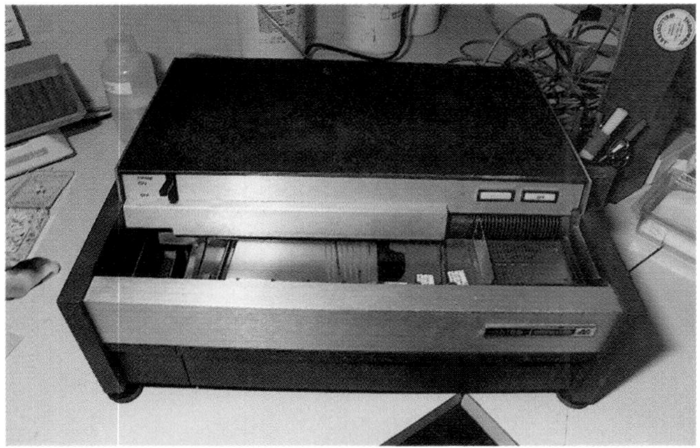

Figure 12–12. *An automated slide stainer may be used to determine a differential blood cell count.*

erally use a manual quick stain method. With this three-step method, the smears are exposed to Wright's stain, buffer, and distilled water in a timed sequence (Fig. 12–13).

Identification of Blood Cells

Much useful information can be gathered from the microscopic identification and evaluation of blood cells in a stained smear. Indeed, a great deal more information can be acquired from the observation of these blood cells than from actual cell counts. In fact, blood smears provide more information about a person's health status than any other laboratory test.

ANALYZE

Essential Features of Blood Cells

- Cell size
- Nuclear appearance
- Cytoplasmic characteristics

These three features are the bases for cell identification. However, much practice is required before one can recognize and classify all the blood cells that may be seen in various disease states.

Cells are examined under the oil-immersion objective of the microscope. The light should be bright to

Figure 12–13. *Manual staining techniques. The slide is immersed first in Wright's stain* (A), *then in buffer solution* (B). *It is then rinsed in distilled water* (C) *and placed in a drying rack* (D).

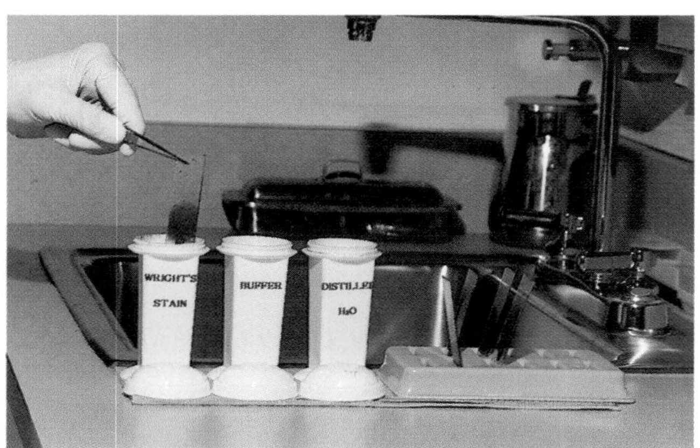

A

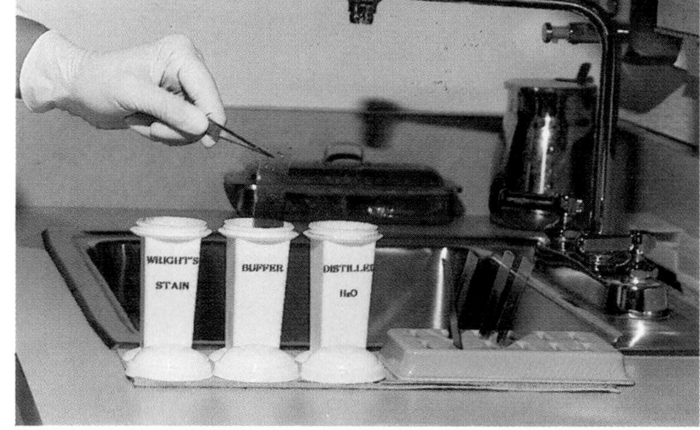

B

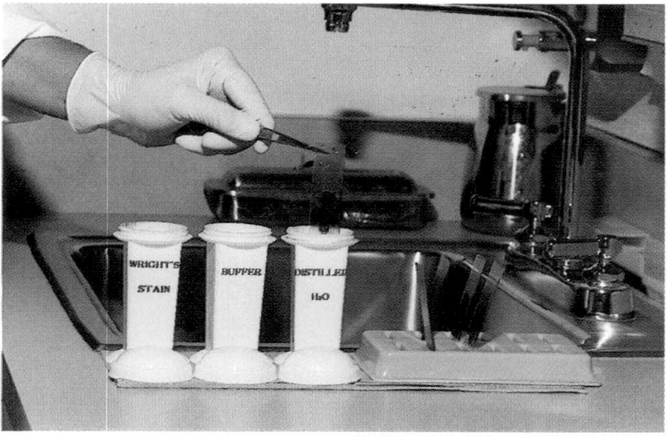

C

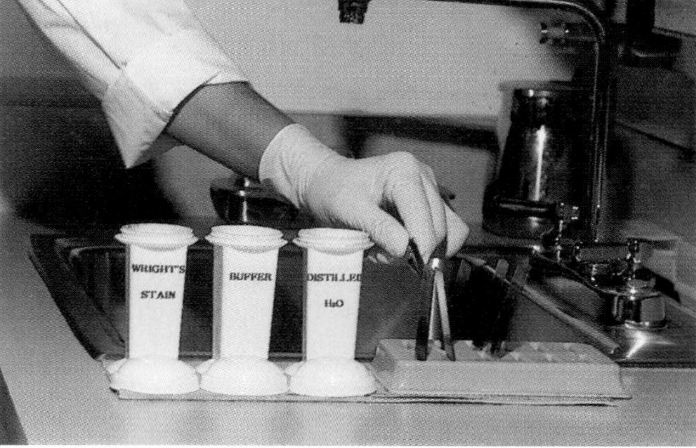

D

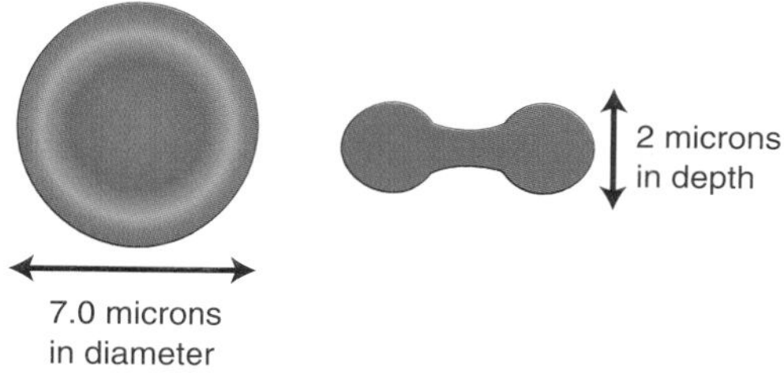

Figure 12–14. *Red blood cell morphology.*

allow visualization of colors and small structures. The slide is examined near the feathered end of the smear, where the cells are barely touching each other and are easiest to identify.

RBCs are the most numerous of the cellular elements, appearing as biconcave discs that have no nucleus (Fig. 12–14). RBCs should stain pinkish-tan owing to the hemoglobin within these cells.

Thrombocytes, or platelets, are the smallest of the cellular elements. They may be round or oval. No nucleus is present, as platelets are just fragments of cytoplasm from large bone marrow cells. They will stain blue.

Leukocytes are the largest of the normal blood cell elements. Each of the five types has a characteristic appearance. The granulocytes include neutrophils, eosinophils, and basophils. Granulocytes contain distinctive granules in their cytoplasm and may have segmented nuclei. The agranulocytes include lymphocytes and monocytes. They have few, if any, granules and nonsegmented nuclei. The nuclei of the leukocytes should stain purple, and their cytoplasm may vary from pink to blue or blue-gray. Neutrophils are known by a variety of names, including polymorphonuclear neutrophils ("polys") and segmented neutrophils, ("segs"), with the latter being the most common name. They are the most numerous of all the WBCs in circulation in adults. Neutrophils are produced in the bone marrow and are released into the circulation, eventually entering tissue to fight off invading microorganisms by engulfing them (*phagocytosis*). Many types of bacterial infections stimulate increased production of neutrophils.

The nucleus of the *segmented neutrophil* (Fig. 12–15*A*) is divided into two to five lobes that are connected by a strand. The nucleus stains a dark purple. The cytoplasm stains pale pink and contains fine pink or lilac granules.

An immature form of the neutrophil is called a *band* or *stab* (Fig. 12–15*B*). Instead of having a segmented nucleus, where the lobes are separated by a thin filament, the band has an unsegmented nucleus shaped like a horseshoe. The results of staining are the same as with the segmented neutrophil. An increase in bands is termed a "shift to the left" and is seen in infections, such as bacterial meningitis, pneumonia, appendicitis, strep throat, and abscesses, and in chronic granulocytic leukemia.

The nucleus of the eosinophil is divided into two or three lobes that stain purple. The cytoplasm stains pink and, upon slowly adjusting the fine focus, is seen to contain large, round or oval, red-orange granules that are refractile. Eosinophils are phagocytic and are associated closely with allergies, such as hay fever and asthma, as well as certain parasitic infestations, such as trichinosis, amebiasis, and schistosomiasis.

The nucleus of the basophil is segmented and stains light purple. The large, dark blue-black granules contain histamine, which is a part of the allergic response. Little is known about the function of the basophil.

Lymphocytes are the second most numerous WBCs in adults. In children, they are usually the most numerous. Their nucleus, which stains purple, is usually smooth and either oval or round. The cytoplasm stains blue. "Lymphs," as they are commonly called, are responsible for the recognition of foreign antigens and the production of circulating antibodies for immunity to disease. Increased numbers of lymphocytes are associated with most viral diseases, some bacterial infections (e.g., syphilis, brucellosis, tuberculosis, and typhoid and paratyphoid fevers), and leukemia, in addition to being found in young children who are actively making antibodies. Stimulated or reactive lymphocytes, called *atypical lymphs,* may be found in many viral infections. These are common in infectious mononucleosis.

Monocytes are the largest of the WBCs in the human circulation. The nucleus may be oval, indented, or horseshoe-shaped. The cytoplasm stains a dull gray-blue and may contain *vacuoles,* which appear as clear spaces in the cytoplasm filled with fluid or air (Table 12–3). Monocytes, also called macrophages, ingest bacteria and the debris of cellular breakdown. Their numbers are increased in certain viral infections, such as Rocky Mountain spotted fever, and in bacterial infections, such as brucellosis, tuberculosis, and typhoid (Table 12–4).

Figure 12–15. *Neutrophilic cells.* A, *Segmented.* B, *Band.*

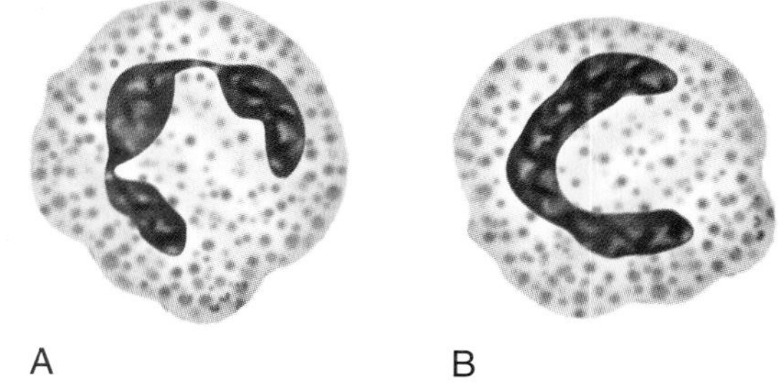

Table 12–3
Characteristics of Leukocytes

	Granulocytes			Agranulocytes		
	Neutrophil Segmented (mature)	*Neutrophil Band (immature)*	*Eosinophil*	*Basophil*	*Lymphocyte*	*Monocyte*
Cell size	10–15 μm	10–15 μm	10–15 μm	10–15 μm	6–15 μm	12–20 μm
Nucleus shape	2–5 lobes connected by thread-like filaments	Band or U-shaped	Bilobed or band	Slightly segmented, granular, or band	Round or oval	Round, indented, or superimposed lobes
Nucleus structure	Coarse	Coarse	Coarse	Obscured by granules	Smudged, lumpy, or clumped	Brainlike convolusions or folded
Cytoplasm amount	Abundant	Abundant	Abundant	Abundant	Scant	Abundant
Cytoplasm color	Colorless to light pink	Colorless to light pink	Colorless to light pink	Colorless to light pink	Sky blue to dark blue	Dull gray to blue-gray
Cytoplasm inclusions	Many tiny tan, pink, or red-purple granules	Many tiny tan, pink with increased red-purple granules	Large rounder oval red to red-orange granules	Large, coarse blue-black granules	None to few round red-purple granules	Ground glass appearance, fine red-purple granules, rare blue granules

Table 12–4
Alterations in Leukocyte Count According to Disease

Cell Type	*Decrease*	*Increase*
Neutrophils	Bone marrow disorders Pernicious anemia Starvation/malnutrition Cancer Folic acid anemia Vitamin B_{12} deficiency Lupus erythematosus Alcohol abuse	Myelocytic leukemia Bacterial infections Rhematoid arthritis Drug reactions Burns and abscesses Uremia Ketoacidosis Toxins and venoms
Bands	None, as bands are present only in small numbers	Bacterial meningitis Appendicitis Strep throat Abscesses Granulocytic leukemia
Eosinophils	Stress Infectious mononucleosis Congestive heart failure Hyperplastic anemia	Asthma and hay fever Parasitic infestations Leprosy Polycythemias Autoallergies Pernicious anemia

(continued)

Table 12–4
Alterations in Leukocyte Count According to Disease *(Continued)*

Cell Type	***Decrease***	***Increase***
Basophils	Normal value = 0–1%	Leukemia Polycythemia vera Nephrosis Hodgkin's disease
Monocytes	None known	Brucellosis Tuberculosis Typhoid fever Rocky Mountain spotted fever Viral infections Lymphomas Moncytic leukemia Polycythemia vera Hemolytic anemias Thrombocytopenia purpura
Lymphocytes	Aplastic anemias Hemolytic disease of the newborn Transfusion reaction Pernicious anemia Pneumonia Bone marrow failure	Lymphosarcoma Malnutrition Lymphocytic leukemia Ulcerative colitis Bacteria and viral infections Infectious mononucleosis

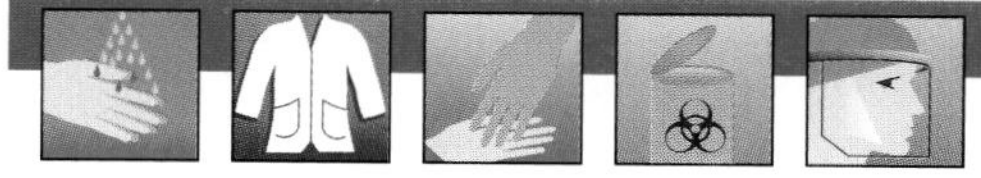

PROCEDURE 12–2

Preparing a Smear Stained With Wright's Stain

Principle

To prepare and stain a blood smear slide to meet the criteria for performing a differential count

Equipment and Supplies

clean glass slides
Wright's stain materials
transfer pipette or capillary tube
EDTA anticoagulant

Procedural Steps

1. Wash and dry hands, following OSHA standards.
2. Assemble all needed equipment and supplies.
3. Don gloves and other protective gear.
4. Mix the blood specimen.
5. Dispense a small drop of blood onto a slide, about ½ to ¾ inch from the right end. Use a transfer pipette or capillary tube.
6. Hold the left side of the slide with your nondominant hand.
7. Using your dominant hand, place the spreader slide in front of the drop of blood at an angle of 30 to 35 degrees.
8. Pull back the spreader slide into the drop of blood, and allow the blood to spread to the edges of the slide.
9. Push the spreader slide forward with a quick smooth motion, maintaining the same angle throughout the maneuver.

(continued)

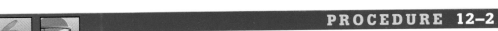

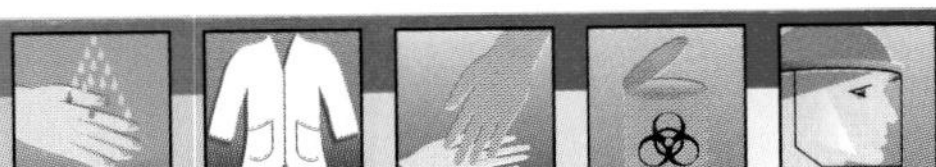

PROCEDURE 12-2

Preparing a Smear Stained With Wright's Stain (Continued)

10. Rapidly but gently wave the smeared slide to accelerate the drying process. **Do not blow on the slide.**
11. Stand the slide with the thick end down, and allow the slide to complete drying.
12. Label the slide when it is dry. Use a pencil to write the patient's name in the thick end of the smear. **Remember: If the slide is not completely dry, artifacts will appear in the cells when the slide is stained.**
13. Stain the slide according to one of the following methods:
    a. *Two-Step Method*
        (1) Place the smeared slide on a staining rack, blood side up.
        (2) Flood the smear with Wright's stain for 1 to 3 minutes.
        (3) Add an equal amount of buffer, drop by drop, on top of the Wright stain.
        (4) Blow gently, mixing the two solutions until a green metallic sheen appears. This should appear within 2 to 4 minutes.
        (5) Rinse the slide thoroughly with distilled water.
        (6) Drain the water from the slide.
        (7) Wipe the back of the smear with gauze.
        (8) Stand the smear to dry.
    b. *Quick Stain Method*
        (1) Place the smear into solutions according to the manufacturer's instructions.
        (2) Proceed with steps (5) through (8) as listed above and perform necessary counts and evaluations.
14. Dispose of blood slides according to OSHA standards.
15. Clean the work area.
16. Remove safety apparel and wash your hands.

Differential Examination

A specific area of the stained smear must be examined when performing a differential cell count. Specifically, this is an area where the RBCs are touching but not clumped, as viewed microscopically. After locating an appropriate area under low-power magnification, the area is then brought into focus under the oil-immersion objective. The differential examination involves counting and classifying 100 consecutive WBCs, proceeding in a serpentine, winding pattern through the blood smear (Fig. 12–16). This pattern must be followed to avoid counting the same cells twice. A tally is kept of the cells observed on a differential cell counter (Fig. 12–17).

Normal values vary with age (see Table 12–2). In addition, many disease states alter the ratios of the different types of leukocytes (see Table 12–4).

Figure 12–16. *Serpentine (winding) pattern used to count cells.*

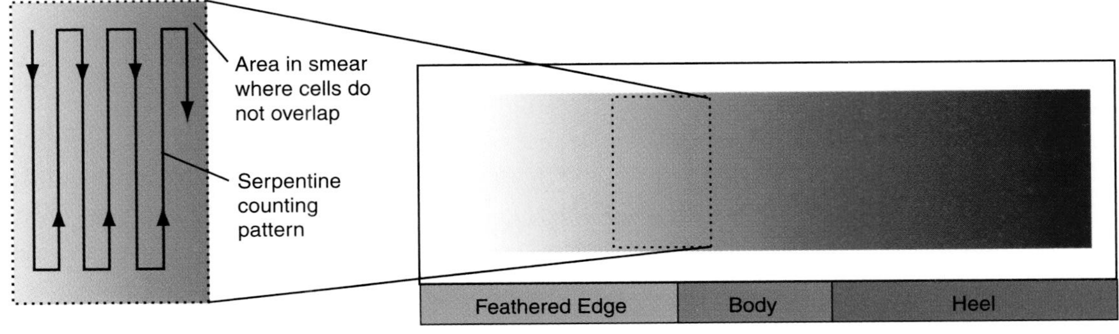

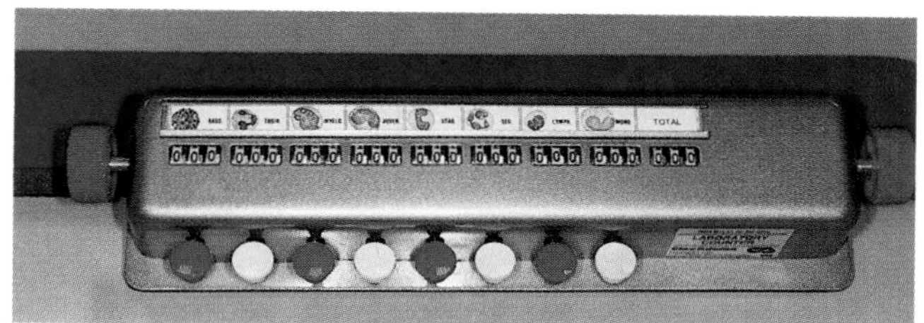

Figure 12–17. *Differential cell counter.*

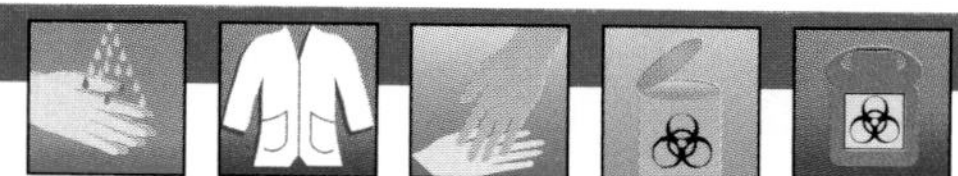

PROCEDURE 12–3

Performing a Differential Examination of a Smear Stained With Wright Stain

Principle

To perform a differential cell count and evaluate RBC, WBC, and platelet morphology

Equipment and Supplies

prepared blood slide
immersion oil
lens tissue and cleaner
differential cell counter

Procedural Steps

1. Wash and dry your hands, following OSHA standards. Don gloves and appropriate safety apparel.
2. Assemble the materials needed.
3. Clean the microscope with lens tissue and lens cleaner.
4. Place the prepared slide on the microscope stage with the smear facing up.
5. Using the low-power objective, locate an area of the smear where the RBCs barely touch each other.
6. Focus the slide under oil immersion using the fine-adjustment knob and increased light.
7. Count 100 consecutive WBCs in a winding (serpentine) pattern, identifying each cell encountered.
8. Record each WBC on the differential cell counter by depressing the appropriate key for each cell.
9. Evaluate the RBCs observed in 10 visual fields located close to the feathered edge. Record any variations in size, shape, and content, using correct terminology.
10. Count the platelets in 10 visual fields, obtain an average, and multiply that average by 15,000 to determine an estimate of the platelet count. Report the count as adequate, decreased, or increased.
11. Clean the microscope with lens tissue and lens cleaner.
12. Clean the work area. Follow OSHA standards for disposal of all contaminated materials.
13. Remove safety equipment and gloves.
14. Wash your hands.
15. Properly record the tests performed and the test results.

RBC Morphology

After determining the differential cell count, the RBCs are observed and evaluated. Normally, stained RBCs have a uniform size and shape, and are well filled with hemoglobin. Any variations from the normal state should be reported.

Size

Normal-sized RBCs are *normocytic*. If the cells are larger than normal, they are described as *macrocytic*. Conversely, if they are smaller than normal, they are *microcytic*. The condition in which different sizes of RBCs are present is called *anisocytosis* (Fig. 12–18).

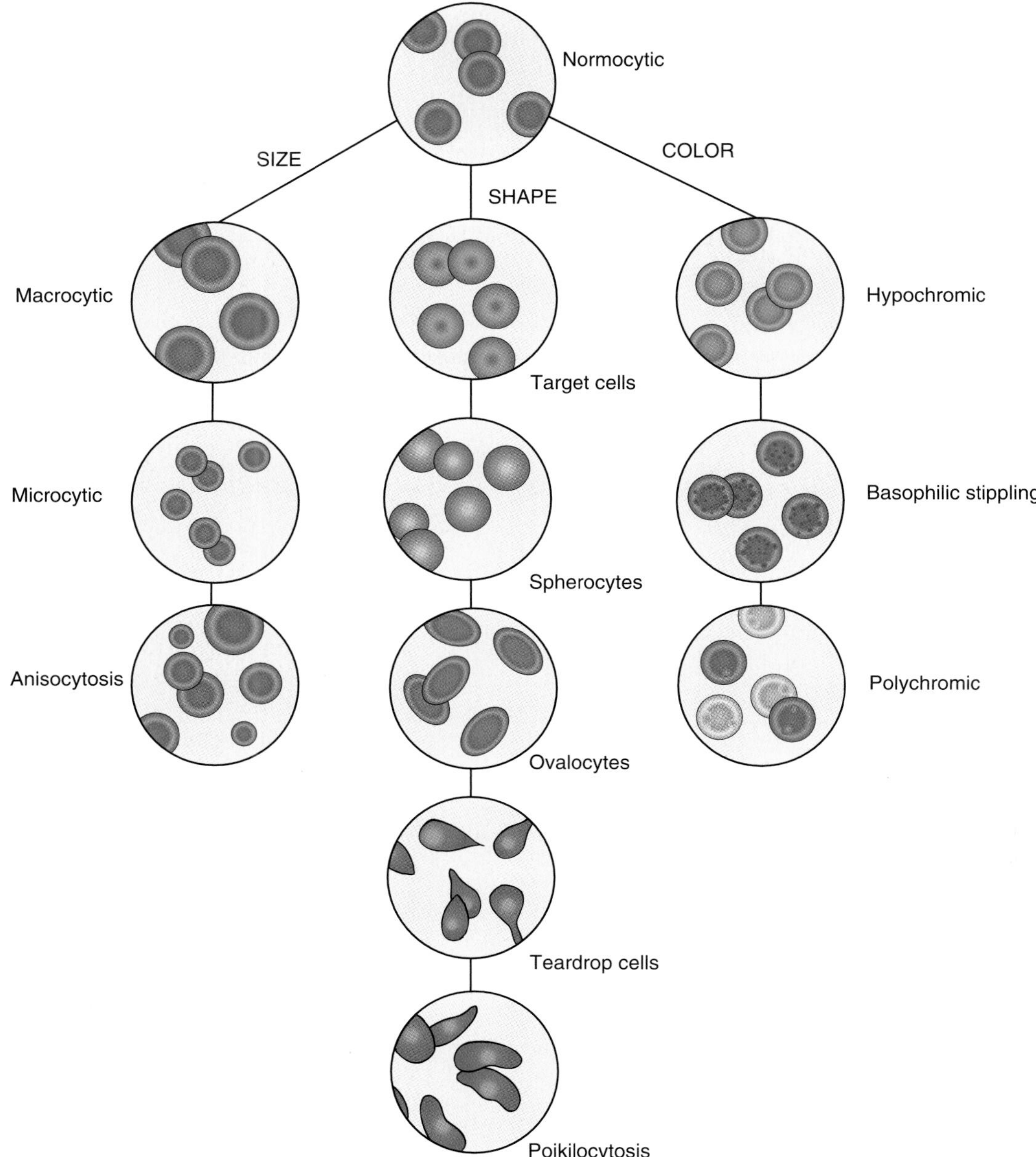

Figure 12–18. *Abnormal erythrocytes.*

Shape

Normal RBCs are round or slightly oval. Cells may be shaped like sickles, targets, spheres, ovals (ellipses), or teardrops. *Poikilocytosis* is the term used for a significant variation in the shape of the RBCs (see Fig. 12–18).

Content (Color)

RBCs with a normal amount of hemoglobin are called *normochromic*. Pale-staining cells are *hypochromic* and have less hemoglobin than normal. Basophilic stippling, which is attributable to precipitation of RNA, causes diffuse or coarse violet-stained particles to appear within the cell. Polychromic cells are a mixed pattern of normochromic, hypochromic, and basophilic cells (see Fig. 12–18).

Characteristics of Platelets

Platelets, or thrombocytes, are formed in the bone marrow from megakaryocytes. As megakaryocytes mature, platelets are shed from the cytoplasm and are released into the circulation, where they function in coagulation.

When damage to a vessel occurs, platelets form a plug at the site; eventually, a fibrin clot seals the leak. On a stained blood smear, the morphology of the platelets is observed for any abnormalities. The platelets are usually small and irregularly shaped, and may vary considerably in size. The average number of platelets seen in 10 to 15 visual fields is the number reported. The normal platelet count is 150,000 to 400,000 per mm^3. An increase in platelets is called *thrombocytosis*, whereas a decrease is called *thrombocytopenia*.

Hemoglobin

Hemoglobin (variously abbreviated as Hb or Hgb) is the main component of erythrocytes (RBCs). The main function of hemoglobin is to transport oxygen from the lungs to the cells and to remove and transport carbon dioxide from the cells to the lungs for elimination. One molecule of hemoglobin consists of a "heme," or iron-bearing portion, and a "globin," the protein portion. It is the hemoglobin molecule that gives blood its characteristic red color. When each heme group is combined with one molecule of oxygen, the hemoglobin is referred to as *oxyhemoglobin* (HbO_2). When the hemoglobin combines with carbon dioxide, it is referred to as *carboxyhemoglobin*. Blood specimens obtained for the measurement of hemoglobin concentration in the blood, or *hemoglobinometry*, may be collected by capillary puncture or venipuncture. Whole blood is required. EDTA is the preferred anticoagulant when collecting specimens for hemoglobin determinations.

Hemoglobin levels are very high at birth, progressively decreasing in childhood. During puberty and adolescence, the level again increases, reaching adult levels. Deviations in hemoglobin concentrations are closely related to deviations in the number of RBCs and the hematocrit level. Increases in hemoglobin level may be seen in patients with burns, certain pulmonary diseases, congestive heart failure, and polycythemia vera. Decreased levels are associated with anemia, leukemia, hemolytic conditions, hyperthyroidism, and liver cirrhosis.

Methods of Measurement

Cyanmethemoglobin Method

The cyanmethemoglobin method for determining hemoglobin concentration in the blood is the most reliable method. It involves photoelectric colorimetric analyses. In the cyanmethemoglobin method, the sample is diluted in Drabkin's reagent. Drabkin's reagent consists of a detergent-modified solution of potassium ferricyanide and potassium cyanide. As it is poisonous, it must be handled with care. Hemoglobin is oxidized by potassium ferricyanide, thereby forming methemoglobin. The methemoglobin then reacts with the potassium cyanide to form cyanmethemoglobin. The blood thus treated changes to a bright, cherry-red. The difference between the color of the solution and the color of normal blood is measured using a photometer (spectrophotometer). The advantage of the cyanmethemoglobin method is that it measures the total hemoglobin level.

Certain substances or conditions may interfere with the reaction, causing an increase in absorbance that is not attributable to the presence of hemoglobin. Turbidity (cloudiness) in the plasma, the presence of lipids, or large numbers of leukocytes are examples of such interfering factors.

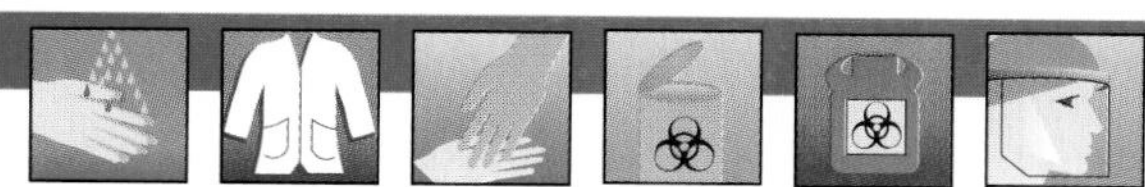

PROCEDURE 12–4

Determining the Hemoglobin Level Using a Nanometer

Principle

To secure an adequate sample and determine the hemoglobin level using the nanometer method

Equipment and Supplies

nanometer
test tubes
Drabkin's solution
5-mL syringe/gradute
blood specimen
mixing sticks

Procedural Steps

1. Wash hands and dry them thoroughly, following OSHA standards.

(continued)

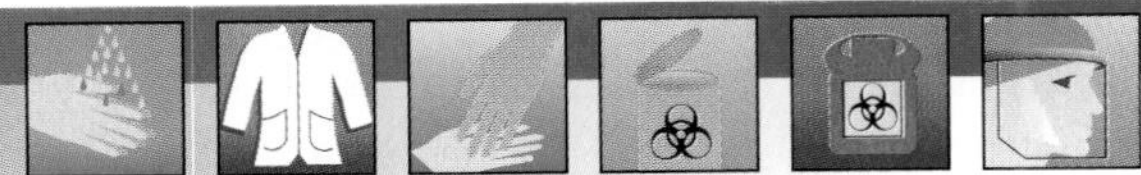

PROCEDURE 12–4

Determining the Hemoglobin Level Using a Nanometer (Continued)

2. Put on gloves and other safety equipment.
3. Assemble equipment and materials.
4. Set the wavelength of the photometer at 540 nm.
5. Label the appropriate number of test tubes for blank, standard (20 gm/dL), controls, and patients.
6. Dispense 5 mL of Drabkin's reagent into each test tube. Add 20 μL (0.02 mL) of sample to the appropriate tube. Mix the tubes thoroughly and let stand for 10 minutes.
7. Transfer the contents of the tubes to the photometer cuvette. Zero the absorbance of the photometer using the blank tube.
8. Read the record the absorbance on the standard, control, and patient samples.
9. Calculate the hemoglobin concentration using the following equation:

$$\frac{\text{absorbance of unknown}}{\text{absorbance of standard}} \times \text{concentration of standard} = \text{concentration of unknown (gm/dL)}$$

10. Record the test results in the laboratory logbook and patient's record.
11. Discard unused specimens according to OSHA standards.
12. Clean the equipment and work area.
13. Remove gloves and wash your hands.

Hemoglobinometer

A hemoglobinometer may be used to estimate the hemoglobin in the blood. This machine consists of a readout device with a chamber located on the side. A graduated slide containing a hemolyzed drop of blood from a capillary puncture or venipuncture is placed in the chamber (Fig. 12–19*A*). Once the slide is in place, the instrument is held at eye level, the light is turned on (Fig. 12–19*B*), and the slide located below the chamber is adjusted until the entire viewing screen is one shade (Fig. 12–19*C*). The hemoglobin level is then determined by reading the slide scale, which is calibrated in gm/100 mL.

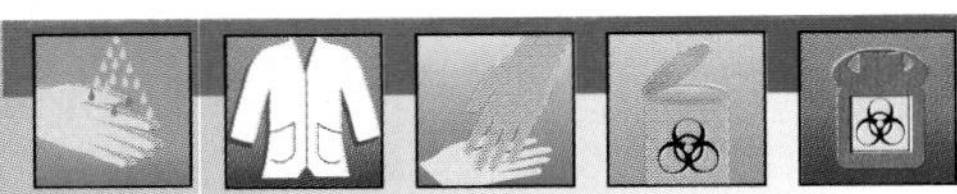

PROCEDURE 12–5

Determining the Hemoglobin Level Using a Hemoglobinometer

Principle

To determine the amount of hemoglobin present in a blood sample using the hemoglobinometer method

Equipment and Supplies

hemoglobinometer
reagent applicators
autolet/blood lancet
alcohol preps
gauze squares

Procedural Steps

1. Wash hands and dry them thoroughly, following OSHA standards.
2. Assemble needed equipment and supplies.
3. Explain the procedure to the patient.
4. Put on gloves.
5. Prepare the clipped chamber by slightly offsetting the cover slide to expose the chamber slide surface.
6. Perform a capillary puncture.
7. Place one drop of blood on the chamber slide.
8. Agitate the blood drop with a reagent stick until the blood is transparent (hemolyzed). This takes approximately 45 seconds.

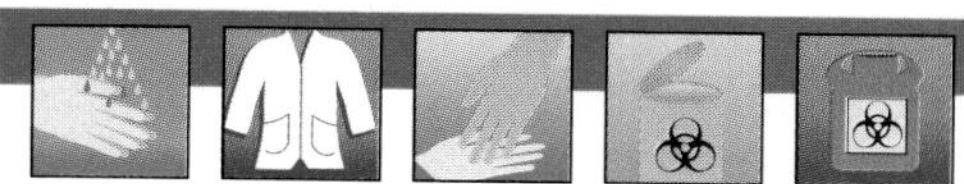

PROCEDURE 12–5

Determining the Hemoglobin Level Using a Hemoglobinometer (Continued)

9. Close the chamber.
10. Insert the chamber completely into the slot on the left side of the hemoglobinometer.
11. Place the device at eye level.
12. Using the left thumb, turn on the light switch located on the bottom of the instrument.
13. Visualize the split green field through the viewer.
14. With the right hand, manipulate the slide on the right side of the instrument until there is no difference in the green field and both sides appear to be the same shade.
15. Read the scale on the top of the slide, which is calibrated in grams of hemoglobin per 100 mL.
16. Clean the work area, dispose of waste, and return the equipment to its proper storage area.
17. Remove gloves and wash your hands.
18. Record the results and enter the test performed in the laboratory log.

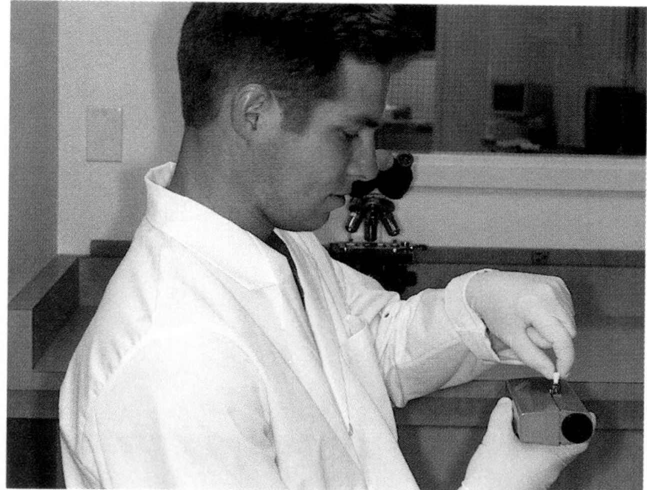

A

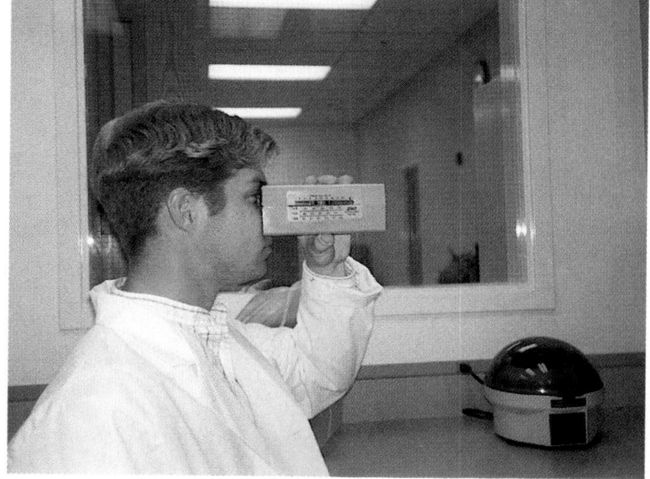

B

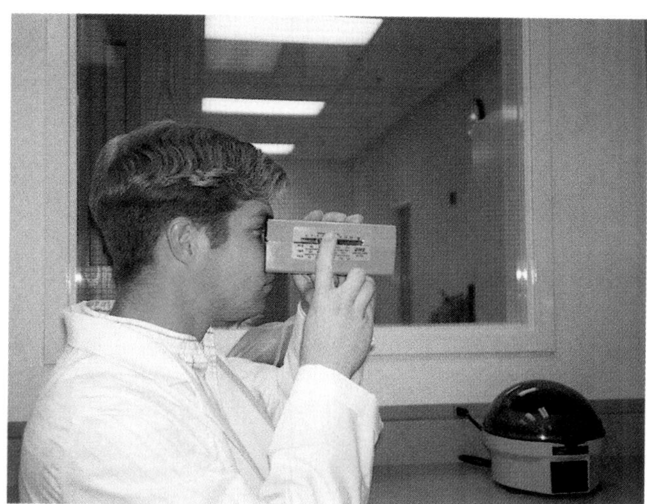

C

Figure 12–19. *Hemoglobinometer reading.* A, *The specimen slide is placed in instrument chamber.* B, *The device is raised to eye level.* C, *A hemoglobin reading is taken.*

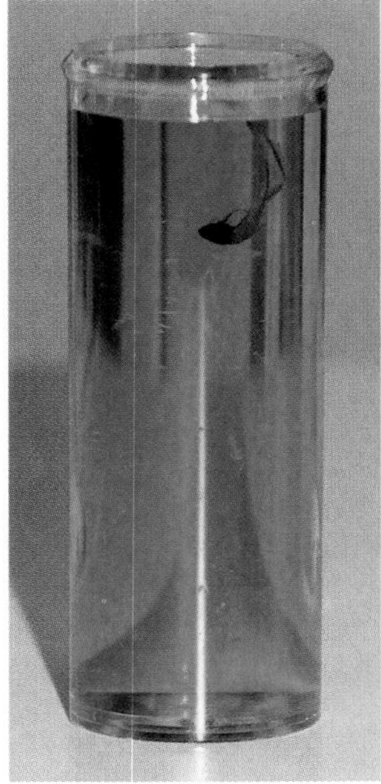

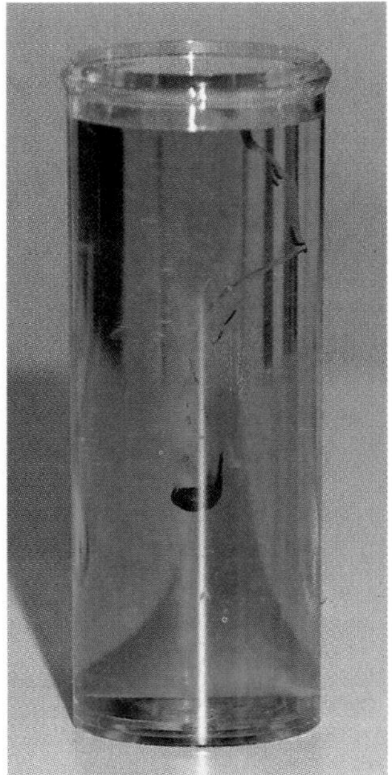

A B

Figure 12–20. *Copper sulfate specific gravity method for determining Hgb.* A, *A drop of the patient's blood is placed in copper sulfate. The rate and distance it drops determine the level of hemoglobin present.* B, *The level indicates that this patient's hemoglobin is within reference range.*

Specific Gravity Method (Copper Sulfate Method)

A simple manual method for the estimation of hemoglobin is the copper sulfate ($CuSO_4$) or specific gravity method. This method is often used to screen blood donors. When blood from a patient with normal hemoglobin values is placed in a copper sulfate solution, the hemoglobin level falls rapidly. However, the hemoglobin level in blood with a low hemoglobin concentration will not decline, or will decline slowly (Fig. 12–20).

Hemoglobin values may be affected by age, gender, altitude, pregnancy, and disease (Table 12–5). Neonates have higher hemoglobin values than do adults, and men have higher hemoglobin values than do women.

Table 12–5
Hemoglobin Reference Values

Age/Gender	***Hgb Level (gm/dL)***
Neonate	17–23
Infant (2 mo of age)	9–14
Adult female	12–16
Adult male	15–18

In anemia, hemoglobin values drop to below-normal levels. Hemoglobin values exceed normal levels in association with dehydration, severe burns, and polycythemia vera.

Hematocrit

The hematocrit (Hct), or packed cell volume, is the ratio of the volume of erythrocytes to that of the whole blood. Hematocrit values are expressed as percentages. As mentioned in Chapter 11, centrifuging a tube of anticoagulated whole blood separates the plasma from the cellular components of whole blood (Fig. 12–21). The erythrocytes (RBCs) collect at the bottom of the tube. Above the packed erythrocytes is a layer of leukocytes and thrombocytes. This layer is called the buffy coat. Above the buffy coat is the plasma, which is free of cellular elements.

Microhematocrit

The microhematocrit is determined by comparing the concentration of RBCs with the total volume of the whole blood sample.

The percentage is determined by placing the specimen tubes on a special microhematocrit reader (Fig. 12–22). Some microhematocrit centrifuges have a built-in readout scale that requires the use of calibrated

Figure 12–21. *Microhematocrit centrifuges.* A, *Clay-Adams.* B, *Damon IEC.*

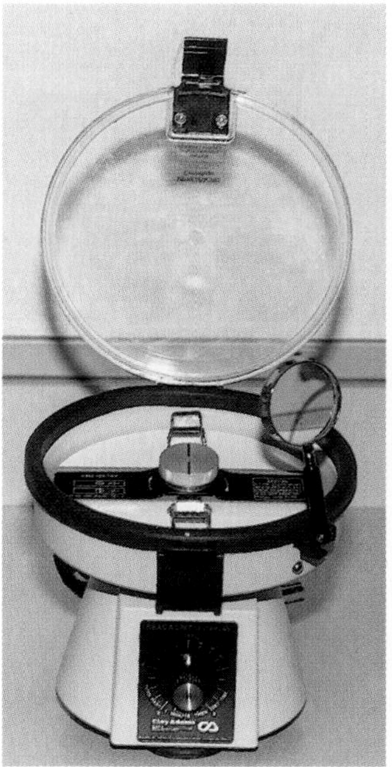

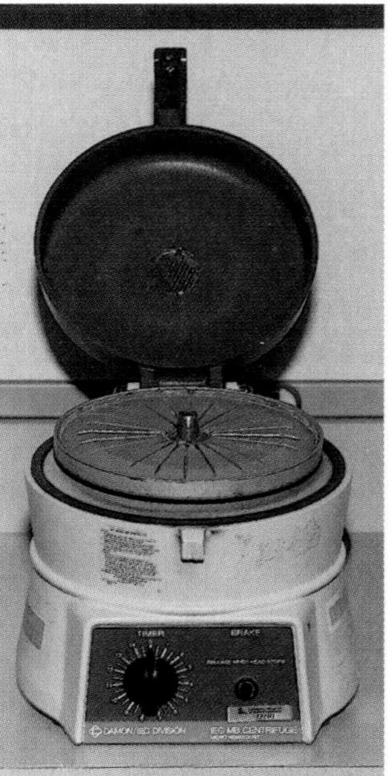

A B

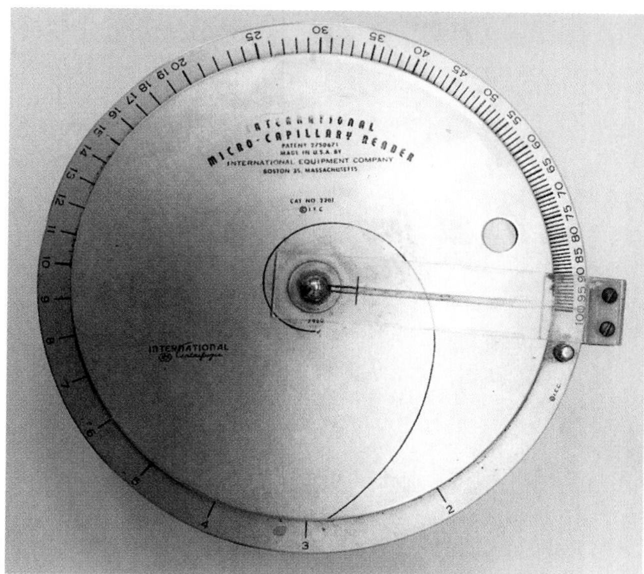

Figure 12–22. *Microhematocrit readout device.*

capillary tubes. Microhematocrit values should be determined by performing duplicate tests and then averaging the two results.

The hematocrit is a test that is commonly requested by physicians. It may be ordered separately, or as a part of a complete blood analysis. Because it is a simple procedure requiring only a small amount of blood, it is an ideal test for monitoring a patient's condition.

Low microhematocrit readings may indicate anemia or a bleeding disorder; high readings may be caused by dehydration or other conditions, such as polycythemia vera. Reference values for the hematocrit vary with the sex and age of the patient (Table 12–6). Values can also be influenced by physiologic or pathologic factors, as well as by collection techniques.

Table 12–6
Hematocrit Reference Values

Age/Gender	*Hct Value (%)*
Neonate	44–64
Infant	
1 mo of age	35–49
6 mo of age	30–40
Child, 1–10 yr of age	35–41
Adult	
Men	42–52
Women	36–45

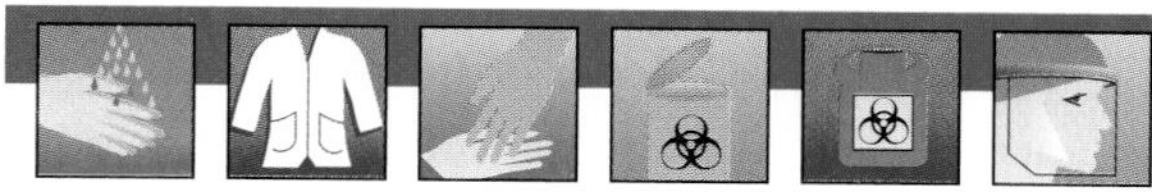

PROCEDURE 12–6

Performing a Microhematocrit Test

Principle

To collect and perform a hematocrit analysis using the microhematocrit method

Equipment and Supplies

EDTA-anticoagulated blood and capillary tubes OR blood obtained from a finger stick and placed in a heparinized capillary tube
sealing clay
centrifuge
microhematocrit reader

Procedural Steps

1. Wash hands and dry them thoroughly, following OSHA standards.
2. Assemble the materials needed.
3. Put on gloves and other safety apparel.
4. Fill two plain (blue-tip) capillary tubes three-quarters full with well-mixed EDTA-anticoagulated blood.
5. Plug the tubes with sealing clay.
6. Place the tubes opposite each other in the centrifuge, with the sealed ends securely against the gasket.
7. To maintain specimen identification, note the numbers on the centrifuge slots and record them.
8. Secure the locking top, fasten the lid down and lock. **SAFETY GLASSES MUST BE WORN WHILE THE CENTRIFUGE IS OPERATING.**
9. Set the timer (usually for 3–5 minutes) and adjust the speed as prescribed.

(continued)

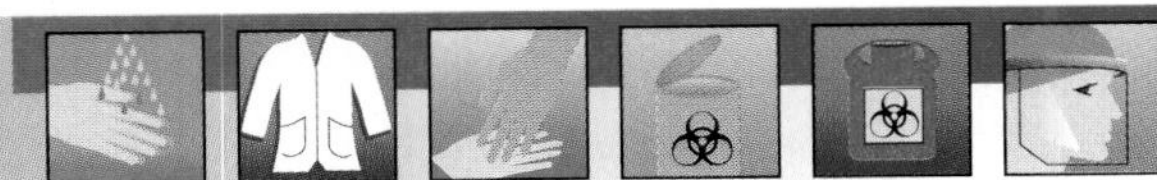

PROCEDURE 12–6

Performing a Microhematocrit Test (Continued)

10. Allow the centrifuge to come to a complete stop. Unlock the lids.
11. Remove the tubes.
12. Determine the microhematocrit value using one of the following instruments/methods.
    a. Centrifuge with built-in reader and calibrated capillary tubes
        (1) Position the tubes as directed in the manufacturer's instructions.
        (2) Read both tubes.
        (3) Report and record the average of the two readings. The two values should not vary by more than ±2%.
    b. Centrifuge without built-in reader
        (1) Carefully remove the tubes from the centrifuge.
        (2) Place a tube on the microhematocrit reader.
        (3) Align the clay-red blood cell junction with the zero line on the reader. Align the plasma *meniscus* with the 100% line. The value is read at the junction of the red cell layer and the buffy coat.
        (4) Read both tubes.
        (5) Report and record the average of the two results. The two values should not vary by more than ±2%.
13. Dispose of the capillary tubes in a biohazard container.
14. Clean the work area according to OSHA standards.
15. Remove gloves and wash your hands.

Red Blood Cell Indices

The RBC (erythrocyte) indices involve calculations to determine the size, content, and hemoglobin concentration of RBCs. These indices, when combined with microscopic analysis of RBC morphology using a stained smear, are helpful in the diagnosis and differentiation of anemias (Fig. 12–23). The RBC indices are calculated using the RBC count, the hemoglobin concentration, and the hematocrit. Most automated hematologic instruments can perform these calculations.

ANALYZE

Red Blood Cell Indices

- Mean cell volume (MCV)
- Mean cell hemoglobin (MCH)
- Mean cell hemoglobin concentration (MCHC)

Normal reference ranges for these indices are presented in Table 12–7.

Mean Cell Volume

Mean cell volume (MCV) is a measure of the average volume of RBCs per liter and is measured in femtoliters (fL) or cubic micrometers (μm^3) of the mean volume.

The formula for MCV is

$$\text{MCV} = \frac{\text{hematocrit} \times 1000}{\text{RBC count in millions}/\mu\text{L}} = \text{fL}$$

Typically, if the MCV is less than 80 mm^3, the red cells are microcytic. If the MCV is greater than 100 mm^3, the red cells are macrocytic. If the MCV is within the normal range of 80 to 100 mm^3, the red cells are normocytic.

Mean Cell Hemoglobin

The mean cell hemoglobin (MCH) is the weight of hemoglobin in the average RBC. The MCH is calculated using the hemoglobin concentration and the RBC count. MCH is measured in picograms (pg). The formula for MCH is

$$\text{MCH} = \frac{\text{hemoglobin} \times 10}{\text{RBC count in millions/mL}} = \text{pg}$$

Table 12–7
Normal Reference Ranges for RBC Indices

	Men	Women	Neonate
MCV	80–94 μm	81–99 μm	96–108 μm
MCH	27–31 pg	27–31 pg	32–34 pg
MCHC	32–36%	32–36%	32–33%

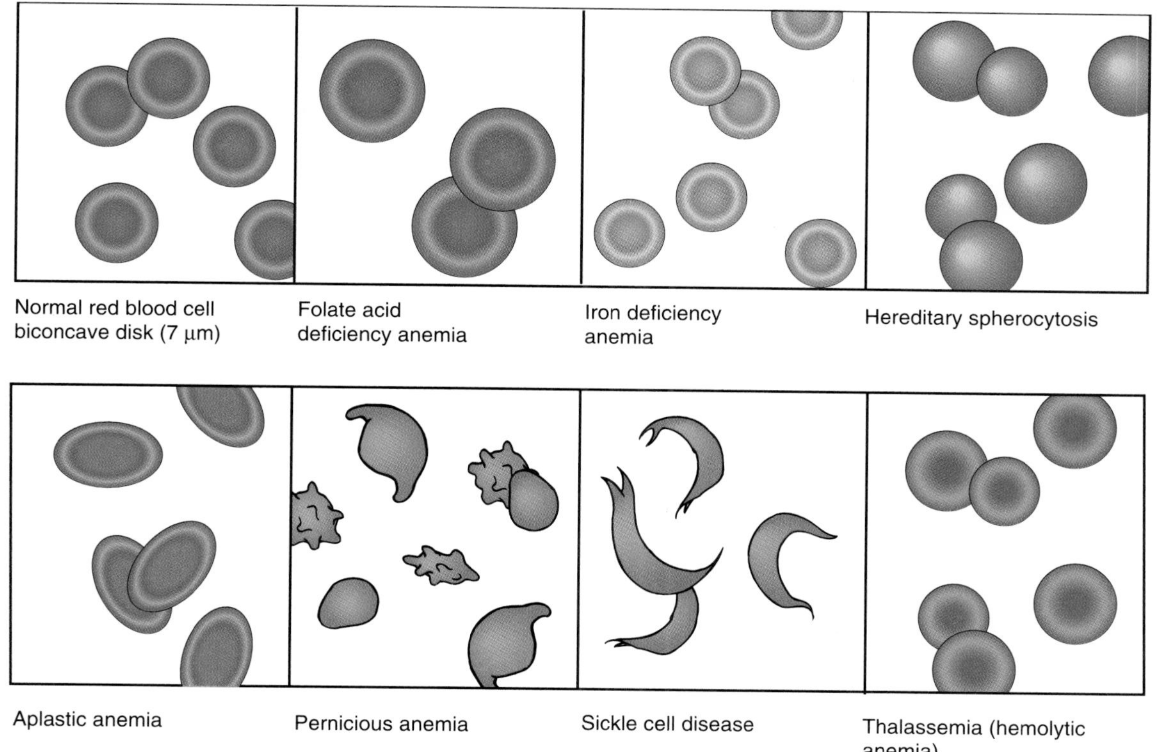

Figure 12–23. *Classification of anemias.*

Normal reference values for MCH may vary, but typically are between 27 and 34 pg. Increased MCH values may be associated with macrocytic anemia, whereas decreased values may be indicative of microcytic anemia.

Mean Cell Hemoglobin Concentration

The mean cell hemoglobin concentration (MCHC) is the average concentration of hemoglobin in a given volume of packed RBCs. It is calculated using the hemoglobin concentration and the hematocrit and is measured in g/dL or percent of volume. The formula for MCHC is

$$\text{MCHC} = \frac{\text{hemoglobin} \times 100}{\text{hematocrit}} = \text{gm/dL or }\%$$

The MCHC is valuable in evaluating anemias because of the accuracy of the hemoglobin and hematocrit measurements used in the calculation. A decreased MCHC value indicates that the RBCs contain less hemoglobin than normal. This is often the case in iron deficiency anemia, chronic blood loss anemias, macrocytic anemias; and **thalassemia.** Increased MCHC values usually indicate spherocytosis. Spherocytes are spherical RBCs that contain more than the normal amount of hemoglobin. *Spherocytosis* is the abnormal presence of spherocytes in the blood. The presence of spherocytes is confirmed by microscopic examination of a stained blood smear. Hypochromic anemias are associated with an MCHC value of 30 or less.

Anemias

Anemias may be classified by cell size (e.g., macrocytic, normocytic, or microcytic anemia) or by cell size and color (e.g., microcytic hypochromic anemia). They may also be classified by the particular deficiency present. Types of anemias include aplastic, folic (folate) acid deficiency, hemolytic, iron deficiency, pernicious, and sickle cell.

Aplastic Anemia

The erythrocyte, leukocyte, and platelet all originate from the stem cell. Aplastic anemia results from a trauma to the stem cells in the bone marrow. This trauma is frequently linked to exposure to toxic substances in the environment, such as radiation, insecticides, benzene, alkylating agents, and specific drugs. In patients in whom diagnosis has been confirmed, all components of the CBC are moderately to markedly decreased.

Folic (Folate) Acid Deficiency

Folic acid is needed for healthy function of both red and white cells. It also promotes normal absorption of the intestinal mucosa. Folates are formed by bacteria in the intestines and are stored in the liver. Folic acid anemia is also known as megaloblastic anemia because it is characterized by an abnormal type of erythropoiesis in the bone marrow. Certain foods, such as eggs, milk, leafy vegetables, yeast, and liver, are rich in folic acid. The folic acid level must remain at a decreased level for 20 weeks or more before anemia develops. Decreased acid levels are associated with alcoholism, liver disease, acute leukemia, ulcerative colitis, and infantile hyperthyroidism (see Fig. 12–23).

Hemolytic Anemia

Hemolytic anemia is characterized by an increased rate of RBC destruction. This destruction is caused either by a defect in the RBCs themselves or by some extrinsic factor that is acting on healthy RBCs. If the defect is in the RBCs, the condition is hereditary. A hereditary cause indicates abnormal hemoglobin formation or synthesis. Thalassemmia and hemoglobinopathies are examples of hereditary anemias. The extrinsic forms are classified as autoimmune hemolytic anemias because the body's own antibodies act on and destroy healthy blood cells. Immunoglobulin G (IgG) and immunoglobulin M (IgM) are the two antibodies that react and cause agglutination and destruction of the RBCs. The cause of the disease is unknown, but it may occur as a complication of systemic lupus erythematosus or lymphoma. In hemolytic anemia, the RBCs are typically normochromic and normocytic. The outstanding feature of the disease is a high reticulocyte count. The reticulocyte count may be 30% of the total cell count (see Fig. 12–23).

Iron Deficiency Anemia

Iron deficiency anemia may be caused by a number of factors. The three major causes of this form of anemia are listed below.

1. Blood loss through hemorrhage
2. Chronic blood loss, such as may accompany bleeding hemorrhoids, bleeding ulcer, and menorrhagia
3. Inadequate iron absorption in the gastrointestinal system, which may be the result of a dietary deficiency or a pathologic defect in the intestine

Regardless of the cause, the effect remains the same. The body easily can replace lost RBCs, but it soon depletes its supply of iron, which is used to manufacture the hemoglobin needed to carry oxygen to the cells. The RBCs become markedly microcytic and hypochromic, and target cells may be present (see Fig. 12–23). All components of the CBC are decreased except the WBC and platelet counts, which either remain normal or increase slightly.

Pernicious Anemia

Pernicious anemia is considered to be a macrocytic anemia because the immature RBCs are macrocytic, misshapen, and fragile. This form of anemia can be caused by a diet deficient in vitamin B_{12} or by autoimmune destruction of the parietal cells in the stomach lining. The CBC shows a gross decrease in hemoglobin and hematocrit values, along with a slight to moderate decrease in the RBC, WBC, and platelet counts. The MCV, MCH, and MCHC are elevated in such cases (Fig. 12–23).

Sickle Cell Anemia

Sickle cell anemia is the result of an abnormal form of hemoglobin known as hemoglobin S. The hemoglobin of patients with sickle cell anemia becomes increasingly viscous and tends to precipitate or bond in such a manner as to cause the RBCs to become sickle-shaped. These abnormal sickle cells are unable to pass through the capillary system. This results in increased viscosity of the blood, which slows the circulation. The increased viscosity and slowed circulation may result in the backup of cells in the capillary system and the stoppage of blood supply to certain organs (Fig. 12–24).

Sickle cell anemia is a genetically transmitted disorder. The sickle cell gene is recessive, and when two recessive genes occur in the same individual, sickle cell disorder results. The sickle cell disorder consists of sickle cell anemia and sickle cell trait. A person with sickle cell trait has inherited a normal hemoglobin gene from one parent and a hemoglobin S gene from the

Figure 12–24. *Sickled cells differ markedly from normal cells.*

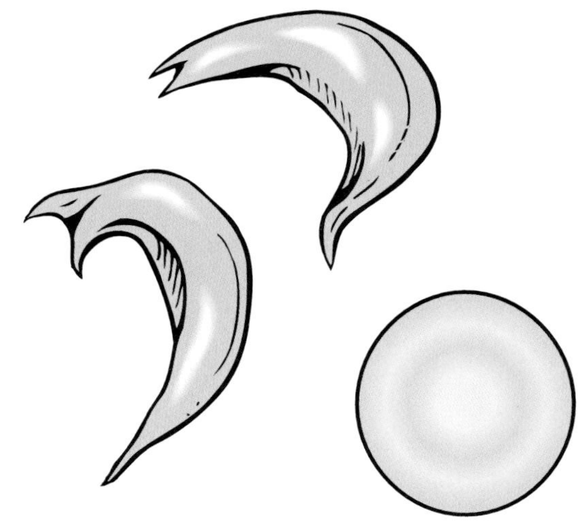

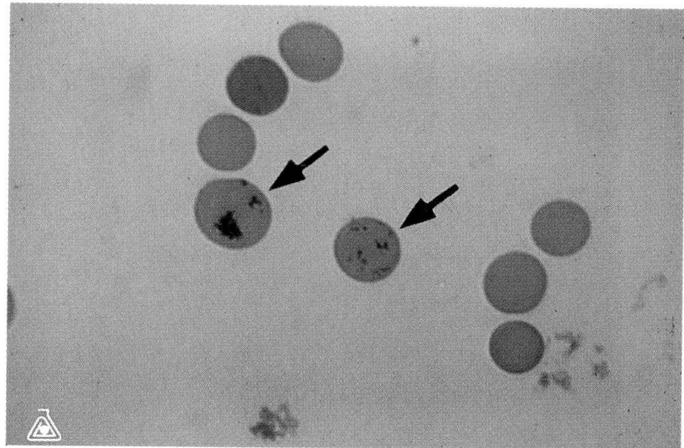

Figure 12–25. *Reticulocytes.*

other parent. This patient does not have any clinical manifestations of the disease, but the offspring of this patient may inherit the disease if the person's mate has the same heterozygous gene pattern. Patients who inherit the hemoglobin S gene from both parents have sickle cell anemia. Patients with sickle cell anemia have all the symptoms of the disease.

Testing for sickle cell disorder is important because positive results have genetic implications. Routine screening tests for sickle cell disorder, such as the Sickledex test, are available. The purpose of the screening test is to detect the presence of hemoglobin S. The test involves removing oxygen from erythrocytes. In erythrocytes with normal hemoglobin, the shape of the erythrocytes is retained. However, in erythrocytes with hemoglobin S, the erythrocytes assume a sickled shape.

A positive Sickledex test result must be confirmed by electrophoresis. Electrophoresis involves the movement of charged, suspended particles through a liquid medium in response to changes in an electric field. The underlying principle is that charged particles of a given substance migrate in an identifiable direction at a characteristic speed.

Polycythemia

Polycythemia is a condition in which the RBC count in a unit volume of blood is raised in the presence of an increased total blood volume. This absolute increase in RBC mass leads to circulatory stagnation, thrombi, and increased blood viscosity. The diagnosis is established with the aid of a CBC, which reveals an abnormal increase in the numbers of RBCs, the hemoglobin level, and the hematocrit value. Leukocyte and platelet counts are also elevated. Periodic venipuncture is a treatment designed to lower the total blood volume. Polycythemia vera is a specific form of polycythemia in which there is a neoplastic proliferation of the blastocyte component of the bone marrow. It is a disease that generally affects late middle-aged or elderly patients, and thrombotic complications are common.

Other Hematologic Tests

Reticulocyte Count

Immature non-nucleated RBCs are known as reticulocytes (Fig. 12–25). Reticulocytes are named for the reticular material that is present inside the cell. As the cells mature, the reticulum disappears. Between 0.5% and 1.5% of the total erythrocytes in a normal adult are reticulocytes. Infants and children have reticulocyte counts that may range from a low of 0.5% to a high of 5.0% of the total erythrocytes. The enumeration of reticulocytes is valuable in providing an estimate of the rate of RBC production. Reticulocyte counts are especially useful in differentiating forms of anemia. Anemia can result from bone marrow dysfunction (Fig. 12–26), blood loss (hemorrhage), or RBC destruction (hemolysis). The reticulocyte count is also used to monitor treatment of pernicious anemia and the recovery of bone marrow function in aplastic anemia.

Reticulocytosis, or an abnormally increased number of reticulocytes, may be attributable to intrinsic RBC anemia, acute blood loss (hemorrhage), or chronic blood loss. Reticulocytopenia, or decreased reticulocyte count, is usually an indication that the bone marrow is producing an insufficient number of erythrocytes (RBCs). Reticulocytopenia occurs in patients with aplastic anemia, iron deficiency anemia, pernicious anemia, and bone marrow tumors.

A reticulocyte count involves the staining of reticulocytes with a supravital stain. In this procedure, the RBCs are stained while still living. The most common supravital dye used in the reticulocyte count is new methylene blue. Some procedures also call for nyal blue sulfate or brilliant cresyl blue. After the supravital staining, the reticulocytes appear as blue-tinged ery-

Figure 12–26. *Wright's stain of bone marrow cells.*

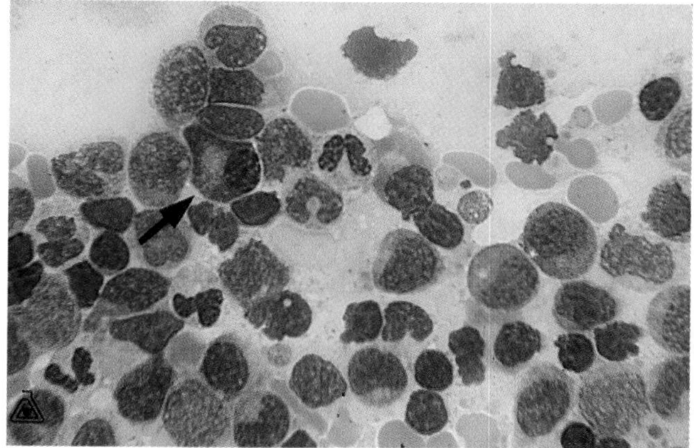

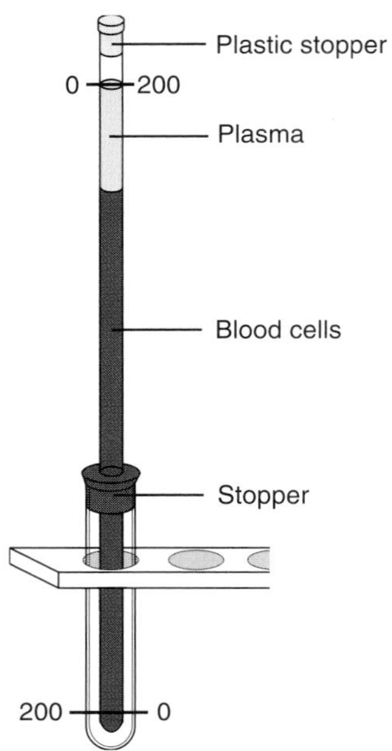

Figure 12–27. *Westergren sedimentation rate system. This is a closed system that protects against exposure to body fluids. In exactly 1 hour, the distance the RBCs have dropped is determined. The tubes used in the Westergren system are much longer than those in the Wintrobe method.*

throcytes with dark bluish granules or filaments within the cell. Mature RBCs appear as blue-stained cells without the dark blue granules or filaments. To perform the reticulocyte count, 3 drops of the supravital stain and 3 drops of EDTA-anticoagulated blood are mixed in a test tube and incubated for 15 minutes at room temperature. When incubation is complete, the test tube is remixed and two blood smears are made on glass slides and allowed to air-dry. The slides are then examined under a microscope using an oil-immersion lens. The number of reticulocytes per 1000 RBCs is recorded. The reticulocyte count is then estimated as a percentage of reticulocytes using the following formula:

$$\text{reticulocyte \%} = \frac{\text{number of reticulocytes counted}}{\text{100 erythrocytes counted}}$$

Care should be taken not to mistake artifacts for reticulocytes.

Eosinophil Smear

Eosinophils are WBCs, or leukocytes, similar to polymorphonuclear neutrophils. The cytoplasm of the eosinophils contain large, round or oval granules and have a strong affinity for acid stains (see Fig. 12–9*B*). The cytoplasm of eosinophils stains light-colored, usually pink, and is filled with large, red-orange granules. Eosinophils are approximately the same size as neutrophils, but are much less numerous. Eosinophils constitute approximately 3% of the total leukocytes in adults.

An increase of eosinophils in the blood, sputum, body fluids, or nasal secretions may indicate allergy. Eosinophils may disappear with biogenic complications. Eosinophils also occur in conditions unassociated with allergy. An eosinophil count of 20% to 25% in a nasal smear is an indication that the patient is allergic. During infectious colds, neutrophils predominate, and eosinophils may disappear completely in the acute stage. To perform an eosinophil differential count, smears of nasal secretions, blood, or other body fluids are prepared and allowed to air-dry. The smears are then stained in the same manner as smears for a differential leukoycte count. The stained smear is then examined under the microscope, and the percentage of eosinophils to total leukocytes is determined.

Erythrocyte Sedimentation Rate

The rate at which RBCs settle out of unclotted blood within 60 minutes is the *erythrocyte sedimentation rate* (ESR). The ESR is often performed as a nonspecific screening test. It is valuable in determining the progress of inflammatory disease and in the diagnosis of inflammatory diseases, such as rheumatic fever, rheumatoid arthritis, acute endocarditis, and certain respiratory infections. In healthy persons, the sedimentation of erythrocytes is a slow process, whereas in certain disease states, the sedimentation rate is quite rapid. In other cases, its rate is proportional to the severity of the underlying disease. The most common method of measuring ESR is the Wintrobe method. Another method frequently used for measuring ESR is the Westergren method. A less frequently performed test is the Zeta sedimentation rate (ZSR). Determination of the

Figure 12–28. *Automated ESR analyzers.*

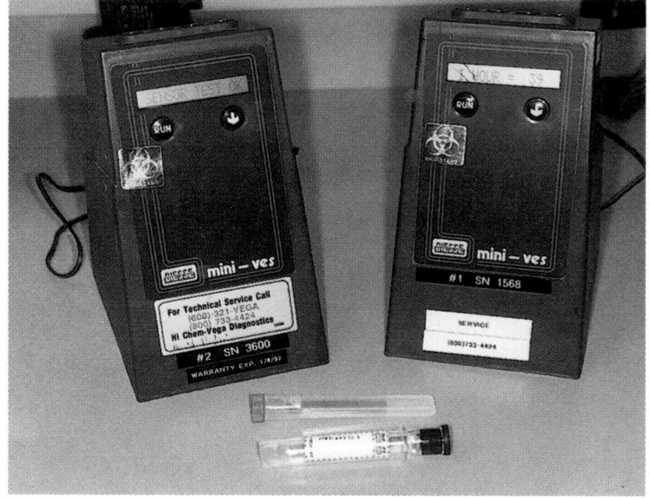

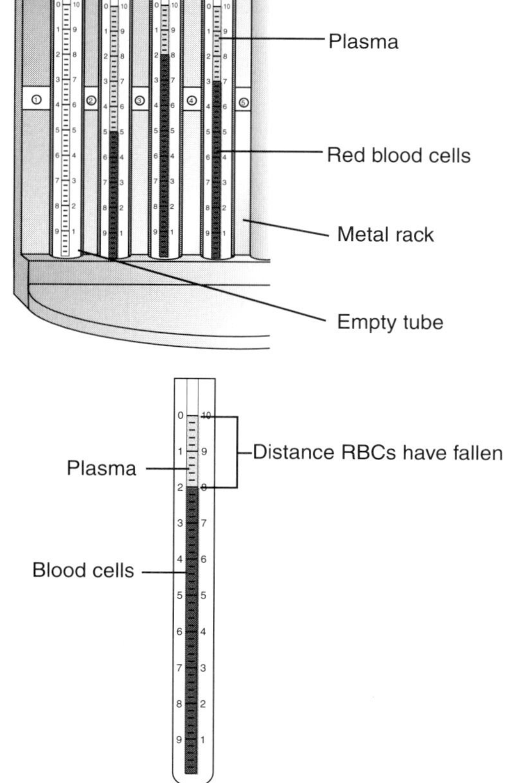

Figure 12–29. *Wintrobe sedimentation rate system. As with the Westergren method, the distance the RBCs have dropped is determined in exactly 1 hour. The enlargement shows a sedimentation rate of 20 mm/hr.*

ZSR involves the centrifugation of capillary tubes in a vertical position.

Westergren Method

The Westergren method of measuring ESR is based on the same principle as the Wintrobe method, and it is currently the preferred method in most hematology, rheumatology, and reference laboratories. Although EDTA-anticoagulated blood is acceptable if diluted with physiologic saline, the preferred specimen for a Westergren ESR test is a citrate-anticoagulated blood specimen collected in a special black-stoppered Westergren sedimentation rate tube. The Westergren method also involves the use of a disposable self-zeroing tube, calibrated from 0 to 200, which is longer than the Wintrobe tube. Once the blood specimen is transferred to the Westergren tube, the tube is inserted into the sedimentation rack and a timer is set for 1 hour (Fig. 12–27).

A modification of the Westergren method allows the use of blood anticoagulated with EDTA. This allows the ESR to be performed on the same tube of blood that may be used for other hematologic analyses.

Technical advances now allow laboratories to perform automated ESR determinations in less than half the time of the standard methods (Fig. 12–28).

Wintrobe Method

In the Wintrobe method, a well-mixed, EDTA-anticoagulated blood specimen is transferred to a disposable Wintrobe tube. Wintrobe tubes are designed with a capacity of 1 mL and are graduated from 0 to 100. Wintrobe tubes are self-zeroing and disposable. The self-zeroing Wintrobe tube is placed in the well-mixed anticoagulated blood and one (1) mL of blood is drawn into the tube using a pipette bulb. A cotton plug in the tube zeroes the blood specimen and avoids the problem of air bubbles. The tube is placed in a special sedimentation rack for 1 hour. After the hour has elapsed, the distance the RBCs have fallen is recorded (Fig. 12–29). This is the sedimentation rate. The ESR is recorded in millimeters per hour. Some procedures require that the sedimentation rate be corrected for the patient's hematocrit level. This is done using a graph or chart that compares the ESR (mm/hour) to the hematocrit value (Table 12–8).

Factors Affecting the ESR

Many factors can affect the ESR. The ESR tube must be properly zeroed with blood and must not contain air bubbles. The tube must sit in the vertical position undisturbed for the full 60 minutes. Tilting of the tube may increase the sedimentation rate. Vibrations may also increase the ESR; thus, it is very important to make sure the tubes are not bumped, jarred, or moved during the testing period. Careful timing is also important. If specimens are not read at 60 minutes, the ESR will be increased. Anticoagulated blood must be tested within 2 hours of collection.

The ESR may be increased under certain conditions, including inflammation, infection, toxemia, pneumonia, and rheumatoid arthritis. The ESR may be decreased in patients with sickle cell anemia, polycythemia vera, or congestive heart failure.

Table 12–8
ESR Reference Values

	Wintrobe Method (mm/hr)	***Westergren Method (mm/hr)***
Men	0–10	≤50 yr of age: 0–15 >50 yr of age: 0–20
Women	1–20	≤50 yr of age: 0–20 >50 yr of age: 0–30

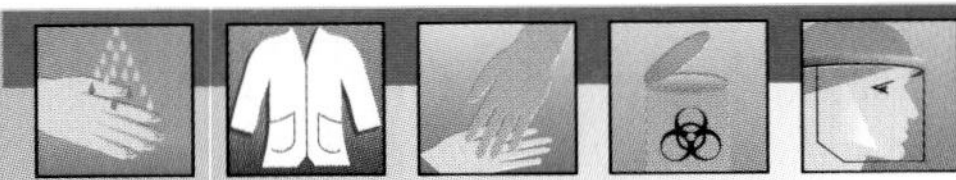

PROCEDURE 12–7

Determining Erythrocyte Sedimentation Rate by the Wintrobe Method

Principle

To achieve skill in properly filling a Wintrobe tube and in observing and reporting the findings of an ESR test using the Wintrobe method

Equipment and Supplies

Wintrobe tube and rack
automatic pipettor
timing device
laboratory tissues
EDTA-treated blood specimen (lavender top)
normal saline

Alert: Continuously mix the blood sample until needed.

Procedural Steps

1. Wash hands and dry them thoroughly, following OSHA standards.
2. Assemble equipment and supplies.
3. Put on gloves and goggles.
4. Dilute 2 mL of blood with 0.5 mL of saline.
5. Using an automatic pipettor, draw the blood into the Wintrobe tube, slightly overfilling it.
6. Cover the top of the Wintrobe tube with your index finger.
7. Bring the tube to eye level and gently allow the meniscus of the blood to drop to the zero mark.
8. Wipe off all excess blood with a laboratory tissue.
9. Place the Wintrobe tube in a rack, making sure it remains vertical.
10. Set the timer for 1 hour.
11. When 1 hour has elapsed, read the level of the meniscus of the blood in the tube.
12. Record the results (mm/hr).
13. Dispose of all biohazardous waste.
14. Clean and return all equipment and supplies to the proper storage area.
15. Remove gloves and wash hands.

ESR Testing Alert

- Results will be inaccurate if the ESR tube is not kept vertical at all times.
- Air bubbles in the tube will interfere with test results.
- The test must be performed within 1 hour after obtaining the blood sample.
- Excess anticoagulant or partially clotted blood will decrease the settling rate.
- The blood and saline **MUST BE THOROUGHLY MIXED** before beginning the test.

Summary

The most important hematologic test is the CBC. Based on the results of a CBC, physicians can often diagnose disease, monitor a patient's prognosis, and evaluate disease conditions. The hemoglobin, hematocrit, and RBC count provide the information necessary for calculating RBC indices (Fig. 12–30). Physicians can classify the various types of anemias and diagnose other disease states in their patients by using these indices and values.

Modern technology has provided instruments for use in the medical office that test for all parameters of the CBC and automatically calculate the RBC indices. This advanced technology allows laboratory assistants to perform a wide range of diagnostic tests in the POL (Fig. 12–31). Whether the test is done manually or by automated methods, accuracy and precision remain paramount.

Chapter Review

True or False

Circle T or F to indicate the correct answers to the following:

T F 1. Peripheral blood is the preferred blood specimen for hematologic testing.

T F 2. Reusable Sahli pipettes are commonly used for dilution of blood cells.

T F 3. The hemacytometer has two raised surfaces surrounded by depressions on three sides.

T F 4. Thrombocytes are the smallest of the formed elements in the blood.

T F 5. Lymphocytes are the most numerous white cell in adults.

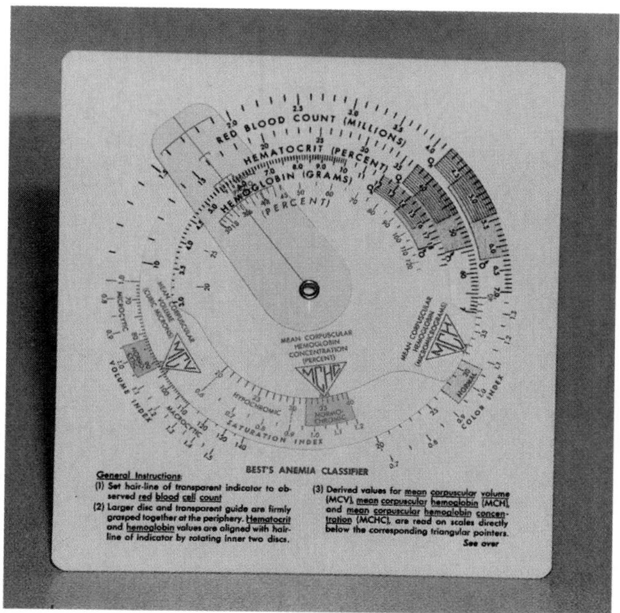

Figure 12–30. *Best's anemia classifier uses the RBC count and hemoglobin and hematocrit values to determine RBC indices.*

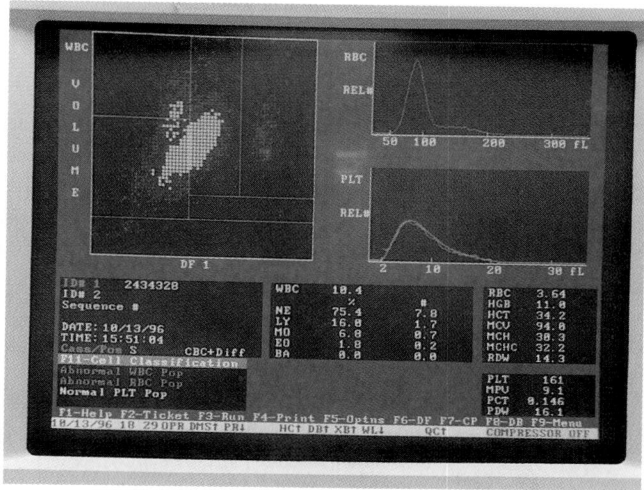

Figure 12–31. *A histogram shows the distribution of WBCs, RBCs, and platelets.*

Fill in the Blanks

Complete the following statements:

6. Lymphocytes are responsible for recognition of

   ______________ and the production of ______________

   ______________ .

7. An immature form of the neutrophil is called a

   ______________ or a ______________ .

8. If the MCV is less than 87 mm, the red cells are

   ______________ .

9. Sickle cell anemia is the result of an abnormal form of

   ______________ known as ______________ .

10. The ESR is recorded in ______________ .

Multiple Choice

Circle the letter that represents the single best answer:

11. In the Neubauer hemocytometer, each of the three millimeter areas is divided into ______________ equal squares.
    a. 3
    b. 6
    c. 9
    d. 12
    e. 15

12. When counting WBCs, the ______________ power objective is used.
    a. 4×
    b. 10×
    c. 40×
    d. Oil immersion
    e. All of the above

13. When counting RBCs, the ______________ power objective is used.
    a. 4×
    b. 10×
    c. 40×
    d. Oil immersion
    e. All of the above

14. The counting pattern used for greatest accuracy and reproducibility is:
    a. Vertical
    b. Horizontal
    c. Lateral
    d. Corner squares only
    e. Serpentine

15. A blood smear enables you to view cellular:
    a. Color
    b. Morphology
    c. Coagulation
    d. Density
    e. Factor VIII

16. Hemoglobin is the main component of:
    a. Leukocytes
    b. Thrombocytes
    c. Erythrocytes
    d. Platelets
    c. Plasma

Vocabulary

ADP: adenosine diphosphate; a product of the hydrolysis of adenosine triphosphate (ATP)
aggregation: the clustering or clumping of blood cells
atherosclerosis: a common condition in which deposits of yellowing plaques containing cholesterol and lipid material form on the inside walls of the arteries
autoimmune: pertaining to an immune response to one's own tissues
catalyze: to cause an increase in the rate of a chemical reaction
diastema: a congenital defect characterized by dwarfing, or changes in bone spacing and clefting
edematous: characterized by excessive fluid accumulation in tissues
embolus: a foreign object obstructing the flow of blood
enzyme: any protein that acts as a catalyst, thereby increasing the rate at which a chemical reaction occurs
fibrinolysis: the continuous process of fibrin decomposition by fibrinolysin; the normal mechanism for the removal of small fibrin clots
fibrometer: an instrument used to perform coagulation tests, such as prothrombin time, that involve detection of the formation of a fibrin clot in plasma
hemophilia: a hereditary disorder resulting from deficiency or absence of factor VIII or factor IX in the blood
hemostasis: the termination of bleeding by mechanical or chemical means
hypersplenism: exaggeration of the hemolytic function of the spleen, resulting in deficiency of peripheral blood elements
in vitro: observable within a test tube; in an artificial environment
in vivo: test performed on a living organism
plaque: a yellowish area within an artery that causes the internal surface to bulge into the lumen
systemic lupus erythematosus: an autoimmune connective tissue disease, affecting more women than men, which produces a high level of autoantibodies, indicating a defect in regulatory mechanisms
thrombocytopenia: a condition in which there is an abnormal decrease in the number of platelets in the circulating blood
thrombocytosis: a condition in which there is an abnormal increase in the number of platelets circulating in the blood
vasculitis: inflammation of a vessel

Chapter Objectives

After reading this chapter, you should be able to:

1. Name the three factors of hemostasis.
2. Compare and contrast clotting factors with natural anticoagulants.
3. List the clotting abnormalities discussed in this chapter.
4. Describe the coagulation pathways in hemostasis.
5. Identify three coagulation tests.
6. List each step of the prothrombin time test.
7. Define disseminated intravascular coagulation (DIC) and describe its importance in coagulation.
8. Outline the Ivy Bleeding Test and the Duke Bleeding Test.

Chapter 13
Coagulation Testing

Hemostasis is the body's mechanism for termination of bleeding. *Coagulation,* or clotting, is the conversion of liquid blood into a semi-solid gel. When damage occurs to the vascular system, several mechanisms function to stop bleeding. *Vasoconstriction,* or the contraction of vascular walls, is the first mechanism for maintaining hemostasis. The blood vessel walls contract, thereby reducing the quantity of blood flow. Next, platelets adhere to each other and to the damaged vascular walls, creating platelet **aggregation.** Platelet aggregation causes the formation of a platelet plug, which provides a surface for the activation of coagulation factors. Once the coagulation factors are activated, they initiate the hemostasis mechanism of coagulation. Coagulation involves a complex, cascading series of reactions that result in the generation of thrombin, a plasma protein, and the formation of a fibrin clot that acts to seal the vascular wall until the body can repair the damaged tissue.

Mechanisms of Hemostasis

Vascular Response

The first mechanism initiated by the body is vasoconstriction. If for any reason this constriction does not occur, the normal body blood pressure will destroy any clot the body attempts to make. The damaged vessel end exposes collagen, which attracts platelets. This decrease in blood flow, combined with the exposed collagen, promotes the aggregation of platelets into a platelet plug.

Platelets

In response to a damaged vessel, platelets change shape, become sticky, and aggregate, forming a platelet plug. As this plug develops, it forms a barrier to close off the break in the vessel. This entire process is completed

Table 13–1
Coagulation Factors

Factor	Name
I	Fibrinogen
II	Prothrombin
III	Tissue factor; thromboplastin
IV	Calcium
V	Labile factor; proaccelerin
VII	Serum prothrombin conversion accelerator; proconvertin
VIII	Antihemophilic factor
IX	Plasma thromboplastin component
X	Stuart-Prower factor
XI	Plasma thromboplastin antecedent
XII	Hageman factor
XIII	Fibrin stabilizing factor
Platelet factor–Cephalin	

within seconds. Once the plug is formed, the platelets release substances that initiate the coagulation cascade.

Substances involved in the coagulation cascade include platelet factors, tissue thromboplastin, and other clotting factors in the circulating blood.

Coagulation Factors

Coagulation factors, which are designated by Roman numerals, include both calcium and plasma proteins (Table 13–1). Two of the most common coagulation factors are fibrinogen (factor I) and prothrombin (factor II). Before coagulation factors can participate in the clotting mechanism, they must first be activated.

Most coagulation factors are produced by the liver. Prothrombin (factor II) is a plasma protein that is produced in the liver. Vitamin K is needed to synthesize prothrombin. Prothrombin, in the presence of thrombokinase, is converted to thrombin. Thrombin is an **enzyme** formed from prothrombin during the clotting process. An enzyme is a protein produced in the body that **catalyzes** an organic chemical reaction. Enzymes facilitate changes in other substances, but are not consumed in the chemical reaction they catalyze. Thrombin, in turn, catalyzes the production of fibrin from the plasma protein fibrinogen (factor I).

Coagulation Pathways

The conversion of fibrinogen to fibrin by the action of thrombin is the end result of a common coagulation pathway. This common pathway is stimulated by an intrinsic (blood) pathway and an extrinsic (tissue) pathway (Figure 13–1). Both intrinsic and extrinsic pathways must work together to activate the common pathway.

When factor XII makes contact with the surface of a damaged vessel, activation of the intrinsic pathway begins. This complex reaction results in the stimulation of the common pathway. It is the intrinsic pathway that is activated during **in vitro** coagulation, as occurs when blood is collected into a red-top tube and a clot forms.

In the extrinsic pathway, tissue damage causes the release of a tissue factor (factor VII) that is predominantly phospholipid. Factor XII, along with factor VII, activate factor X, which stimulates the common pathway, the end result of which is formation of a fibrin clot.

Once the clot has served its function and bleeding has stopped, fibrinolysis and clot retraction occur. This requires platelets, adenosine triphosphate (ATP), and factor XIII, and it involves layering of the fibrin threads, which effectively pulls the edges of the injured vessel wall closer together. The clot thus retracts as the size of the injured area is reduced. As the healing process begins, the clot begins to dissolve, a process referred to as **fibrinolysis.**

Figure 13–1. *Coagulation pathways.*

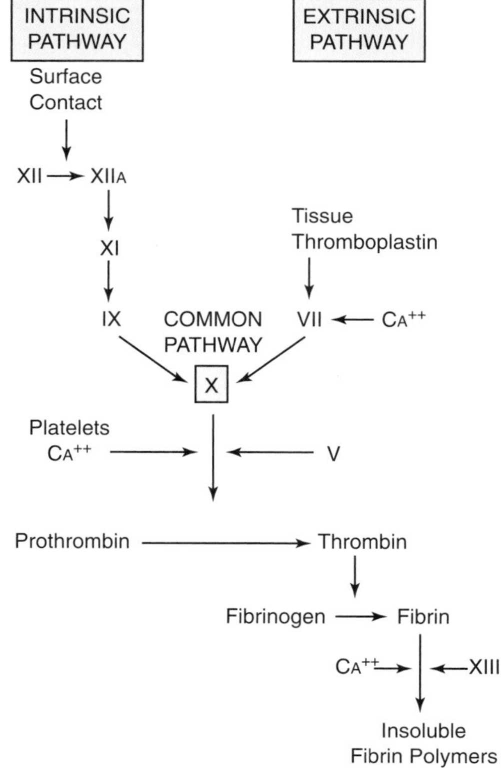

Fibrinolysis

Fibrinolysis involves the activation of plasminogen, which is then converted into plasmin. The conversion of plasminogen, a plasma protein, activates the dissolution of the fibrin clot. The removal of the fibrin clot is part of the complex process of hemostasis.

Natural Anticoagulants

The action of clotting factors is opposed by the action of natural anticoagulants, the most important of which are heparin, antithrombin, and plasminogen. Heparin acts on several steps of the coagulation cascade to counterbalance clot formation. Heparin may be administered to patients to prevent clotting. Antithrombin inactivates thrombin, preventing the activation of fibrinogen. In the body, the primary function of antithrombin is to prevent formation of blood clots. Plasminogen is activated to form plasmin, which lyses fibrin, and is used in the body to dissolve clots.

Bleeding, by itself, is not an indication of an abnormality in hemostasis. Platelet deficiency is the most common cause of such an abnormality. Normally, a blood clot seals the damaged blood vessel, stopping blood loss. An abnormality occurs when clotting is insufficient to stop the flow of blood from the damaged vessel, or when there is unnecessary clotting.

Clotting Abnormalities

Vascular Disorders

Thrombosis and Embolism

Thrombosis is the abnormal formation of a clot, or thrombus. A thrombus can cause damage when pieces of it break loose and enter the circulating blood of the vascular system. A free-floating clot in the vascular system is called an **embolus.** Emboli cause damage when they travel through the vascular system and block small vessels (a process referred to as an embolism), particularly those in vital organs, such as the heart, brain, lungs, and kidneys. An embolus is a serious, potentially life-threatening complication. The vessels of some patients have a buildup of **plaque** along their walls, resulting in a rough and irregular surface. This condition is called **atherosclerosis.** This buildup of plaque can cause a thrombus to form, thereby increasing the risk of an embolus.

Vessel Integrity

Small bruises and hematomas of the blood vessels, caused by the mechanical trauma of everyday injuries, are the most common causes of hemorrhage. Some individuals have an increased tendency to bleed and cannot withstand vessel stress as well as others. This disorder can be manifested as vessel wall weakness. Other causes of vessel wall weakness are age, metabolic disorders, or congenital disorders of the connective tissue. This vessel weakness may cause spontaneous or trauma-induced hemorrhages.

Vessel inflammation and congestion is known as **vasculitis.** It may be associated with infection, septicemia, or ingestion of drugs.

Platelet Disorders

Most platelet abnormalities may be either quantitative or qualitative. Quantitative abnormalities, such as thrombocytopenia or decreased platelet count, are sometimes caused by decreased production, **hypersplenism,** or increased use or destruction of platelets. **Thrombocytosis,** or increased platelet count, occurs in association with iron deficiency anemia, hemorrhage, splenectomy, or inflammation. An increased platelet count increases the risk of unwanted clot formation. In many diseases, such as polycythemia vera or granulocytic leukemia, platelet counts are extremely elevated and the platelets do not function properly.

Qualitative platelet abnormalities may be congenital or hereditary, or may be caused by drug use, dialysis, or the use of aspirin or other anti-inflammatory drugs.

Platelet disorders involve either a decreased number of platelets or an abnormality in platelet structure and function. Most hemorrhage (bleeding) disorders involve platelet abnormalities. Vascular platelet abnormalities are difficult to detect with common laboratory coagulation tests.

The average normal platelet count is approximately 200,000/μL. When this count drops below 70,000, the condition is termed **thrombocytopenia.** This low platelet count leads to spontaneous bleeding within the tissues, which produces visible bluish areas on the skin. These areas of discoloration are known as purpura. Tissue hemorrhaging can also occur in the gastrointestinal and urinary systems.

Decreased Platelet Production

As discussed in Chapter 10, platelets develop from megakaryocytes in the bone marrow. They are anuclear fragments of megakaryocytes, and upon entering the peripheral blood, survive for only 2 to 3 days. Any disease or condition that affects megakaryocytes will cause thrombocytopenia (Table 13–2). Affected patients develop bleeding tendencies and require transfusions of whole blood and/or platelets.

Table 13–2
Disorders/Agents Affecting Megakaryocytes

Disorders/Agents	***Laboratory Findings***
Aplastic anemia	Loss of all hematopoietic cells
Leukemia	Replacement of normal hematopoietic cells with tumor cells
Drugs	Megakaryocyte damage
Infectious agents	Interference with megakaryocyte production

Increased Intravascular Consumption

Many **autoimmune** disorders are associated with platelet destruction. Antibodies to platelets are formed in certain conditions, such as **systemic lupus erythematosus,** some hemolytic anemias, and in drug-induced hematologic disorders. This type of antibody malfunction is also the major feature in *idiopathic thrombocytopenia purpura (ITP).* It may develop after major blood transfusions because of platelet-specific antigens that are capable of producing antibodies. Aspirin use may affect the aggregation of platelets for 7 to 10 days after ingestion. This is because of the effect aspirin has on the platelet release reaction.

Disseminated Intravascular Coagulation

In disseminated intravascular coagulation (DIC), platelets are consumed at an accelerated rate. DIC might be triggered by infection, tumors, or some form of shock or severe stress. The disorder occurs when intravascular coagulation causes small thrombi to form in the small vessels. The plasma clotting factors are exhausted by the formation of these thrombi. Fibrinolysis occurs, dissolving the thrombi and resulting in spontaneous bleeding. The bleeding cannot be controlled because the coagulation factors have been totally depleted. These factors must be replaced by transfusion or the patient will bleed to death.

Congenital Disorders

Congenital disorders are rare, and their diagnosis requires extensive laboratory testing and investigation. *Thrombasthenia* is a congenital disorder in which the platelet is abnormally characterized by defective clot retraction and impaired adenosine diphosphate (**ADP**)–induced platelet aggregation. It is characterized by excessive bruising, post-traumatic tissue bleeding, nosebleeds, excessive menstrual flow, and, in severe cases, intracranial bleeding. The platelet count, morphology, and adhesion remain within normal limits.

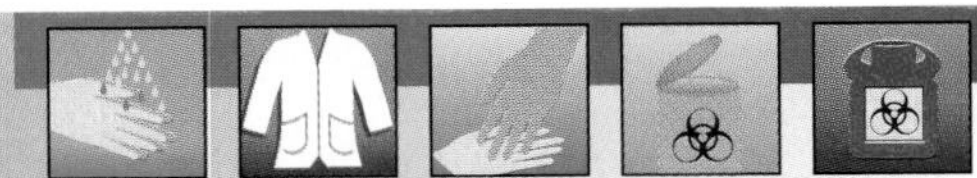

PROCEDURE 13–1

Performing a Manual Platelet Count: Unopette Method

Principle

To determine the number of platelets per cubic millimeter to assist in disease prognosis and therapy

Equipment and Supplies

Neubauer ruled hemocytometer
hemocytometer coverslip
lint-free tissue or gauze
70% alcohol
Unopette System (reservoir containing 1.98 mL of diluent mixture; capillary pipette 20 µL)
microscope
hand tally counter
Petri dish lined with moist filter paper
ethylenediaminetetra-acetic acid
(EDTA) blood specimen or capillary puncture

Procedural Steps

1. Wash and dry hands. Put on gloves.
2. Assemble the necessary equipment and supplies.

Filling a Unopette

3. Remove a Unopette reservoir from the storage container and recap the container tightly.
4. Use the pipette shield to puncture the diaphragm

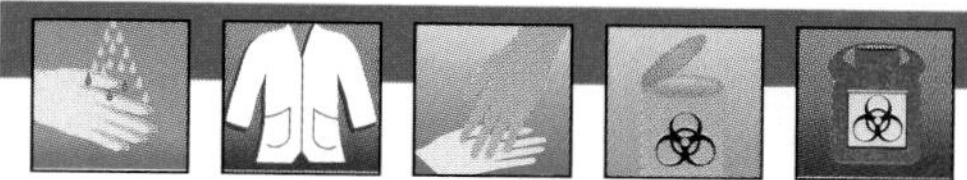

PROCEDURE 13–1

Performing a Manual Platelet Count: Unopette Method (Continued)

of the Unopette reservoir. The hole must be large enough to allow the pipette to enter freely.

5. Remove the pipette shield.
6. Hold the pipette nearly horizontal.
7. Place the tip of the pipette into a well-mixed tube of EDTA-anticoagulated blood, and allow the pipette to fill by capillary action until the blood reaches the end of the pipette, or do a finger stick and fill the capillary tube.
8. Place a finger over the hole in the pipette to prevent loss of any portion of the sample, and carefully wipe the outside of the pipette with gauze to remove all traces of blood.
9. Squeeze the reservoir gently with one hand to force out air, but do not expel any liquid. Maintain pressure on the reservoir.
10. While holding the index finger over the hole in the top of the pipette, insert the pipette in the reservoir with a firm twisting motion.
11. Release the pressure on the reservoir and remove the finger from the top of the pipette. The sample will be drawn into the reservoir. You may place the shield at the open end of the pipette to prevent spilling of the contents and possible contamination.
12. Gently squeeze (so that the cells will not be destroyed) and release the reservoir several times to rinse all blood from the pipette into the reservoir. The reservoir fluid should rise to the overflow chamber, but should not be forced out of the top of the pipette.
13. Gently mix the contents of the Unopette by inversion or by rolling the Unopette between the palms of the hands.
14. Label the Unopette with the appropriate information.
15. Allow the Unopette to sit for 10 minutes.
16. Make sure the Unopette reservoir is capped with a Unopette pipette shield to prevent evaporation.

Charging (Filling) a Hemocytometer

17. While the Unopette System is sitting, clean the hemocytometer with 70% alcohol and lint-free tissue. Dry thoroughly.
18. Place the coverslip on the counting chamber.
19. Convert to dropper assembly by withdrawing the pipette from the reservoir and reseating it securely in the reverse position.
20. To clean the capillary bore, invert the reservoir, gently squeeze the sides, and discard the first three or four drops of blood.
21. Controlling the flow, gently fill the chamber with diluted blood in one smooth motion. Fill slowly and smoothly to avoid air bubbles and overfilling.
22. Fill both sides of the hemocytometer.
23. Allow the chamber to sit undisturbed for approximately 10 minutes so that the cells can settle to prevent the sample from evaporating. The hemocytometer can be placed in a clean Petri dish humidified by moist filter paper or gauze.
24. Once the cells have settled, carefully place the hemocytometer on the microscope stage for viewing.

Counting and Calculating

25. Under 40× magnification, using bright light or phase microscopy, count the platelets in all 25 small squares within the large center square using a serpentine pattern.

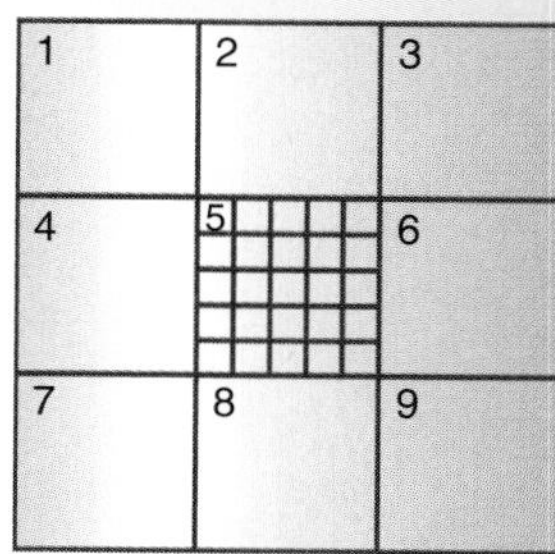

26. Count the second side of the chamber in the same manner. Average the counts from both sides.
27. Multiply the number of platelets counted by 1000 to determine the total platelet count/mm^3.
28. Record/report the test and the results.
29. Clean the work area. Follow OSHA standards for proper disposal of all used materials.
30. Remove your gloves and wash your hands.

Clotting Factor Disorders

Congenital clotting factor defects are relatively common. Each of the proteins participating in the coagulation cascade is encoded by a distinct gene. Mutation or deletion of these genes results in a bleeding disorder. Congenital coagulation abnormalities, such as **hemophilia,** result from defects in the coagulation cascade. Acquired vascular abnormalities are more common and are often associated with drugs, vitamin C deficiency, or an allergic response to infection. Acquired coagulation abnormalities include defects in circulatory anticoagulant activity, vitamin D deficiency, and liver disease, among others.

Hemophilia

Hemophilia is an inherited, sex-linked, recessive disorder associated with a gene causing a clotting factor deficiency. The gene is carried on the X chromosome; because men inherit both the X and Y chromosome, this disorder almost always affects male offspring. It occurs in two forms: *hemophilia A,* which is characterized by a deficiency of factor VIII, and *hemophilia B* (also known as Christmas disease), which is characterized by a deficiency of factor IX. The clinical symptoms are the same for both deficiencies. Female patients are carriers of the recessive gene, but rarely develop the disease.

Affected males tend to bruise easily and often develop subcutaneous hematomas, hemarthritis, and joint deformities. The most significant abnormality is a prolonged partial thromboplastin time (PTT). The bleeding time and prothrombin time will remain within normal limits. Genetic molecular testing techniques are used to characterize the nature of the defect and the extent of the disorder.

Common Coagulation Tests

Coagulation tests are useful in determining the cause of all disorders of hemostasis. The normal clotting time is between 5 and 10 minutes. When the clotting time is prolonged, there is a strong likelihood that there is a

Table 13–3
Reference Values for Selected Coagulation Tests

Test	*Reference Values*	
Bleeding time (Ivy)	1–8.5 min (average, 3–6 min)	
Platelet count	150,000–400,000/mm^3 (average, 250,000/mm^3)	
Platelet aggregation	Aggregation visible within <5 min	
Capillary fragility	Normal: <10 petechiae/2-in circle	
	Grade 1: 0–10 petechiae/2-in circle	
	Grade 2: 10–20 petechiae/2-in circle	
	Grade 3: 20–50 petechiae/2-in circle	
	Grade 4+: >50 petechiae/2-in circle	
Activated clotting time (ACT)	70–120 sec	
Partial thromboplastin time (PTT)	30–45 sec	
Prothrombin time	11.0–13.0 sec	
Thrombin time	7.0–12.0 sec	
Fibrinogen assay	200–400 mg/dL or 2.0–4.0 g/L	
Clot retraction	50% in 2 hr; 90% in 4 hr	
Factor assays		
Factor II	Extrinsic pathway	70–130 mg/100 mL
Factor V	Extrinsic pathway	70–130 mg/100 mL
Factor VII	Extrinsic pathway	70–150 mg/100 mL
Factor VIII	Intrinsic pathway	50–200 mg/100 mL
Factor IX	Intrinsic pathway	70–130 mg/100 mL
Factor X	Extrinsic pathway	70–130 mg/100 mL

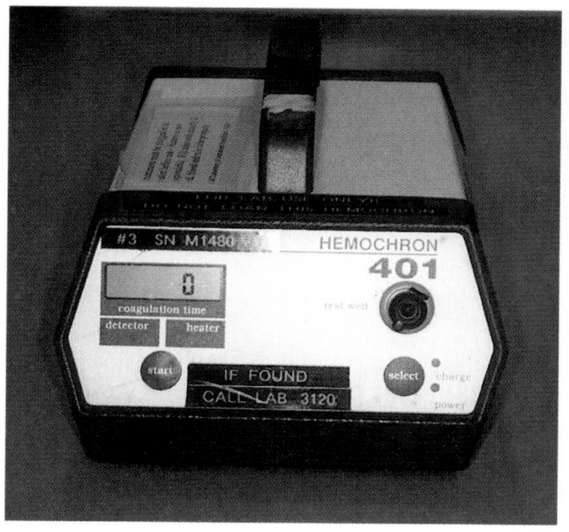

A

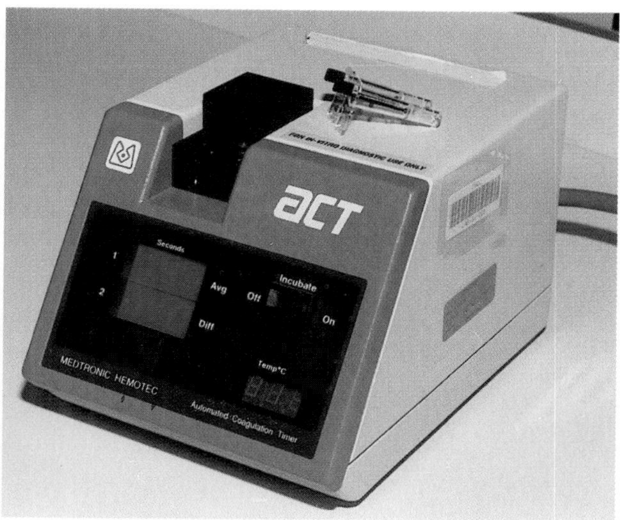

B

Figure 13–2. A, *Hemochron instrument for determining activated clotting time.* B, *Medtronic Hemotec instrument for determining activated clotting time.*

deficiency in one or more of the clotting factors, or in the intrinsic or common pathway (Table 13–3).

Prothrombin Time

The prothrombin time (PT) is one of the most common and important screening tests used in laboratory coagulation testing. PT directly measures defects in the clotting mechanism involving the coagulation factors by measuring prothrombin, factor V, fibrinogen, factor VII, and factor X. A PT test is usually ordered to monitor sodium warfarin (Coumadin) anticoagulant therapy, as well. Prothrombin is produced in the liver and is vitamin K–dependent. In patients with liver disease, the prothrombin content of the blood will be increased. Reference ranges for PT are usually established by each laboratory. However, typically, PT (also called protime) values range from 11 to 14 seconds. A PT test is performed by adding tissue thromboplastin to the patient's plasma. Calcium is then added to initiate coagulation. The PT, which is the time elapsed from the initiation of coagulation until the appearance of fibrin strands, is measured and compared to a control.

Partial Thromboplastin Time

Partial thromboplastin time (PTT) is based on the time required for fibrin clot formation in a glass tube. PTT determinations are used to monitor heparin therapy and to measure the factors of the common pathway. Typical reference ranges for PTT are 30 to 45 seconds.

Activated Coagulation Time

The activated coagulation (clotting) time (ACT) test screens for coagulation deficiencies using whole blood. It is also used to monitor heparin therapy. The ACT test is a bedside test that must be performed by a medical technologist. Reference ranges are typically between 70 and 120 seconds.

The Hemochron is a battery-operated device designed to perform the whole blood ACT test in vitro at any patient location (Fig. 13–2). The Hemochron clot detection mechanism consists of a precision-aligned magnet within a test tube and a magnetic detector located within the test well. When a test tube is inserted into the well, the magnetic detector senses a magnet within the test tube as the tube slowly rotates. When the clot begins to form, it causes the magnet to lift within the tube. Because the magnet has been displaced, it is no longer detected by the instrument's magnetic detector. At that point, the instrument gives an audible beep and displays the ACT.

PROCEDURE 13–2

Performing the Activated Clotting Time: Hemochron Method

Principle

To achieve proficiency in performing and reporting ACT testing using the Hemochron

Equipment and Supplies

Hemochron blood coagulation timing instrument and blood coagulation test tubes (CA 510 black rubber stopper)
5-mL syringe mot siliconized and nonheparinized Syringe needle, 21- or 23-gauge (A vacutainer may NOT be used.)
tourniquet
alcohol preps
bandaids
timing device
gloves and goggles or face mask
biohazard waste container

Procedural Steps

1. Wash hands and put on safety equipment and gloves.
2. Assemble needed equipment and supplies.
3. Explain the procedure to the patient.
4. Depress the "pre-warm" button on the Hemochron instrument to pre-warm the test well for 3 seconds. **The test well will warm to and maintain 37°C for 5 minutes.**
5. Perform venipuncture as quickly as possible.
6. Inject exactly 2.0 mL of blood into the Hemochron tube.
7. Press the "start" button.
8. Agitate the Hemochron test tubes vigorously from end to end 10 times to disperse activator.
9. Insert the ACT tube in the Hemochron test well.
10. Gently rotate the tube clockwise until the green "detector" light is illuminated.
11. Continue to rotate the ACT tube one more full turn after the green detector light comes on.
12. The end of the test is signalled by an audible tone.
13. Read the ACT tube (in seconds) at the conclusion of the test.
14. Record and report the test results.
15. Clean the work area and return the equipment to proper storage.
16. Remove safety equipment and wash hands.

Bleeding Times

Bleeding times are determined in the laboratory to measure constriction of the vascular wall and platelet function, as well as the interaction of these mechanisms, which are both involved in the formation of the platelet plug. A bleeding time is defined as the time it takes for a standardized skin wound to stop bleeding. Upon vessel injury, platelets adhere and form a hemostatic platelet plug. Bleeding time measures the ability of these platelets to arrest bleeding and, therefore, measures platelet number and function. Bleeding times may be slightly affected by capillary contractibility, as well as disorders of the intrinsic and the extrinsic pathways. Bleeding time determination is a screening procedure used to asses **in vivo** platelet function.

Bleeding times are significant indicators in patients with vascular abnormalities. The two most commonly used bleeding tests are the Ivy bleeding time test and the Duke bleeding time test.

Ivy Bleeding Time Test

In the Ivy bleeding time test, a vessel-free area below the antecubital space on the forearm is cleansed with alcohol and allowed to dry. A blood pressure cuff is then placed on the arm, above the elbow, and inflated to 40 mm Hg. Avoiding surface vessels, scars, bruises, and **edematous** areas, an incision is then made in the cleansed area of the forearm using a Surgicutt bleeding time device (Fig. 13–3*A*). The bleeding time device makes an incision that measures 5 mm long and 1 mm deep (Fig. 13–3*B*). A stopwatch is started at the time of incision. After 30 seconds, the flow of blood is blotted with filter paper (Fig. 13–3*C*). It is important not to touch the filter paper directly to the incision, so as not to disturb the formation of the platelet plug. The incisional area is blotted every 30 seconds thereafter until blood no longer stains the paper. Once the blood no longer stains the paper, the stopwatch is stopped. The blood pressure cuff is then removed, and a hypoallergenic bandage is applied to the site. In normal patients, the Ivy bleeding time is between 1 and 8.5 minutes.

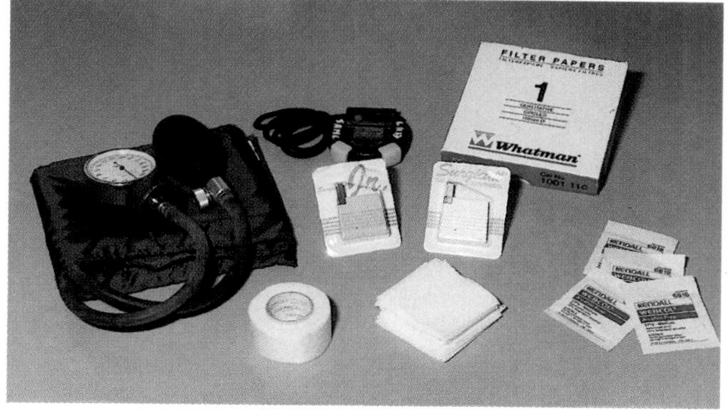

A

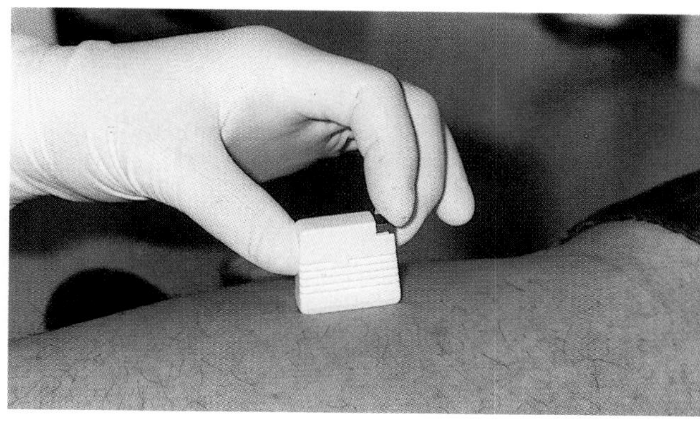

B

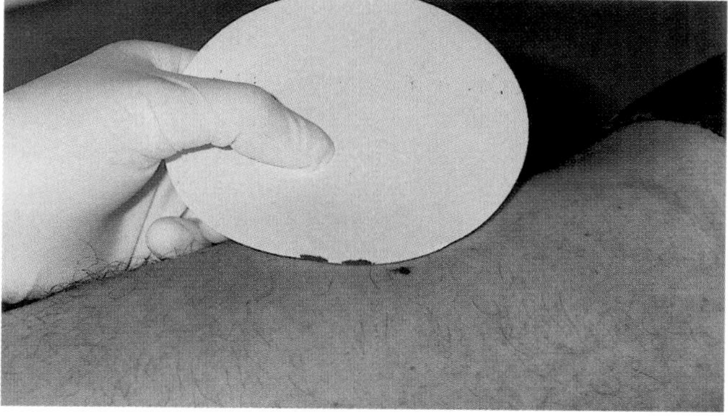

C

Figure 13–3. A, *Surgicutt bleeding time device.* B, *Incision with Surgicutt device.* C, *Blotting with filter paper.*

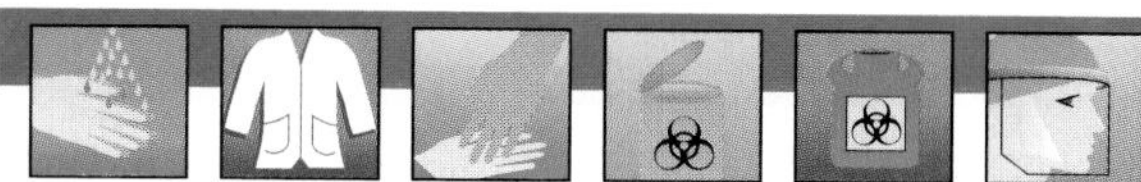

PROCEDURE 13–3

Ivy Bleeding Time Test (Surgicutt)

Principle

To understand the need for and become familiar with IVY bleeding time tests

Note: This test may not be performed by a medical/laboratory assistant in all states. Check your state protocols. If an assistant cannot perform the test, a laboratory technologist can perform the procedure while the student observes.

Equipment and Supplies

sphygmomanometer
stopwatch with readout of seconds
filter paper disk, Whatman #1
alcohol sponge
butterfly bandage or Steri-strip (sterile)
disposable razor
Surgicutt instrument

Patient Preparation

Instruct the patient not to take aspirin or aspirin-containing drugs for 1 week prior to testing. If this is not possible, notify the physician for testing recommendation.

Procedural Steps

1. Wash hands and put on gloves.
2. Assemble necessary equipment.
3. Check the patient's platelet count. If it is less than 40,000, DO NOT perform the bleeding time test. Notify the physician.

(continued)

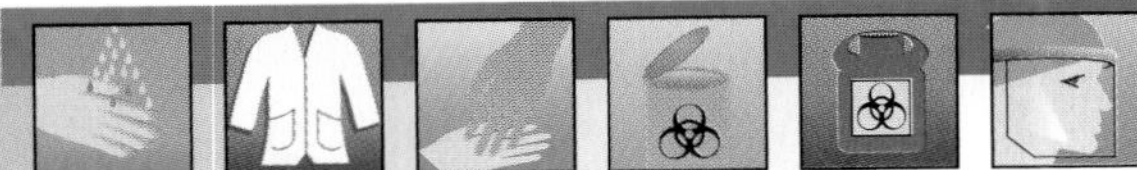

PROCEDURE 13–3

Ivy Bleeding Time Test (Surgicutt) (Continued)

4. Explain the procedure to the patient.
5. Seat the patient so that one arm rests on a steady support with the forearm surface exposed.
6. Taking care to avoid surface veins, scars, and bruises, select an area on the forearm distal to the antecubital fossa. If the patient has a considerable amount of hair, lightly shave the area.
7. Place a sphygmomanometer cuff on the upper arm.
8. Cleanse the area with an alcohol sponge and allow it to air dry for at least 30 seconds.
9. Remove the Surgicutt from the blister pack, being careful not to contaminate the instrument by touching it.
10. Remove the safety clip. **DO NOT PUSH THE TRIGGER OR TOUCH THE BLADE SLOT.**
11. Inflate the sphygmomanometer cuff to 40 mm Hg.
12. Allow 45 seconds to elapse.
13. Gently rest the Surgicutt on the patient's forearm and apply minimal pressure so that both ends of the instrument are lightly touching the skin.
14. Make a horizontal incision approximately 5 cm below and parallel to the antecubital crease.
15. Depress the trigger of the Surgicutt and simultaneously start the timer.
16. Remove the Surgicutt IMMEDIATELY after triggering.
17. After 30 seconds, bring the filter paper close to the incision, without touching the edges of the wound, and blot the area.
18. Blot every 30 seconds using the same technique until blood no longer stains the filter paper.
19. Stop the timer.
20. Remove the cuff, clean the arm, and apply butterfly bandages or Steri-strips, bringing the edges of the cut together to prevent scar formation.
21. Cover the incision with a Band-Aid. Inform the patient that the bandage should be kept in place for 24 hours and that a faint scar may occur.
22. Record the bleeding time to the nearest 30 seconds. (Report the results in minutes.)
23. Return the Surgicutt to the opened blister pack and discard in a biohazard sharps container.
24. Clean the area and equipment and return the equipment to the proper storage area.
25. Remove safety equipment and wash your hands.

Normal Range

Expected Range: 1–8.5 minutes.

Duke Bleeding Time Test

In the Duke bleeding time test, the site of puncture is the highly vascularized earlobe. After cleansing the earlobe with alcohol, a sterile lancet, or Hemolet, is used to puncture the earlobe. A stopwatch is started when the first drop of blood first appears. The earlobe is then allowed to bleed freely, with the blood being blotted every 30 seconds with filter paper, until all bleeding has stopped. As with the Ivy bleeding time test, care should be taken not to disturb the platelet plug. Normally, patients have a Duke bleeding time of between 1 and 3 minutes.

Bleeding times may be prolonged when there is a quantitative or qualitative platelet abnormality. Bleeding time abnormalities may also occur when there are defects or abnormalities in the capillaries and small blood vessels.

Coagulation Test Performance

All coagulation tests are difficult to perform and should only be attempted by medical technologists or, when allowed, by competent laboratory technicians/assistants. In addition to the tests just described, some laboratories may perform thrombin time tests. Thrombin times are often determined to monitor streptokinase and heparin therapy. Fibrinogen studies are often done in combination with other coagulation tests, particularly when abnormal test results have previously been obtained. The quantity of platelets is best determined by a platelet count. However, when there is some question about the quality or functional ability of the platelets, a clot retraction evaluation may be helpful. Clot retraction provides an estimate of both platelet quantity and quality. Normally, clot retraction is normal and complete when approximately half the total vol-

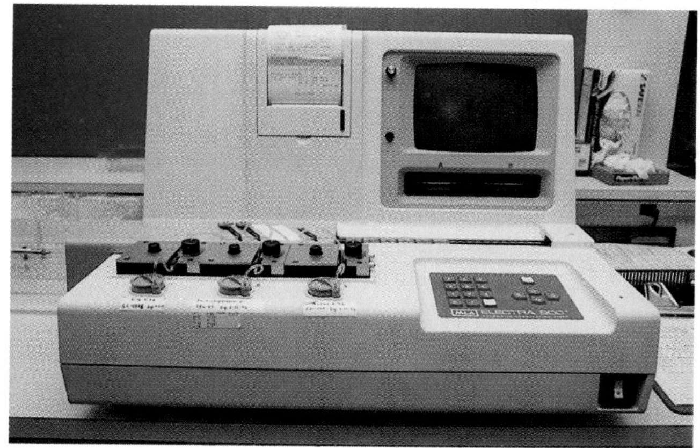

A

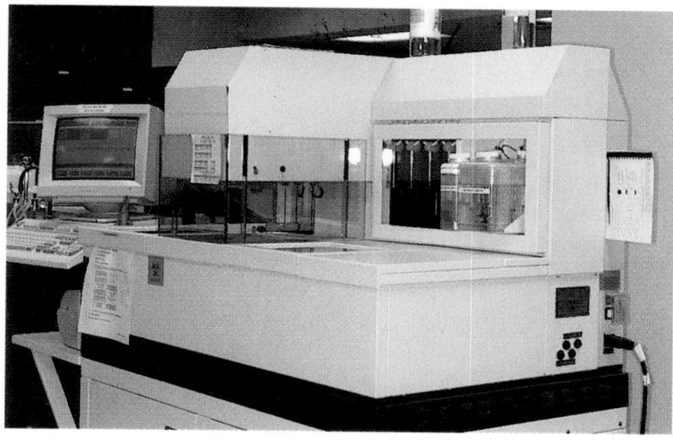

B

Figure 13–4. A, *An MLA Electra 900 device used for automated coagulation testing.* B, *Automated coagulation instrument (Organon MDA).*

ume of the blood is clot and half the total volume of the blood is serum. This complete retraction usually occurs within 4 to 24 hours. Decreased or defective clot retraction is often seen in patients with abnormal platelet quantity or quality. Prolonged clot retraction may be observed in patients with severe anemia. It is important to note that, when there is increased fibrinolysis, clot retraction may be normal but will appear to be decreased. This is because of the rapid destruction of the clot as a result of increased fibrinolysis.

Coagulation Studies

Coagulation studies, such as PT, PTT, thrombin time, and fibrinogen time determinations, are used to detect disorders of coagulation factors I, II, V, VII, and X. They are also useful in monitoring oral Coumadin anticoagulant therapy. These tests may be performed using automated equipment, such as the MLA, Electra 900 automated coagulation instrument (Fig. 13–4). Plasma from blood drawn in a blue-top tube (citrate) is needed for these tests. Bleeding time and clot retraction tests are performed manually. Before the advent of automation, coagulation studies, such as PT, PTT, thrombin time, and fibrinogen time were done manually using a tilt-tube method. The tests were performed using small test tubes that were tilted at timed intervals until the first appearance of a clot. Manual coagulation studies are rarely performed today and should only be attempted by highly trained and qualified medical laboratory personnel. Some laboratories have continued to use semi-automated procedures for coagulation studies, such as those involving the **fibrometer. Always check your laboratory procedure manual to determine the protocols established for the laboratory in which you are employed.**

Coagulation Abnormalities

Abnormalities of coagulation may be difficult to diagnose and may have serious consequences. In DIC, uncontrolled bleeding is caused by numerous abnormalities in hemostasis. DIC is a syndrome characterized by the massive depletion of coagulation factors, resulting in uncontrolled bleeding. DIC may be the result of a transfusion reaction, trauma, **diastema,** or cancer. The underlying condition or disease must be treated for DIC to be effectively managed. Heparin anticoagulant therapy is usually the preferred treatment for controlling bleeding secondary to DIC. Thrombin formation is halted by heparin, which blocks the activation and depletion of other clotting factors.

Summary

Coagulation or clotting involves the conversion of fibrinogen to fibrin. The mechanism for coagulation has been described. It is sufficient to note that coagulation can be initiated by clotting factors derived from either blood or damaged tissue. Antithrombin III and its cofactor heparin are naturally occurring anticoagulants, and the constant bathing of the area by a flow of blood prevents excessive accumulation of clotting factors.

It is important for you to understand the delicate balance of these clotting factors in the human body. When performing an analysis of clotting factors, precision and attention to detail are extremely important. Even a small deviation in the testing procedure may cause erroneous results.

The importance of this finely balanced hemeostatic mechanism has led to much research into the coagulation mechanism, the properties of platelets, and precision testing procedures.

Always check with your state and local laboratory guidelines to be certain that you can legally perform the tests discussed in this chapter.

Chapter Review

True or False

Circle T or F to indicate the correct answers to the following:

T F 1. A foreign object circulating in the blood is called an embolus.

T F 2. The clumping or clustering of blood cells is called edema.

T F 3. Fibrinolysis is part of the complex process of hemostasis.

T F 4. The reference range for PTT is 30 to 45 seconds.

T F 5. Coagulation or clotting involves the conversion of thrombin to prothrombin.

Fill in the Blanks

Complete the following statements:

6. Three common coagulation factors are ______________, ______________, and ______________.

7. Vasoconstriction is the first mechanism in maintaining ______________.

8. Prothrombin (Factor II) is a plasma protein that is ______________ dependent.

9. Abnormalities in hemostasis may be either ______________ or ______________.

Multiple Choice

Circle the letter that represents the single best answer:

10. Most coagulation factors are produced by the:
    a. Bone marrow
    b. Liver
    c. Kidney
    d. Lymph system
    e. Plasma
11. The most common cause of an abnormality in hemostasis is:
    a. Hemorrhage
    b. Erythrocyte deficiency
    c. Leukemia
    d. Platelet deficiency
    e. Thrombocytopenia
12. When performing the Ivy bleeding time test, inflate the blood pressure cuff to:
    a. 40 mm Hg
    b. 100 mm Hg
    c. 140 mm Hg
    d. 160 mm Hg
    e. Never use a blood pressure cuff

Unit IV
Clinical Chemistry

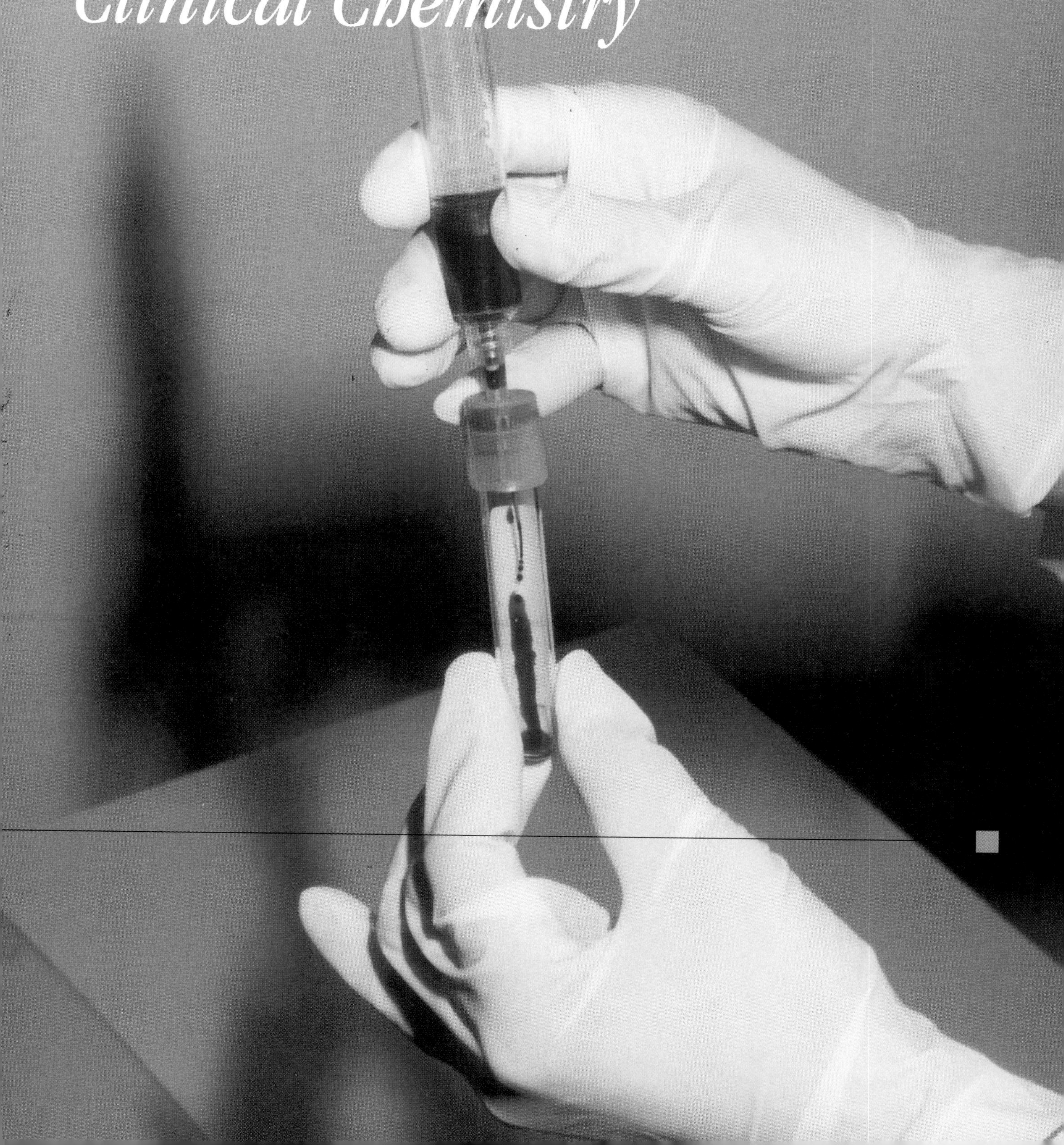

Vocabulary

aerosols: nebulized particles suspended in a gas or air

aliquot: a sample that is representative of the whole

anaerobic: absence of air and oxygen

analytes: any component in blood or other body fluid that can be measured

bilirubin: an orange bile pigment produced by the breakdown of heme

diurnal variation: normal variation in blood cells in the body throughout a 24-hour period

feces: body waste discharged from the large intestine

heme: the nonprotein, insoluble, iron protoporphyrin constituent of hemoglobin

hemolytic: capable of breaking down red blood cells

homeostasis: the maintenance of relatively constant conditions in the body's internal environment

hyperlipidemia: abnormally high level of fat in the blood

icterus: jaundice caused by a high level of bilirubin

inversion: the reversal of the normal position of the specimen

myocardial infarction: death of all or part of the heart muscle

opaque: neither translucent nor transparent; impervious to light

serum: liquid portion of coagulated blood

supernatant: the liquid lying above the insoluble cell layer

synovial fluid: the transparent viscid fluid found in joint cavities, bursae, and tendon sheaths

turbid: cloudy, not clear

Chapter Objectives

After reading this chapter, you should be able to:

1. Define the vocabulary words.
2. List the eight human fluids that may be used in chemical analysis.
3. Identify the three substances most frequently measured in the physician's laboratory.
4. Give the ideal temperature for refrigerators and freezers used in specimen storage.
5. Indicate the tube-top color that is appropriate for collecting blood for serum analysis, for plasma, and for whole blood.
6. Explain why a lavender-top tube is not used for plasma chemical analysis.
7. Describe the abnormal appearance of serum or plasma and indicate the probable cause.
8. List the materials and equipment needed when a urine chemistry is ordered.
9. Describe the regimen for a 24-hour urine collection.
10. Indicate the urine chemistries that can be run on a random urine specimen.
11. Specify the reasons for recording the time of collection on all specimens.
12. Explain the meaning of "panic results," and describe the manner in which such results are handled.

Chapter 14
Introduction to Clinical Chemistry

Clinical chemistry is the study and analysis of the chemical constituents in the human body. In the healthy human body, regulatory mechanisms monitor and adjust internal conditions to maintain a constant balance or equilibrium. This constant internal balance, regardless of external changes, is called **homeostasis,** a Greek word meaning "staying the same."

A healthy person, for instance, will maintain an approximate body temperature of 98.6°F (37°C) whether sunbathing on a tropical island or trekking over a polar ice cap. Likewise, the body's salt balance and blood glucose level remain within normal limits regardless of diet.

When this delicate balance is challenged, the body's reaction is characterized by abnormal elevations or decreases in various chemical constituents. It is the study of these **analytes** that aids the clinician in assessing a patient's status.

Chemical analyses may be performed on any fluid found in the body, such as blood, urine, cerebrospinal fluid (CSF), **synovial fluid,** pleural fluid, pericardial fluid, gastric contents, or **feces.** The substances most frequently measured in the physician's laboratory are usually part of the basic assessment of body metabolism. These substances include carbohydrates, lipids, and proteins.

Chemistry Panels

Chemistry tests are frequently ordered in "panels" (Fig. 14–1). A panel is a group of tests designed to evaluate several body systems simultaneously. In using the panel, the physician is able to get a better idea of what is happening to the patient, and the multiple tests provide a much better overview of the patient's general health. Although panels involve multiple tests, they require only a small amount of blood (Fig. 14–2).

Different laboratories may use different measuring instruments, which can cause slight variations in the normal chemistry ranges. Always use the

PHYSICIAN'S MEDICAL CENTER
77332 E. CAPITAL DRIVE
ANYTOWN, USA 11123

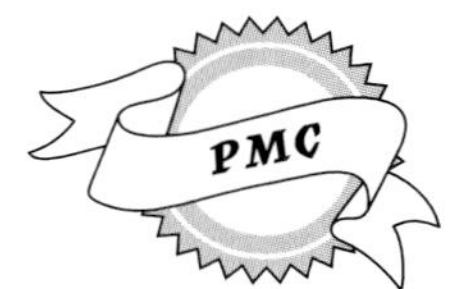

Ronald J. Haldor M.D.
Kaye M. Jones M.D.
Nicholas C. Stepp M.D.

PATIENT – PLEASE NOTE

☐

If this box is checked, don't eat or drink anything, except water, for 14 hours before going to the lab.

PATIENT NAME ______ LAST ______ FIRST ______ M.I.

ADDRESS ______ DOB ______

CITY ______ STATE ______ ZIP ______ SEX: M F

TELEPHONE # ______ SOCIAL SECURITY # ___ – ___ – ___

ORDERING PHYSICIAN ______ DATE ______

BILLING: ☐ HMO ☐ MEDICARE ☐ MEDI-CAL ☐ OTHER # ______
(Please attach copy of eligibilty card.)

GUARANTOR (If other than patient) ______

☐ PHONE RESULTS TO ______

☐ SEND ADDITIONAL COPIES OF REPORT TO ______

Patient Diagnosis ______

☐ 906 ARTERIAL BLOOD GASES
ROOM AIR ______
RESP. ASSIST ______
☐ 105 BLOOD CELL PROFILE (Hgb + Hct)
☐ 862 BILIRUBIN (NEONATAL)
☐ 868 BILIRUBIN (TOTAL & DIRECT)
☐ 100 CBC (Complete Blood Count & Diff)
☐ 3000 ELECTROLYTES
☐ (NA, K, CO2, Cl)
☐ FANA
☐ GLUCOSE
☐ 915 GLUCOSE, PRE-NATAL DIABETIC SCR.
(1 Hour Post-Glucola)
☐ GLUCOSE TOLERANCE TEST
OF HOURS ______ DOSE ______
☐ 3398 HEPATITIS PANEL
(B-Surf Ag/Ab, B-Core Ab, A-Ab)
☐ 988 LIPID PROFILE
(Chol, Trig, HDL, LDL, Cardiac Risk)
☐ 3380 LIVER PANEL
(Alk Phos, Bili, TP, Alb, GGT, SGOT (AST) SGPT (ALT), & Consult)
☐ 3006 METABOLIC 7
(Na, K, CO2, Cl, Glu, Mg)

☐ 3035 PANEL 17
(Panel 13 + Na + K + Cl + CO2)
☐ 3020 METABOLIC 10
(Na, K, CO2, Cl, Glu, BUN, Creat)
☐ 3015 METABOLIC 11
(Met 10 & Phos)
☐ 3160 OBSTETRICAL PANEL 1
(CBC, UA, ABO/Rh, Antibody Screen, Rubella, RPR)
☐ 3172 OBSTETRICAL PANEL 3
(CBC, ABO/Rh, Antibody Screen, Rubella, RPR)
☐ 3445 OBSTETRICAL PANEL 7
(ABO/Rh, Antibody Screen, Rubella, RPR)
☐ 3447 OBSTETRICAL PANEL 7A
(ABO/Rh, Antibody Screen, Rubella, RPR, Hepatitis B Surt Ag)
☐ 3025 PANEL 13
(Glu, BUN, Creat, Uric Acid, Ca, Tp, Alb, Bili, Chol, Alk, Phos, SGOT (AST), LDH, Phos)
☐ 3030 PANEL 15
(Panel 13 + Na + K)

☐ 3010 METABOLIC 8
(Na, K, CO2, Cl, Glu, BUN)
☐ 3040 PANEL 20 - SMAC
(Panel 17 + SGPT (ALT) + GGT + Osmolality)
☐ 3043 S-1 Panel (Panel 20 + Triglyceride)
☐ 500 PROTHROMBIN TIME (PT)
☐ 505 Partial Thromboplastin Time (PPT)
☐ 7500 RPR
☐ 7515 RUBELLA
☐ 2030 THYROID SCREEN
(T4, T3, Uptake, Adj T4)
☐ 704 URINALYSIS

BACTERIOLOGY

SPECIMEN SOURCE **(REQUIRED)**
______
COLLECTION DATE ______
☐ ______ ROUTINE CULTURE
☐ 8919 AFB CULTURE
☐ 8921 FUNGAL CULTURE

ADDITIONAL LABORATORY TESTS:

LABORATORY OUTPATIENT REQUEST

2804 (4/93)

OFFICE USE ONLY

Telephone Order per ______

Order Received by ______

Figure 14–1. *Panel request form.*

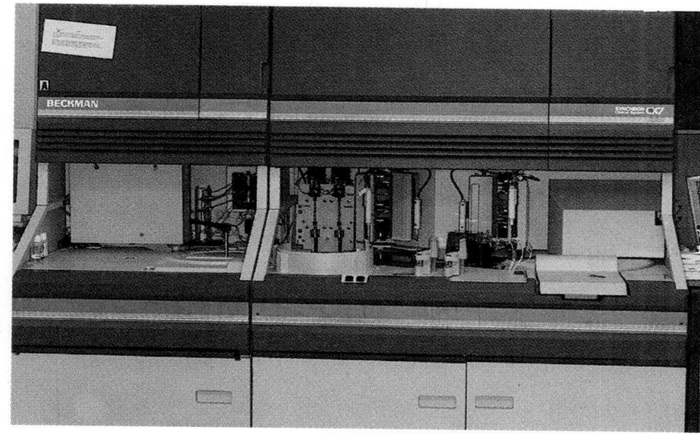

Figure 14–2. *Automated equipment for chemistry panels.*

ranges recommended by the testing laboratory or the equipment manufacturer (Fig. 14–3). It is also wise to remember that, because of rapid advances in technology and research concerning the body, both in health and disease, it is impossible to remain current in all aspects of clinical chemistry. Therefore, all personnel should use testing guides and manuals to ensure that the tests are performed correctly and the results are reported according to the guidelines outlined.

Blood Specimen Requirements

It is important to remember that a laboratory result is only as good as the specimen sent to be tested. Some of the chemicals to be tested may continue to break down, even after collection. For this reason, it is extremely important to follow **ALL** of the guidelines for collecting and preserving the specimen. In the balance of the chapters in this unit, you will be given these guidelines as they apply to each test.

SUPPLIES AND EQUIPMENT

Equipment Required for Collecting Blood Specimens

- Vacutainers:
  - Red-top or tiger-top tube for coagulated blood
  - Green-top tube (lithium heparin) for uncoagulated blood
  - Dark blue–top tube (specialty tube for trace metals)
  - Grey-top tube (fluoride) used for blood glucose or blood alcohol (optional)
- Syringe and needle (optional)
- Aliquot vial/tube
- Stoppered tubes for serum or plasma (SST Tube)
- Labeling tape for patient identification
- Centrifuge capable of speeds of 2000 rpm to 3500 rpm. The ground and speed must be verified and documented biannually by the facility's engineers.
- Refrigerator for specimen storage. The refrigerator temperature must be monitored, and the results documented daily. The ideal temperature is 4°C (allowable limits: 2°–8°C).
- Freezer for specimen storage. The freezer temperature must be monitored, and the results documented daily. The ideal temperature is –20°C (allowable limits: –15° to –25°C).
- Personal safety equipment. Disposable latex gloves, eye protection, and laboratory coats must be worn when handling all laboratory specimens. In special circumstances, it may be necessary to wear a mask for protection against **aerosols.**

Fluid Collection

Serum

Most chemical procedures are performed on **serum.** Blood is drawn from the patient into a red- or tiger-top Vacutainer tube, or with a syringe and needle, after which the sample is carefully transferred to a clean culture tube. Most tiger-top tubes now contain a clot activator, which requires gentle **inversion** two or three times, after which the tube is allowed to stand. The blood should be allowed to stand undisturbed for 15 to 30 minutes at room temperature to allow for a solid clot formation. The sample is then centrifuged at 2500 rpm to 3500 rpm for 5 or 10 minutes, which results in separation of the clear **supernatant** from the clot (Fig.

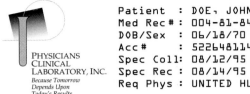

PHYSICIANS CLINICAL LABORATORY, INC.
1925 E Oregon Avenue, Our Town, US 65432 FINAL
(800)000-0000
Ronald B. Woodman M.D., Medical Director

32497
To:UNITED HLTH CENTER—HEALTH FAIRE
1925 Oregon Ave.
Our Town, US 65432

Patient : DOE, JOHN
Med Rec # : 004-81-8408
DOB/Sex : 06/18/70 25 YRS MALE
Acc # : 5226481140 Non-Fasting
Spec Coll: 08/12/95 Loc: CV01
Spec Rec : 08/14/95
Req Phys : UNITED HLTH CENTER - HEAL

LOCATION	TEST	RESULTS WITHIN RANGE	RESULTS OUT OF RANGE	REFERENCE RANGE	UNITS
	— CHEMISTRY —				
C	Chemistry Panel				
	Glucose	94		70-110	mg/dL
	Sodium	138		135-145	mmol/L
	Potassium	4.6		3.5-5.1	mmol/L
	Chloride	100		98-110	mmol/L
	BUN	18		7-22	mg/dL
	Creatinine	1.2		0.5-1.5	mg/dL
	BUN/Creat Ratio	15		8-24	Ratio
	Uric Acid	7.1		3.5-7.2	mg/dL
	Bili, Total	0.7		0.2-1.2	mg/dL
	GGT		55 H	11-51	IU/L
	AST (SGOT)	16		0-40	IU/L
	ALT (SGPT)	24		0-45	IU/L
	LD	146		100-210	IU/L
	Alkaline Phos	67		31-102	IU/L
	Calcium	10.0		8.6-10.1	mg/dL
	Phosphorus	3.5		2.5-4.6	mg/dL
	Total Protein	7.4		6.0-8.0	g/dL
	Albumin	4.9		3.5-5.0	g/dL
	Globulin	2.5		1.5-4.0	g/dL
	A/G Ratio	2.0			
	Iron	126		65-175	ug/dL
	Cholesterol		239 H	0-200	mg/dL
	Triglyceride	115		10-140	mg/dL
C	HDL	51		30-85	mg/dL
C	CHOL + LDL Group				
	CHOL/HDL Ratio	4.7			mg/dL
				Male / Female	
	1/2 Average Risk			3.4 / 3.3	
	Average Risk			5.0 / 4.4	
	2x Average Risk			10.0 / 7.0	
	3x Average Risk			24.0 / 11.0	
	LDL		165 H	0-130	mg/dL

Printed: 08/15/95 8:02AM

Figure 14–3. *Test result form showing normal ranges and results.*

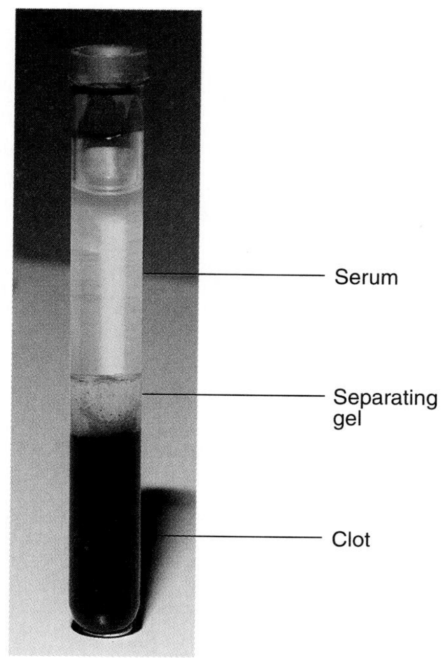

Figure 14–4. *Centrifugation separates supernatant from clot.*

14–4). The serum is then transferred, using a Pasteur pipette, to a clean sample tube. All patient information on the label from the original tube must be transferred to the sample tube. It is at this point that most specimen misidentification occurs. **Always double check the patient information for total accuracy.**

Plasma

Heparinized plasma may be used for most chemical analyses. Plasma is the fluid portion of uncoagulated blood. Heparin is an anticoagulant used to prevent blood from clotting. Vacutainer tubes labeled "lithium heparin" should be used, as sodium heparin is unsuitable for routine chemical procedures. Lavender-top Vacutainer tubes containing the anticoagulant ethylenediaminetetra-acetic acid (EDTA) are appropriate for hematologic or toxicologic testing, but unsuitable for most chemical procedures.

Blood is drawn from the patient into a green-top Vacutainer tube containing heparin, or it is drawn with a needle and syringe and transferred to a heparinized tube. In either case, the tube is gently inverted six times to ensure that the blood is adequately mixed with anticoagulant (Fig. 14–5). If the blood is to be transported, place it in the designated area for pick-up. If testing is done on site, centrifuge the specimen for 5 minutes. Remove the clear supernatant from the specimen with a Pasteur pipette and place it in a sample

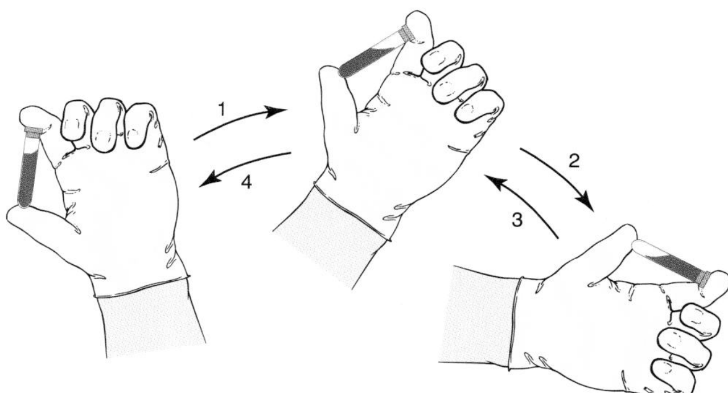

Figure 14–5. *Inversion technique.*

container. Transfer all patient information on the label from the original tube to the sample tube, and double check the label for accuracy.

The advantage of plasma over serum is speed, as the sample may be processed immediately. This is a prerequisite for stat or emergency room laboratory requests.

Whole Blood

Whole blood is heparinized blood that is unclotted and unseparated. The blood is drawn from the patient into a green-top tube containing heparin, and gently inverted to mix. No further handling is indicated. Whole blood is used for tests such as arterial blood gas determinations.

Arterial Blood

Specimen collection and handling are very important in the analysis of arterial blood gases. For arterial blood studies, blood collection is **anaerobic,** using a plastic syringe and needle (no Vacutainer). Liquid heparin is the anticoagulant of choice, and no tourniquet is used. The specimen must be kept on ice, be free of clots and air bubbles, and be delivered promptly to the laboratory for testing (Fig. 14–6).

Arterial blood procedures vary slightly according to the method used to obtain the sample. Specialized training is required to draw arterial specimens, and such procedures should not be attempted unless this training is completed. In addition, not all states allow the medical or laboratory assistant to perform arterial procedures. Check your state and laboratory regulations and protocols regarding eligibility to perform arterial techniques.

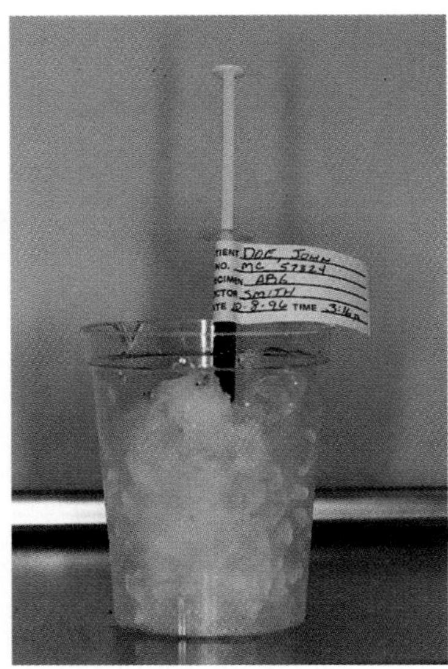

Figure 14–6. *Arterial blood is readied for transport to a laboratory.*

Specimen Appearance

The normal appearance of serum or plasma is a clear, pale yellow color (Fig. 14–7, #1). The appearance of serum or plasma may be altered artificially by improper collection or handling of a specimen, or by a disease state, such as **hyperlipidemia** or liver disease.

Hemolysis

Hemolysis is the destruction of red blood cells (RBCs) in the blood, which involves rupture of RBCs. The serum or plasma will have a pink or red appearance (Fig. 14–7, #2). This is usually caused by drawing the sample too slowly, inserting the needle only partially into a vein, or improper handling, such as allowing the sample to sit too long before centrifugation, excessive centrifugation, shaking, or freezing. The pink or red appearance may also be an indication of **hemolytic** disease. Hemolyzed blood is not suitable for most analyses. Certain substances, such as potassium and many enzymes, are released from the RBCs into the serum or plasma, causing false elevations of the test results.

Lipids

Lipids are fats, such as cholesterol, triglycerides, and other related compounds. Lipids are a good source of stored energy for the body and are used as structural materials in the cells. Hyperlipidemia will give the serum or plasma a milky or **turbid** appearance (Fig. 14–7, #4). Specimens collected shortly after eating may appear lipemic; however, lipemia may also be seen in patients with lipid metabolism disorders. Such specimens may require special treatment to remove the lipids before testing.

Icterus

Specimens from patients with **icterus** appear deep yellow to orange (Fig. 14–7, #3). This color change is attributable to elevations of **bilirubin** in liver disorders.

Pale Serum

Occasionally, serum or plasma will have a pale, watery appearance. This may be an indication of protein disorders and kidney disease.

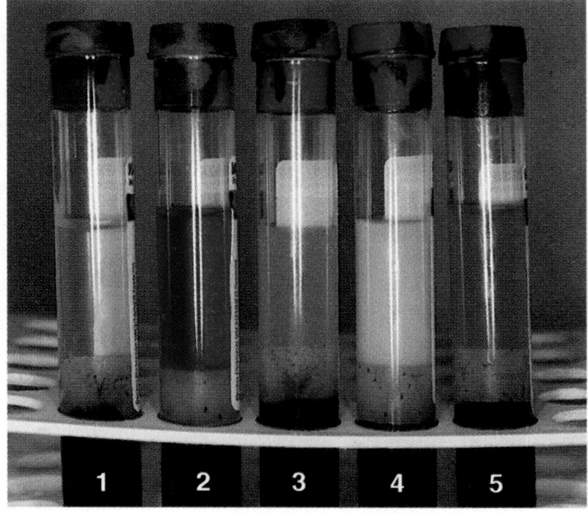

Figure 14–7. *The appearance of normal serum and various types of abnormal serum:* 1, *normal;* 2, *hemolyzed;* 3, *icteric;* 4, *lipemic;* 5, *bilirubin.*

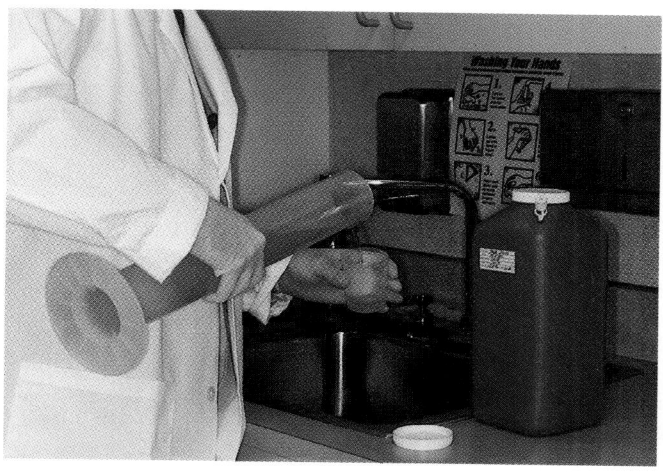

Figure 14–8. *Materials and equipment required for 24-hour urine collection.*

Green Serum

A definite green tint may be seen in serum or plasma (Fig. 14–7, #5). This is thought to be attributable to **heme** (a metal complex consisting of an iron atom in hemoglobin), which is released from the RBCs into the blood and which may be seen in patients with certain types of malignant disease.

Urine Specimen Requirements

Most urine chemistries done in the physician's office laboratory are performed with automated equipment and reagent strips. However, an outside laboratory is sometimes needed for testing. The outside laboratory usually provides a container (often plastic) to which a preservative has been added. The container should first be labeled, and the patient should be instructed to collect a urine specimen into a cup and then transfer it carefully into the laboratory container. If acid has been added to the container, this must be included on the label. **In such cases, you MUST instruct the patient not to touch the acid preservative, as it will burn the skin upon contact.**

When the specimen is brought to the office, it should be handled with caution. It is recommended that all urine specimens be treated as if they are infected and that Universal Precautions be observed.

Urine Specimen Collection

SUPPLIES AND EQUIPMENT

Equipment Required for Collecting Urine Specimens (Fig. 14–8)

- A 1-L (1000-mL) graduated cylinder for measuring urine output
- A 50- or 100-mL graduated cylinder for measuring the preservative
- Litmus or pH paper for verifying the pH of the urine specimen
- Urine collection containers (provided by the testing laboratory): 3-L (3000-mL) volume for 24-hour collections and 4-oz volume for random collections (e.g., for routine urinalysis)

Do not accept a specimen that has been collected in a container from home. Even trace amounts of a substance, such as pickle juice, in a collection jar will alter test results, making them unreliable.

Urine Preservatives

A 24-hour urine sample is required for most assays. For assays that require acidified urine, 20 to 30 mL of 6NHCl (6 normal hydrochloric acid) should be placed in the collection container so that the urine will be acidified as it is collected. The pH should remain between 1 and 2.

Some laboratories prefer using 30 gm of boric acid as a preservative, but the pH is not low enough for many assays, such as the urinary amine determinations. Table 14–1 lists the preservatives required for a number of urine tests.

If an alkaline specimen is required, sodium carbonate may be added to an **aliquot** after collection, as is done for some porphyrin assays. This test also requires that the specimen be protected from light. Most collection containers are an **opaque** brown, but the aliquot vial is not. Brown paper or foil wrapped around the vial provides sufficient protection (Fig. 14–9).

Some assays require no preservative; however, the urine should be kept refrigerated between excretions. Always indicate on the specimen label the preservative

Table 14–1
Summary of Urine Preservatives

Assays	*Collection Time*	*Refrigeration/ No preservative*	*Boric Acid*	*6NHCl*	*Freezing*	*Other*
Aldosterone	24 hr	–	A	–	P	pH 4
Amino acids	24 hr	A	–	30 mL	P	pH 3–5
Aminolevulinic acid (ALA)	24 hr	–	–	A	P	Protect from light
Amylase	2 hr	P	–	–	–	–
Arsenic	24 hr	–	–	20 mL	–	–
β_2-Microglobulin	Random/high diuresis	–	–	–	P	pH 6–8
Cadmium	24 hr	P	–	–	–	–
Calcium	24 hr	–	–	30 mL	–	pH <3
Catecholamines	24 hr	–	–	25 mL	P	pH 2–4
Chloride	24 hr	P	–	–	–	–
Chorionic gonadotropin (hCG)						First AM specimen
Qualitative	Random	P	A	–	–	
Chromium	Random	P	–	–	–	Acid-washed container
Citric acid	24 hr	A	10 gm	–	P	–
Creatinine	24 hr	P	A	A	A	–
Glucose	24 hr	–	1 gm	–	–	–
17-Ketosteroids	24 hr	A	1 gm	–	–	–
Lipase	24 hr	P	–	–	–	–
Magnesium	24 hr	–	–	25 mL	–	pH <2
Microalbumin	24 hr	P	–	–	–	–
Nitrogen	24 hr	–	–	P	–	pH <4
Osmolality	Random	A	–	–	P	–
Oxalate	24 hr	–	–	40 mL	–	pH 2–3
Porphyrins	24 hr	–	–	–	–	Protect from light
Potassium	24 hr	P	A	A	–	–
Protein	24 hr	P	–	–	–	–
Sodium	24 hr	P	A	A	–	–
Substance abuse panels	Random	P	–	–	A	–
Urea nitrogen	24 hr	A	10 gm	A	–	–
Uric acid	24 hr	A	–	–	–	5 gm of sodium carbonate
Urobilinogen	2 hr	–	–	–	P	Protect from light

P, preferred method of storage and/or collection; A, acceptable method of storage and/or collection; –, unacceptable or unproven method.

used, if any. Remember to caution the patient to avoid contact with skin.

When more than one assay requiring different preservatives is requested, urine must be collected on two separate days.

Urine Aliquot Containers

An aliquot of a specimen is a portion, a representative sample, of the whole. After the 24-hour urine specimen is mixed and measured, an aliquot of the specimen (approximately 50 to 100 mL) is poured into a smaller vial, labeled with the collection time period and the total volume, and sent to the laboratory for analysis (Fig. 14–10).

Urine Collection

Reliable test results are based on the accuracy of the urine collection method, use of the proper preserva-

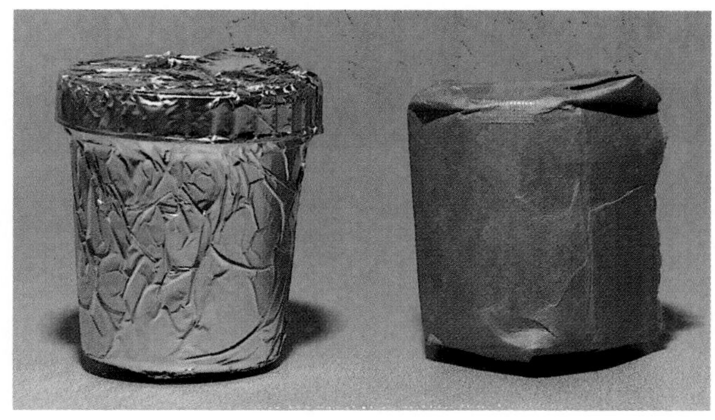

Figure 14–9. *Brown paper or aluminum foil may be used to protect the specimen from light.*

CENTRAL VALLEY MEDICAL CENTER

INSTRUCTIONS TO THE PATIENT
24 HOUR URINE COLLECTION
FOR VMA

Abstain from Coumadin, Tetracycline, aspirin, bananas, chocolate, caffeine, coffee, tea, vanilla, and foods with vanilla in them for one week prior to and during the 24-hour urine collection.

1. On the morning of the test, at 7:00 a.m., completely empty bladder. Discard this urine.
2. Collect all urine until the next morning at 7:00 a.m. (24 hours later) and pour into the provided container. Void at 7:00 a.m. and add this urine to the collection.
3. Be sure to pool all specimens into the container provided and refrigerate.
4. Bring the urine collection to the Lab immediately.
5. If you have any questions during the urine collection, call 449-3451 or 449-3120.
6. Please return this form with your urine collection.

PATIENT'S NAME: ______________________

HEIGHT: ____________ WEIGHT: ____________

URINE STARTED: DATE: ________ TIME: ________ AM PM

URINE ENDED: DATE: ________ TIME: ________ AM PM

7722 South Wisconsin Avenue, Chicago, Utah 56789

Figure 14–10. *Printed form of patient instructions.*

tive, appropriate storage, and accurate measurement of volume. As mentioned earlier, most urine assays are performed on 24-hour urine specimens. Printed instructions, indicating the proper method of collection, should be given to the patient or caregiver to increase compliance with the collection regimen.

Collection Regimen

A set of instructions should be given to the patient, such as the following:

1. Discard the first morning specimen on Day 1 and record the time.
2. Collect all specimens during the remainder of the day and night.
3. Collect the first morning specimen of Day 2 at the exact time the first morning specimen on Day 1 was discarded.

Label the collection container with pertinent patient information, the preservative used, and acid warnings if applicable. Ask the patient or caregiver to record the starting and ending date and time of the collection.

The urine collection should be sent to the laboratory as soon as possible. The specimen must then be well mixed by inversion. If an acidified specimen is required, check the pH using litmus or pH paper. Accurately measure the volume, using a graduated cylinder. Results are based on the 24-hour urine volume, so accurate measurement is critical. One aliquot must be poured into a specimen vial for analysis and another preserved for storage in the event that additional testing is indicated. Transfer all the information from the original collection container to the aliquot vial.

Urinary clearance tests require a body surface estimate. In such instances, the patient's height and weight must be included on the label.

PROCEDURE 14–1

Calculating Body Surface Area

Principle

To learn to calculate body surface mass using the nomogram

Equipment and Supplies

balance scale with measuring bar
pencil
paper
ruler

Procedural Steps

1. Remove your shoes.
2. Check to see that the balance barpointer points to the middle of the balance frame when all weights are at zero.
3. Step on the scale.
4. Move the large weight to the closest estimated weight.
5. Slide the small upper weight until the pointer balances to the center of the balance frame.
6. Read your weight from the scale.

Ask your laboratory partner to assist you in determining your height.

7. Stand up straight and look straight ahead.
8. Adjust the height bar so that it just touches the top of your head.
9. Step off the scale.
10. Record your weight and height from the scale.
11. Return weights and measuring bar to zero.

Calculating Body Surface Area

12. Using the nomogram for determination of body surface area, locate your height (in feet) on the lefthand scale and mark it.
13. Now locate your weight (in pounds) on the right-hand scale and mark it.
14. Using a ruler, draw a straight line across the nomogram from your height mark through the mark indicating your weight.
15. Using the surface area scale located in the center of the nomogram, locate the point on the scale where your height/weight lines intersect. This is your body surface area.
16. Record your body surface area.

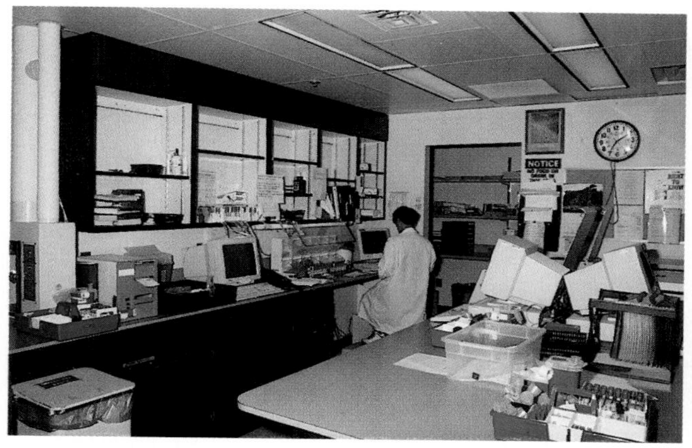
A

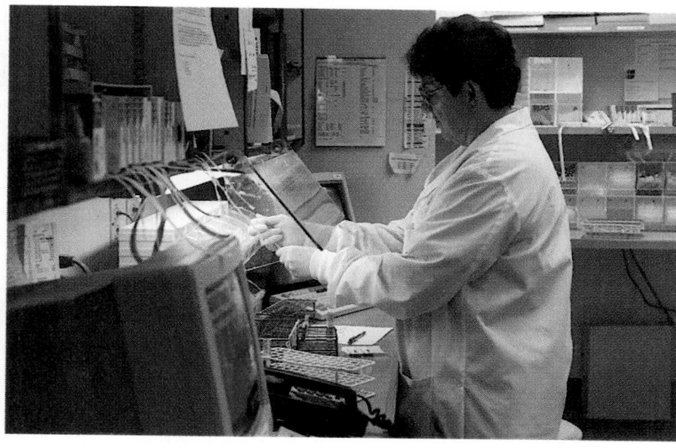
B

Figure 14–11. A, *Laboratory specimen processing area.* B, *A laboratory assistant processes a specimen behind a safety shield.*

A random urine specimen is a collection of urine from a single excretion. This type of sample is often used to test for urine glucose levels, either after fasting or at periodic intervals.

Refer to your laboratory's specimen collection manual for instructions on storage or shipping of specimens.

Specimen Storage

For most routine tests, specimens may be stored at room temperature for a few hours. If testing is to be delayed or performed elsewhere, however, refrigeration or freezing may be indicated. Refer to your laboratory's specimen collection procedure manual for appropriate storage instructions.

General Considerations

The importance of proper collection, handling, storage, and labeling of specimens cannot be overemphasized, as test results are dependent upon the integrity of the specimen (Fig. 14–11). Misdiagnoses have occurred, some with catastrophic results, owing to errors in collection or preservation procedure.

Diurnal Variations

Changes may occur in a specimen depending on the time of day it is collected. These are referred to as **diurnal variations.** Some analytes, such as the corticosteroids, exhibit different concentrations at various times of day. Other tests, such as cardiac enzyme tests (CK-MB and LD-1), may be performed at specified times for the diagnosis of **myocardial infarction.** It is essential that the time of collection be recorded for these assays; indeed, it is a good practice to record the time of collection on all specimens.

Given the current economic constraints under which laboratories operate, many assays are now being referred to reference laboratories. Always consult the reference laboratory's specimen requirements before collecting a specimen, and follow the guidelines exactly. Reliable test results can only be obtained if proper methods for specimen collection and handling are employed.

Reference Ranges

Reference ranges refer to the expected range of test results in a normal healthy population. A normal range has been established for each test. Test results below that range are considered to be decreased, whereas those that exceed that range are elevated; in both cases, they are considered to be abnormal.

Abnormal results that are life-threatening are called *panic results.* Panic levels require immediate attention by a physician. It is the responsibility of the laboratory to notify the physician promptly. If you are a medical laboratory employee and you attempt to phone in panic results but the physician is unavailable, the results may be conveyed to an assistant or a nurse employed by the physician. If this is done, record in the

Table 14–2
Chemistry Test Reference Ranges

Test	Infants	Children	Adults
Serum sodium (NA)	134–150 mEq/L	135–145 mEq/L	135–145 mEq/L
Serum potassium (K)	4.1–5.3 mEq/L	3.4–4.7 mEq/L	3.5–5.0 mEq/L
Serum chloride (Cl)	95–110 mEq/L	98–105 mEq/L	95–105 mEq/L
Serum calcium (Ca)	5.0–6.0 mEq/L	<6.0 mEq/L	4.5–5.5 mEq/L
Serum phosphorus (P)	4.5–6.7 mg/dL	4.5–5.5 mg/dL	2.4–4.7 mg/dL
Serum magnesium (Mg)	1.4–2.9 mEq/L	1.6–2.6 mEq/L	1.5–2.5 mEq/L
Serum glucose	30–60 mg/dL	60–105 mg/dL	70–110 mg/dL
Blood urea nitrogen (BUN)	4–18 mg/dL	5–18 mg/dL	6–20 mg/dL
Creatine	0.3–0.6 mg/dL	0.4–1.2 mg/dL	0.5–1.3 mg/dL
Uric Acid	—	2.5–5.5 mg/dL	2.7–8.5 mg/dL

This chart is only an example of chemistry test ranges. It is designed to illustrate the difference between the ranges in adults and children.

laboratory log the name of the person informed of the results, the date, and the time of day of the phone call.

Reference ranges (normal ranges) are often established on the basis of the sex or age of the patient (Table 14–2). Ranges for children are called pediatric ranges, and these are often very different from those appropriate for adults. Some institutions establish their own reference ranges based on their particular geographic region and population. Different test methods and instrumentation may yield dissimilar ranges, and, in some cases, may involve different units of measure.

When phoning test results to a physician or physician's office, always include the unit of measure and the reference range of the test that is appropriate for the patient in question.

Summary

Throughout this chapter, great emphasis has been placed on accuracy. The laboratory is an area that requires your constant attention to ensure that every collection is done correctly, safely, and in a timely manner. Remember, testing labs have precise specimen guidelines and thus may reject a testing sample that does not meet testing criteria. It is not only the patient who is relying on your precision, but also the physician, who must base treatment decisions on the test results provided.

Check Appendix A for rejection policy and procedure.

Chapter Review

True or False

Circle T or F to indicate the correct answers to the following:

T F 1. Homeostasis is considered your internal balance.

T F 2. The optimal temperature of a freezer used for laboratory specimens is between –25° and –35°C.

T F 3. A lavender-top tube is used for serum collection.

T F 4. EDTA is an anticoagulant.

T F 5. Hemoptesis is the destruction of RBCs in the blood.

Fill in the Blanks

Complete the following statements:

6. Two examples of lipids are ______________ and ______________ .

7. An icteric specimen will appear ______________ in color, which usually indicates an elevated ______________ .

8. All urine specimens should be treated as if they were ______________ .

Multiple Choice

Circle the letter that represents the single best answer:

9. If a 24-hour acidic urine specimen is collected, the following preservative should be added to the collection container:
   a. Sodium carbonate
   b. Boric acid
   c. Hydrochloric acid

   d. A and C
   e. B and C
10. When reporting "panic results" to a physician, you should always document:
   a. The name of the person to whom you reported the results
   b. The date and time you called
   c. The name of the person who witnessed your call
   d. A and B
   e. A, B, and C

Vocabulary

accuracy: an indication of how close the obtained answer or test result is to the true value
control: a serum solution with a known range for the serum being tested
critical measurement: a measurement in which accuracy is vitally important
estradiol: the most potent naturally occurring estrogen hormone in humans
leaching: separating soluble from insoluble matter by slowly running water over it
lyophilization: the creation of a stable preparation of a biologic substance by rapid freezing and dehydration of the frozen product under high vacuum
mean: average of all values in a set of numbers that are distributed equally on both sides of a symmetrical curve
meniscus: convex surface of a liquid in a tube or pipette
noncritical measurement: a measurement in which estimated accuracy is acceptable
precision: the extent to which a measurement yields the same results when repeated under identical conditions
quantitate: to measure or determine the quantity of mass
radiant: capable of emitting rays, such as light or heat
reliability: an indication of the reproducibility of a measurement
standard: a solution with an exact known value for the constituent being tested
TC: a pipette marking indicating *to contain*
TD: a pipette marking indicating *to deliver*

Chapter Objectives

After reading this chapter, you should be able to:

1. Identify the nine functional units in a chemical analyzer.
2. Write test results using the International System of Nomenclature.
3. List the six common methods of analysis in blood chemistry.
4. State Beer's law.
5. Define critical and noncritical measurement.
6. Differentiate between volumetric, Pasteur, and graduated pipettes.
7. Identify different types of labware.
8. Discuss quality control measures.

Chapter 15
Basic Chemistry Laboratory Instrumentation

Each constituent in clinical chemistry has its own unique properties, such as molecular weight, solubility, and binding capacity. Moreover, each constituent requires specific chemicals or reagents to measure these analytes, as well as a method to accomplish the task. This chapter illustrates types of methods used to analyze and **quantitate** constituents.

To follow instructions for testing procedures accurately, it is always necessary to use correct measurements. The type of labware used and the instruments selected for measuring amounts into a container are critical factors in terms of accuracy. Decisions as to whether to use, for example, a tube or flask, or a graduated or total volume, Pasteur or volumetric pipette, all have a bearing on test results; and thus should be considered carefully. Accordingly, critical and noncritical measuring protocols, as well as their importance in laboratory testing, are discussed in this chapter.

As testing procedures increase in complexity, so does the importance of quality control. Reliability of results is directly linked to the accuracy and precision of the testing procedure and instrumentation. To ensure an acceptable degree of accuracy and precision, continuous quality control measures must be implemented.

Chemistry Analyzers

It is not necessary for the laboratory worker to understand the chemical or electronic basis for each testing method or to know all of the intricate details of each. Rather, exposure to the meaning of a particular method of testing is generally sufficient. Most routine tests are performed on a laboratory chemistry analyzer. Each analyzer is set up to accommodate certain methods for testing the analyte.

Special chemistry techniques, however, require special instruments dedicated to certain methods or tasks (e.g., a gamma counter for radioim-

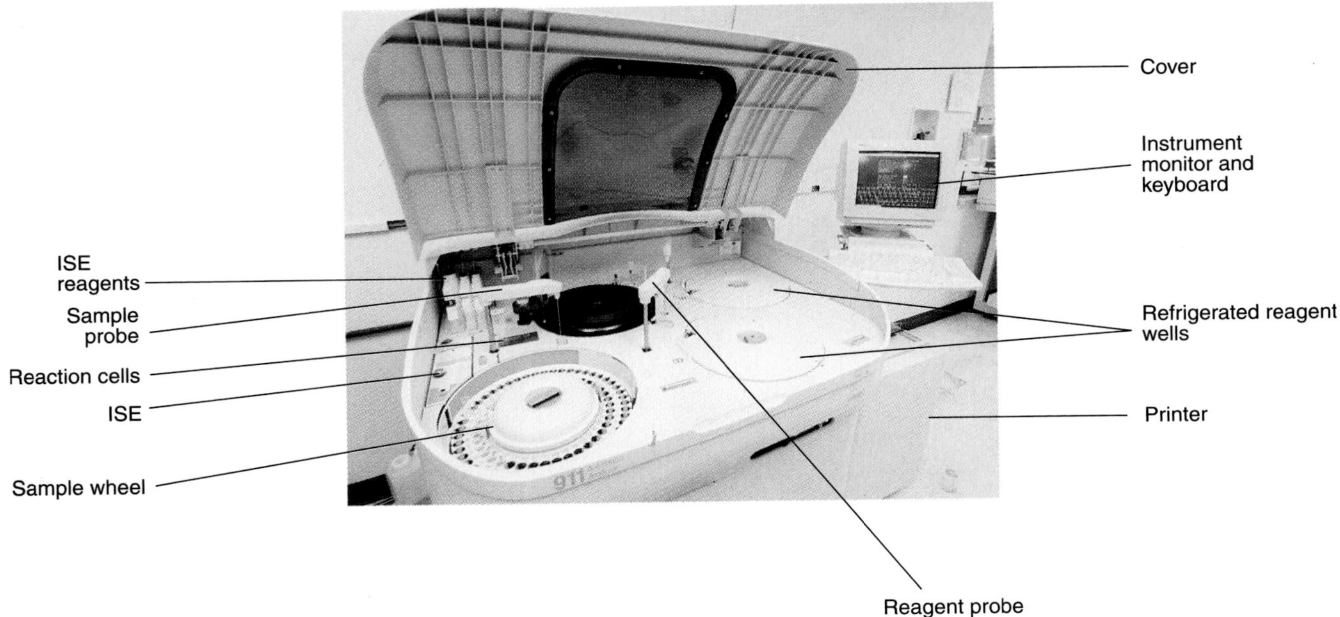

Figure 15-1. *Laboratory chemistry analyzer.*

munoassay (RIA), or a fluorometer for fluorometric procedures).

All modern chemistry analyzers have at least the following basic functional units (Fig. 15–1):

1. A power source
2. A signal source, such as a photometric lamp
3. A reagent compartment
4. A sample compartment
5. A reaction compartment where the sample is mixed with the reagent, and where the reaction takes place at a given time and temperature
6. A signal processing unit (computer)
7. A monitor or cathode ray tube (computer screen) that gives the operator instructions and displays test results
8. A keyboard or keypad for entering patient identification and making test requests
9. A printer or tape, which prints final results

Units of Measurement

Test results in clinical chemistry are expressed in metric units using the International System of Nomenclature. For example, 80 mg/dL of glucose is 80 mg (0.0080 of 1 gm or 0.00000080 μg) of weight in 1 dL (100 mL) of blood volume (Table 15–1).

Urine test measurements are expressed in metric units of measurement (gm, mg, μg, mEq, etc.) per 24-hour collection volume. For example, a normal urine calcium level may be expressed as 200 mg/24 hr, and a normal urine potassium level may be expressed as 100mEq/24 hr.

Common Methods of Testing

Spectrophotometry (Photometry)

Spectrophotometry is one of the oldest and simplest testing methods. It is based on the Beer-Lambert law, commonly referred to as *Beer's law*, which states that "the concentration of a substance is proportional to the amount of **radiant** energy absorbed." This means that, as light passes through a substance, the amount of light absorbed depends on the number of absorbing molecules in its path (Fig. 15–2).

Colorimetric Method

The colorimetric method may be used in some chemical analyzers. This method involves adding serum to a reagent to cause a color reaction. A wavelength of light, specific to the color of the solution, is then passed through the solution; as this light passes through, it is absorbed by molecules in its path. Thus, the darker the reaction color becomes, the greater the amount of that particular absorbing substance present.

Kinetic Method

The kinetic method, commonly used to measure enzymes, is based on a changing reaction measured at its

Table 15–1
International System of Nomenclature

Measurement	***Common Analyte Uses***
gm/dL (grams per deciliter)	Serum protein, albumin
mg/dL (milligrams per deciliter)	Glucose, cholesterol
μg/dL (micrograms per deciliter)	Serum iron, copper
mg/mL (milligrams per milliliter)	Used in toxicology
ng/mL (nanograms per milliliter)	Serum folate, therapeutic drugs (e.g., digoxin)
pg/mL (picograms per milliliter)	Vitamin B12, **estradiol**
mEq/L (milliequivalents per liter)	Electrolytes
mmol/L (millimoles per liter)	A measurement that is interchangeable with mEq/L
U/L (units per liter)	Enzyme assays
IU/L (international units per liter)	Enzyme assays
mm Hg (millimeters mercury)	Arterial blood gases (oxygen pressure measurement)

point of optimal activity. For example, when an enzyme is added to a reagent or reagents (there are usually two), a reaction begins. When the reaction peaks, an instrument records the absorbance and processes it to calculate the enzyme's activity.

Enzymatic Method

The enzymatic method is widely used in chemistry analyzers. With this method, serum is added to a solution containing specific enzymes, thereby freeing the analyte being analyzed. The mixture is then incubated at a given time and temperature, and the end product (color) is measured photometrically.

Ion-Specific Electrodes

Ion-specific electrodes (ISEs) are used to measure the electrolytes sodium, potassium, and chloride. Each electrode has properties of permeability that are specific for only one ion. As the sample flows through the system, it interacts with the electrode membrane and diffuses through the interface, creating an impulse. This impulse is measured and processed by an instrument which then generates a report of the test results.

Flame Photometry

Flame photometry is rapidly being replaced by ISEs for electrolyte measurements. With this method, propane and air are used to produce a flame. Certain elements, when exposed to sufficient heat energy (as supplied by the flame), will readmit that energy at given wavelengths specific for that element. The energy level is then measured and processed by an instrument that reports the test results. This method requires a flame photometer, which is not usually included in a routine laboratory analyzer.

Figure 15–2. *Spectrophotometer components.*

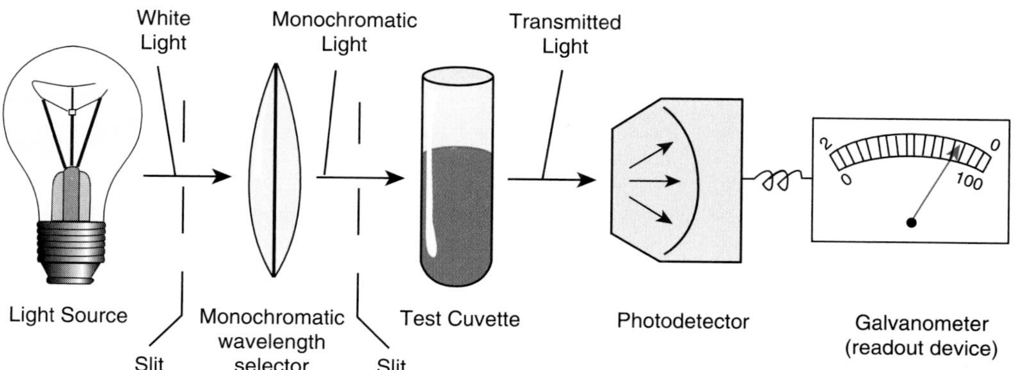

Atomic Absorption

The atomic absorption method is used primarily to assay certain metals. It is only mentioned here because some laboratories still use this method to test for serum iron, or as a back-up procedure for measuring electrolyte levels.

A photometer measures the absorption of light from a hollow-cathode lamp, specific for each metal or family of metals. The instrument measures and processes this information and translates it into test results. This method also requires a special instrument.

Laboratory Equipment

Labware

Glassware or some type of receptacle is frequently used in the laboratory to measure, transfer, and/or prepare reagents. Labware comes in five basic shapes and a variety of sizes (Fig. 15–3). Each type has been designed for a specific purpose. Many laboratory containers are made of plastic and are designed to be discarded after use. Glass containers are more expensive and require care in cleaning to prevent breakage and scratches, but they have the advantage of not **leaching** or binding solutes.

To ensure accuracy, all laboratory glassware is calibrated to 20°C. In choosing a receptacle, the assistant should select the container that most closely approximates the total volume that it will need to hold. The choice must also reflect whether the solution being measured is **critical** or **noncritical. Remember that all fluid readings are at the meniscus, and that the meniscus must rest on the desired calibration line (See Chapter 8).**

Common labware includes tubes, pipettes, Petri dishes, beakers, bottles, cylinders, and flasks (Table 15–2), each of which is designed for certain uses. These items may be graduated, have specific volume markings, have only total volume or capacity noted, be designed for either **noncritical** or **critical measurement,** or be heat-resistant (Pyrex or Kimax).

Pipettes

Pipettes are used primarily for measuring small quantities. They are available in both glass and plastic. Graduated pipettes have metric measurement markings.

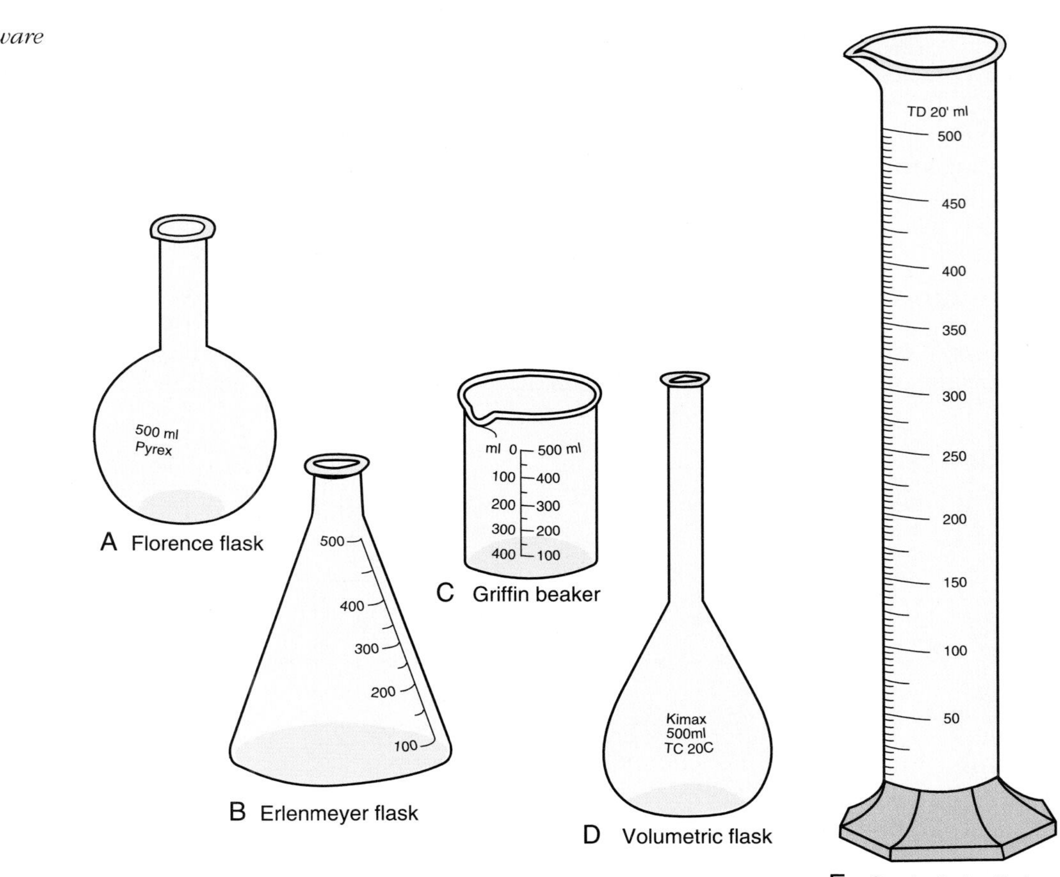

Figure 15-3. *Common labware items.*

Table 15–2
Common Labware Items

Container	***Description***	***Use***
Beakers	Deep glass containers with wide mouths	To measure and transfer noncritical solutions
Bottles	Containers of varying sizes and types, either plastic or glass, and clear or brown in color	To hold all reagents
Cylinders	Containers that are graduated, upright, and straight-sided, with an octagon base	To hold 24-hour urine volume; noncritical volumes
Flasks		
Florence	Flat-bottomed container with sloping sides; marked only for total volume	For noncritical measurement
Volumetric	Container with rounded sides; a long, slender neck; and calibration lines etched into the neck	For critical measurement
Petri dishes	Flat, covered, clear plastic or glass dishes	For bacterial cultures
Pipettes		
Volumetric	Tube of varying size having a wide open upper end, a round or oval bulb at the center, and a tapered tip at the lower end	For critical measurement of liquids
Graduated	A long, tapered tube of varying size having an open upper end and tapered tip	For transfer and noncritical measurement of liquids
Test tubes	Containers of varying size having rounded bottoms and open, stoppered, or screw-on tops; usually disposable	To hold specimens

Pipettes are identified by their markings and/or shape. There are three basic types of pipettes; volumetric, graduated, and Pasteur (Fig. 15–4).

Volumetric pipettes are designed to dispense a specific amount of fluid in a precise time frame and are used primarily when accuracy of a transferred volume is critical. To use the volumetric instrument, a bulb is fixed to the upper end and squeezed. The fluid to be transferred is drawn up into the pipette by releasing the squeeze on the bulb, allowing the fluid to fill to the designated amount marking on the stem above the center. The pipette tip is then wiped clean with a laboratory tissue, and placed at a vertical angle, with the tapered tip resting on the surface of the receptacle into which the fluid is being transferred. The suction on the bulb is then released to allow the fluid to flow into the designated receptacle. One must be certain that all of the measured fluid has drained from the pipette before it is removed from the receptacle.

Graduated pipettes have a total capacity mark near the upper end and a frosted band around the top. The graduations allow measurement of differing volumes and may vary according to their designated purpose. Two of the most frequently used pipettes are the serological pipette, with graduations extending to the tip, and the Mohr pipette, on which graduations end before the tip. Both are used for noncritical measurement and transfer of liquids from one container to another. There is also a micropipette available which is calibrated for a volume of 0.5 mL or less. All graduated pipettes are

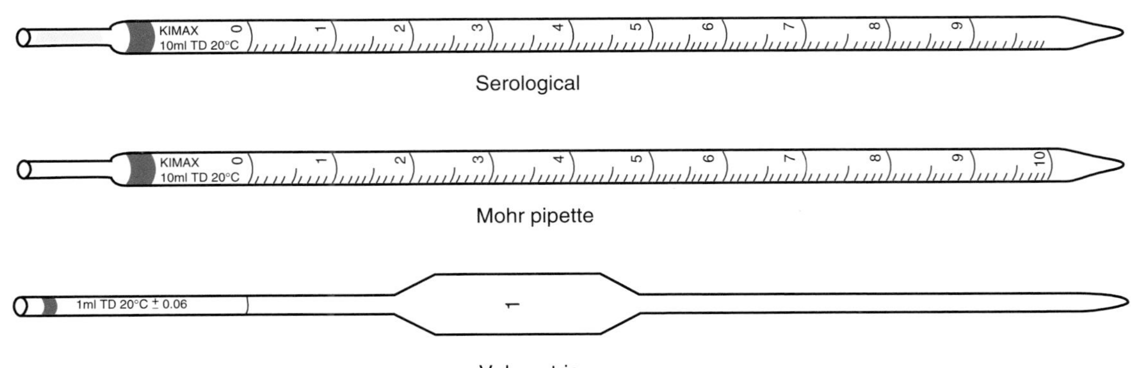

Figure 15-4. *Basic types of pipettes.*

available in manual or semi-automated models (Fig. 15–5).

Pasteur pipettes are used to add small, unmeasured quantities of fluid to receptacles. They are disposable and are available in both glass and plastic. To use the glass version one must first attach a rubber bulb to the upper end. The plastic version comes with a small bulb molded to the upper end of the pipette. This type of pipette has no markings on it.

Pipette Markings

With the exception of the Pasteur pipette, all pipettes have markings. At the upper end of the pipette, the total volume and the increments of graduation are indicated. In addition, TD and TC markings may be found. **TD** means *to deliver;* these pipettes are allowed to drain by gravity and need not be rinsed in order to secure the entire desired amount of fluid. **TC** means *to*

Figure 15-5. *Semi-automatic micropipettes.* A, *A set of graduated semi-automatic pipettors.* B, *Large semi-automatic pipettors.*

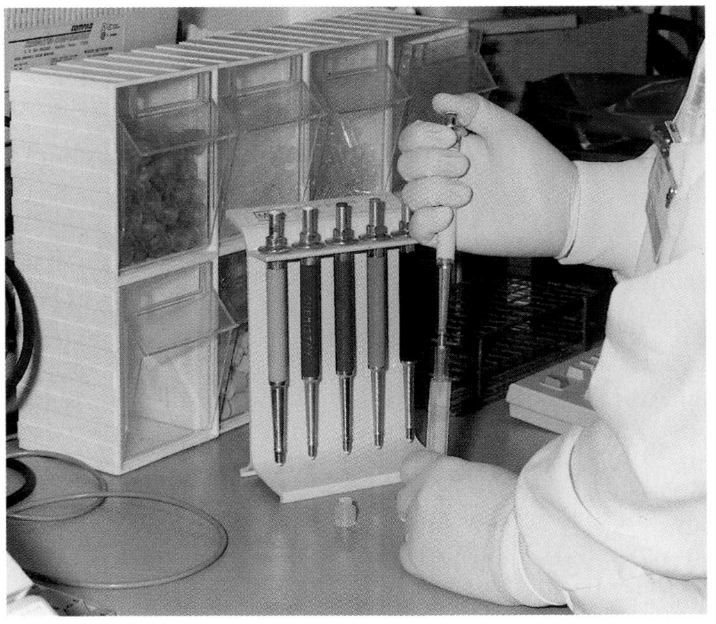

A

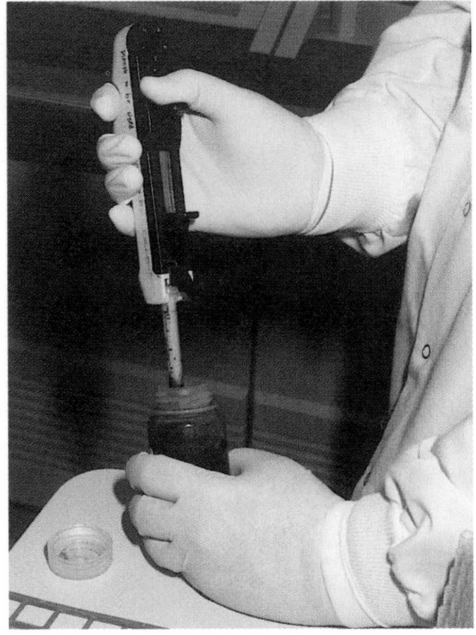

B

contain; in order to obtain the entire volume of fluid from this type of instrument, the interior of the pipette must be rinsed with the recommended diluent after all the fluid has drained.

Some pipettes may also have an etched or frosted ring around the upper end. This ring indicates that the last drop of fluid must be expelled from the pipette after draining. This marking is found on serological pipettes, but not on volumetric and Mohr.

Care and Cleaning

All labware must be either washed with an authorized laboratory detergent or discarded after use. If an item is labeled "disposable," do not attempt to clean it for another use. The term "disposable" means exactly what it says. Glassware and reusable items are to be thoroughly washed in detergent, using a brush if needed, and then rinsed several times in tap water. After rinsing with tap water, the labware is then rinsed with distilled water. Depending on the sensitivity of the test procedure for which the receptacle will be used, the required number of distilled water rinses may range from 3 to 12.

When washing labware by hand, always wear gloves and a protective apron. It is preferable to wash pipettes in a commercial pipette washer. When the washing process is completed, glassware is placed in a drain rack in an inverted position and allowed to dry. Alternatively, a drying oven may be used.

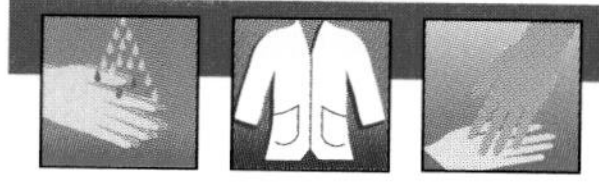

PROCEDURE 15-1

Using a Pipette to Transfer Fluid

Principle

To recognize the different types of pipettes; to achieve success in transfering fluids; to obtain skills that will be necessary to ensure testing accuracy

Equipment and Supplies

volumetric pipette
pipette bulb or pump
laboratory tissue
graduated serological pipette
colored water in 250- to 500-mL flask or beaker
beaker or large test tube (50–100 mL)

Procedural Steps

1. Wash your hands and put on gloves.
2. Assemble equipment and supplies.
3. Attach the pipette bulb or pump to a 1-mL serological pipette.

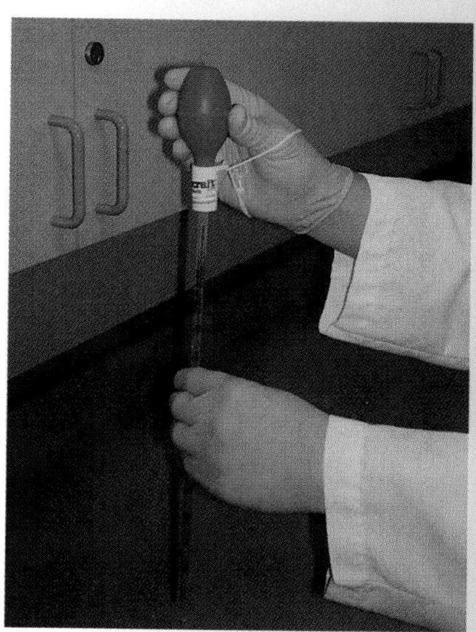

(continued)

PROCEDURE 15-1

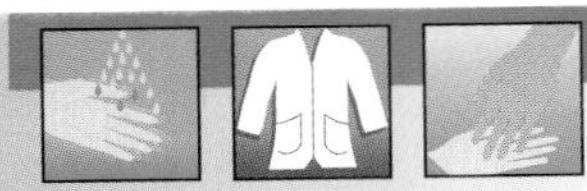

Using a Pipette to Transfer Fluid (Continued)

4. Squeeze the bulb before placing the tip of the pipette into the colored water.

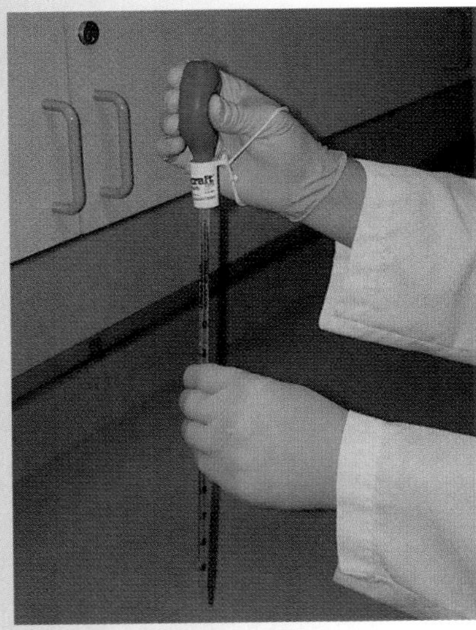

5. Slowly release the bulb, allowing the water to be drawn up into the pipette.

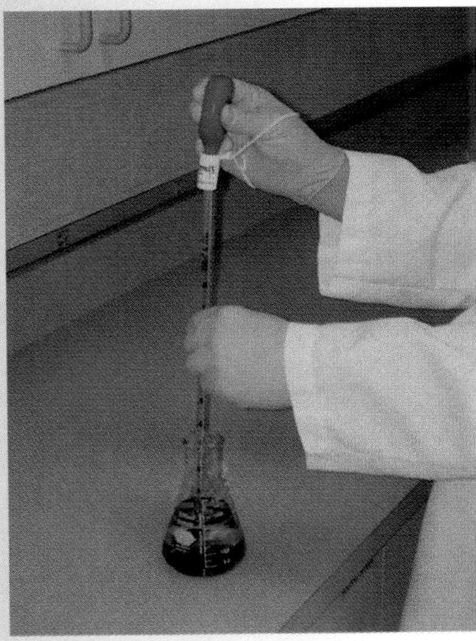

6. Continue to draw the water until the level is slightly above the 1-mL mark.

7. Remove the bulb and quickly place your index finger over the upper end of the pipette.

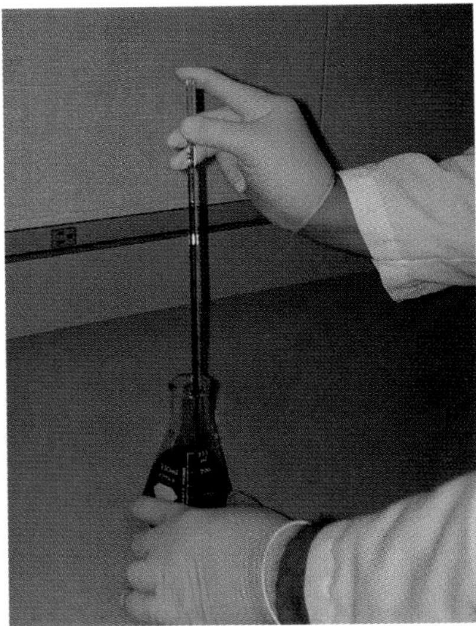

8. With the pipette held vertically, carefully and slowly begin to release the pressure of your index finger on the top of the pipette.
9. Carefully wipe the outside of the pipette with laboratory tissue to remove all excess fluid.

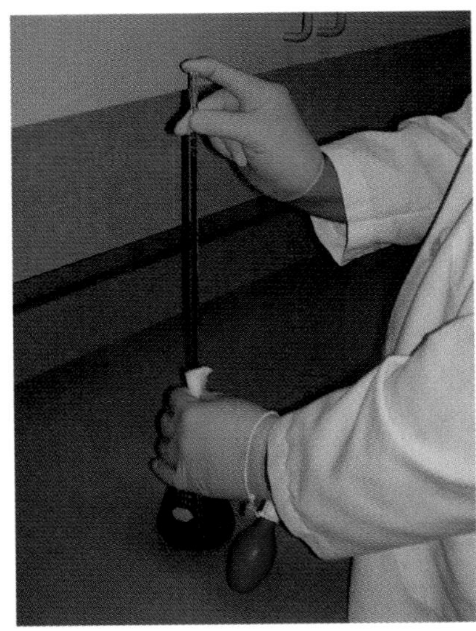

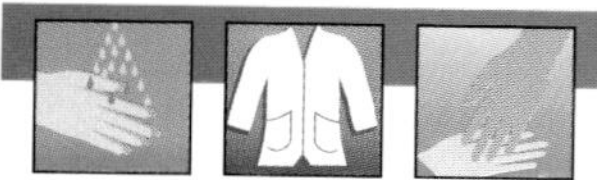

PROCEDURE 15-1

Using a Pipette to Transfer Fluid (Continued)

10. Allow the colored water to drain from the pipette until the meniscus rests on the 1-mL mark.
11. Dispense the colored water into the test tube or clean small beaker, allowing the liquid to drain by gravity.

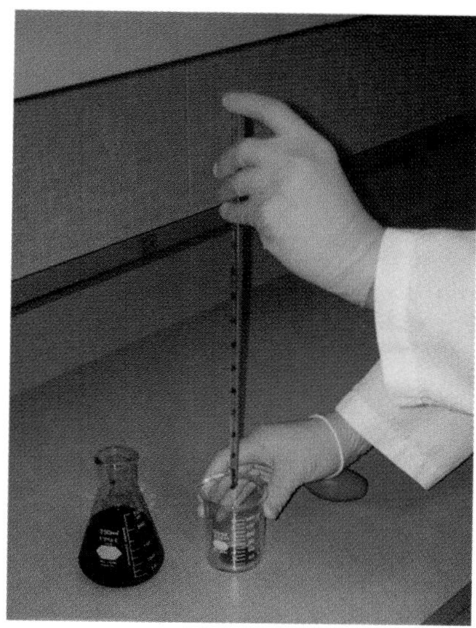

12. If the pipette has a frosted ring, use the pipette bulb to blow the last drop of liquid out of the pipette.
13. Repeat this procedure using various sizes of volumetric and serological pipettes.

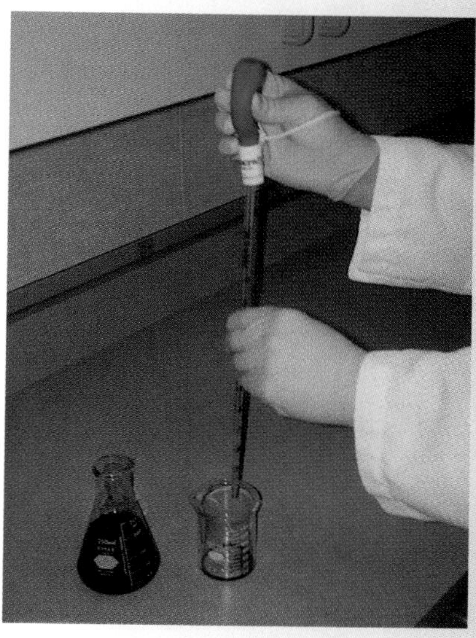

14. Clean the equipment and work area.
15. Remove and discard gloves and wash hands.

Remember when using a volumetric pipette, DO NOT blow out the last drop of fluid in the pipette. Instead, touch the tip of the pipette to the side of the container. A small amount of the colored water will drain; the remainder should be left in the pipette.

Quality Control

Many clinical laboratories perform thousands of tests each day. A large number of test results are generated in conjunction with these tests. Laboratory methods of quality control ensure that these data are reliable, accurate, and precise.

Quality control is practiced daily in the clinical laboratory. This is important because laboratory test results are used to diagnose, treat, and monitor patients. Only with a good quality assurance program can these results have any **reliability.**

The Clinical Laboratory Improvement Act (CLIA) of 1988 requires clinical laboratories to implement and maintain quality assurance programs. To this mandate, individual states have added their own requirements for laboratory operation. The standardized quality assurance programs provided for by CLIA 88 affect laboratories of all sizes, from the physician's office laboratory (POL) to large hospital laboratories.

To guarantee reliability, patient samples are tested alongside standards and control samples. **Standards** are commercially prepared solutions with exact known values for the constituent being tested. Standards are used to calibrate instruments and are essential to the reporting of reliable, accurate, and precise results.

Controls are usually commercial solutions that contain the constituents being tested. Controls are

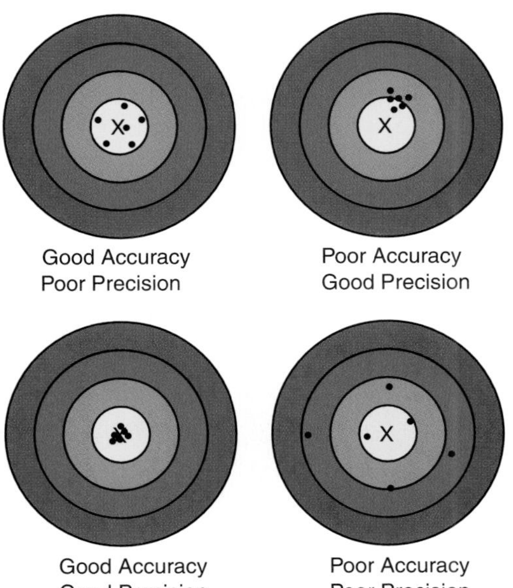

Figure 15-6. *Relationship between accuracy and precision.*

made from the **lyophilization** of sera with an expected range of values for each constituent in the control. Controls may be specific to the constituent being tested, or they may contain every constituent tested by multitest analyzers.

Most tests require that two different controls be tested with each test on a patient sample. These controls are usually a high-value sample and low-value sample. Occasionally, a normal value is required.

Accuracy is an indication of how close the answer obtained (the test result) is to the true value. The closer to the exact value a test result is, the more accurate it is. Accuracy and **precision** are independent from one another, so a test may be accurate but not precise and vice versa (Fig. 15–6).

The reference range (normal range) of any test result is a reflection of the expected range of testing results that would be obtained in a defined population with no obvious clinical problems. Both testing methodology and the instrumentation used will affect the reference range.

Quality assurance programs are based on the monitoring of statistical data. Reproducibility can only be determined by performing many assays for the specific constituent. The results from these assays are then plotted on a graph, which should yield a symmetrical, bell-shaped curve. The location of values on this curve is called *Gaussian* distribution (Fig.15–7). *Errors* may be preanalytical, analytical, or postanalytical. Preanalytical errors include errors in patient identification and specimen collection and processing. Analytical errors may be systemic or random. Systemic analytical errors cause defined variance in all testing results, meaning that all the results will be consistently higher or lower than the actual value. This type of error is usually caused by reagent problems or analyzer malfunction. An error whose cause cannot be identified is considered to be a random error. Random analytical error may produce a variance on the high or low side of the **mean.** Air bubbles or inconsistencies in technique may cause random error. Postanalytical errors are similar to preanalytical errors in that they are man-made errors. Reporting and transcription errors are two common causes of postanalytical problems.

Summary

There are numerous methods of testing, and many require special instrumentation to accommodate these procedures, however most chemistry analyzers on the market today can test 20 or more analytes in 15 to 20 minutes.

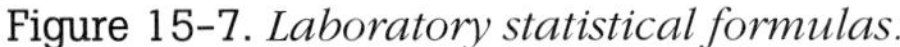

Figure 15-7. *Laboratory statistical formulas.*

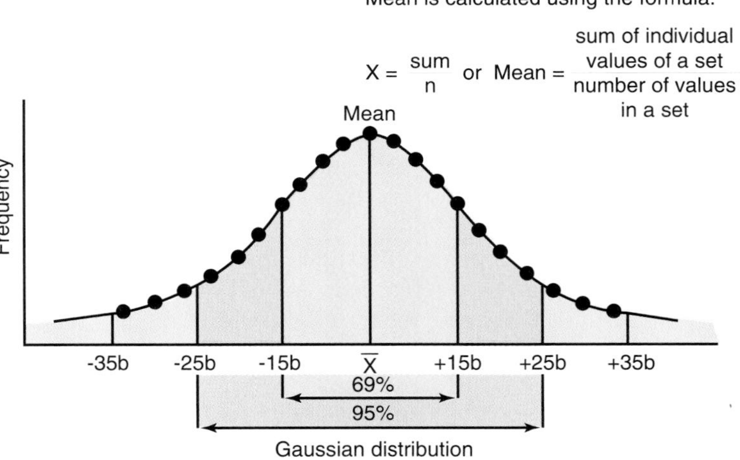

The reliability of laboratory results can only be guaranteed when a quality assurance program is properly implemented and maintained. Maintenance of proper quality control records is time consuming. Chapter 3 contained an outline for program implementation to assist with the establishing of these programs.

Chapter Review

True or False

Circle T or F to indicate the correct answers to the following:

T F 1. A routine chemical analyzer has a processing unit.

T F 2. Serum protein measurements are expressed in gm/mL.

T F 3. Nanograms per milliliter can also be written ng/mL.

T F 4. Millimeters of hemoglobin is usually abbreviated mm/Hg.

T F 5. Volumetric pipettes are primarily used when the accuracy of a transferred volume is critical.

Fill in the Blanks

Complete the following statements:

6. Spectrophotometry is one of the oldest methods of testing and is based on ____________ law.
7. The method that is commonly used to measure enzymes is called ____________ .
8. The end product of an enzymatic mixture is measured ____________ .
9. Ion-specific electrodes are used to measure ____________ .

Multiple Choice

Circle the letter that represents the single best answer:

10. To use flame photometry, you need __________ to produce the flame.
    a. Oxygen and helium
    b. Propane and air
    c. Nitrous and oxygen
    d. Propane and oxygen
    e. Helium and nitrous
11. Atomic absorption is used to test for:
    a. Electrolytes
    b. Iron
    c. Proteins
    d. a and b
    e. All of the above
12. To ensure accuracy, all laboratory glassware is calibrated to:
    a. 10°C
    b. 20°C
    c. 30°C
    d. 40°C
    e. 50°C
13. The volumetric pipette tip is placed at a __________ angle when fluid is being transferred.
    a. Transverse
    b. Horizontal
    c. Reverse
    d. Vertical
    e. Lateral
14. Preanalytical errors in quality assurance may be caused by errors in:
    a. Patient identification
    b. Specimen collection
    c. Speciman processing
    d. b and c
    e. a, b, and c

Vocabulary

dehydration: a condition that results from undue loss of water from the body or body tissues

diabetes mellitus: a disturbance in the oxidation and utilization of glucose caused by malfunctioning pancreatic beta cells, which are responsible for the secretion of insulin

fast: abstinence from food

gout: a hereditary form of arthritis characterized by excessive quantities of uric acid in the blood

hydrational: relating to the absorption of water or combination with water

ketoacidosis: the accumulation of fatty acids, called ketone bodies, in the blood

urea: the chief nitrogenous end product of protein metabolism, formed in the liver and excreted in urine

Chapter Objectives

After reading this chapter, you should be able to:

1. Describe the two divisions of clinical chemistry testing.
2. Define *reference ranges.*
3. List four disease states that can be confirmed by electrolyte testing.
4. Identify three tests that can assist in the management of diabetes mellitus.
5. Explain why protein analyses are conducted.
6. List the minerals that are frequently included in chemistry panels.
7. Identify the waste product derived from the breakdown of hemoglobin and the form in which it is excreted.
8. List the lipids assayed in a routine chemistry panel.

Chapter 16
Routine Clinical Chemistry Procedures

In the clinical laboratory setting, a number of clinical chemistry tests are routinely performed. These tests are performed in all hospital laboratories and independent laboratories, as well as in physician's office laboratories. These tests are important in assessing, diagnosing, managing, and treating a variety of disease states in patients.

Occasionally, your laboratory may be asked to take part in a regional health fair, and you may be asked to obtain blood for glucose and/or cholesterol screening tests. The *Screening Consent and Referral Form* must be completed and signed by the individual before you can legally obtain blood for any testing procedure (Fig. 16–1).

In this chapter, you will study some of the most frequently performed clinical chemistry tests.

Chemistry Tests

Clinical chemistry tests are divided into two groups: routine and special chemistry. The special chemistry tests will be discussed in Chapter 19.

Routine tests are those that may be performed quickly and inexpensively. Special chemistry tests are those that require more elaborate techniques, equipment, or expertise.

A test may be ordered in a panel or as a single test. Many laboratories offer routine panels, which assess the general health of a patient, as well as special panels, which target a specific suspected disease or condition, such as a liver or cardiac disorder. Panel tests are usually less expensive than if each test were performed individually.

Single tests or test groups, such as electrolytes, may be used to monitor a particular disease or the progression of an illness. When laboratory tests are ordered, the results may assist the physician in establishing a diagnosis. A diagnosis cannot be established solely on the basis of one test or test panel, but such tests can be instrumental when used in conjunction with additional procedures and clinical evaluation.

SCREENING CONSENT AND REFERRAL FORM

Please Print:

Name: ____________________

Address: ____________________

Phone: ____________________

Sex (circle one) M F Date of Birth: ____________________

Physician's Name: ____________________

Physician's Address: ____________________

Date of Test: ____________ Time of Day: ____________

Cholesterol Level: ____________ Glucose Level: ____________

PLEASE READ CAREFULLY:

I hereby consent to a fingerstick blood sample drawing for determining my total blood ____________ level. I understand that there may be some discomfort, possible bruising, and/or potential for infection from the fingerstick. If signs of infection (redness, swelling, warmth, pain, and/or pus) develop and persist for more than 24 hours, I will seek medical care. I release ____________, their employees, or volunteer staff from any and all liability arising from or in any way connected to the blood drawing and testing. I understand that:

1. To my knowledge, I do not suffer from any bleeding disorder or similar condition.
2. The screening will be administered by ____________ personnel.
3. The results of this screening will be kept confidential.
4. The results of this screening are to be considered preliminary only, and are in no way conclusive.
5. The responsibility for initiating follow-up examination to confirm high blood cholesterol or glucose levels and to obtain advice and treatment is mine, and not that of the organizations associated with this screening.

Operator ID ____________________ Instrument No.____________

Site ____________________ Referral: Y N

Figure 16–1. *Sample form used for consent and referral of patients.*

Reference ranges (normal ranges), listed on the laboratory forms or in reference tables, are the expected ranges for a particular testing facility, taking into consideration the average healthy patient, the patient's gender and age, and the testing methodology. The physician evaluates the test results received using the reference range on the merit of the patient's history and physical state. When assessing data obtained on a patient, care must be taken to determine whether the results are within normal or abnormal ranges (Table 16–1). Test results can be considered to be normal by one laboratory's standards/methods and abnormal by another. Ultimately, it is the physician's decision to determine the merit of the test results in terms of the treatment of the patient.

Routine Chemistry Tests

Electrolytes

Electrolytes are substances which, when placed in water, separate into charged particles called ions. Posi-

Table 16–1

Normal Ranges for Common Blood Chemistry Tests

Name of Test	***Specimen Required***	***Normal Range***		
Albumin (ALB)	Serum	Neonates: 2.6–3.6 g/dL Adults: 3.8–5.0 g/dL		
Albumin/globulin ratio (A/G ratio)	Serum	1.5:1 to 2.5:1 or ≥1		
Alkaline phosphate (ALP)	Serum	30–115 mU/mL		
Amylase	Serum	Neonates: 6–65 U/L Adults: 25–125 U/L Elderly: 21–160 U/L		
Anion gap or R factor (AG)	Serum	< ± 12 mEq/L <16 mEq/L if potassium concentration is used to calculate		
Alanine transaminase (ALT)/serum glutamic-pyruvic transaminase (SGPT)	Serum	Adults: 7–56 U/L Children: 10–35 U/L Neonates: 6–50 U/L		
Aspartate transaminase (AST)/ serum glutamic-oxaloacetic transaminase (SGOT)	Serum	Adults: 5–40 U/L Children: 10–50 U/L Infants: 20–60 U/L		
Bicarbonate (HCO_6)	Serum	Peripheral vein: 19–25 mEq/L Arterial: 22–26 mEq/L		
Blood urea nitrogen (BUN)	Serum	8–25 mg/dL		
Total bilirubin (T Bili)	Serum	0.2–1.0 mg/dL		
Direct bilirubin (D Bili)	Serum	0.0–0.2 mg/dL		
Indirect bilirubin (I Bili)	Serum	0.3–1.1 mg/dL		
Calcium (Ca)	Serum	8.5–10.5 mg/dL		
Chloride (Cl)	Serum	96–110 mEq/L		
Cholesterol (CH or Chol)	Serum	Adults: Desirable, <200 mg/dL Borderline, 200–239 mg/dL High, >240 mg/dL		
Low-density lipoprotein (LDL)		Children (Ages 12–18 yrs.): Desirable, <170 mg/dL Borderline, 170–199 mg/dL High, >200 mg/dL		
High-density lipoprotein (HDL)		Males: 37–70 mg/dL Females: 40–85 mg/dL		
Creatinine (Creat)	Serum	0.4–1.5 mg/dL		
Creatine phosphokinase (CPK)	Serum	Males: 38–174 U/L Females: 96–140 U/L		
Globulin (Glob)	Serum	1.0–3.5 g/dL		
Glucose	Serum			
Fasting blood sugar (FBS)		FBS: 70–110 mg/100 mL		
Postprandial blood sugar (PPBS)		2-hr PPBS: <140 mg/dL (mg/100mL)		
Glucose tolerance test (GTT)		**NORMAL**		**DIABETIC**
		Adult—FBS:	70–110	>120
		30-min:	110–170	>200
		1-hr:	120–170	>200
		2-hr:	70–120	>140
		3-hr:	<120	>140
		Child—FBS:	<130	>140
		1-hr:	<140	>200
		2-hr:	<140	>200
Iron (Fe)	Serum	50–165 µg/dL		
Lipase	Serum	Adults: 10–140 U/L		
Lactic acid dehydrogenase (LD or LDH)	Serum	100–225 mU/mL		
Magnesium (Mag)	Serum	1.2–2.4 mg/dL		
Phosphorus (P)	Serum	2.5–4.5 mg/dL		
Potassium (K)	Serum	3.5–5.5 mEq/L		
Sodium (Na)	Serum	135–145 mEq/L		
Thyroxine (T_4)/free thyroxine (FT_4)	Serum	1–2.3 mg/dL		
Total protein (TP)	Serum	6.0–8.0 g/dL		
Triglycerides (Trig)	Serum	20–180 mg/dL		
Uric acid	Serum	Males: 3.5–7.2 mg/dL Females: 2.6–6.0 mg/dL		

Table 16–2
Serum Electrolyte Panel: Adult Reference Ranges

Electrolyte	*Reference Range*	*Critical Value**
Sodium (Na)	135–145 mEq/L	<120 mEq/L or >160 mEq/L
Potassium (K)	3.5–5.5 mEq/L	<2.5 mEq/L or >6.5 mEq/L
Chloride (Cl)	96–110 mEq/L	<80 mEq/L or >115 mEq/L
Osmolality (Osm)	280–300 mOsm	<240 mOsm or >360 mOsm

*Notify the physician of the results immediately.

tive charged ions are called *cations,* whereas negative charged ions are called *anions.*

In blood, the positively charged ions or cations are sodium (Na^+), potassium (K^+), calcium (Ca^{++}), and magnesium (Mg^{++}). The negatively charged ions or anions include chloride (Cl^-), bicarbonate (HCO_3^-), phosphate (HPO_4^-), and sulfate (SO_4^{--}).

The electrolytes commonly measured in an electrolyte panel, and the ones most frequently tested, are sodium, potassium, and chloride (Table 16–2), along with carbon dioxide content. Total carbon dioxide content is measured by determining the total of carbonic acid and bicarbonate.

Anion Gap

Based on calculations derived from these electrolytes, the unmeasured cations and anions—called the anion gap—can be estimated. Elevations in the anion gap aid in the diagnosis of types of metabolic acidosis (Table 16–3).

Electrolytes are also indicative of water balance (Table 16–4), changes in respiratory and metabolic acid–base balance (see Table 16–3), and **hydrational** status, and can aid in the diagnosis of **dehydration** and **ketoacidosis** in patients with diabetes mellitus or other disorders.

The method most commonly used for electrolyte studies in the modern laboratory is the ion-specific electrode (ISE) technique. However, some laboratories may still use flame photometry or atomic absorption techniques. Each of these methods requires unique instrumentation (Fig. 16–2).

Renal Tests

Renal tests and renal panels are the most frequently ordered tests in the laboratory. A renal panel can quickly assess the general health of a patient, as well as monitor the progression of kidney disease or complications of **diabetes mellitus,** including diabetic nephropathy (kidney disorders).

Renal panels may be performed in a physician's laboratory or emergency laboratory setting. Additionally, as a result of new technology now available, these tests may be performed at the patient's bedside in the hospital or in the patient's home.

Tests Included in the Renal Panel

Many analytes are affected in patients with kidney disease, and these can be of significant diagnostic value. In the physician's office, testing usually includes determinations of creatinine, blood urea nitrogen (BUN), uric acid, and glucose levels.

Renal tests are usually performed on a laboratory chemistry analyzer (Fig. 16–3). The methods used vary according to whether ordinary colorimetric, enzymatic

Table 16–3
Acid–Base Disorders (pH)

Disorder	*Cause*
Acidosis (blood pH <7.35)	
Metabolic	Hydrogen production
Respiratory	Carbon dioxide buildup
Alkalosis (blood pH >7.45)	
Metabolic	Base intake
Respiratory	Carbon dioxide loss

Table 16–4
Sources of Body Water

Source	*24-Hr Amount*
Drink	1000 mL
Food	1000–1200 mL
Metabolism/oxidation	
Carbohydrate	60 mL/100 gm eaten
Fat	100 mL/100 gm eaten
Protein	44 mL/100 gm eaten

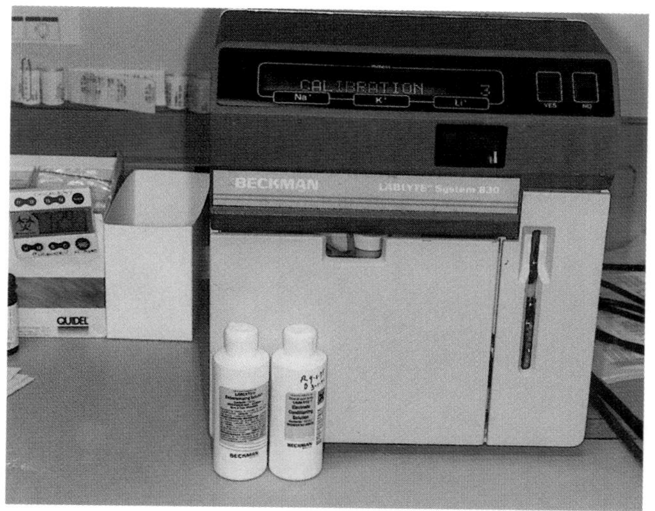

A

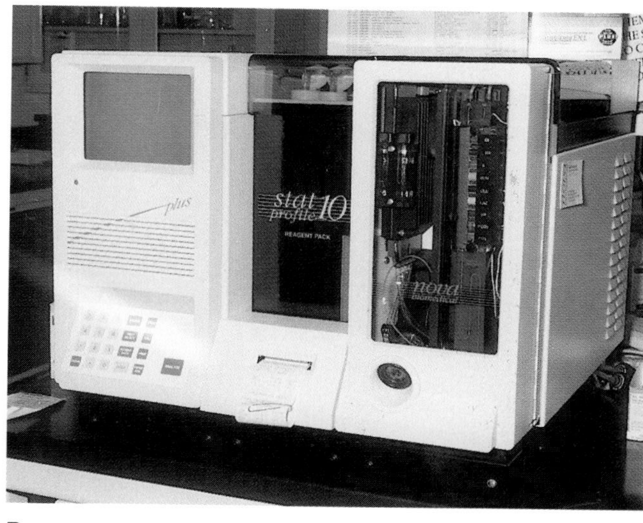

B

Figure 16–2. A, *Electrolyte analyzer.* B, *Chemical analyzer for performance of electrolyte, BUN, glucose, and arterial blood gas analysis.*

reactions, or specific electrode assays are performed. Reference ranges will also vary slightly according to the method (see Table 16–1).

Common Blood Chemistry Tests

Creatinine

Creatinine is a compound that is derived from muscle creatine and excreted in the urine. When the rate of production exceeds the rate of excretion, creatinine levels become elevated in the blood.

Increased serum creatinine levels occur in patients with renal diseases or renal insufficiency with decreased glomerular filtration. The creatinine level is only elevated when approximately half the nephrons have stopped functioning. A decreased serum creatinine level has no clinical significance.

Urea Nitrogen

Urea nitrogen is often referred to as BUN (blood urea nitrogen). The reference range (normal range) for BUN levels is 5 to 18 mg/dL.

Figure 16–3. A, *Multitest chemical analyzer (Hitachi Mfg.).* B, *Beckman Synchron CX7 Clinical System chemistry analyzer.*

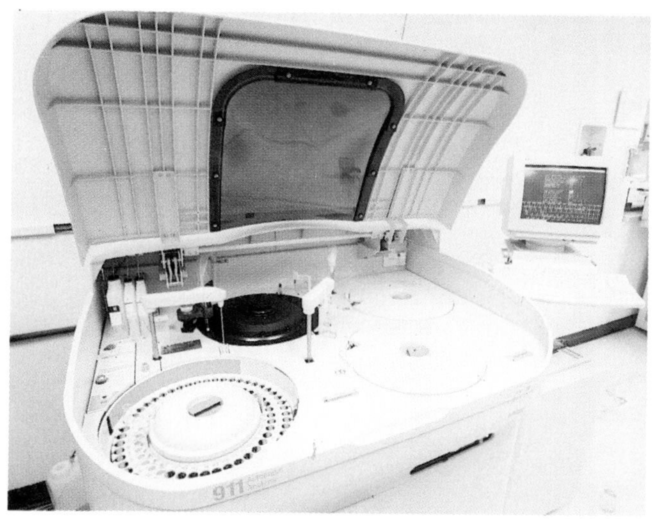

A

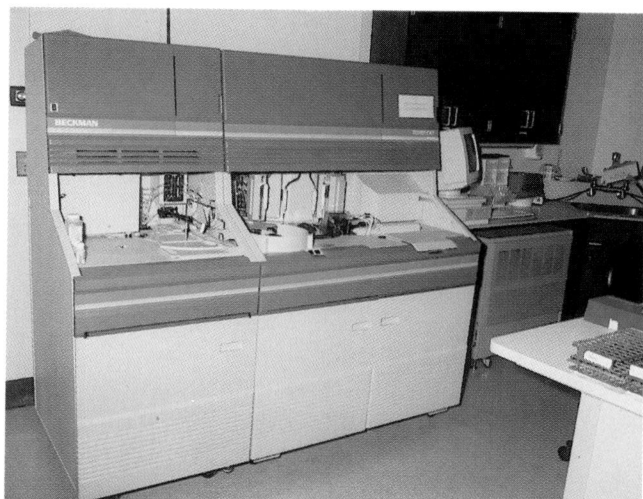

B

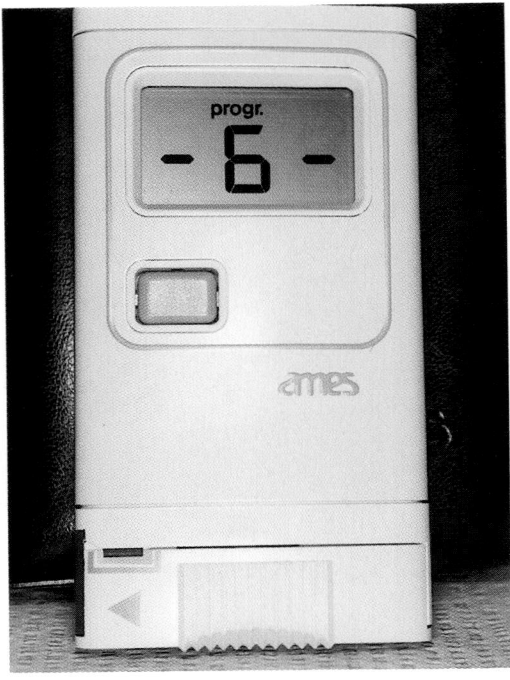

A

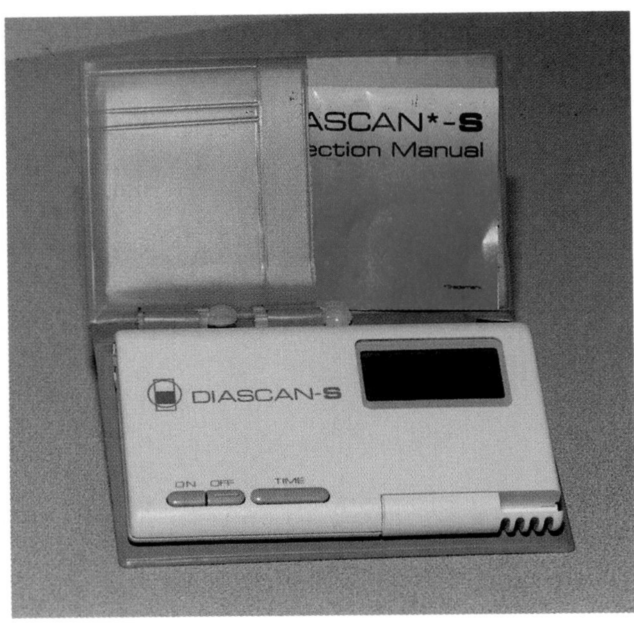

B

Figure 16–4. A, *Ames glucometer used for blood glucose monitoring.* B, *Diascan S blood glucose monitor.*

In patients with impaired renal function, the kidneys do not effectively excrete or convert surplus amino acids to **urea.** The result may be high concentrations of urea in the blood. Some conditions associated with elevated BUN levels include impaired renal function, chronic glomerulonephritis, acute renal failure, and urinary tract obstruction. High concentrations of urea are also seen in congestive heart failure.

Decreased BUN concentrations may be seen in pregnant patients or those with severe liver insufficiency or malnutrition.

Blood Glucose

Elevated blood glucose levels are associated with diabetes mellitus. This is a disorder of carbohydrate metabolism that results in elevated blood and urine glucose levels secondary to the inability of the pancreas to produce sufficient insulin. Other possible causes for increased blood glucose levels include pancreatitis, endocrine disorders, and chronic renal failure. Decreased blood glucose levels may occur in patients with hypoglycemia, insulinoma, or severe liver disease.

Glucose is used as a fuel by many cells of the body, and it is the only substance used by the brain under normal circumstances. Therefore, the maintenance of blood glucose levels within narrow limits is an important homeostatic mechanism. This explains why glucose is the urine analyte most frequently tested in the laboratory.

To perform a glucose tolerance test, a fasting patient previously receiving an adequate carbohydrate diet is given 100 gm of glucose by mouth. (The amount may be adjusted according to the weight of the patient.) If normal, the patient's blood glucose level should not exceed 100 gm/dL at the start of the test, or 180 gm/dL 1 hour later. If the blood glucose level exceeds 200 gm/dL, glucose escapes into the urine because the renal tubules are no longer able to absorb the excessive amount present in the glomerular filtrate (Fig. 16–4).

In the fasting state, the liver and insulin-dependent tissues (resting muscle and fat) show little glucose uptake. The insulin-independent tissues, particularly the brain, show continued glucose uptake, and the normal blood glucose level is maintained by release of glycogen from the liver. Reference ranges for blood glucose level are listed in Table 16–1.

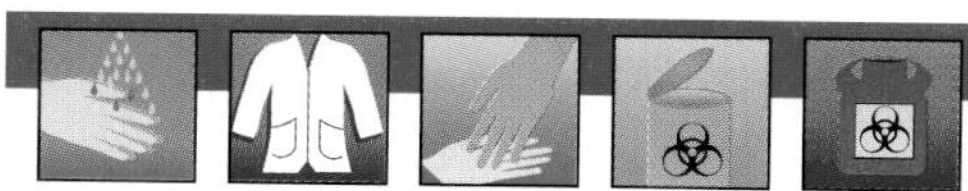

PROCEDURE 16–1

Performing a Blood Glucose Accu-Chek Test

Principle

To perform and report with accuracy abnormalities of carbohydrate metabolism blood that may occur in diabetes mellitus using an Accu-Chek or similar automated equipment

Equipment and Supplies

Accu-Chek Monitor that has been properly coded
Accu-Chek Glucose Test Strip Vial
finger stick device loaded with a new lancet
alcohol wipes
rayon ball

Procedural Steps

1. Wash your hands and put on gloves.
2. Ask the patient to wash his/her hands in warm soapy water, rinse them, and **dry them completely.** Warming the fingers can help increase blood flow.
3. Ask the patient to be seated.
4. Select a finger and site for testing.
5. Turn on the Accu-Chek monitor by pressing the ON button.

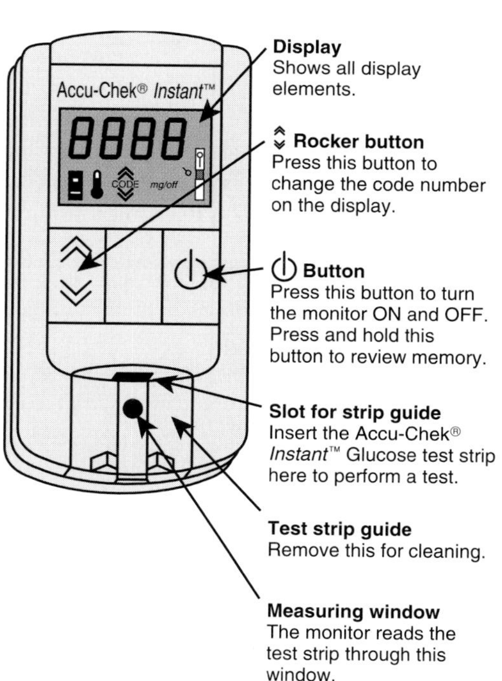
Accu-Chek® Instant™
8888
CODE
mg/off
Display
Shows all display elements.
Rocker button
Press this button to change the code number on the display.
Button
Press this button to turn the monitor ON and OFF. Press and hold this button to review memory.
Slot for strip guide
Insert the Accu-Chek® Instant™ Glucose test strip here to perform a test.
Test strip guide
Remove this for cleaning.
Measuring window
The monitor reads the test strip through this window.

6. Make sure the code number on the display matches the code number for the Accu-Chek monitor in the box on the side of the vial of test strips. If the code numbers do not match, recode the monitor before proceeding.
7. Remove a test strip from the vial. Immediately replace the vial cap. Check the strip for discoloration by comparing the color of the round window on the back of the test strip with the color designated "unused" on the color chart provided on the test strip vial label. **Do not touch the yellow test pad or round window on the back of the strip when handling the strip.**
8. When the symbol of the test strip flashes in the lower right-hand corner of the display screen, insert the test strip into the slot of the test strip guide until it locks into place. When the test strip is inserted correctly, the arrows on the test strip should be facing up and pointing toward the monitor.

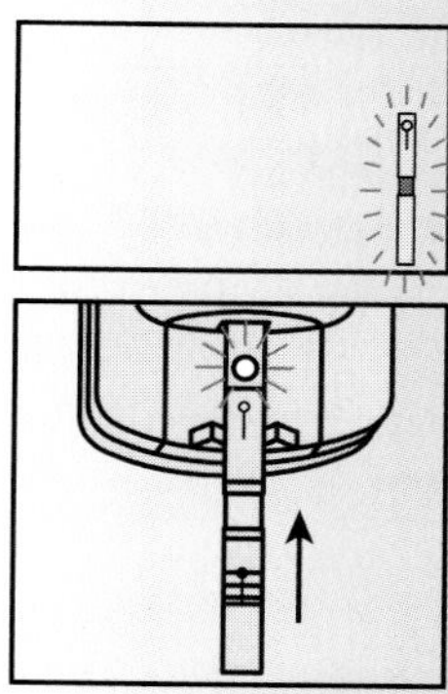

9. Cleanse the patient's fingertip with an alcohol wipe.
10. Prick the fingertip with the prepared lancet device.
11. Apply a hanging drop of blood to the center of the yellow test pad. **DO NOT touch the pad with the finger. DO NOT apply a second drop of blood to the test pad. DO NOT smear the blood with your finger. NOTE: The yellow test pad MUST be completely covered with blood without smearing the blood.**

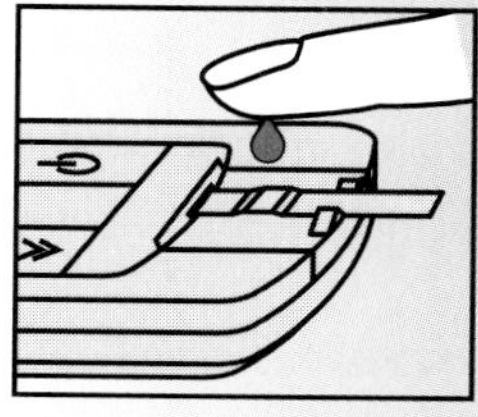

(continued)

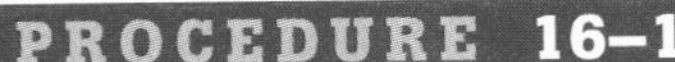

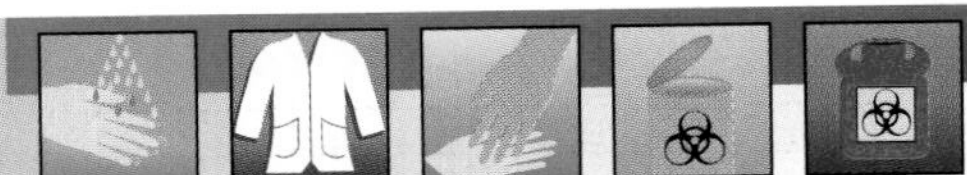

Performing a Blood Glucose Accu-Chek Test (Continued)

12. Give the patient a clean rayon ball or gauze square to hold over the puncture site.
13. The monitor automatically begins measurement as soon as it senses the drop of blood.
14. The test result, displayed on the readout, is expressed in mg/dL.
15. Turn off the monitor by pressing the "O" button.
16. Record the test results.
17. Excuse the patient.
18. Clean the work area and discard all used test strips and lancets in a puncture-proof sharps container.
19. Remove and discard gloves and wash your hands.

Figures reprinted courtesy of Boehringer Mannheim Corp.

PROCEDURE 16–2

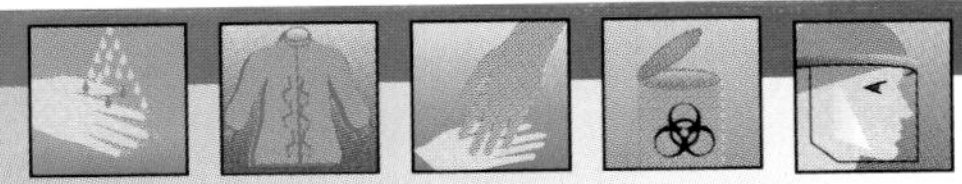

Preparing a Patient for a 2-Hour Postprandial Test

Principle

To adequately prepare a diabetic patient for and to perform a postprandial test designed to monitor the patient's disease state

Equipment and Supplies

neddle, syringe, and specimen tubes or a Vacutainer needle (single-draw or multiple-draw)*
green- or gray-top tube for first draw
green- or gray-top tube for second draw
red-top tube if other tests are ordered
70% isopropyl alcohol
sterile gauze pads
tourniquet
nonallergenic bandage
permanent marking pen

*Two green- or gray-top tubes or red-top if other chemistry tests are ordered

Procedural Steps

When the Appointment Is Made

1. Inform the patient of the date and time the postprandial test is scheduled and instruct him/her to take medication(s) as usual on that day.
2. Instruct the patient to eat a **test meal** (usually breakfast) of 100 gm of carbohydrates and to report to the laboratory 2 hours later for a blood specimen to be drawn. Discuss a sample meal plan with the patient and provide him/her with a printed set of instructions, including a menu guide.

Instructions and Menu Guide for a 2-Hour Postprandial Glucose Test

PLEASE FOLLOW ALL INSTRUCTIONS PRECISELY.

1. Follow as closely as possible one of the menus listed below, or use the suggested meal planning guide to make up your own.
2. After you have finished your meal, take nothing by mouth (except water) and refrain from smoking until a blood sample has been drawn.
3. Exactly 2 hours after you finish eating, a blood sample is to be drawn at the laboratory. Plan to arrive at the laboratory about 10 to 15 minutes prior to the time that blood must be drawn.

100-gm Carbohydrate Test Meal

Description: The 100-gm carbohydrate test meal is used when determining a 2-hour postprandial blood glucose level.

Suggested Guide for Planning a Meal:

Food Group	*No. of Servings*	*Approx. Carbohydrate Content (gm)*
Fruit or juice	2	20
Milk	1	12
Bread	3	45
Meat	1	–
Sweets	6	28
		Total 105 gm

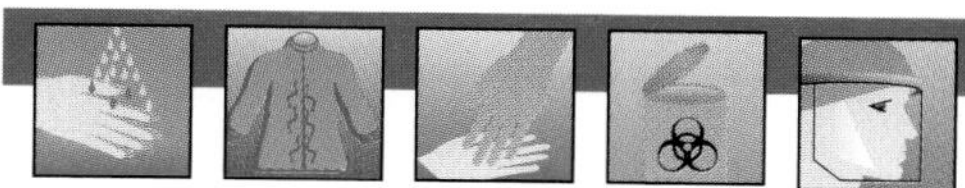

PROCEDURE 16–2

Preparing a Patient for a 2-Hour Postprandial Test (Continued)

Sample Menus

2 peach halves (canned) ½ cup Cream of Wheat 1 poached egg 2 slices toast 1 tbsp. jelly coffee or tea	OR	1 banana 1 cup cornflakes 1 scrambled egg 1 sweet roll 1 cup milk coffee or tea	OR	1 cup orange juice 2 small pancakes 3 tsp. margarine 2 tbsp. syrup coffee or tea

3. After finishing the test meal, the patient is to take nothing by mouth (although water is allowed) and is to refrain from smoking until the blood specimen has been drawn.
4. The blood specimen is to be obtained *exactly* 2 hours after the patient has finished eating. Advise the patient to arrive at the laboratory 10 to 15 minutes prior to the appointed time for drawing blood.

At the Time of Testing

5. Wash hands and put on gloves.
6. Assemble necessary equipment.
7. Prepare the patient's arm in the usual manner for a venous blood sample (Procedure 11–2).
8. Exactly 2 hours after the patient has finished eating, draw a blood specimen using a green- or gray-top tube.
9. Process the specimen according to laboratory protocol.
10. Remove and discard gloves and wash your hands.

PROCEDURE 16–3

Preparing a Patient for a Glucose Tolerance Test

Principle

To understand the preparation and procedure for the glucose tolerance test, which is used to establish a diagnosis of diabetes mellitus or hypoglycemia

Equipment and Supplies

standard venipuncture supplies (Procedure 11–2)
1 bottle oral glucose beverage
4 midstream urine collection kits
urine glucose reagent test strips
paper and pencil

Preparation Guidelines

Discuss the following with the patient when the appointment is made or prior to the day of testing.

1. Dietary considerations should be discussed thoroughly with the patient.
   A. The patient should observe a dietary regimen that includes at least 150 gm of carbohydrates (preferably, 300 gm of carbohydrates) per day for the 3 days preceding the test. A dietary list should be provided. (These are generally available upon request from the laboratory processing the test specimens.)

(continued)

PROCEDURE 16–3

Preparing a Patient for a Glucose Tolerance Test (Continued)

B. The patient should fast for a least 8 hours, but not longer than 16 hours, before the test. Water is permitted.

2. At the time of the test, the patient should not be acutely ill; recovering from recent stress, trauma, or surgery; or taking drugs that are likely to interfere with the testing protocol, including oral contraceptives, salicylates, nicotinic acid, diuretics, insulin, oral hypoglycemia drugs (tolbutamide [Orinase]), dilantin, cortisone, spironolactone, dyazide, ethanol, or estrogens.
3. The test should be conducted between 7:00 AM and 9:00 AM. The doctor should specify the amount of glucose to be administered (75 gm is the usual dose).
4. The patient is permitted to walk about the office during the test, but should remain calm. The patient may also remain seated if he/she prefers.
5. Neither coffee nor smoking is permitted during the testing period.

Procedural Steps

1. Obtain a fasting urine specimen from the patient and perform a "dipstick" test for glucose. At the same time, obtain a blood specimen for an immediate serum glucose determination. If the serum glucose level is at or below 140 mg/dL, proceed with the glucose tolerance test. The test should be canceled if the serum glucose value exceeds 140 mg/dL.

A. Draw blood from the patient using a green-top tube (heparin) and label it "fasting." Include on the label all necessary patient information.

2. Administer 75 gm of glucose or the amount ordered by the physician.
3. The glucose should be consumed within 5 minutes. The time the patient begins drinking the liquid is the starting time for the test.
4. At exactly 60-minute intervals from the starting time, collect a blood sample (fluoride or heparinized) and a urine sample. Label the specimens with the appropriate patient information and the specific time interval (e.g., 1 hour, 2 hours, 3 hours, etc.). *All specimens will be processed at one time.*
5. If the patient becomes nauseated and vomits, the test must be discontinued and rescheduled for another day.
6. If the patient exhibits hypoglycemic symptoms, such as tachycardia, sweating, or tremor, a blood specimen should be drawn and tested for glucose immediately. If the blood glucose level is less than 50 mg/dL, the test should be discontinued and the patient given orange juice or something to eat. **Document all of the patient's responses and reactions.**
7. When the test is completed, the patient should be given any previously withheld medications and some refreshments before being allowed to leave.
8. Properly dispose of or clean and store all equipment and supplies.

PROCEDURE 16–4

Preparing a Patient for a 2-Hour Oral Glucose Test

Principle

To understand the preparation and procedure for a 2-hour oral glucose test, which is used to monitor the status of borderline or known diabetics.

Equipment and Supplies

standard venipuncture supplies (Procedure 11–2)
1 bottle oral glucose beverage
2 midstream urine collection kits
urine glucose reagent test strips
paper and pencil

Procedural Steps

When the Appointment Is Made

1. Inform the patient of the date and time of the test, and instruct him/her to take medication(s) as usual

PROCEDURE 16–4

Preparing a Patient for a 2-Hour Oral Glucose Test (Continued)

on that day. Instruct the patient to **fast** for at least 8 hours prior to the test.

At the Time of Testing

2. Obtain a random urine sample to be tested for glucose.
3. Prepare the patient for a venous blood draw.
4. Obtain one 5-mL green-top tube of blood to be tested for glucose.
5. Have the patient's urine and blood tested to determine glucose levels. If the urine tests negative for glucose and the blood glucose level is within normal range, proceed with the test. If the urine tests positive or the blood glucose level is not within normal limits (74–115 mg/dL), consult the physician or pathologist for guidance.
6. If it is appropriate to proceed with testing, administer 225 mL (75 gm) of oral glucose beverage, or the amount ordered by the physician, to the patient. The oral glucose beverage should be consumed within 5 minutes. Note the time the patient begins drinking the oral glucose beverage, as the blood specimen must be drawn exactly 2 hours after that time.
7. Inform the patient that it is necessary to remain NPO (to consume nothing by mouth) for the next 2 hours, and that you should be informed if he or she feels nauseated or if vomiting occurs.
8. Obtain one 5-mL green-top vial of blood from the patient exactly 2 hours after the starting time for glucola consumption.
9. Inform the patient that the test is now completed and that he/she may eat and take any medications that were withheld during testing. It is advisable to offer the patient something to eat and drink before they leave.
10. Clean work area and properly dispose of or clean and store equipment and supplies.

Uric Acid

In patients with kidney disease, uric acid is similar to BUN and creatinine in that it is produced by the breakdown of nucleic acids and excreted in the urine. It is primarily used to diagnose **gout,** an accumulation of uric acid in the joints.

Uric acid levels are elevated in patients with gout, renal failure, or ketoacidosis and are decreased with some therapeutic drug regimens and renal tubular disease.

Proteins

Proteins represent the largest constituent routinely measured in the blood. Unlike most other analytes whose values are reported in milligrams, protein levels are reported in grams (1000 mg).

Total protein is the sum of all the body proteins, which include chains of amino acids occurring as free molecules or linked to other compounds, such as lipoprotein (Table 16–5). Protein levels are used to assess many disease states and are included in most comprehensive chemistry panels. The two main components of protein are albumin and globulin, the sum of which is total protein. Total protein and albumin levels are measured colorimetrically on a routine chemistry analyzer; globulin levels are calculated by subtracting the albumin value from the total protein value. A ratio of albumin to globulin (A/G ratio) is calculated, which is the amount of albumin divided by the amount of globulin. When this ratio is reversed (i.e., when the globulin level exceeds the albumin level), it is indicative of kidney disease, certain liver diseases, myeloma, or severe infection or inflammatory disease. Dehydra-

Table 16–5
Functions of Protein

Type of Protein	*Function*
Antibody	Neutralizes foreign bodies (antigens)
Contractile	Causes muscle contraction
Enzyme	Catalyzes biochemical reactions
Hormone (peptide)	Regulates metabolism
Structural	Provides cellular or body support
Transport	Conveys molecules

tion is associated with elevated albumin levels, whereas decreased levels are characteristic of renal disease, liver insufficiency, malnutrition, acute or chronic inflammation, malignant disease, and burns. The total protein value is elevated in patients with dehydration, chronic inflammation, or myeloma and is decreased in those with nephrosis, protein-losing diseases, hepatic insufficiency, malignant disease other than melanoma, and malnutrition.

Testing for Pancreatitis

The pancreas is a gland with two primary purposes. It functions both as an endocrine gland, synthesizing glucagon, insulin, and gastrin, and also as an exocrine gland, producing the digestive enzymes amylase and lipase.

The two most definitive tests for pancreatitis are amylase and lipase tests. However, owing to the analytical difficulties involved in testing for lipase, only amylase testing is offered in the routine chemistry laboratory, and then only when clinical symptoms (e.g., severe abdominal pains) suggest pancreatitis.

Amylase Test

Amylase is an enzyme in the exocrine pancreas. Its function is to break down starches into dextrin and maltose during the digestive process.

The methods and instrumentation for assaying amylase vary greatly, as do the reference ranges and units of measurement. Because the reference range is method-dependent, results must be carefully recorded and the reference range clearly documented. Increased amylase levels may occur in patients with a perforated ulcer, salivary gland disease, obstruction of the pancreas duct, pancreatic cancer, and many other conditions. An amylase level that is elevated more than three times the upper limit of normal is indicative of acute pancreatitis. Decreased amylase levels are seen in patients with extensive destruction of the pancreas and hepatic insufficiency.

Minerals

Assays of the minerals calcium, phosphorus, magnesium, and iron are frequently included in chemistry panels or ordered as single test requests. Elevations or decreases in mineral levels may occur in any number of diseases. It is wise to remember that calcium is essential for bone formation, muscle function, blood coagulation, and numerous other functions. Iron is necessary for hemoglobin production and is essential in many biological and chemical reactions throughout the body.

Calcium, phosphorus, and magnesium determinations are obtained using a routine chemistry analyzer, usually by the calorimetric method. Iron levels may also be determined by a routine chemistry analyzer, but nephelometric and atomic absorption methods may be used.

Calcium Analysis

Calcium analysis results are used to assess thyroid and parathyroid function, calcium metabolism, and malignant disease (Table 16–6). The reference range for calcium is 9.0 to 10.5 mg/dL. When the level is increased, it may indicate hypothyroidism, hyperparathyroidism, myeloma, or metastatic carcinoma. Decreased calcium levels suggest hyperthyroidism, hypoparathyroidism, chronic renal disease, acute pancreatitis, malnutrition, or vitamin D deficiency.

Phosphorus Analysis

Phosphorus analysis can be useful in properly evaluating and interpreting calcium levels, and it is used to detect disorders of the endocrine system, bone diseases, and kidney dysfunction. The normal reference ranges for phosphorus are found in Table 16–1. Phosphorus levels are increased in renal insufficiency, hypoparathyroidism, and hyperthyroidism, and are decreased in hypothyroidism, hyperparathyroidism, vitamin D deficiency, and malabsorption.

Iron Analysis

Iron levels are increased in hemochromatosis, various hemoglobin abnormalities, and certain genetic disorders. When test results reveal decreased iron levels, iron-deficiency anemia, chronic infection, or nephrosis may be responsible.

Magnesium Analysis

Increased magnesium levels may indicate renal disease, whereas a decrease may be attributable to alcoholism, malnutrition, malabsorption, or related conditions. Severe deficiencies can cause neuromuscular disorders, such as tremors or convulsions.

Liver (Hepatic) Tests

The liver is the largest organ in the body, performing 500 or more functions. It is the hepatic cell, however, that is responsible for most of the liver's vital accom-

Table 16–6
Disorders Affecting Blood Calcium Levels

Causes of Hypercalcemia	*Causes of Hypocalcemia*
Acidosis	Renal failure
Hyperparathyroidism	Excessive use of laxatives
Metastatic bone cancer	Cytotoxic drugs
Paget's disease of bone	Pancreatic dysfunction
Hodgkin's disease	Acute pancreatitis
Tuberculosis	Malabsorption syndrome
Hyperthyroidism	Burns
Multiple myeloma	Osteomalacia
Lymphoma	Peritonitis
Polycythemia vera	Pregnancy
Leukemia	Alkalosis (calcium ions bound to protein)
Excessive intake of vitamin D	Vitamin D deficiency
Prolonged immobilization	Alcoholism
Milk/antacid intoxication	Liver cirrhosis
	Prolonged use of adrenocorticosteroids

plishments, including the secretion of glucose, proteins, fats, and vitamins. The liver also produces bile and processes hemoglobin. It is estimated that there are more than 300 billion of these cells.

Owing to the complex nature of the liver, a battery of liver function tests (LFTs) is used to evaluate liver function. A liver panel or profile is a group of tests that can be used to assess the general condition of the liver, as well as a particular functional disorder or disease.

The tests included in a liver battery may vary. Some of the commonly used tests include total bilirubin, direct bilirubin, and enzyme tests.

Bilirubin is a waste product from the breakdown of hemoglobin that is formed in the liver and excreted in the bile. Total bilirubin levels can be broken down into direct (conjugated) bilirubin, which is excreted primarily via the intestinal tract, and indirect (free) bilirubin, which circulates primarily in the blood. Total bilirubin levels rise with any type of jaundice, whereas direct and indirect levels rise depending on the *etiology* of the jaundice. Some laboratory tests involving total and direct bilirubin determinations help to evaluate liver function and to detect hemolytic anemia. There is no specific laboratory test for indirect bilirubin; rather, it is calculated by subtracting direct bilirubin from total bilirubin.

Tests on liver enzymes include alkaline phosphatase (ALP), alanine aminotransaminase (ALT), serum glutamic-pyruvic transaminase (SGPT), asparatate aminotransaminase (AST), serum glutamic-oxaloacetic transaminase (SGOT), and gamma-glutamyltransferase (GGT) (Table 16–7). SGOT and SGPT are now referred to as ALT and AST (see Table 16–7). Liver enzyme tests are performed using a laboratory chemistry analyzer. Bilirubin is generally assayed by a colorimetric method, whereas liver enzymes are tested by a kinetic procedure.

The reference ranges for enzyme values vary depending on the analyzer, the time and temperature of the reaction, and the particular chemical analysis being done.

Generally, one or more liver tests will show mild to marked elevations, suggesting liver insufficiency, hepatitis, alcoholism, or bile obstruction. Because of this, a diagnosis cannot be established on the basis of the test results alone; rather, these test results must be interpreted in conjunction with other diagnostic assessments. Decreased liver values have little clinical significance.

Table 16–7
Liver Enzymes

Enzyme	*Clinical Utility*
ALP	Increased in obstructive liver disorders
ALT & AST	Increased in a variety of liver diseases; early indicators of cellular damage
GGT	Increased in patients with liver damage secondary to alcohol consumption
LDH	Increased in patients with metastatic cancer; isoenzyme LD-5 is general indicator of liver damage

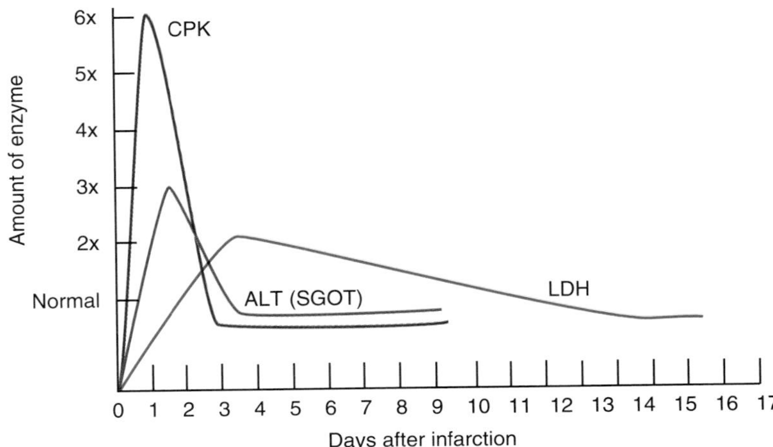

Figure 16–5. *Cardiac enzyme pattern typical of patients with myocardial infarction.*

Cardiac Circulation

The heart is a muscle, consisting of two pumps. The right side of the heart receives blood that is partially depleted of oxygen and pumps it into the lungs, where it is replenished with oxygen. The left side of the heart takes this oxygenated blood from the lungs and pumps it to the rest of the body.

Both the right and left sides of the heart have large veins and arteries. The pulmonary artery takes blood containing depleted amounts of oxygen and carbon dioxide to the lungs. The lungs then oxygenate the blood. This blood is carried via the pulmonary veins to the left side of the heart, where it is pumped to the arteries and on to the rest of the body. Arterial blood is bright red in color. In the event of a myocardial infarction (heart attack), the heart muscle is damaged, and part of it may die. In such instances, the enzymes lactic dehydrogenase (LDH) and creatine phosphokinase (CPK) are released from tissue and muscle into the blood. Although levels of these enzymes may be increased in any muscle or tissue disorder, such elevations are a significant tool in diagnosing cardiac damage (Fig. 16–5).

Cardiac Enzyme Tests

The isoenzymes of LDH and CPK (LDH-1 and CPK-MB) are definitive indicators of myocardial infarction, but are not considered to be routine chemistry tests. Thus, they will be discussed in Chapter 19.

CPK and LDH

CPK and LDH levels are measured by a routine chemistry analyzer using a kinetic method. The reference ranges are dependent upon the instrument, chemistry, and the time and temperature of the reaction used. Myocardial infarction causes elevations of CPK in the blood before LDH levels increase. CPK levels are also increased in patients with muscular dystrophy and in those undergoing surgery or engaging in strenuous exercise. CPK levels are decreased in patients who are physically inactive and in those with decreased muscle mass. LDH levels are increased in myocardial infarction, hemolytic diseases, malignant disease, progressive muscular dystrophy, and hepatic disorders. Decreases in LDH levels are not clinically significant.

Lipid Tests

Lipid tests have become a popular tool for assessing cardiac risk. Cholesterol, triglyceride, high-density lipoprotein (HDL), and low-density lipoprotein (LDL) levels, as well as calculations of cardiac risk factors, based on sex and age, are frequently assessed as part of a routine physical.

Dietary fats and oils are synthesized in the liver and stored in adipose tissue. Both diet and genetic predisposition play an important role in the concentrations of body fats.

The most common coronary heart disease is arteriosclerosis (hardening of the arteries). This condition is caused by the accumulation of fatty deposits on the wall of the coronary arteries (atherosclerosis), which leads to obstruction of normal blood flow (Fig. 16–6).

Cholesterol and triglycerides are usually the only lipids assayed in a routine chemistry panel. Pretreatment is required before HDLs can be measured, so such determinations are considered to be special chemistry procedures.

In the modern laboratory, cholesterol and triglyceride levels are assayed by an enzymatic method using a routine laboratory chemistry analyzer.

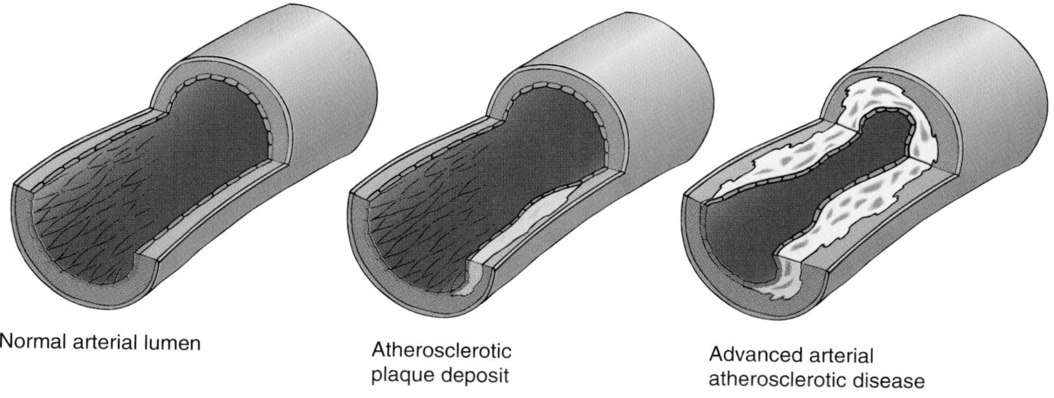

Figure 16–6. *The appearance of a normal artery compared to that of a fatty artery.*

Cholesterol

Reference ranges for cholesterol are listed in Table 16–1. Increases suggest familial (hereditary) hypercholesterolemia (high cholesterol), biliary obstruction, nephrotic syndrome, and hypothyroidism. Decreased cholesterol levels are seen in patients with severe liver insufficiency, malnutrition, hyperthyroidism, chronic anemia, or thyroiditis.

Triglycerides

Increases above the normal reference range for triglycerides may indicate a familial (hereditary) hypertriglyceridemia (high triglyceride level), nephrotic syndrome, diabetes, pancreatitis, pregnancy, liver disease, or alcoholism. Triglyceride levels are decreased in patients with malnutrition and a betalipoproteinemia.

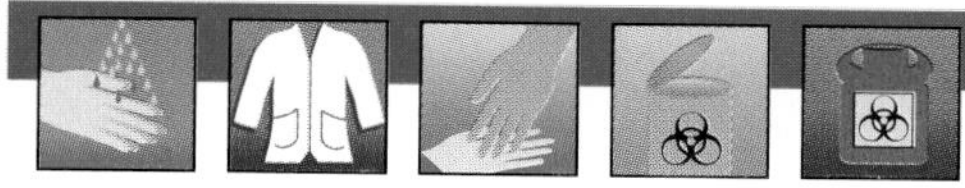

PROCEDURE 16–5

Testing Cholesterol Levels Using a ProAct Instrument

Principle

To execute and report with accuracy ProAct test for cholesterol level

Equipment and Supplies

ProAct instrument
capillary pipettor
capillary tube
alcohol wipes
adhesives bandages
lithium heparin capillary tubes
lancets and lancet device
sterile gauze or cotton balls

Procedural Steps

Obtaining the Specimen

1. Have the client sit down at the table for approximately 5 minutes prior to the finger stick. Explain the purpose of the test and the steps of the testing procedure to reassure the patient.
2. Assemble needed equipment.
3. Put on clean, disposable gloves.
4. Load the lancet device with a sterile lancet.
5. Cleanse the patient's ring or middle finger with an alcohol wipe. Allow it to air dry.
6. Puncture the side of the fingertip. Wipe away the first drop of blood with a sterile gauze pad.
7. Hold the capillary tube horizontally by the colored end and fill the capillary tube to the black line. Do not allow air bubbles to enter the tube. If this occurs, discard the tube and continue drawing the sample with a new tube.
8. Have the patient apply pressure against the puncture with a clean gauze pad or cotton ball to stop bleeding. Place an adhesive bandage on the patient's finger. Dispose of the gauze pad and cotton ball in an approved waste container.

Performing the ProAct Test

1. If gloves were removed, reglove with clean disposable gloves.

(continued)

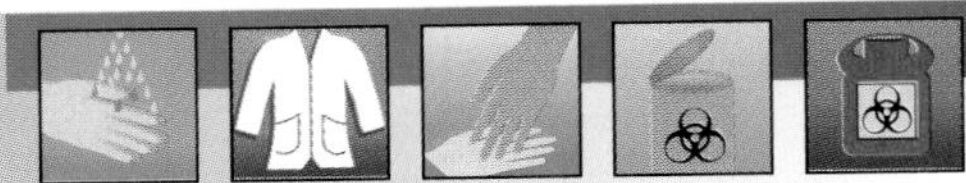

PROCEDURE 16–5

Testing Cholesterol Levels Using a ProAct Instrument (Continued)

2. Take a cholesterol test strip out of the vial. Close the vial immediately with the desiccant stopper. (Make sure the strips are at room temperature before testing.)

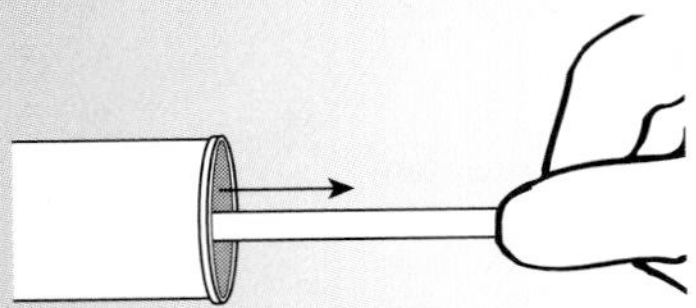

1. Remove strip from vial

3. Remove the foil protecting the test area of the strip and place the strip on a dry, hard, flat surface.

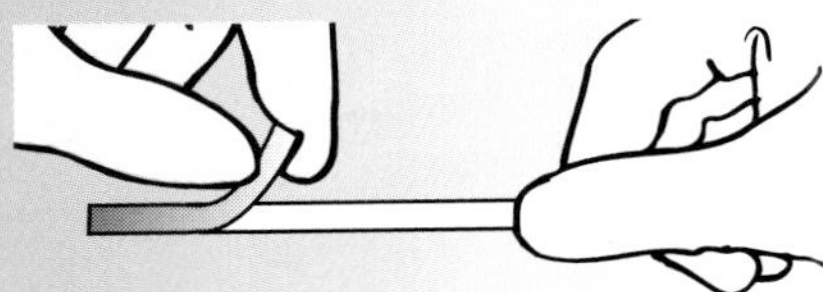

2. Remove protective layer from strip

4. Secure the capillary tube filled with blood in the pipettor.
5. Depress the plunger of the pipettor securely and smoothly to allow a drop of blood to form at the end of the capillary tube.
6. Apply the drop to the center of the red mesh application zone. Make sure that the tip does not touch the test strip and that all blood is dispensed.

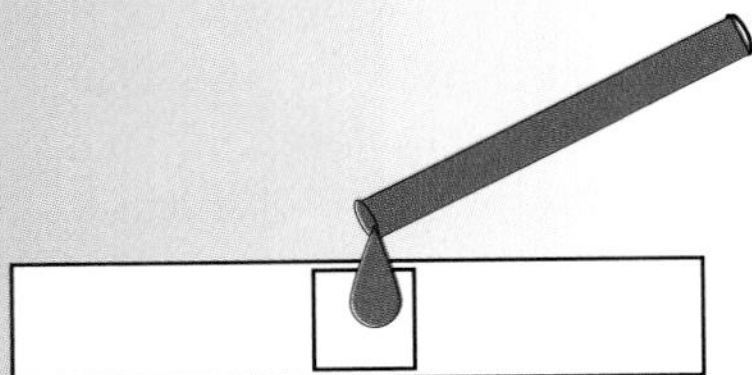

3.Add blood to strip using micropipettor

7. Allow the sample to soak into the red mesh for at least 3 seconds, but no longer than 15 seconds.
8. Insert the cholesterol test strip into the test port. The ProAct device will count down approximately 160 seconds.

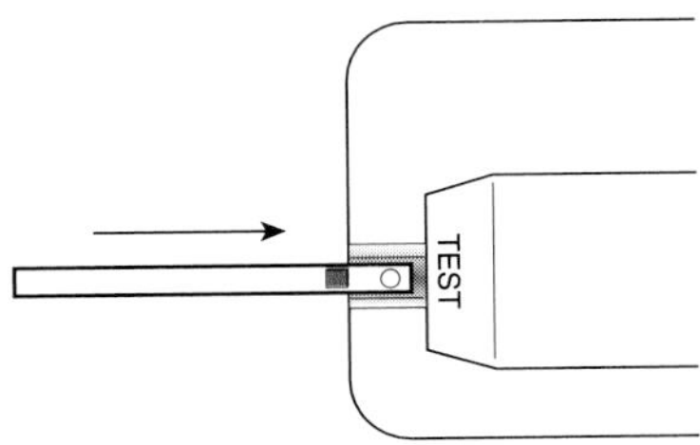

4. Add strip to test port of ProAct system

9. Remove the capillary tube from the pipettor and discard it in a biohazard container.
10. When the measurement is complete, REMOVE STRIP will appear in the display. Remove the used test strip. The test result will appear on the display.

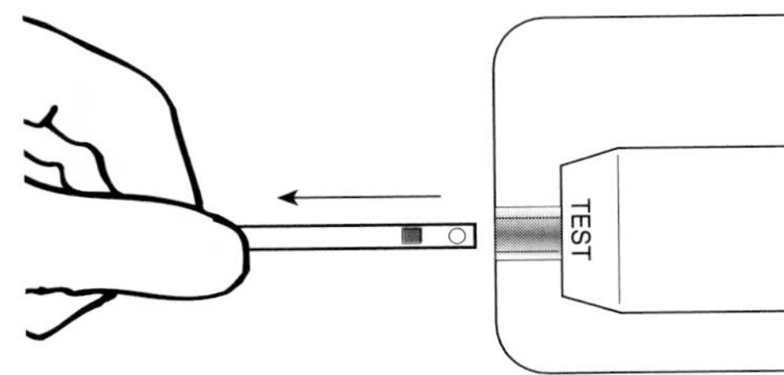

5. Remove strip when testing complete

11. Examine the test area of the used test strip for uneven color development before discarding it in a biohazard container. If the color appears mottled, repeat the test.
12. Clean the testing area and any equipment used, and discard all disposable supplies in biohazardous/sharp containers.
13. Remove gloves and wash hands.
14. Record the date and time, the test performed, and the testing results in the patient's chart or on the appropriate log (per laboratory policy). Initial the entry.

Comparing Results Against Expected Values

Assessing blood cholesterol values using ProAct:

<200 mg/dL	Desirable blood cholesterol level
200–239 mg/dL	Borderline-high blood cholesterol level
≥240 mg/dL	High blood cholesterol level

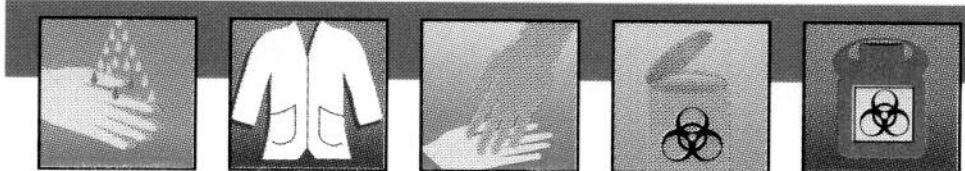

PROCEDURE 16–5

Testing Cholesterol Levels Using a ProAct Instrument (Continued)

15. Note the appropriate risk category in the patient's chart, and inform the doctor of the results. Instruct the patient to wait until the doctor has told you how to proceed. The physician may have a standard set of protocols for you to follow when test results indicate a high blood cholesterol level (see Appendix B).
16. If a value is obtained that is less than 100 mg/dL or greater than 300 mg/dL, test results should be confirmed by repeating the entire procedure.

Routine Urine Chemistry Tests

Glucose

Glucose is the urine analyte most frequently analyzed in the laboratory. Glucose determinations are usually done on a random urine specimen as part of a urinalysis, or as part of a glucose tolerance or fasting blood test. Urine glucose levels are seldom quantitated, but rather are reported qualitatively as negative, +1, +2, +3, or +4.

Protein

Although urine protein levels are part of a routine urinalysis, they are often quantitated on a chemistry analyzer. This test requires collection of a 24-hour urine specimen, refrigerated during the collection period and with no preservative added. Elevated urine protein levels are commonly found in patients with renal disease or myeloma.

Urine protein output is 30 to 100 mg/24 hr. A normal random urine protein level is less than 10 mg/dL.

PROCEDURE 16–6

Preparing a Patient for Timed/24-Hour Urine Collection

Principle

To prepare a patient for a urine specimen collection that will be used to assess hepatic or renal function

Equipment and Supplies

24-hour urine collection container
instructions for collection

Procedural Steps

Prior to urine collection, a request form will be received from the testing lab that will include a summary of urine preservative protocols. The laboratory technologist checks this summary and prepares the collection container accordingly (see Appendix A). The container is then released to you to give to the patient.

1. Determine whether the patient must observe any restrictions in dietary or medication regimen prior to timed urine sample collection. Check to see whether specific preservatives have been added to the specimen container prior to urine collection, or if they must be added after the collection period.
2. Make sure that the specimen container bears a label specifying the patient's name, height, and weight; the time interval for specimen collection; the test(s) to be performed; and any preservatives used. All containers should have a biohazard label, and a CAUTION label should also be added if a preservative has been used.
3. Prior to the start of the urine collection period, instruct the patient to abstain from any food or medications that will affect test results. Provide written instructions regarding restrictions and the proper collection procedure to the patient (see chart), along with the specimen container.

(continued)

PROCEDURE 16–6

Preparing a Patient for Timed/24-Hour Urine Collection (Continued)

Dietary/Medication Restrictions Imposed Prior to and During Timed Urine Collections

Specific Test	*Restrictions*	*Time Interval for Restriction*
5-hydroxyindoleacetic acid (5-HIAA) (serotonin)	Bananas, avocados, phenothiazine tranquilizers, pineapples, walnuts	3 days prior to and during test period
Vanillylmandelic acid (VMA)	Warfarin (Coumadin), tetracyclines, aspirin, bananas, chocolate, caffeine, coffee, tea, vanilla, food containing vanilla	1 week prior to and during test period

Instructions for Collecting a Timed Urine Sample

1. On the morning of the test, at 7:00 AM, completely empty your bladder. Discard this urine. Note the date and time of voiding on the section of the form attached to the urine collection container labeled "Urine Started" (see form below).
2. Collect ALL urine voided until the following morning at 7:00 AM (24 hours later), pouring specimens into the provided container. KEEP THE SPECIMEN REFRIGERATED THROUGHOUT THE COLLECTION PERIOD UNTIL IT IS DELIVERED TO THE LABORATORY. Void at 7:00 AM and add this urine sample to the collection container. Note the date and time on the section of the accompanying form labeled "Urine Ended."
3. Remove the urine specimen from the refrigerator and bring it to the laboratory *immediately* with the attached form specifying dates and times.
4. If you have any questions during the urine collection period, call 000–0000 or 000–0000.

Patient Information Form

PATIENT'S NAME ______________________________

HEIGHT: ______________WEIGHT: _____________

URINE STARTED: DATE: _____ TIME: _____ AM PM

URINE ENDED: DATE: _____ TIME: _____ AM PM

4. When the patient returns the collected urine specimen, check to be sure that all the necessary information is provided. Immediately send the specimen to the Chemistry Department of the laboratory.
5. Record the date and type of specimen collected on the patient's chart or in the laboratory logbook (per protocol). Be sure to initial the entry.

Creatinine, Sodium, and Potassium

Creatinine, sodium, and potassium levels are also indicators of renal function. The creatinine test is performed on either a 12- or 24-hour urine sample. The reference range for creatinine is 1.0 to 2.0 gm/24 hr; however, it may be reported in milligrams, in which case the range is 1000 to 2000 mg/24 hr. Sodium levels are usually assessed to evaluate acute renal failure, and potassium levels are used to evaluate acid–base balance.

Urine creatinine excretion is fairly constant for a given individual; for different individuals, it is approximately proportional to body surface area. It is nearly independent of diet.

PROCEDURE 16–7

Preparing a Patient for a Creatinine Clearance Test (24-Hour Urine Specimen)

Principle

To prepare a patient for a urine specimen that will be used to assess the filtering rate of the glomerulus

Equipment and Supplies

24-hour labeled urine collection container
instructions for collection
low-protein diet guidelines
venous blood-drawing tray (Procedure 11–2) stocked with 5-mL red-top tube

Procedural Steps

1. Prior to the start of the urine collection period, instruct the patient to abstain from meat, coffee, tea, and drugs from 10:00 PM the night before beginning urine collection until the end of the urine collection period. The patient should also be instructed to consume a low-protein diet during the urine collection period (see table). Explain the testing procedure to the patient and provide a specimen container and a written set of instructions (see chart).
2. When the patient returns with the collected urine specimen, check the accompanying form to be sure that all necessary information is included.
   A. Proper labeling—urine-started section
   B. Correct preparation
   C. Label completion—urine-ended section
3. Prepare the patient for a venous blood draw.
4. Obtain a specimen of clotted blood, using one 5-mL red-top tube, for creatinine clearance testing.
5. If the urine specimen will not be tested on the day that specimen collection is completed, it should be stored at a temperature of 2° to 8°C. No preservatives should be added to the specimen.

Guidelines for a Low-Protein Diet

Type of Food	*Foods Allowed*	*Restrictions*
Soups	Clear broth, tomato (if water is used), vegetable	No meat soups or cream soups
Eggs	2 per day, either eaten as such or used in cooking	Not to exceed the limit stated
Meat	NONE	Avoid all meat
Milk and milk products	1 cup of milk, either consumed as such or used in cooking, plus 1/2 cup of cottage cheese	Not to exceed the limit stated
Vegetables	Any vegetable, as desired, cooked or eaten raw	None prepared with milk or cheese
Fruits	Any fruit or fruit juice, as much as desired; may be consumed in large quantities	No restrictions
Salad	Any nonmeat salad, with dressing as desired.	No cheese in salad, unless within the limits stated
Cereals	Any kind, any way (1 serving)	No restrictions
Breads	Any kind, as desired (3 servings)	No restrictions
Desserts	Fruit dessert, cake, sherbet, fruit pies if prepared without milk or eggs or if the limits stated are not exceeded	No ice cream, puddings, cream pies, angel food cake, or sponge cake
Concentrated Sweets	Sugars, jams, jellies, syrup, honey, hard candy, eaten as desired	
Fats	Butter as desired	
Peanut Butter	Limit of 2 tbsp.	Not to exceed the limit stated
Beverages	Water, fruit juice, or vegetable juice	No coffee or tea

(continued)

PROCEDURE 16–7

Preparing a Patient for a Creatinine Clearance Test (24-Hour Urine Specimen) *(Continued)*

Instructions for Collecting a 24-Hour Urine Sample

1. On the morning of the test, at 7:00 AM, completely empty your bladder. Discard this urine. Note the date and time of voiding on the section of the form attached to the specimen container labeled "Urine Started."
2. Collect ALL urine voided until the following morning at 7:00 AM (24 hours later), pouring specimens into the provided container. KEEP THE SPECIMEN REFRIGERATED THROUGHOUT THE COLLECTION PERIOD UNTIL IT IS DELIVERED TO THE LABORATORY. Void at 7:00 AM and add this urine sample to the collection container. Complete the "Urine Ended" section of the form accompanying the specimen container.
3. Remove the urine specimen from the refrigerator and bring it to the laboratory *immediately* with the attached form. A blood specimen will be drawn when you return to the laboratory with your urine specimen.
4. If you have any questions during the urine collection period, call 000–0000.

Patient Information Form

PATIENT'S NAME ____________________________

HEIGHT: ______________WEIGHT: ____________

URINE STARTED: DATE: _____ TIME: _____ AM PM

URINE ENDED: DATE: _____ TIME: _____ AM PM

Other Frequently Ordered Tests

The tests described in this chapter are only the routine tests that can be performed quickly and inexpensively. However, as previously mentioned, many more tests and test panels are frequently ordered that require special methodology and instrumentation.

These tests include the thyroid panel, hepatitis panel, electrophoresis, arterial blood gas studies, hormone studies, fluorescent antibody studies, osmolality, radioimmunoassay, prostatic acid phosphatase, urinary amines, and paternity tests or genetic studies. These test are described in Chapter 19.

Summary

This chapter has provided an overview of clinical chemistry, described various tests and how they relate to both health and disease, and underscored the importance of these tests as aids to diagnosis and treatment of individual patients.

Proper specimen collection for such tests begins with adequate patient preparation. Once the patient has been prepared, it is extremely important that you collect specimens in the appropriate container, which ensures that you will have the correct additive to secure valid testing information (Table 16–8). In addition, it is important to understand the meaning of reference ranges, units of measurement, common testing methods used, and some of the more frequently ordered routine tests and their diagnostic value.

Chapter Review

True or False

Circle T or F to indicate the correct answers to the following:

T F 1. Routine chemistry tests are costly to perform.

T F 2. A physician can make a diagnosis solely on the results of an accurate test panel.

T F 3. Ultimately, it is the physician's decision to determine the merit of the test results as they relate to the treatment of the patient.

T F 4. Positively charged ions are called anions.

T F 5. A negatively charged ion is HOP_4.

Fill in the Blanks

Complete the following statements:

6. Elevations in the anion gap help to diagnose

   ______________ .

7. One test that can assist in the management of diabetes mellitus is ______________ .

Table 16–8
Characteristics of Various Blood Collection Tubes

Color	Optimum Volume (mL)	Minimum Volume (mL)	Additive
Blue	4.5	4.5	Sodium citrate
			No additive (for trace metals)
Blue-navy	7	NA	Heparin (for trace metals)
Fibrinogen split products (FSP) (blue top) inhibitor	2	2	Thrombin, trypsin
Gray	10	10	Potassium oxalate, sodium fluoride
Green	10	3.5	Heparin
Lavender	7	2	EDTA
Orange	10	NA	Thrombin
Red	10	NA	None
Red (for tissue typing)	10	NA	Heparin added
Red/gray (gel) activator	10	NA	Inert barrier clot
Yellow	5	NA	ACD
Yellow/black	7	NA	Thrombin
PEDIATRIC TUBES			
Blue	2.7	2.7	Sodium citrate
Yellow (culture)	3.3	3.3	SPS
Green	2	2	Heparin
	2	0.6	
Lavender	3	0.9	EDTA
	4	1	
	2	NA	
Red	3	NA	None
	4	NA	

NA, not applicable; *EDTA,* ethylenediaminetetra-acetic acid; *ACD,* acid-citrate-dextrose; *SPS,* sodium polyanetholesulfonate.

8. Serum creatinine levels increase in ______________ .

9. The normal range for BUN level is ______________ .

Multiple Choice

Circle the letter that represents the single best answer:

10. Increases in blood glucose levels may be caused by:
    a. Chronic renal failure
    b. Pancreatitis
    c. Endocrine malfunction
    d. Defective carbohydrate metabolism
    e. All of the above

11. A uric acid test may be ordered to help diagnose:
    a. Diabetes mellitus
    b. Gout
    c. Cancer
    d. Jaundice
    e. Prostatitis

12. Albumin levels are elevated in:
    a. Renal disease
    b. Malnutrition
    c. Dehydration
    d. Burns
    e. Heart attack

13. Lipid tests include all of the following EXCEPT:
    a. HDL
    b. Bilirubin
    c. LDL
    d. Triglycerides
    e. Cholesterol

14. Two enzymes that are helpful in diagnosing a heart attack are:
    a. Glucose and CPK
    b. CPK and LDL
    c. CPK and LDH
    d. Glucose and LDH
    e. LDL and LDH

Vocabulary

cholinesterase: an enzyme that is present throughout the body and is released when a nerve impulse reaches the myoneural junction
decongestant: an agent that reduces swelling
glaucoma: disease of the eye resulting in pathologic changes in the optic nerve
index: the numerical ratio produced when measuring any part in comparison with a fixed standard
indices: plural of index
idiosyncrasy: an abnormal susceptibility to a drug or other agent that is peculiar to the individual
psychosis: a state in which a person's mental capacity to recognize reality is impaired
qualitative: pertaining to a precise measurement that determines the amount of a substance that is present or absent
quantitative: pertaining to a precise physical measurement of energy or mass
solvent: a substance capable of dissolving another material
STAT: immediately
suppressant: an agent that stops secretion, excretion, or normal discharge

Chapter Objectives

After reading this chapter, you should be able to:

1. Define and elaborate on therapeutic index.
2. Define therapeutic drug monitoring.
3. List two tests used in environmental toxicology laboratories for the detection of pesticides and herbicides in the blood.
4. Identify four poisonous metals and cite a possible source for each.
5. List 10 poisonous plants that may be ingested.
6. Explain the effects of inhaling carbon monoxide.
7. Describe the most widely used and abused drug (ethanol).
8. List the most common illicit drugs used in the United States today.
9. Identify the types of specimens commonly used for drug testing.
10. Outline the most common methods of testing for drugs.
11. Explain why urine specimens are so good for drug screening tests.
12. Explain a positive test result.

Chapter 17
Toxicology

Toxicology is the study of poisonous substances and their effects on living organisms. There are huge numbers of potentially toxic substances, many of which can be beneficial medicines when properly used. Some examples of toxic substances that can be beneficial medicines include pesticides, plants, animal toxins, gases, ethanol, and tobacco. Depending on the particular substance and conditions being considered, laboratory tests may be of either great or little use in care of the patient. Furthermore, the legal and social implications of testing for toxic substances must be given serious consideration.

Therapeutic Drug Monitoring

Some medicines, such as digoxin (a cardiac stimulant) and theophylline (an asthma medicine), have narrow therapeutic **indices.**

The *therapeutic **index*** is the range of blood levels of a drug, beginning at the point at which the drug begins to have a significant medicinal effect and terminating at the point where toxic effects begin to occur. Therapeutic drug monitoring (TDM) is useful for such drugs. This subject is discussed in detail in Chapter 18.

Monitored Substances

Pesticides and Herbicides

Pesticides and herbicides may be highly toxic, but blood levels are rarely measured, and then only in special environmental toxicology laboratories. The **cholinesterase** test is commonly performed in clinical laboratories to detect poisoning by organophosphate pesticides, such as Malathion, that lower both serum and red blood cell (RBC) cholinesterase levels. The RBC cholinesterase test is important for long-term monitoring of pesticide exposure, but it is difficult to perform and so is only conducted in large research laboratories. Serum cholinesterase levels, which are generally available on a **STAT** basis at many hospitals, are satisfactory for diagnosis of acute poisoning.

Metals

Poisonous metals include iron, arsenic, mercury, and lead. Iron (typically in the form of adult iron pills) is toxic for infants and very young children whose bodies cannot yet regulate iron uptake from the intestine. At many clinical laboratories, STAT serum iron levels can be performed. Arsenic and mercury were once widely used as pesticides and herbicides, and are still so used to some extent. They can persist in the environment for decades. Chronic lead exposure is a significant public health problem, especially in areas with old housing. This is because paint containing white lead-based pigments was once widely used. Lead is particularly dangerous for growing children because the damage can be permanent and irreversible if not discovered and treated promptly. Poisoning with lead, mercury, and arsenic is usually chronic, so the tests are not normally available on a STAT basis.

Plants

Plants produce a wide range of physiologically active materials, and some of these are strong poisons. Blood levels are not generally available; diagnosis and treatment are normally based on history and symptoms.

Common plant poisons include castor beans, wisteria seeds, morning glory seeds, jimsonweed, foxglove, oleander, and peach leaves, among others. Tobacco, cocaine, marijuana, and opiates are discussed in subsequent sections of this chapter.

Animal Toxins

Fewer toxic substances are derived from animals than from plants. Again, laboratory tests are not generally available for these toxins. The parotid secretions of toads, the secretions of "poison arrow" frogs (when given their natural diet), snake venom, and spider and insect venom are examples of animal toxins. Hospital emergency rooms may stock antivenins for locally significant animal toxins.

Poisonous Gases

Many toxic gases may be encountered in industrial settings, but there is only one to which people are commonly exposed: carbon monoxide. Carbon monoxide is formed whenever fuels are burned with insufficient air. It is a particular problem during the winter, when people are likely to be inside closed houses that are heated by fuel. Modern automobiles produce very little carbon monoxide, but can still produce enough to kill, especially if the pollution control devices are not working properly. Carbon monoxide displaces oxygen from hemoglobin to form *carboxyhemoglobin,* which prevents the blood from carrying sufficient oxygen. Even a small percentage of carbon monoxide in the air can, in time, bring about death, but prompt treatment with 100% oxygen quickly restores the patient. The respiratory therapy department or the laboratory of a hospital may be equipped to measure carboxyhemoglobin or carbon monoxide on a STAT basis.

Volatile Hydrocarbons

Acetone, ethanol, isopropanol, and methanol are the four toxic substances that constitute the toxicology volatile group. Whenever persons are newly unconscious, for unknown reasons, a toxicology screening test for volatiles is routinely ordered. This test detects the presence of any of these four substances.

These chemicals are found in many household products, such as cleaning solutions, nail polish removers, disposable lighters, and various types of glue. Spray products, such as hair spray, paint, and lacquers, use hydrocarbons as the propellant. Because they are relatively inexpensive and legal to purchase, the inhaling of a volatile hydrocarbon has become popular among teens and those who cannot afford other illegal drugs. "Huffing" is a street term used to describe inhalation of a volatile hydrocarbon.

Determination of the acetone level by a volatile screening test helps to identify isopropanol alcohol (rubbing alcohol) ingestion and/or toxicity because, when ingested, isopropanol is converted to acetone. Isopropanol is also a major component in perfumes, aftershaves, and antifreeze.

Methanol, also known as wood alcohol, is an ingredient in antifreeze and "moonshine" liquor. Methanol and isopropanol may be consumed by alcoholics who are accustomed to grain alcohol but who, for one reason or another, cannot obtain it.

Ethanol, also known as grain alcohol, is found in beer, wine, and distilled liquors, and is the most widely used and abused drug in most societies (Table 17–1). This substance depresses the central nervous system and may lead to coma, progressing to death at panic levels (Table 17–2). Most societies permit the use of alcohol but at the same time attempt to limit alcohol abuse. Alcohol is one of the few drugs for which there is an established correlation between blood levels and impaired driving ability. Testing of the blood of accused drunk drivers for alcohol is strictly regulated by law when it is to be used for prosecution.

Table 17–1
Approximate Ethanol Content in Alcoholic Beverages

Beverage	*Ethanol Content (%)*
Beer	3–6
Ciders	4–5
Wines	8–15
Sherry, madeira, port	18–20
Whiskey, gin	40–45
Vodka	40–50
Brandy	45–50
Rum	50–70

From Calbreath, D. F., *Clinical Chemistry* (Philadelphia: W. B. Saunders, 1992), p. 426.

Both blood and urine levels of these substances are important. Blood levels reflect the level of substances that have been ingested recently, whereas urine levels are indicative of substances that may have been ingested over a longer period of time. Blood and urine alcohol tests, when performed for medical reasons, are regulated like any other clinical laboratory tests. For legal purposes, a level of alcohol, above which a person is presumed to be too impaired to drive, is established by law. Forensic laboratories usually measure the amount of alcohol in whole blood, whereas clinical laboratories usually measure alcohol in plasma or serum, which contains about 10% more alcohol than whole blood.

Table 17–2
Volatile Hydrocarbon Panic Levels

Substance	*Blood Panic Level (μg/mL)*	*Urine Panic Level (μg/mL)*
Acetone	>500	>500
Ethanol	>2000	>1600
Isopropanol	>500	>500
Methanol	>500	>500

Sufficient blood is drawn to allow for immediate testing and for analysis by the defendant if requested by the defense attorney. In addition, the balance must be retained for 1 year after the date of collection for forensic needs. If the case is being handled by the coroner, the blood samples should be retained for at least 90 days. The time for specimen retention may differ from state to state.

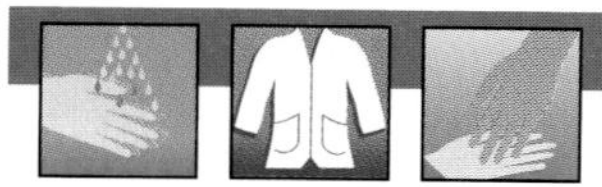

PROCEDURE 17–1

Assisting With Blood Alcohol Testing

Principle

To prepare testing equipment and assist with the testing protocols

Equipment and Supplies

gray-stoppered tubes
nonvolatile disinfectant (e.g., benzalkonium [Zephiran] or aqueous thimerosal [Merthiolate])

Patient Preparation

The patient will probably still be "under the influence" of alcohol. An officer of the law will be present to act as a witness to the procedure. Explain to the patient what you will be doing in as brief and concise a manner as possible. Do not allow yourself to become irritated by the speech and/or mannerisms of your patient. Treat this patient with the respect and dignity with which you treat all your patients.

Procedural Steps

The Department of Justice for each state has established uniform standards for the collection, handling, and preservation of blood samples prior to analysis. If you are authorized to obtain specimens for forensic analysis, check your laboratory's procedure manual so that you perform the collection *exactly* as required by the uniform standards established for your state.

1. Wash hands, dry them thoroughly, and don gloves.
2. Label two gray-stoppered tubes with the following information:
   a. Full name of patient
   b. Date and time of blood draw

(continued)

PROCEDURE 17-1

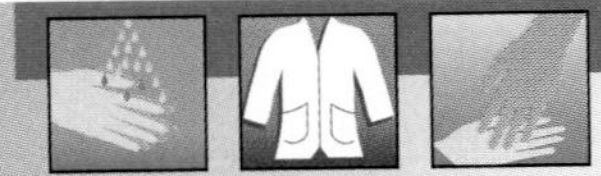

Assisting With Blood Alcohol Testing (Continued)

   c. Your initials (as the person drawing the blood)
   d. Initials of the witnessing officer
3. Prepare the draw site using Zephiran, aqueous Merthiolate, or another suitable aqueous disinfectant. **DO NOT USE alcohol or other volatile organic disinfectant to clean the skin site.**
4. Complete the blood draw, filling both labeled tubes. Sufficient blood should be collected to permit duplicate blood alcohol determinations.
5. Give the blood samples to the officer present, who will immediately complete the required information on the envelope/container label and seal the container or envelope securely. Information on the envelope/container should include:
   a. The full name of the patient
   b. Whether the patient is alive or dead
   c. The submitting agency
   d. The geographical location where the blood was drawn (e.g., hospital, clinic, or jail)
   e. The name of the person drawing the blood sample
   f. The date and time the blood sample was drawn
   g. The signature of the witnessing officer
6. Once the envelope/container is sealed, it must not be opened except for analysis. Each person who subsequently is in possession of the sealed sample must sign his or her name in the space provided on the envelope/container label. The integrity of the example MUST be safeguarded.
7. Remove gloves and wash hands.

Problem Solving Exercise

Break into groups of three. Each member of the group should assume one of the following roles: officer, patient, authorized laboratory assistant. Role play the specimen collection procedure without referring to the written procedure. When finished, refer to the written procedure and analyze what you did as a group to determine whether the procedure you followed would be valid in a court of law.

Tobacco

Tobacco use is legal, but increasing concerns about its health effects have led to regulations designed to discourage its use and to make it illegal for anyone younger than 21 years of age to buy tobacco. It is undoubtedly an addictive stimulant, and it is associated with well-known and potentially very serious toxic effects. Research has shown that the use of tobacco frequently diminishes a person's normal respiratory response to elevated carbon dioxide levels, causing the patient to experience difficulty in ventilating the lungs and thus limiting the free exchange of respiratory gases.

Tobacco has been labeled a "gateway drug;" that is, many people believe that the use of it often precedes the use of illicit drugs. This has not been proven, however, and studies have been conducted that both support and deny this claim. Tobacco use is known to be directly and indirectly associated with a large number of deaths, but until very recently, it has only been tested for as cotinine, which is the metabolite of nicotine. Now it is being tested for primary and secondary smoke inhalation also.

Over-the-Counter and Prescription Drugs

There are thousands of over-the-counter (OTC) drugs and prescription drugs that can make patients ill. Individuals may have a drug **idiosyncrasy** or sensitivity, they may take too much of a drug, or they may suffer ill effects from incompatible drugs. People may also become ill when they do not take a prescribed medicine or OTC drug as directed. People have a tendency to overmedicate themselves, applying the old adage "If a little is good, a whole lot is better." Alternatively, they may discontinue use of a drug before it is appropriate to do so ("I feel so great, I don't need this prescription any more."). Tests for a particular drug, or for drugs in general, may be ordered in any of these cases. Patients may also tend to forget that OTC medications are drugs, and that the use of these drugs should be re-

Table 17–3
Time Interval for Detecting Drugs in Urine

Drug	Time Interval
Amphetamines	4 hr
Cannabinoids	1 hr to 3 days
Codeine	4 hr
Methaqualone	7 days
Barbiturates	24 hr to 7 days
Cocaine	2–3 days
Methadone	3 days
Morphine	4 hr

ported to their physician when laboratory tests are to be performed (Table 17–3).

Drugs of Abuse

Any drug can be abused, but "drugs of abuse" are nowadays often understood to be illegally obtained drugs used for recreational purposes or to satisfy an addiction. In some cases, these drugs have legitimate legal uses. Patterns of drug abuse vary greatly with place and time, but the most common illicit drugs used in the United States today are methamphetamine, cocaine, opiates, phencyclidine, and marijuana. Testing for these drugs is common in clinical laboratories; however, such tests are seldom performed in the physician's office laboratory (POL).

Methamphetamine

Methamphetamine (also known as "crank" or "speed") is a synthetic stimulant that was developed as a substitute for ephedrine (a natural product). Methamphetamine is available by prescription, but is nowadays rarely used for legitimate medical purposes. In addition to its powerful stimulatory effects, methamphetamine is a **decongestant** and an appetite **suppressant.** Chronic use of even therapeutic doses can induce paranoid **psychosis,** and abuse can result in extreme restlessness, anxiety, and violent behavior, among other symptoms. Heart failure is a common cause of death in methamphetamine addicts.

Cocaine

Cocaine is a natural stimulant, vasoconstrictor, and anesthetic. It has remained the anesthetic of choice for certain types of oropharyngeal surgery. There was an epidemic of cocaine abuse in the United States in the late 19th and early 20th centuries, and in the latter 20th century, another such epidemic began. Out of this latest epidemic has come new forms of the same drug, such as "rock cocaine" and "crack." Chronic abuse of cocaine produces lesions in the heart muscle that can lead to sudden heart failure.

Opiates

Opiates are derived from the opium poppy, *Papaver somniferum*. Opium and its derivatives—morphine, codeine and heroin—are very potent pain medicines. Up until the late 1960s, there were no painkillers that were even comparable in strength. Hospitals still use morphine and codeine, and both of these remain under lock in every institution that carries them. Some people will become addicted to these drugs when they have ready access to them; thus, access to these substances is carefully controlled.

Phencyclidine

Phencyclidine piperidine (PCP) was developed as a general anesthetic, but its legal use was discontinued because of the very disturbing hallucinations suffered by some patients. In low doses, its effects are similar to those of alcohol (including driving impairment). With overdoses, patients may exhibit maniacal violence, sudden behavioral changes, and other behavioral/psychological abnormalities.

Marijuana

Marijuana (cannabis) is a widely used drug which has a long history of both recreational and medical use throughout much of the world. However, its possession and use is generally illegal in the United States at this time. The main active ingredient of marijuana is tetrahydrocannabinol (THC). Recent scientific studies supported and published by the U.S. government indicate that marijuana does not seem to impair driving ability significantly, and many of the claims that marijuana induces aberrant behavior or illness seem to be ill-founded. It is reasonable to assume that smoking marijuana would have an effect on one's health. It is very important to remember that marijuana is an illegal drug, and that buying or using it is prohibited by law. Medical uses of marijuana have included general anesthesia, pain relief; treatment of **glaucoma,** and treatment of chemotherapy side effects (notably, nausea and loss of appetite). When used medically, it is prescribed under the same precautions as cocaine and morphine.

Methadone

One method for treating narcotic addiction is by administration of methadone (Dolophine). Methadone is a synthetic narcotic which prevents withdrawal symptoms and satisfies the craving for the narcotic. The potential problem with methadone treatment lies in the duration of therapy, as it, too, is an addicting substance. Once the person is free from the use of the original narcotic addiction, the methadone addiction must be overcome.

Why Test for Drugs?

Drug testing has become very widespread, and it is done for a variety of purposes. Physicians may order drug tests as an aid to diagnosis and treatment. Police may order drug tests to establish whether a person's abnormal behavior or impaired driving are the result of drug abuse. Employers may require drug screens because they want to avoid hiring users of illicit drugs or to rule out drugs as the cause of on-the-job accidents or impaired performance. Courts may impose drug testing as a condition of probation or as a condition of visitation rights. Newborn children may be taken from their mothers by government agencies if the babies test positive for certain drugs. Schools may impose drug testing as a condition of students' participation in certain activities.

We are seeing many attempts to control the use of illegal drugs in the hopes of avoiding the dependency that accompanies their usage. Many of the methods used have been widely criticized, and the controversy within this area will likely continue for years.

Types of Specimens Used for Drug Testing

Clinical laboratories commonly test serum, plasma, and urine for drugs. Forensic laboratories often test whole blood. Availability is the first consideration. For instance, a patient in renal failure cannot produce a urine specimen, so blood is the only specimen that can be tested. Coroners' laboratories may have to test solid tissues for drugs. If a phlebotomist is not available, urine may be the only available specimen.

The second consideration is the intended use of the specimen. Urine specimens are very good for **qualitative** drug screening, because most drugs that are present in the blood will be present in the urine, normally at far higher concentrations. It is relatively simple to test a urine specimen for hundreds of common drugs within less than an hour. Furthermore, because urine is essentially a protein-free filtrate, it is far easier to test than blood or serum. However, correlating urine concentrations of drugs or drug metabolites with the patient's clinical condition is difficult or even impossible. Serum and blood are satisfactory for specific **quantitative** drug tests, and for correlation with a subject's clinical condition. Thus, it makes no sense to order simultaneous serum and urine general drug screens. It does make sense, however, to order a urine drug screen and to collect a blood specimen at the same time if quantitation of any drugs detected could be of use to the attending physician. Law enforcement agencies may request screening of blood for a small number of specific illicit or commonly abused drugs, with confirmation and quantitation of positive test results. This is also practical for instances in which a specific drug is strongly suspected or known to be present, in which case it would be reasonable to proceed directly to a blood test (see Table 17–2).

Methods of Testing for Drugs

There are many different methods of testing for drugs. There is no single best method. In selecting the testing method that will produce the best analyses, three factors are considered:

1. The drug being tested
2. The type of specimen used for the test
3. The testing circumstances

Immunoassays

Immunoassays are common in clinical laboratories. Some of those most frequently used include latex agglutination tests (which are read visually), radioimmunoassay (RIA), fluorescence polarization immunoassay (performed on the Abbott TDx and related instruments), and enzyme-multiplied immunoassay technique (EMIT), a trademark of the Syva Corporation. These tests are not completely specific.

Latex Agglutination

Latex agglutination tests are examples of tests that can conveniently be performed on an occasional basis in a POL. They are too expensive for large-volume work, but require no instrumentation. Their use is generally confined to urine specimens.

Radioimmunoassay

Radioimmunoassay is usually a manual test. It is satisfactory for use on blood as well as other body fluids, and is widely used in forensic toxicology laboratories.

Fluorescence Polarization Immunoassay

Fluorescence polarization immunoassay is an automated test. It can be used for both quantitative analysis of therapeutic drugs and for urine screening for specific drugs of abuse.

EMIT

EMIT is very widely used for testing urine specimens for drugs of abuse. It is fully automated and can be performed with ordinary clinical chemistry analyzers, along with alcohol tests.

Chromatography

Thin-Layer Chromatography

Thin-layer chromatography is well suited for simultaneous screening of urine specimens for hundreds of drugs. Results are qualitative only, and the test is not extremely sensitive. It is best used for testing specimens from hospital emergency rooms, but is not widely available because of the technical expertise required to perform the test. Drugs are extracted from the specimens to be tested, concentrated, and applied to the bottom of a strip of paper or other permeable material. The bottom of the strip is then immersed in a **solvent** inside a closed container. As the solvent travels up the paper, drugs are carried along at different rates and separated. After drying the chromatogram, the drugs (if present) may be visualized as colored spots by spraying with various chemicals (Figs. 17–1 *A–G* and 17–2).

High-Pressure Liquid Chromatography

High-pressure liquid chromatography (HPLC) is generally used for the analysis of certain therapeutic drugs. As in thin-layer chromatography, drugs are extracted from a sample of blood, injected into an instrument, as in gas chromatography, and carried by a flowing liquid through a heated tube filled with porous material. The drugs are separated from one another and detected at the end of the tube or column by one of several types of detectors (Fig. 17–3). Figure 17–4 shows a chromatogram of the benzodiazepine (Valium and Librium) standards and Figure 17–1*E* depicts the ultraviolet spectra of nordiazepam.

Gas Chromatography

Gas chromatography is the method of choice for forensic blood alcohol tests and is the basis of gas chromatography–mass spectrometry (GC/MS). A sample of blood is pretreated, injected into the testing instrument, and carried by a flowing gas through a heated tube filled with porous material. Volatile components, including alcohol, are separated from one another and detected at the end of the tube or column by one of several types of detectors. In the case of alcohol, the detector is usually a flame ionization detector (FID) (Fig. 17–5).

Gas Chromatography/Mass Spectrometry

GC/MS is now the method of choice for many drug tests, including the common drugs of abuse. It is not satisfactory for screening purposes. Extensive and sometimes complicated preparation of samples is often required, followed by very careful separation of components by gas chromatography. The detector is a mass spectrometer, which works by ionizing and fragmenting the compounds that come through the gas chromatograph, and then measuring the amounts of the various fragments. **If done very carefully, this is a method of unparalleled specificity.** It is very complicated, and is only performed at a small number of reference and specialty laboratories. In order to test positive for a drug by GC/MS, a specimen must contain a substance that:

1. is extracted from the specimen under the same conditions as an established standard
2. undergoes the same derivatization as an authentic standard
3. produces a derivative that is extracted under the same conditions as that of an established standard
4. passes through a gas chromatograph in the same length of time as an established standard
5. when ionized, produces fragments of the same size as an established standard
6. produces those fragments in the same proportions as an established standard

It would seem that meeting these requirements would ensure that all positive tests by GC/MS were reliable, but as previously stated, one test alone should never be considered sufficient to establish a positive result. GC/MS tests are considered to be very reliable, but they are so long and complicated, and operation of the instrument is so demanding, that errors may be made. If the analyst does not realize that an error has occurred, an erroneous report may be issued, perhaps with terrible consequences for the person being tested. For this reason, GC/MS results are normally confirmed by some other method (Figs. 17–6 and 17–7).

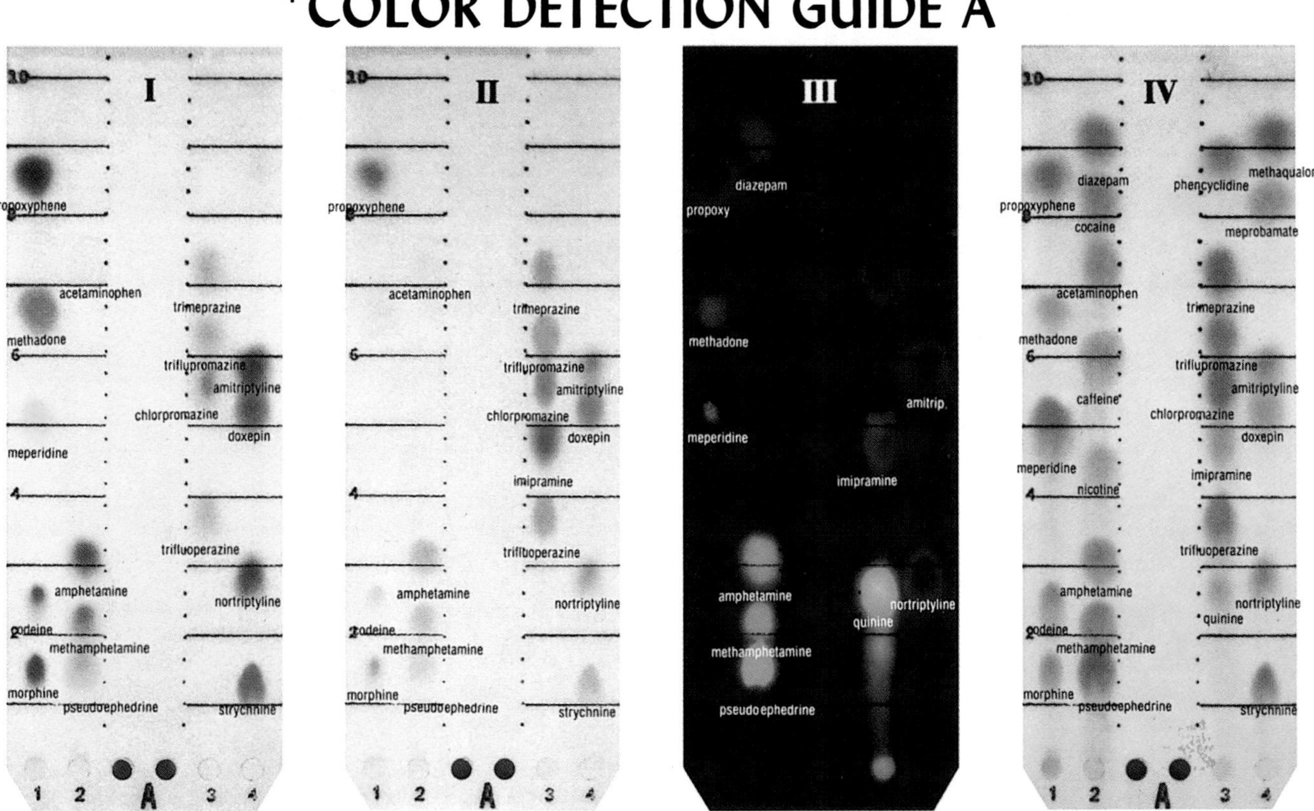

* Some variation in the color and position of the drug spots is normal.

A

Figure 17–1. *See legend on opposite page.*

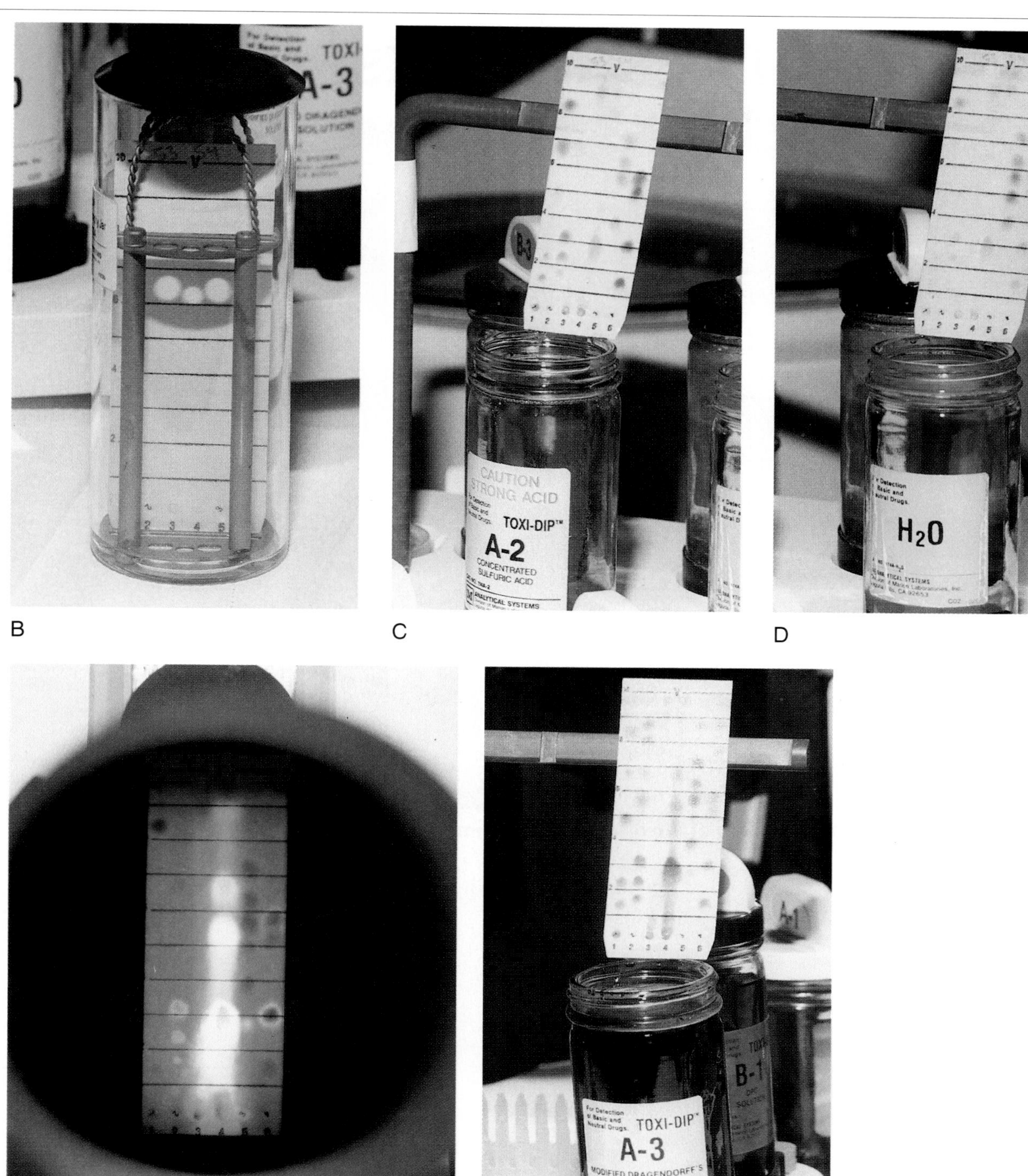

Figure 17–1. *Thin-layer chromatography.* A, *Color Detection Guide A.* B, *Chromatogram in the solvent.* C, *Developing the chromatogram.* D, *Rinsing the chromatogram.* E, *Chromatogram under ultraviolet light.* F, *Final step in the development of the chromatogram.* G, *Toxic lab worksheet used for recording results. (Courtesy of Toxi-Lab, A Division of Ansys, Inc.)*

Figure continued on followiing page

TOXI-LAB® A WORKSHEET

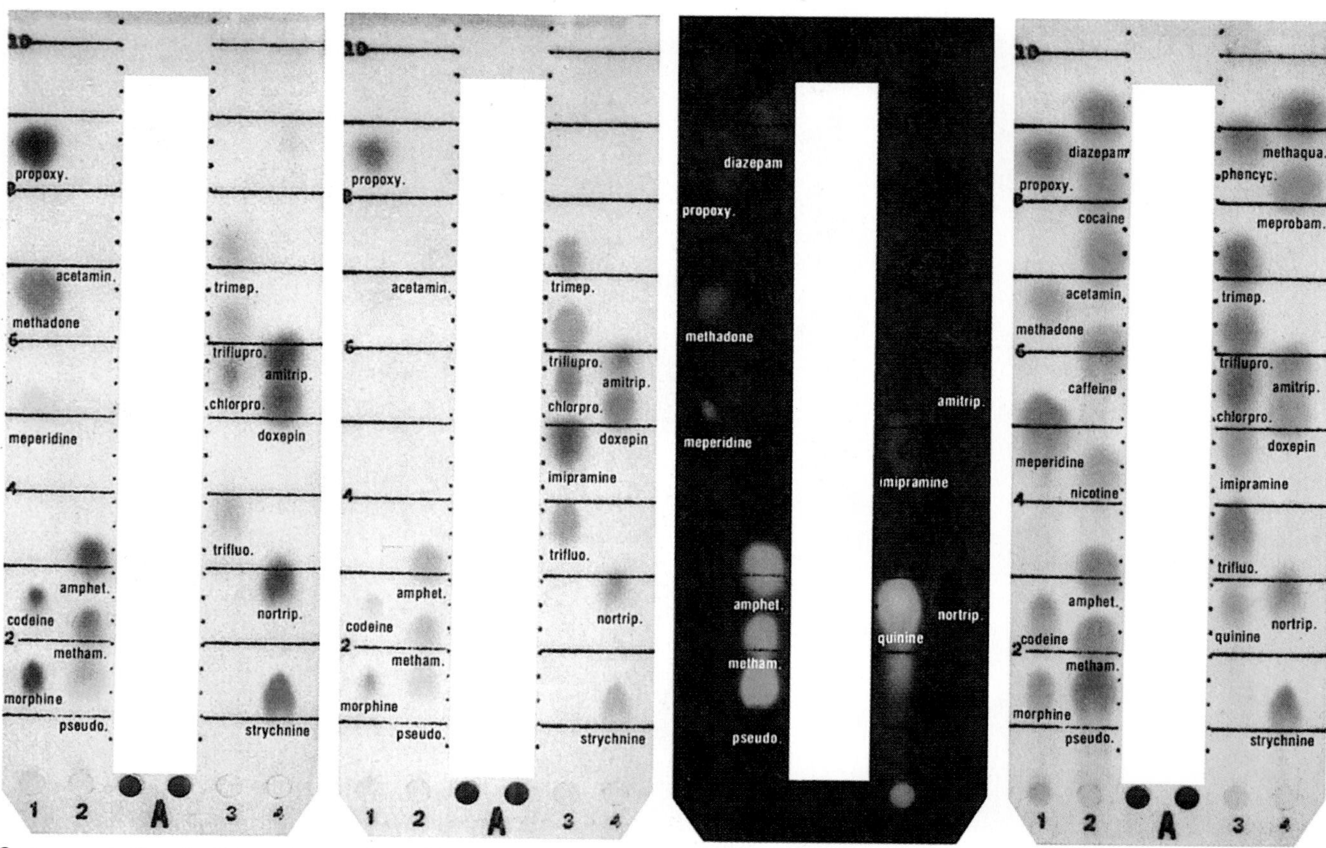

Some variation in the color and position of the drug spots is normal.

Notes: ______________________________

____

____

____

TUBE LOT NO: __________

QUALITY CONTROL CRITERIA MET? Yes: _____

No: _____ Refer to Out of Control Procedure.

Analyst: ______________________________

Specimen information

I.D.: ______________________________

Date: __________ Time: __________

Specimen Type: ______________________

Specimen History: ____________________

____

____

____

____

H86a

Cat. No. 187A

G

Figure 17–1 *Continued*

*COLOR DETECTION GUIDE B

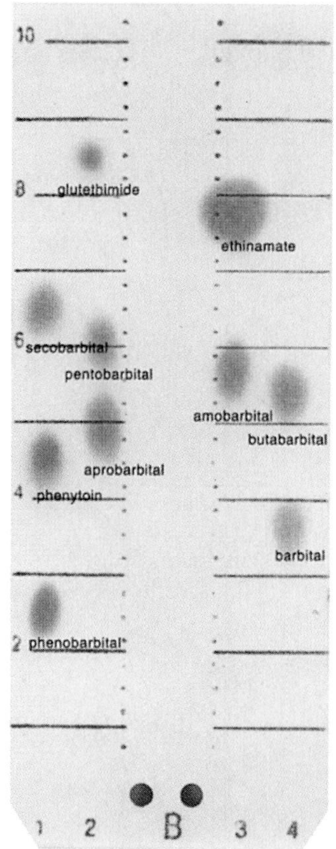

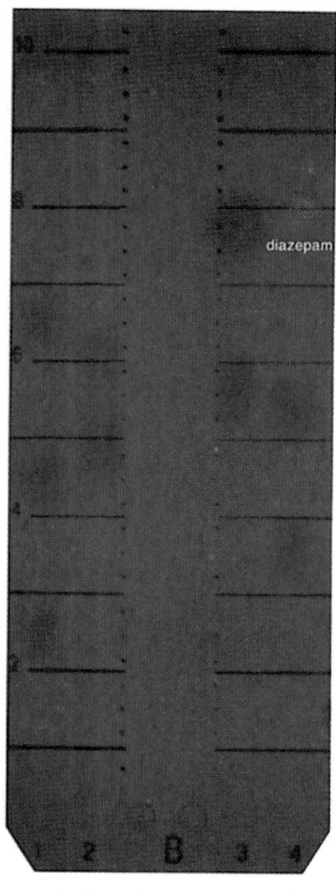

*** Some variation in the color and position of the drug spots is normal.**

Figure 17–2. *Color Detection Guide B, used for detection of barbiturates. (Courtesy of Toxi-Lab, A Division of Ansys, Inc.)*

Screening and Confirmation

It is a general principle of analytical chemistry that if the same result is obtained when specimens are analyzed by multiple methods, the result is reliable. The tests selected must be based on different physical or chemical properties; otherwise they would essentially be repetitions of the same test. Some laboratories, upon obtaining a positive drug screen result, will repeat the same test and report a positive result if the repeat test is also positive. If there was an interfering substance present, however, it will still be present, and the test will still yield a false-positive result. Repeating the same test may rule out clerical errors, but not erroneous testing. For example, neonates will sometimes have a substance in their urine that yields a positive result by any immunoassay. When GC/MS barbiturate tests are performed on these same specimens, however, the results are negative. Likewise, use of a certain type of decongestant will produce a positive test for methamphetamine by many immunoassays, and some GC/MS assays will indicate a positive test result for methamphetamine on these same samples, even in the absence of any methamphetamine. In cases where history and/or physical presentation can be considered and time is of the essence in saving a life, a drug test may be ordered by the physician without laboratory confirmation.

Figure 17–3. *High-pressure liquid chromatograph.*

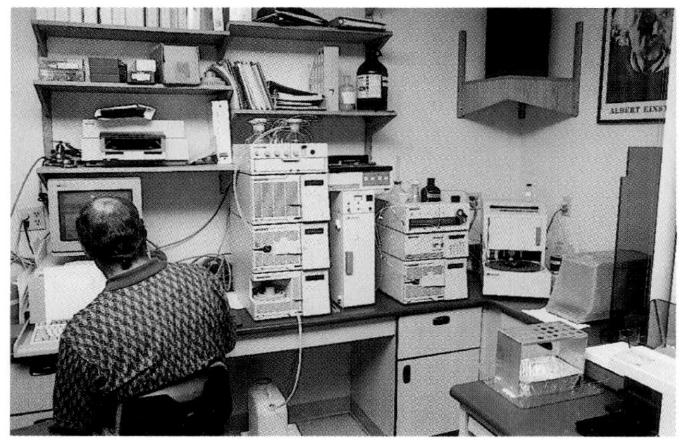

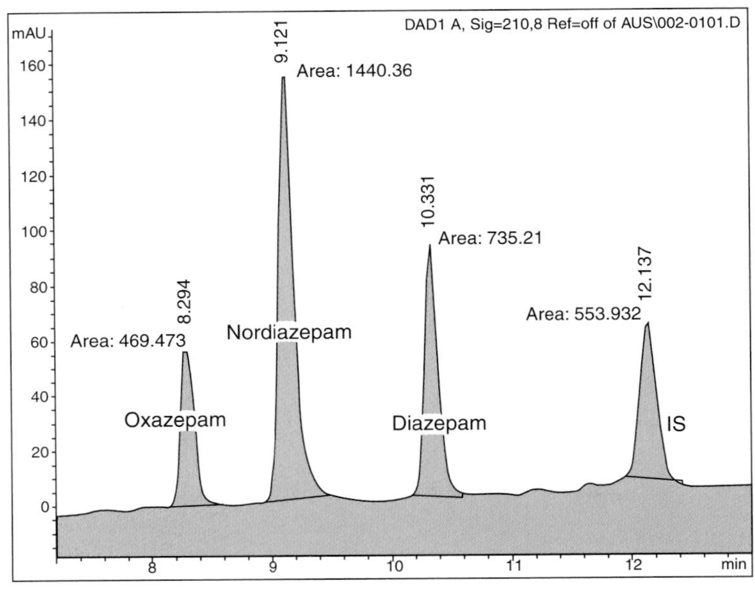

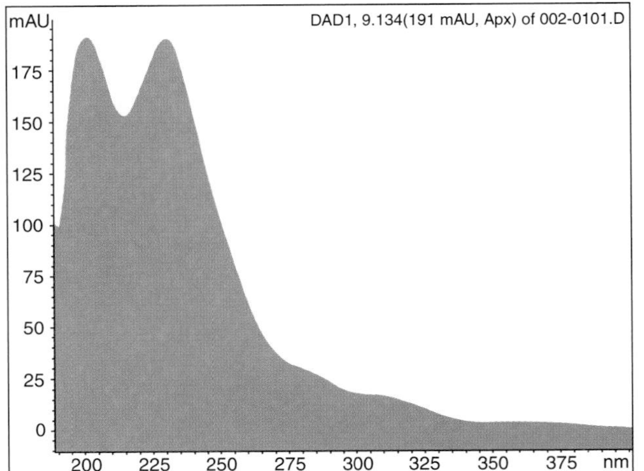

Figure 17–4. *High-pressure liquid chromatogram.*

Figure 17–5. *Gas chromatograph with flame ionization detector.*

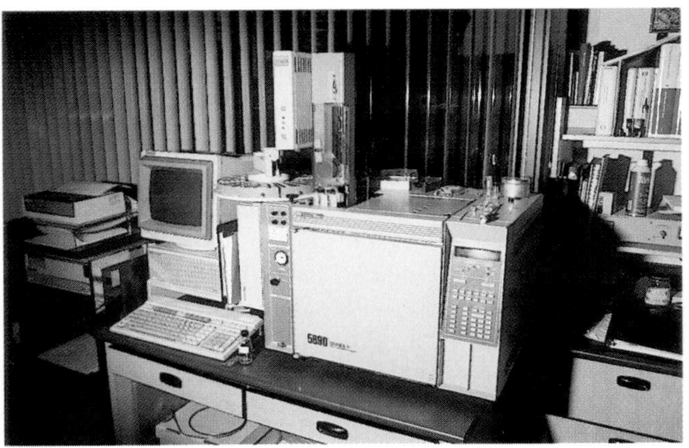

Figure 17–6. *Gas chromatograph/mass spectrometer.*

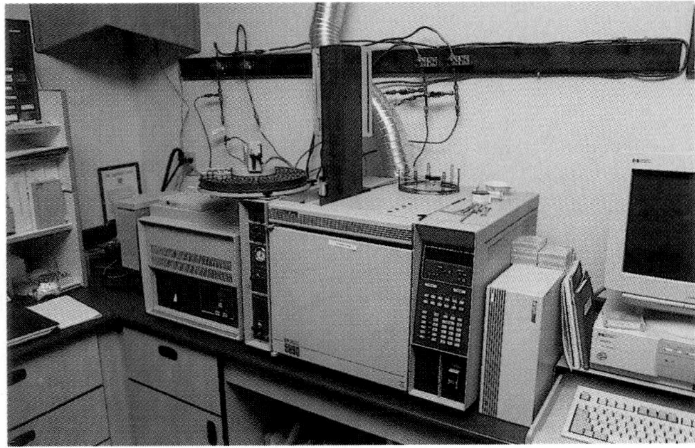

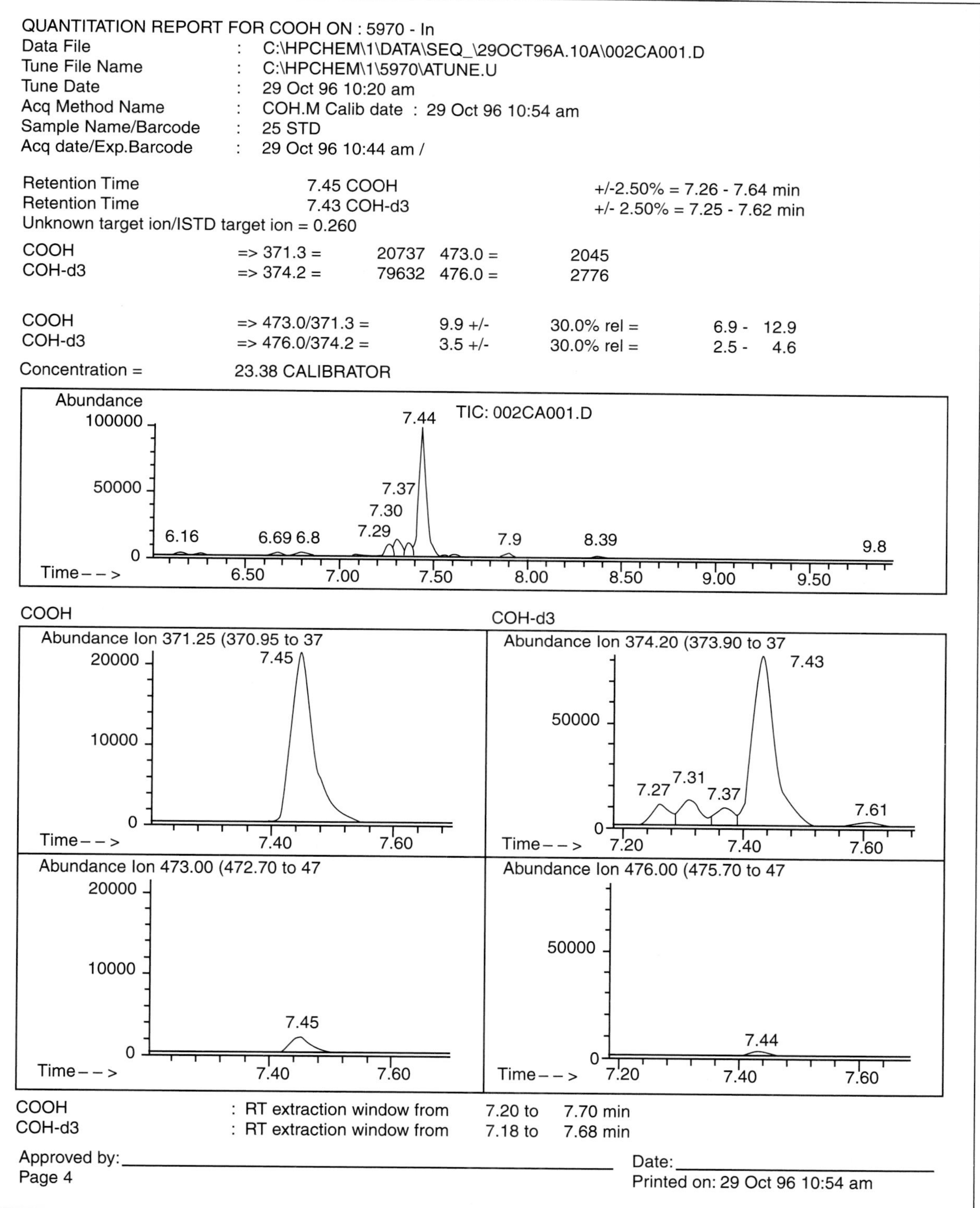

QUANTITATION REPORT FOR COOH ON : 5970 - In

Data File	:	C:\HPCHEM\1\DATA\SEQ_\29OCT96A.10A\002CA001.D
Tune File Name	:	C:\HPCHEM\1\5970\ATUNE.U
Tune Date	:	29 Oct 96 10:20 am
Acq Method Name	:	COH.M Calib date : 29 Oct 96 10:54 am
Sample Name/Barcode	:	25 STD
Acq date/Exp.Barcode	:	29 Oct 96 10:44 am /

Retention Time 7.45 COOH +/-2.50% = 7.26 - 7.64 min
Retention Time 7.43 COH-d3 +/- 2.50% = 7.25 - 7.62 min
Unknown target ion/ISTD target ion = 0.260

COOH	=> 371.3 =	20737	473.0 =	2045
COH-d3	=> 374.2 =	79632	476.0 =	2776

COOH	=> 473.0/371.3 =	9.9 +/-	30.0% rel =	6.9 - 12.9
COH-d3	=> 476.0/374.2 =	3.5 +/-	30.0% rel =	2.5 - 4.6

Concentration = 23.38 CALIBRATOR

COOH : RT extraction window from 7.20 to 7.70 min
COH-d3 : RT extraction window from 7.18 to 7.68 min

Approved by:__________ Date:__________
Page 4 Printed on: 29 Oct 96 10:54 am

Figure 17–7. *GC/MS ion fragmentation spectogram for detecting marijuana.*

PROCEDURE 17–2

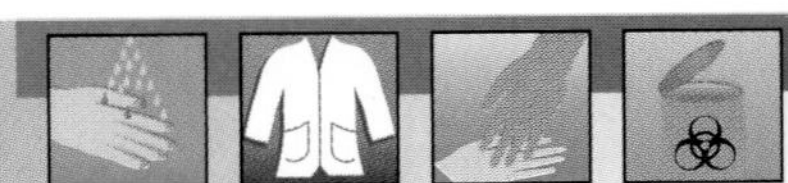

Assisting With Urine Drug Screening

Principle

To assist with accuracy a drug screening procedure on urine

Equipment and Supplies

100-mL urine container (labeled)
consent forms
lab plastic sealed sack
chain of custody documents

Procedural Steps

1. Wash hands thoroughly, dry them, and put on gloves.
2. Explain to the patient the purpose of the test and the procedure to be followed for specimen collection.
3. Follow laboratory and OSHA guidelines for safe, effective testing.
4. A trained individual must witness the actual voiding of a 50-mL random urine sample. After collection, label the sample in the same manner as you labeled the blood sample in Procedure 17–1.
5. Obtain a signed consent form from the testee (patient).
6. Place the sample in a plastic, sealed sack, and mark it with a notary-style seal or with tamper-proof tape to protect the integrity of the sample.
7. Originate a "chain of custody" document at the time of the sample collection. The person who witnessed the voiding must sign the document, as must every other person who handles the sample.
8. Inform the technologist that you are obtaining a specimen for screening. If you are trained/qualified to do the testing, proceed with the testing according to laboratory/state regulations.
9. After both initial and confirmatory testing, mark the urine sample, reseal it, and securely store it for a minimum of 30 days or for the length of time specified by laboratory protocols.
10. Enter all information relating to all tests performed in the laboratory records. Carefully maintain the chain of custody report according to laboratory protocols.
11. Clean/discard all equipment and supplies according to safety guidelines.
12. Remove gloves and wash hands.

Problem Solving Exercise

Practice this procedure with another laboratory student. You may role play the actual collection of the specimen. After completion, check the written procedure to determine whether you completed every step, and whether your techniques would hold up under forensic scrutiny.

Chain of Possession

Name	Time Received	Date
Name	Time Received	Date
Name	Time Received	Date

Interpretation of Drug Screening Results

In the case of the false-positive methamphetamine test mentioned earlier, there was no amphetamine present. Because amphetamine is a metabolite of methamphetamine, the material that appeared to be methamphetamine was not, and the test should be reported negative.

Certain prescription drugs are metabolized to methamphetamine, so a person may have methamphetamine detected in urine without ever having taken the drug. The laboratory can report that methamphetamine is present, but cannot confirm how it got there.

If a person takes heroin, it is quickly metabolized to morphine. Morphine is present in poppy seeds as well. A person who eats a poppyseed bread of some sort will have measurable amounts of morphine in his or her urine. Presence of morphine does not necessarily indicate opiate abuse.

Government-mandated drug screens for truck drivers require that the tests be reported as negative unless the amount of drug detected is above a certain cutoff level. Except for marijuana (cannabis), the cutoff level is well above the level at which the drug can actually be detected and positively identified, so some tests of specimens that truly contain illicit drugs are reported as negative. In the case of marijuana, cutoff levels are so low that residual marijuana from use months before can be detected.

It sometimes happens that undiagnosed or uncontrolled diabetics (who have sugar in their urine) have urinary tract yeast infections. The yeast can turn sugar in the patient's urine into alcohol, either in the bladder or in the specimen collection bottle. Thus, a patient may have alcohol in his or her urine without having consumed any. The point of these examples is that drug screen results should not merely be taken at face value, nor should they be overinterpreted. Not only must the laboratory tests be performed with the utmost care and attention, they must be interpreted with caution and in conjunction with a history and physical examination. When doing, assisting, or reporting the results of drug testing, it is vitally important that you remember the rules of confidentiality. **Never give out test results without explicit WRITTEN instructions from the physician or laboratory supervisor.**

Summary

We are constantly exposed to harmful and poisonous substances. Even prescription medications may be harmful if not used as ordered. Toxicology is the study and monitoring of these substances. Improper use of common household products can be hazardous, even deadly, when improperly used or abused. The physician needs to know whether the drug the patient is using is at therapeutic level or whether the drug needs to be adjusted to allow the patient maximum benefit. If the patient has been exposed to a harmful substance, before a successful treatment can be designed, the medical team must know what the substance causing the problem is and how great was the exposure. This information is secured through testing procedures done in toxicology.

Chapter Review

True or False

Circle T or F to indicate the correct answers to the following:

T F 1. Plants are one form of toxic substances.

T F 2. TDM stands for therapeutic drug monitoring.

T F 3. The RBC cholinesterase test is used for long-term monitoring of pesticide exposure.

Fill in the Blanks

Complete the following statements:

4. Poisonous metals may include ____________, ____________, ____________, and ____________.

5. The most common gas people are exposed to is ____________.

6. The most widely used and abused drug in society is ____________.

7. Methamphetamine is also known as ____________ or ____________.

8. Two examples of opiate-derived drugs are ____________ and ____________.

Multiple Choice

Circle the letter that represents the single best answer:

9. The test that most hospital emergency rooms use to screen for drugs is:
   a. HPLC
   b. Gas tomography
   c. TLC
   d. RIA
   e. BUN

10. Forensic laboratories often prefer ____________ for qualitative drug testing.
    a. Urine
    b. Serum
    c. Plasma
    d. Whole blood
    e. Breath

Vocabulary

absorption: passage of a substance through the surface of the body into body fluids and tissues
liberation: the release of a prescribed drug from its dosage
metabolite: a substance produced by the metabolism of a drug in the body
toxicity: the level at which a drug becomes poisonous in the body

Chapter Objectives

After reading this chapter, you should be able to:

1. Describe the five steps in pharmacokinetics.
2. Discuss the meaning of "drug half-life."
3. List the five dependencies of the half-life cycle.
4. Describe the five different dosing regimens.

Chapter 18
Therapeutic Drug Monitoring

Therapeutic drug monitoring (TDM) is a means by which the physician can measure the effects or levels of a drug being administered to a patient. There are different ways by which medications can be monitored. When giving insulin, a physician can measure the blood glucose level to determine what effect the insulin is having on the body. The efficacy of medications to control blood pressure can be monitored simply by obtaining a blood pressure measurement. There are also drugs whose effects can only be assessed by actual measurement of drug levels in the body (Fig. 18–1). One example of such a drug is digoxin. To a certain degree, the effects of digoxin can be monitored by determining the heart rate. However, digoxin has a narrow therapeutic range, which means that it can quickly become toxic to the patient. Thus, the aim of digoxin therapy is to give enough medication to be effective, but not enough to produce symptoms of **toxicity** (Table 18–1). On the basis of pharmaceutical studies, therapeutic ranges for different drugs have been established, which gives the physician guidelines for prescribing medications. The "fine tuning" required to prescribe the exact effective amount of medication can be accomplished by determining the drug level.

For certain drugs, it is very important to collect a blood sample for TDM at a certain time either before or after administering the drug. Otherwise, the test results will be useless and unreliable, or even worse, they may prompt the physician to initiate inappropriate treatment. Digoxin is a good example of one such drug. Shortly after a dose of digoxin (the period depends on the method of administration), the blood levels are high, but the patient shows no sign of intoxication. After this, the drug is taken up by the target tissue (the heart) and blood levels become quite low. At that point, the blood levels are in equilibrium with the levels in the target tissue, correlating with clinical status.

Measurement of blood levels for certain therapeutic drugs and in certain situations may be useless. In some cases, the drug's therapeutic index may be so wide that toxic overdoses are extremely rare. In other cases, the drug may have an active **metabolite** that cannot readily be measured. The patient's status and prognosis may correlate much better with indirect mea-

Table 18–1
Therapeutic Drug Levels

Drug	*Therapeutic Range*	*Toxic Level*
ANTIBIOTICS		
Ampicillin	20–25 μg/mL	35 μg/mL
Gentamicin	4–8 μg/mL	12 μg/mL
Kanamycin	20–25 μg/mL	35 μg/mL
Tobramycin	2–8 μg/mL	12 μg/mL
ANTICONVULSANTS		
Carbamazepine (Tegretol)	2–10 μg/mL	12 μg/mL
Ethosuximide (Zarontin)	40–80 μg/mL	100 μg/mL
Phenobarbital	10 μg/mL	>55 μg/mL
Phenytoin (Dilantin)	10–20 μg/mL	>20 μg/mL
Primidone	1 μg/mL	>10 μg/mL
ANTIDEPRESSANTS AND ANTIPSYCHOTICS		
Amitriptyline (Elavil)	100–250 ng/mL	>300 ng/mL
Diazepam (Valium)	5–70 ng/mL	>70 ng/mL
Imipramine (Tofranil)	100–250 ng/mL	>300 ng/mL
Lithium (Lithonate)	0.8–1.4 mEq/L	1.5 mEq/L
ANTIRHEUMATICS		
Salicylate (aspirin)	2–30 mg/dL	>40 mg/dL
Acetaminophen (Tylenol)	0–25 mg/mL	>150 μg/mL
BARBITURATES		
Amobarbital (Amytal)	7 μg/mL	30 μg/mL
Pentobarbital (Nembutal)	10 μg/mL	55 μg/mL
Secobarbital (Seconal)	3 μg/mL	10 μg/mL
CARDIOTONICS		
Digoxin	0.5–2 μg/mL	>2.5 μg/mL
Disopyramide (Norpace)	2–4.5 μg/mL	>9 μg/mL
Lidocaine	2–6 μg/mL	>9 μg/mL
Procainamide (Pronestyl)	4–8 μg/mL	>12 μg/mL
Quinidine	2.3–5 μg/mL	>5 μg/mL

surements of the drug's effect, such as an electrocardiogram (EKG). There are also cases in which a substance can alter or impair testing, as may occur with the use of digoxin prior to EKG testing. Sometimes, the attending physician must treat the patient on the basis of history and symptoms because there is not enough time to measure the blood level of the drug before deciding on treatment (Fig. 18–2).

Pharmacokinetics

How do we know when to collect blood for TDM? To determine when it is appropriate to collect a sample, one must first understand the pharmacokinetics of the drug administered. *Pharmacokinetics* is the mechanism of the drug's action in the body from the time of introduction to elimination.

A number of steps are involved in pharmacokinetics, including liberation, absorption and distribution, and metabolism and elimination.

Liberation

Liberation is the release of a drug from its dosage. In order for a drug to be liberated, it must first go into solution. For example, eye drops go into solution in the tears of the eye. Swallowed medication goes into solution in the gastric fluid.

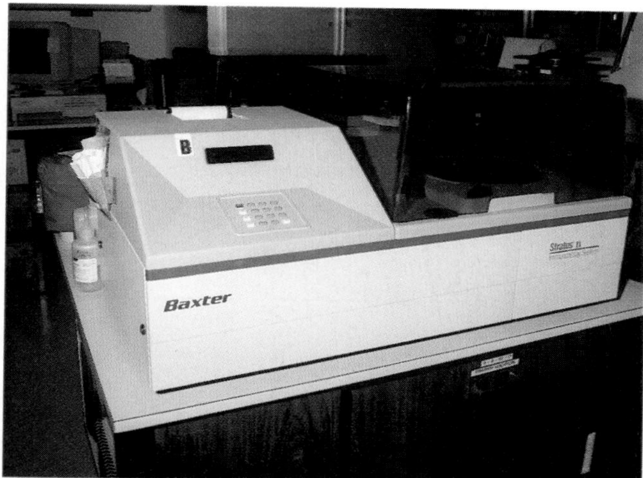

Figure 18–1. *Digoxin analyzer.*

Absorption and Distribution

Absorption is the movement of a drug from some body surface, through the tissue to the blood, also known as uptake. The blood then distributes the drug *(distribution)* throughout the body, where it can work on its target. As the drug circulates through the body, it begins to break down.

Metabolism and Elimination

Most of the breakdown (*metabolism*) of a drug occurs in the liver. After the drug is broken down, it must be eliminated. Most of the drug is *eliminated* by the kidneys in urine, but some is eliminated by the liver and converted to bile, which ends up in the stool. The drug may also be excreted through the skin (sweat), the lungs (expired air), or the salivary or mammary glands.

Figure 18–2. *Therapeutic drug level analyzer.*

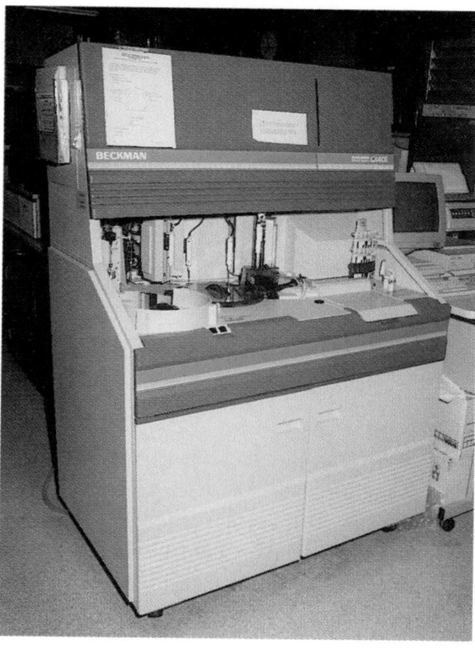

Table 18–2
Elimination Half-Lives

No. of Half-Lives	% of Drug Remaining in Body	% of Drug Eliminated
1	50	50
2	25	75
3	12.5	87.5
4	6.25	≅94
5	3.125	≅97
6	1.5625	≅98.5
7	0.78125	≅99.2
8	0.3906	≅99.6
9	0.195	≅99.8
10	0.097	≅99.9

From Kaplan, L. A., and Pesce, A. J., *Clinical Chemistry: Theory, Analysis, and Correlation,* 2nd ed. (St. Louis: Mosby-Year Book, Inc., 1989).

Drug Half-Life

The time it takes to eliminate 50% of a drug is called its half-life. The drug literature refers to *half-life* when considering the disposition of a drug (Table 18–2). As can be seen in this chart, the half-life of drugs varies.

Half-Life of Specific Drugs

Drug	Half-Life
Digoxin	1–2 days
Digitoxin	6–7 days
Lidocaine	1–2 hours
Procainamide	3–4 hours
Propranolol	3–6 hours
Quinidine	6–8 hours
Theophylline	3–6 hours
Gentamicin	2–4 hours
Amikacin	2–5 hours
Phenobarbital	80–110 hours
Primidone	3–12 hours
Carbamazepine	10–60 hours
Ethosuximide	40–100 hours

This half-life cycle varies for each individual depending upon sex, age, body weight, and health status. Each of the steps of pharmacokinetics can also be altered by other factors. Figure 18–3 illustrates how drug levels can be affected by different variables. Thus it can

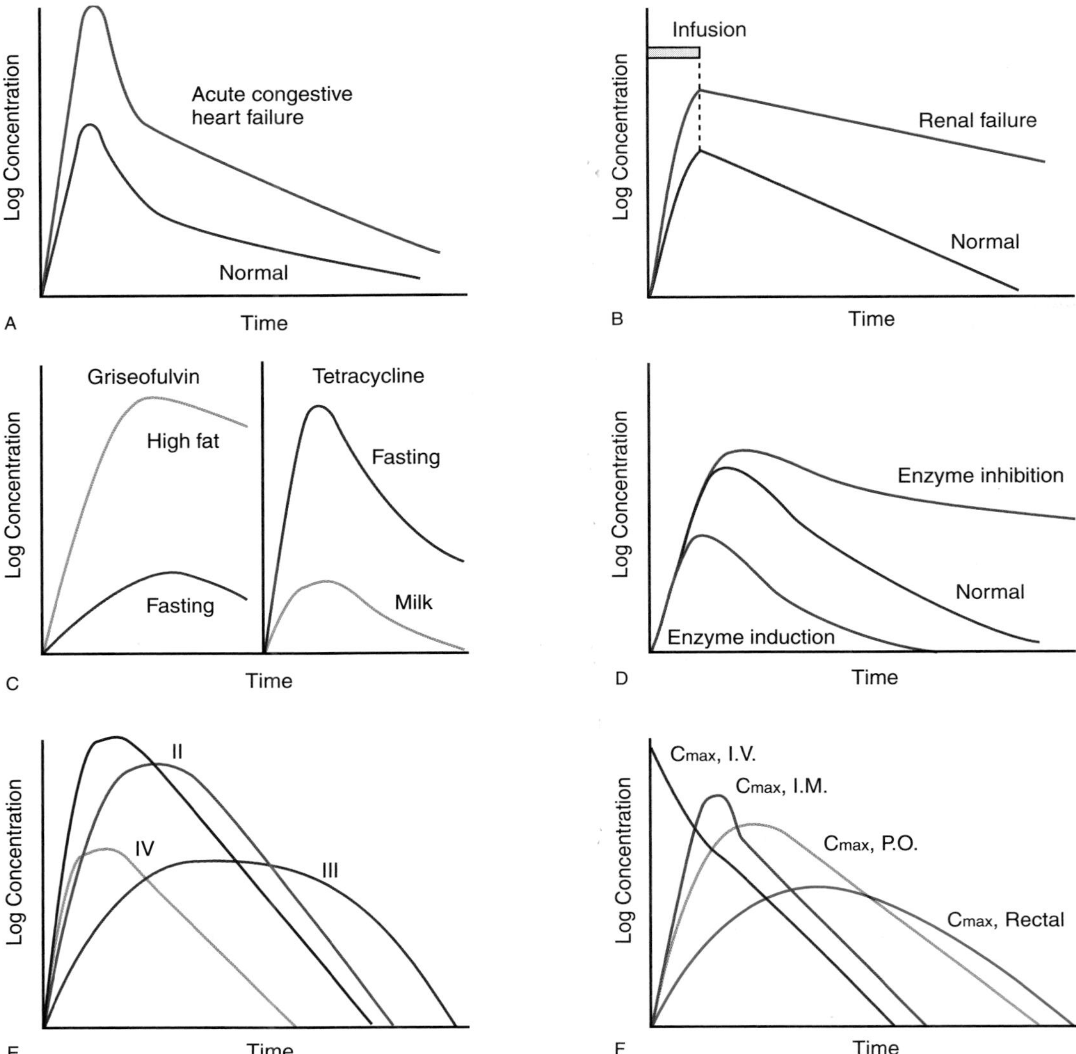

Figure 18–3. *Blood level time curves in humans.* A, *Influence of distribution process on course of blood level time curves of digoxin. In congestive heart failure a higher blood level is observed because of decreased volume of distribution.* B, *Influence of elimination processes on course of blood level time curve of gentamicin. In the presence of renal failure, blood level remains elevated, with a longer elimination half-life.* C, *Influence of absorption process on course of blood level time curves of griscofulvin and tetracycline. High-fat meals result in increased absorption of griscofulvin. Milk causes decrease in blood level of tetracycline.* D, *Influence of metabolism processes on blood level time curves. Enzyme inhibition and liver damage may greatly increase blood level; however, enzyme induction may decrease it.* E, *Influence of liberation process on course of blood level time curves. I, Fast-dissolving tablet. II, Tablet with slower dissolution rate. III, Sustained-release tablet. IV, Tablet with poor bioavailability.* F, *Blood level time curves of a hypothetical drug given by different routes. (From Kaplan, L. A., and Pesce, A. J.,* Clinical Chemistry: Theory, Analysis, and Correlation, *3rd ed. [St. Louis: Mosby-Year Book, Inc., 1996].)*

be seen that different people will react differently to the same drug given in the same dosage.

The ideal situation would be to measure the drug level at the site of action. Because this is not practical, however, and because blood circulates through the entire body and thus is representative of the target area, the drug level in blood samples is assumed to reflect the drug level in the target area. Thus, the blood level should be an indicator of the patient's clinical response. As the blood level increases, so should the clinical response increase. Likewise, as the level increases, the toxicity of the drug increases. This means that the *therapeutic range* of a drug is the range within which a clinical response is achieved without toxic ef-

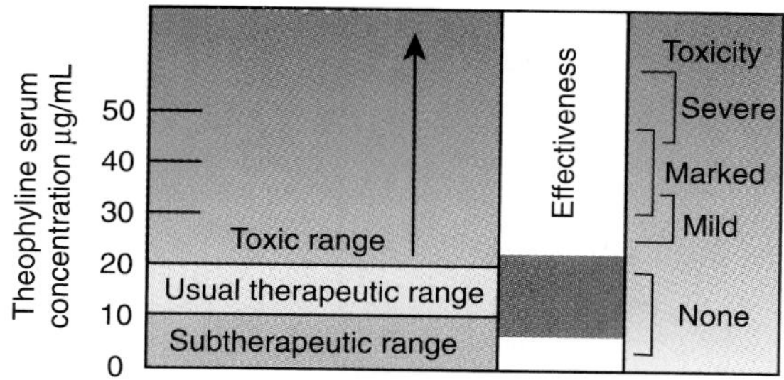

Figure 18–4. *Therapeutic range graph showing the relationship between theophylline serum concentration and effectiveness and toxicity. (From Kaplan, L. A., and Pesce, A. J.,* Clinical Chemistry: Theory, Analysis, and Correlation, *3rd ed. [St. Louis: Mosby-Year Book, Inc., 1996].)*

fects. Drug levels below this therapeutic range are ineffective (Fig. 18–4).

There are five different dosing regimens. Dosages for bacteriostatic antibiotics and sulfonamides, which have a large therapeutic index, are based on a minimum effective concentration (MEC) or minimum inhibitory concentration (MIC) (Fig. 18–5).

Among the drugs that need to be evaluated by a steady-state peak concentration are bactericidal drugs that work on proliferating organisms. These include penicillins, cephalosporins, gentamicin, and kanamycin (Fig. 18–6). A maximum to minimum steady-state concentration (limited fluctuation) dosage regimen is used for drugs with a narrow therapeutic range, such as gentamicin, kanamycin, streptomycin, isoniazid, and theophylline. If a patient has hepatic or renal impairment,

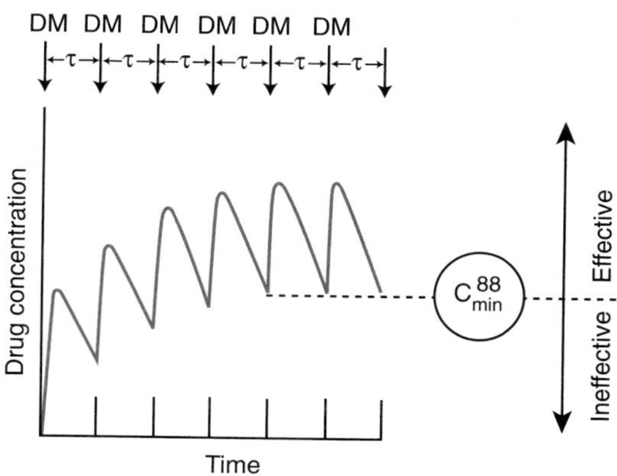

Figure 18–5. *Method of calculating a dosage regimen based on MEC or MIC. (From Kaplan, L. A., and Pesce, A. J.,* Clinical Chemistry: Theory, Analysis, and Correlation, *3rd ed. [St. Louis: Mosby-Year Book, Inc., 1996].)*

drug levels may be monitored using this regimen (Fig. 18–7).

Mean or steady-state dosing is used for drugs that respond according to the peak height of the drug. In other words, as the peak of the drug increases, so does its effect and toxicity. Drugs included in this category are digoxin, procainamide, theophylline, quinidine, bacterial antibiotics, analgesics, antipyretics, and hypoglycemic agents (Fig. 18–8).

Some drugs have a so-called therapeutic window upon which the dosage is based. If you administer too little of such a drug, there is no effect, but if the drug is

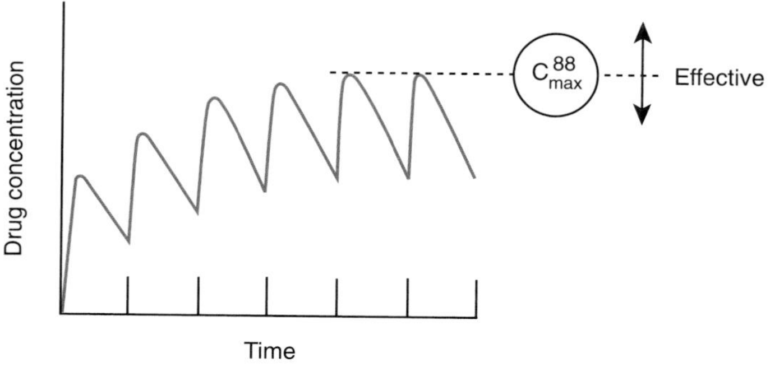

Figure 18–6. *Method of calculating a dosage regimen evaluation of a steady-state peak. (From Kaplan, L. A., and Pesce, A. J.,* Clinical Chemistry: Theory, Analysis, and Correlation, *2nd ed. [St. Louis: Mosby-Year Book, Inc., 1989].)*

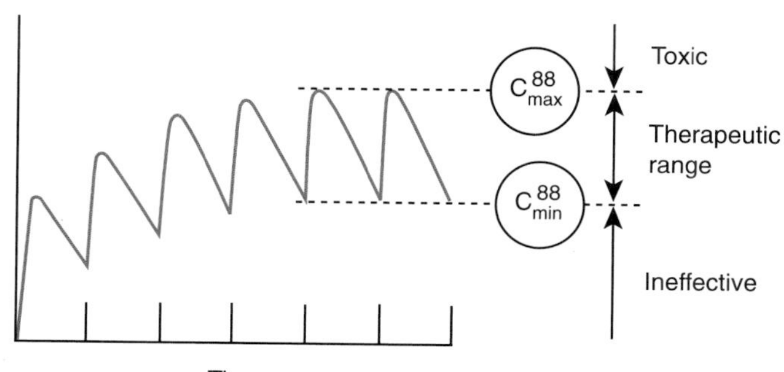

Figure 18–7. *Method of calculating a dosage regimen indicating limited fluctuation dosage. (From Kaplan, L. A., and Pesce, A. J.,* Clinical Chemistry: Theory, Analysis, and Correlation, *3rd ed. [St. Louis: Mosby-Year Book, Inc., 1996].)*

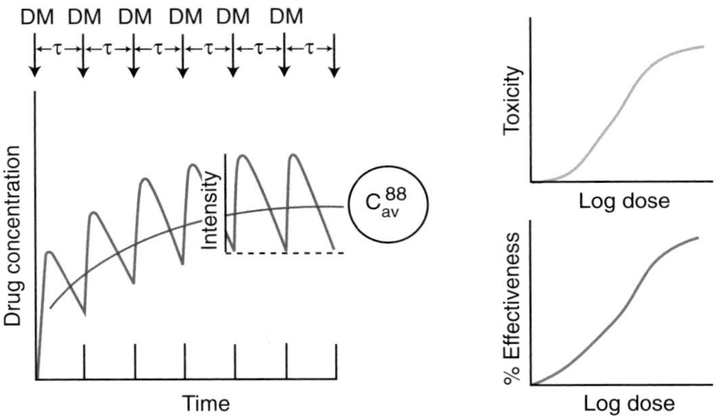

Figure 18–8. *Method of calculating a dosage regimen showing response based on peak height of the day. C_{av}^{88} = mean or average steady-state concentration. (From Kaplan, L. A., and Pesce, A. J.,* Clinical Chemistry: Theory, Analysis, and Correlation, *2nd ed. [St. Louis: Mosby-Year Book, Inc., 1989].)*

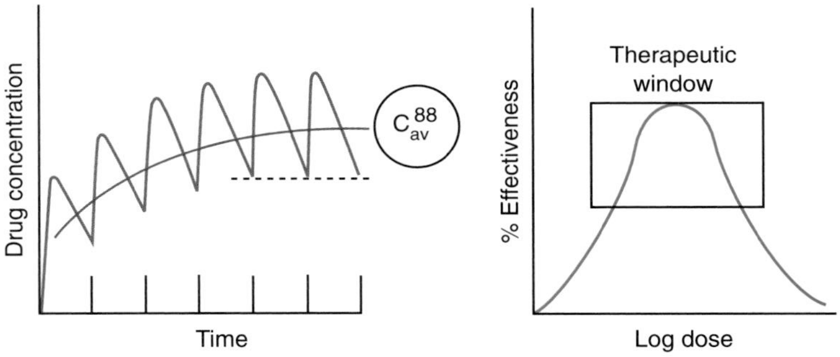

Figure 18–9. *Method of calculating a dosage regimen based on therapeutic window. (From Kaplan, L. A., and Pesce, A. J.,* Clinical Chemistry: Theory, Analysis, and Correlation, *2nd ed. [St. Louis: Mosby-Year Book, Inc., 1989].)*

administered in a dose that exceeds the therapeutic range, there is a diminishing effect, hence the therapeutic window. Antidepressants and antipsychotics belong to this category (Fig. 18–9).

GUIDELINES

Monitoring Drug Levels

- The dosage size, form, and means of administration must be known.
- There must be compliance with the dosage regimen.
- The time of the last dose of medication prior to blood sampling must be known.
- The blood sampling time must be recorded.
- The blood sample must be drawn at the optimal time for the drug being tested.

Figure 18–10 illustrates appropriate sampling times for the five different dosing regimens.

Recommended Drug Sampling Times

Figure 18–11 illustrates a scheme for determining when drug monitoring is necessary. When drug sampling is required, it is important to draw the blood sample at the recommended sampling time for that particular drug (Table 18–3).

Figure 18–10. *Optimal sampling times for monitoring different methods used for calculating dosage regimens. (From Kaplan, L. A., and Pesce, A. J.,* Clinical Chemistry: Theory, Analysis, and Correlation, *3rd ed. [St. Louis: Mosby-Year Book, Inc., 1996].)*

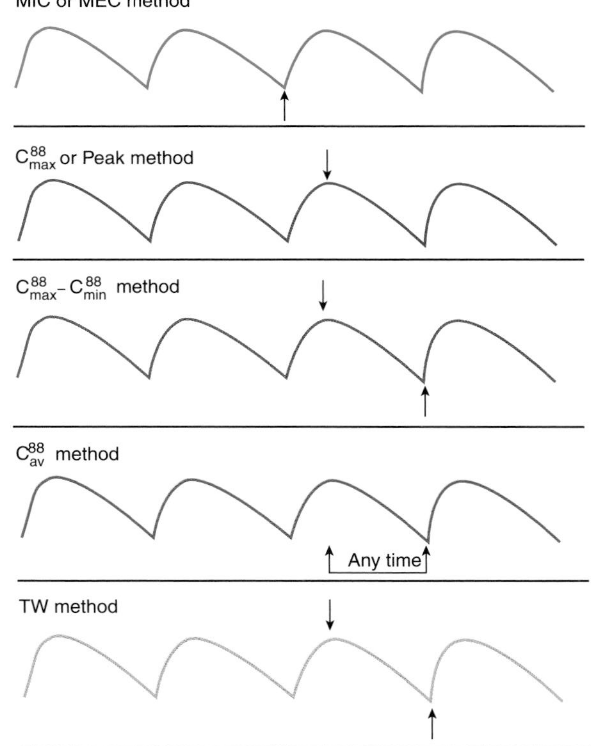

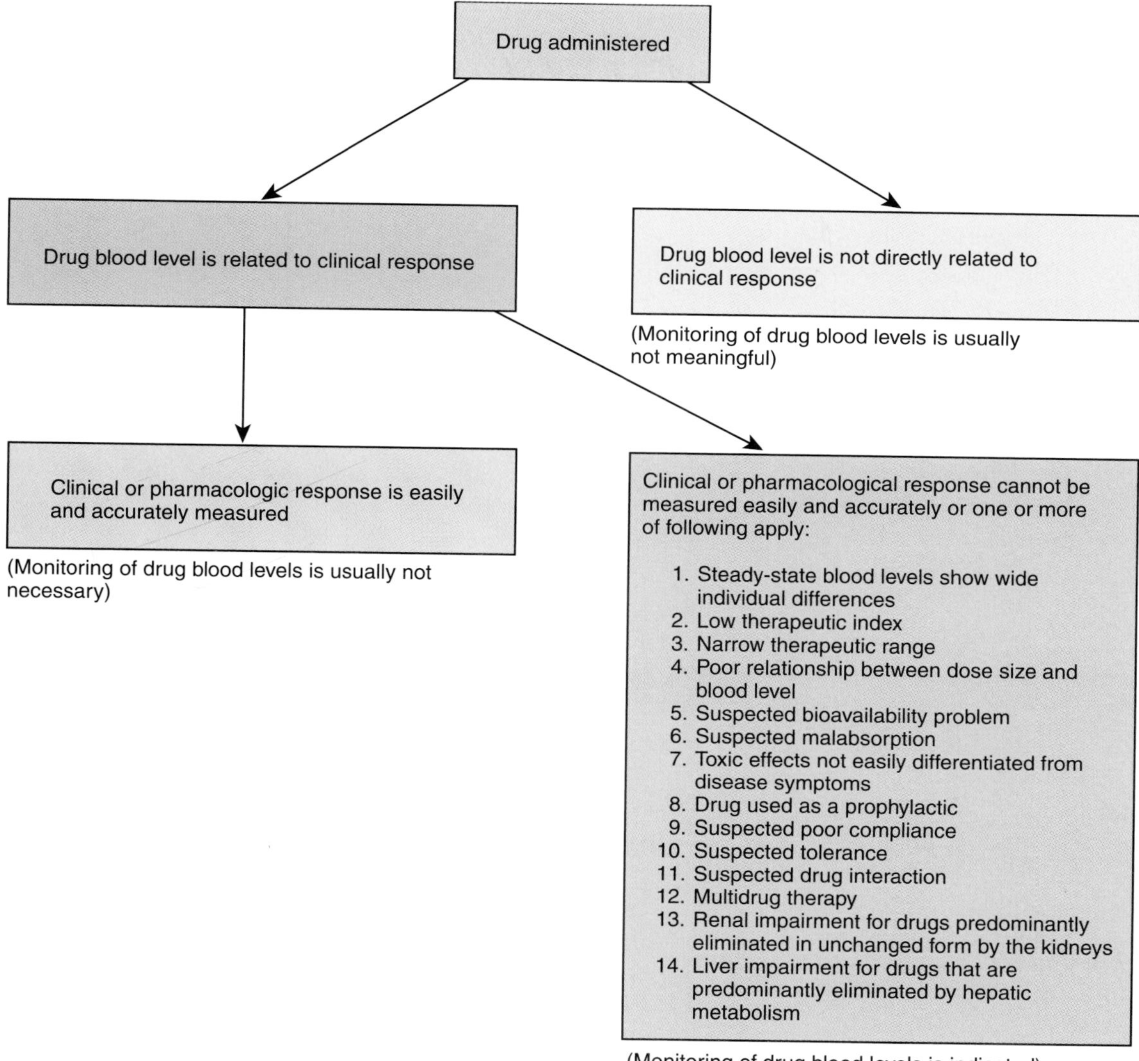

Figure 18–11. *Optimal drug sampling time. This scheme identifies situations in which monitoring of drug blood levels is indicated. (From Kaplan, L. A., and Pesce, A. J.,* Clinical Chemistry: Theory, Analysis, and Correlation, *3rd ed. [St. Louis: Mosby-Year Book, Inc., 1996].)*

Table 18–3
Recommended Sampling Times for Commonly Monitored Drugs

Drug	*Recommended Sampling Time*	*Drug*	*Recommended Sampling Time*
Amikacin	0.5 to 1 hour after dose and end of dosing interval	Digitoxin	Any time at least 6 hours after dose
Carbamazepine	End of dosing interval	Digoxin	Any time at least 6 hours after dose
Clonazepam	3 to 5 hours after dose	Dipropylacetate	1 to 2 hours and 8 hours after dose
Diazepam	3 to 5 hours after dose	Ethosuximide	2 to 5 hours after dose
Desmethyldiazepam	3 to 5 hours after dose		

(continued)

Table 18–3
***Recommended Sampling Times for Commonly Monitored Drugs** (Continued)*

Drug	Recommended Sampling Time
Gentamicin	0.5 to 1 hour after dose and end of dosing interval
Lidocaine	24 hours after start of infusion
Lithium	End of dosing interval
Oxazepam	1 to 3 hours after dose
Phenobarbital	End of dosing interval
Phenytoin	End of dosing interval
Primidone	End of dosing interval
Procainamide	End of dosing interval
Salicylate	1 to 3 hours after dose
Theophylline	Intravenous infusion: 24, 48, and 72 hours after start of infusion Oral or intravenous injection: 2 hours after dose or end of dosing interval, or both Oral sustained release: 6 hours after dose and end of dosing interval
Tobramycin	0.5 to 1 hour after dose and end of dosing interval

From Kaplan, L. A., and Pesce, A. J., *Clinical Chemistry: Theory, Analysis, and Correlation,* 3rd ed. (St. Louis: Mosby-Year Book, Inc., 1996).

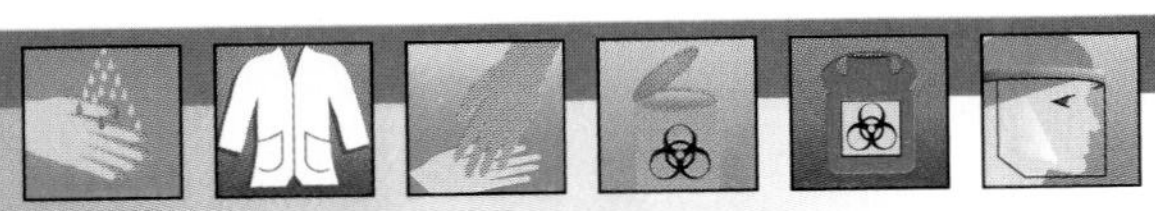

PROCEDURE 18–1

Sampling Procedure for Determining Peak and Trough Levels of Aminoglycosides (Amikacin, Gentamicin, and Tobramycin)

Principle

To understand the timing and procedure for obtaining venous blood samples to determine peak and trough levels of a particular drug

Prolonged high serum concentrations of aminoglycoside may result in renal toxicity and/or ototoxicity. Aminoglycosides reach a serum steady state in 3 to 4 doses. Once the steady state has been reached, peak and trough levels of the drug are determined. The peak level is the highest concentration of the drug present in the serum. The trough level is the lowest concentration present in the serum. These levels must be monitored to ensure that therapeutic levels are maintained and toxic levels are avoided.

The sampling procedure for determining aminoglycoside levels involves a simple venous specimen draw. The important factor is to know the appropriate time to obtain the blood sample. To ascertain this, you must find out the exact dosing schedule the patient is following for the drug to be tested. For example, if the drug is being taken every 4 hours at 0800, 1200, 1600, 2000, 2400, and 0400, you would have to draw a sample for trough levels immediately prior to the dose on the schedule, or 5 minutes before the patient takes the next dose. If the dose is intramuscularly given (IM), you would draw the sample for peak levels exactly 60 minutes after the injection. If the dose is given intravenously (IV), you would draw the peak level specimen 30 minutes after onset of the infusion.

Equipment and Supplies

appropriately stocked phlebotomy tray
timing device
appropriate requisition and laboratory forms

Procedural Steps

Intramuscular (IM) Administration

Blood samples are drawn in red-top tubes using standard venipuncture techniques.

1. *Trough Level.* The trough level sample is drawn immediately prior to the next dose. The specimen is processed by the laboratory and held for the peak level sample.

NOTE: Whether testing is done on site or sent to an outside testing facility, the trough sample is held until the peak sample is available. Both samples are then tested and reported simultaneously.

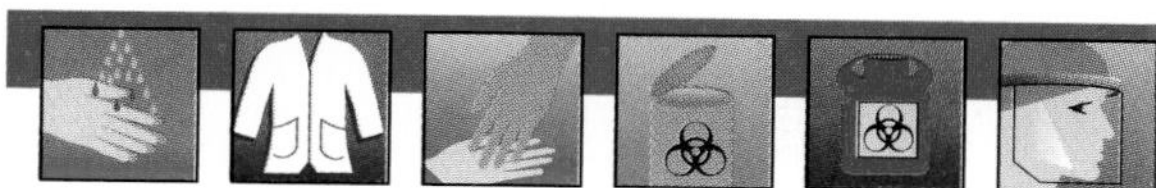

PROCEDURE 18–1

Sampling Procedure for Determining Peak and Trough Levels of Aminoglycosides (Amikacin, Gentamicin, and Tobramycin) (Continued)

2. *Peak Level.* The peak level sample is drawn 60 minutes after the injection of the medication.*

Intravenous (IV) Administration

1. *Trough Level.* The trough level sample is drawn immediately prior to the next dose.
2. *Peak Level.* The peak level sample is drawn 30 minutes after a 30-minute IV piggyback (IVPB) infusion or 15 minutes after a 60-minute IVPB.

Sampling should be closely coordinated with the person responsible for medication administration. *Timing* of the draws and correct *labeling* of the specimens are *critical.

Problem Solving

List testing concerns and possible steps you can take to ensure that this procedure is done correctly and efficiently.

Summary

Therapeutic drug monitoring is the quantitative study of drug disposition in the body. For most drugs, we can show a relationship between the drug concentration in blood, plasma, or serum. Through the use of drug monitoring, the physician can mathematically predict the pharmacokinetics of a drug upon administration in a given dosage form by a given route of administration. It is also possible to compare one drug with another or one dosage regimen with another. Sometimes, in treating a disease, the physician must be able to predict blood levels achieved by a single dose, or by multiple dosages under varied conditions. It is through laboratory drug monitoring tests that this information can be supplied, enabling the physician to effectively monitor the patient's response to treatment.

Chapter Review

True or False

Circle T or F to indicate the correct answers to the following:

T F 1. Therapeutic drug monitoring is a way for the physician to measure the effects of a drug.

T F 2. Pharmacokinetics is the study of drugs.

Fill in the Blanks

Complete the following statements:

3. ____________ is the term meaning the release of the drug from its dosage.

4. The movement of a drug from solution to the blood is called ____________ .

5. The distribution of a drug throughout the body via the blood is called ____________ .

6. The term for the breakdown of a drug within the body is ____________ .

7. The two main organs that eliminate drugs are the ____________ and the ____________ .

8. The time it takes to eliminate 50% of any drug is called its ____________ .

Multiple Choice

Circle the letter that represents the single best answer:

9. An example of a drug that has a narrow therapeutic range is:
   a. Gentamicin
   b. Cloxacillin
   c. Oxacillin
   d. Ethosuximide
   e. Salicylate
10. Drugs may be excreted through all of the following EXCEPT:
    a. Skin
    b. Sweat
    c. Stool
    d. Tears
    e. Lungs

Vocabulary

ankylosing: characterized by immobility or stiffening of a joint
antidiuretic hormone (ADH): a hormone secreted by the posterior lobe of the pituitary gland that suppresses the secretion of urine
isoenzymes: forms of enzymes that catalyze the same reaction but that may differ in reaction rate
MN blood group: a blood grouping system discovered by Landsteiner and Levine that is based on M and N antigens, which are products of paired genes; it is helpful in paternity testing, but rarely clinically significant
myasthenia gravis: an autoimmune disease manifested by fatigue and exhaustion of the muscles
neurotransmitter: a substance that is released from a nerve when it is excited by an impulse
sclerosis: abnormal hardening
spondylitis: inflammation of the vertebrae

Chapter Objectives

After reading this chapter, you should be able to:

1. List 10 specialized chemistry tests.
2. Identify the test done to isolate serum protein enzymes.
3. Define distinct forms of isoenzymes.
4. Describe the type of patient for whom arterial blood gas studies (ABGs) are used to guide treatment.
5. Describe the function of hormones in the body.
6. Explain how fluorescent antigen studies are used.
7. Compare osmolality and specific gravity.
8. Describe the procedure for prostatic acid phosphatase testing.
9. Elaborate on the procedure for paternity testing.
10. Identify the genetic diseases that human leukocyte antigen(HLA) testing can help diagnose.

Chapter 19
Specialized Testing

Today, physicians have thousands of clinical laboratory tests to choose from to help them diagnose and treat their patients. Some of these tests are so specialized and used so rarely that the procedures are performed only by large reference laboratories, government-sponsored laboratories, or university-affiliated laboratories. However, a number of tests, although not routine, are more commonly performed in private laboratories and hospital laboratories. These procedures are generally called special procedures. Special procedures can be performed by any department in the clinical laboratory, but because of the technology involved, they are usually performed in the clinical chemistry department. Thyroid studies, hepatitis panels, electrophoresis, arterial blood gas studies, radioimmunoassays, fluorescent antibody studies, osmolality determinations, prostatic studies, paternity testing, and gene studies are some of the more common special procedures performed.

Thyroid Panel

The thyroid gland is part of the endocrine system. It covers the larynx and produces the prominence on the neck known as the Adam's apple. The hormones secreted by the thyroid gland— thyroxine (T_4) and tri-iodothyronine (T_3)—are activated by the anterior lobe of the pituitary and stimulated by thyrotropin (also known as thyroid-stimulating hormone or TSH). Both hormones are synthesized in the thyroid gland from iodine; their function in the body is to maintain a normal level of metabolism in all body cells. In addition, thyroglobulin compound is also produced in the thyroid gland and is utilized in the immune system.

These hormones increase metabolism; regulate protein, fat, and carbohydrate catabolism; affect body temperature; maintain growth hormone secretion; assist with skeletal maturation; stimulate the cardiac and nervous systems; promote enzyme synthesis; and maintain muscle tone and vigor.

Laboratory tests are an important tool in the diagnosis of thyroid abnor-

Table 19–1
Normal Values for Thyroid Tests

Category	*Normal Range*
Free thyroxine (T_4)	0.8–2.4 ng/dL or 10.3–31.0 pmol/L
Free tri-iodothyronine (T_3)	260–480 pg/dL or 4.0–7.4 pmol/L
Thyroglobulin (Tg)	3–42 ng/mL or µg/L
Neonate at 48 hours	36–48 ng/mL
Thyrotropin (TSH)	0.2–5.4 µU/mL
Neonate	3–20 µU/mL by 3 days of age

Table 19–2
Epidemiologic Features of Specific Types of Viral Hepatitis

Type	*Characteristics*
Hepatitis A	This form of hepatitis is caused by the hepatitis A virus. Formerly called infectious hepatitis, it is usually spread by the fecal-oral route when improper personal hygiene methods are used or when contaminated foods, such as shellfish, are eaten. It is a very common form of viral hepatitis, with approximately 22,000 cases reported in 1993 in the United States. However, it is estimated that the infection rate is actually much higher, approaching 143,000 cases in the U.S.
Hepatitis B	This form of hepatitis, formerly called serum hepatitis, is caused by the hepatitis B virus. Hepatitis B virus may be found in blood and other body fluids, such as urine, tears, semen, vaginal secretions, saliva, and breast milk. Hepatitis B is usually spread by contact with infected blood or blood products (e.g., through illicit injectable-drug use). Transmission of the disease can also occur through close interpersonal contact, including sexual contact and the sharing of razors or toothbrushes. Although most patients recover, the disease can be very serious and can even be fatal.
Hepatitis C	The hepatitis C virus is the primary cause of another form of parenterally (non-orally) transmitted hepatitis, formerly called non-A, non-B hepatitis. Like the hepatitis B virus, the hepatitis C virus may be spread through contact with contaminated blood or through household or sexual contact with an infected person. Transfusion recipients, dialysis patients, and intravenous drug users are among those at greatest risk for contracting hepatitis C infection.
Hepatitis D	The delta virus, also know as the delta agent, is not a complete virus in and of itself; it can infect and cause illness only in persons who are already infected with the hepatitis B virus. When it does become active in the presence of hepatitis B virus, however, it is extremely pathogenic. Persons who are immune to hepatitis B viral infection should also be immune to delta virus infection.
Hepatitis E	This form of hepatitis was known as enterically (gastrointestinally) transmitted non-A, non-B hepatitis. Hepatitis E is usually acquired by consuming contaminated food or water. It is not known whether the hepatitis E virus is present in the United States or Western Europe; however, since epidemics and sporadic cases have been reported in parts of Asia, North and West Africa, and Mexico, travelers may be at increased risk.

Adapted with permission from Fischbach, F., *Laboratory and Diagnostic Tests,* 5th ed. (Philadelphia: J. B. Lippincott, 1995), p. 530.

malities. The thyroid panel test commonly includes T_3, T_4, and their components; TSH, and sometimes, thyroglobulin (Table 19–1). This battery of tests assists the physician in differentiating between euthyroidism (normal thyroid function), hyperthyroidism (increased function), and hypothyroidism (decreased function). It should be kept in mind that values obtained in the assessment of thyroid function can be influenced by factors other than disease, such as age, current illness, binding capacity of serum proteins, and certain drugs.

Hepatitis Panel/Profile

Hepatitis, or inflammation of the liver, can be caused by bacteria, drugs, toxins, alcohol, or viruses. Viral hepatitis is caused by one of five major types of hepatitis, classified as hepatitis A, B, C, D, and E (Table 19–2).

Hepatitis is highly contagious. Thus, rapid diagnosis is essential so that precautionary measures can be initiated to prevent the spread of the disease. As health care workers are at increased risk for hepatitis B, it is crucial that the guidelines for safe, effective pretest care be adhered to (Table 19–3). Health care workers should be tested periodically for hepatitis exposure. In many states, it is mandatory for all health care personnel to be vaccinated for the virus.

Table 19–3
Standard Precautions for Viral Hepatitis

1. After the onset of symptoms and/or jaundice, observe enteric (intestinal) precautions as well as universal guidelines. Hepatitis A is most contagious before symptoms or jaundice occur.
2. Use universal blood and body fluid precautions for type B hepatitis and hepatitis B antigen carriers. Avoid sharp injuries, such as needle sticks. Immediately report any such incidents to the proper person and follow the necessary interventions.
3. Universal precautions must be observed in all cases of suspected hepatitis until the diagnosis and hepatitis type are confirmed.
4. Immunization of persons exposed to the infection should be done as soon as possible. For hepatitis, the vaccine should be administered within 24 hours of skin break.
5. It is strongly advised that all health care workers, including those working in a laboratory setting, be immunized for hepatitis as soon as employment is secured. It is also recommended that workers undergo periodic testing for the disease, or assessment of titer levels, or both.

Because the symptoms of the various forms of hepatitis are so similar, diagnosis of the specific viral agent responsible is difficult and cannot be established by clinical examination alone. Performing a battery of serologic tests for the specific type of hepatitis helps to pinpoint the diagnosis and is the only definitive method for defining the category.

This battery of tests is called a hepatitis panel or profile. The panel includes radioimmunoassay (RIA) and enzyme-linked immunosorbent assay (ELISA).

Test Results. The results of RIA and ELISA testing are read as negative for hepatitis A, B, C, and D. A positive result would indicate that a patient had the disease or has the antigens present in his/her body.

Electrophoresis

Electrophoresis is a technique used to isolate and identify serum proteins, enzymes, and other substances on the basis of the substance's ability to migrate in an electrical field. The substance being tested is placed in a medium, usually a liquid or a gel, and an electrical field is applied. The substance then migrates in a predictable direction and speed and this pattern of migration can be recorded. This allows the identification and quantification of the substance being tested. Electrophoresis is very important in enzyme studies. Many enzymes, such as creatine kinase (CK) (also known as creatine phosphokinase, or CPK) and lactate dehydrogenase (LOL) occur in chemically distinct forms called **isoenzymes.** In the case of both CK (CPK) and LDL, the isoenzymes of each are important in the diagnosis and treatment of patients who have had cardiac arrest. Electrophoresis is also routinely performed for alkaline phosphatase and protein (Fig. 19–1).

Figure 19–1. *Electrophoresis.*

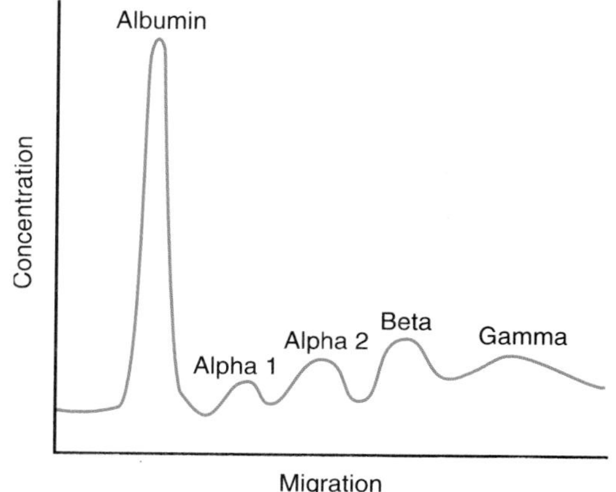

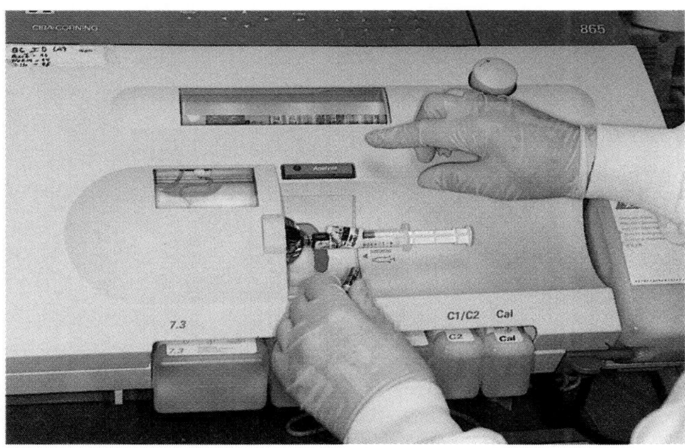

Figure 19–2. *ABG analyzer.*

Arterial Blood Gas Studies

Arterial blood gas studies (ABGs) are valuable tools in the treatment of critically ill patients. As the name suggests, ABGs are one of the few clinical laboratory procedures performed on arterial blood. Arterial blood gas analyzers quantitate ABG components using special electrodes (Fig. 19–2). ABGs help assess a patient's ventilation, oxygenation, and acid–base balance. ABGs are also used to monitor the condition of critically ill patients, to diagnose electrolyte imbalances, to monitor oxygen flow rates, and to complement other pulmonary function studies (Table 19–4). **It should be remembered that any arterial puncture should not be attempted by anyone who is not trained and licensed to perform this procedure.**

The pH is a determination of the acidity or alkalinity of the blood. The body requires that the pH remain within a narrow range (7.35–7.45). The pH is regulated by the kidneys and the lungs. The partial pressure of oxygen (PO_2) is the amount of oxygen dissolved in the plasma and is a reflection of the status of alveolar gas exchange with inspired air. Oxygen saturation (SO_2) is the amount of oxygen bound to hemoglobin and available for transport in the blood. The partial pressure of carbon dioxide (PCO_2) is a reflection of alveolar ventilation based on the pressure carbon dioxide exerts in the blood.

Other parameters frequently tested as part of an ABG analysis are CO_2 content, total CO_2, bicarbonate (HCO_3), oxygen content, and base excess/deficit. Deviations in any of the parameters tested by ABGs can indicate a life-threatening condition; thus, results must be reported immediately to the physician.

Table 19–4
Reference Ranges for Frequently Ordered ABG Tests

Tests	*Reference Range*
pH	7.35–7.45
O_2 content	15–22 vol%
PO_2	≥80 torr*
SO_2	≥95% of capacity
CO_2 content	23–30 nmol/L
PCO_2	35–45 torr*
HCO_3	24–28 mEq/L
Base excess	>3 mEq/L
Base deficit	<3 mEq/L

*torr = a unit of pressure equal to exactly 1/760 atmosphere and nearly equal to 1 mm Hg.

Hormone Studies

Hormone studies are another category of clinical laboratory testing performed in the special procedures section of the laboratory. Hormones are complex chemical substances that are produced in a specific organ or part of the body and that regulate or initiate the activity of another organ or tissue. Certain hormones are carried by the blood to the organ to be regulated. Other hormones, such as those released by organs in the digestive tract, have a localized effect. Hormones are regulated by other hormones, by **neurotransmitters** and by negative feedback. Negative feedback means that the organ being stimulated by the hormone signals to the producing organ that the need for the hormone is diminishing (Table 19–5).

Fluorescent Antibody Studies

Fluorescent antibody studies are another category of important special diagnostic procedures. The fluorescent antibody test most routinely performed is the fluorescent antinuclear antibody (ANA or FANA) test, which is useful in the diagnosis of certain autoimmune diseases. Autoimmune diseases occur when the body's own immune system ceases to protect the body from invading organisms. The diagnosis of these diseases, an example of which is systemic lupus erythematosus (SLE), is complicated by the number of antibodies directed at different tissues and organs, the variations in the clinical setting for each patient, and symptoms that mimic other diseases. The ANA test detects the presence of antinucleoprotein factors, which form identifiable patterns that are indicative of specific autoimmune diseases. These patterns are observed using a fluorescent microscope. Although ANA testing is a useful di-

Table 19–5
Common Hormones and Their Effects

Gland	*Hormone*	*Effect*
Pituitary		
Anterior Lobe	Growth hormone (GH)	Stimulates growth of all body tissue
	Thyroid-stimulating hormone, or thyrotropin (TSH)	Stimulates production of thyroid hormones
	Adrenocorticotropic hormone (ACTH)	Stimulates the adrenal cortex to produce cortical hormones
	Follicle-stimulating hormone (FSH)	Stimulates the growth of ovarian follicles, testes, and sperm
	Luteinizing hormone (LH)	Aids in development of corpus luteum
	Interstitial cell–stimulating hormone (ICSH)	Stimulates testosterone secretions
Posterior Lobe	Antidiuretic hormone (ADH)	Stimulates reabsorption of water in the renal tubules
	Oxytocin	Stimulates uterine contractions and mammary gland milk
Pineal	Melatonin	Function unknown in humans
Thymus	Thymosin	Aids in development of antibodies
Thyroid	Thyroxine (T_4) and triiodothyronine (T_3)	Regulates metabolic rate; required for normal growth
	Thyrocalcitonin	Regulates calcium phosphate levels in the blood
Parathyroids	Parathormone	Controls calcium and phosphate levels in the blood
Adrenal		
Medulla	Epinephrine/norepinephrine	Prepares the body in times of stress; increases heart rate and blood pressure
Cortex	Mineralocorticoids	
	Cortisol	Stimulates antibody production; regulates response to stress
	Aldosterone	Regulates sodium reabsorption
	Sex hormones	Influences secondary sex characteristics
Pancreas		
Islets	Insulin	Regulates cellular metabolism; decreases blood glucose levels
	Glucagon	Increases blood glucose levels
Sex Glands		
Testes	Testosterone	Stimulates growth and development of male sex organs; maturation of sperm
Ovaries	Estrogen	Regulates development of female sex organs and sexual characteristics
	Progesterone	Prepares the uterine lining for egg implantation; pregnancy maintenance

Table 19–6
Positive FANA Test in Selected Clinical States

Disease	***Percentage of Positive Results***
Systemic lupus erythematosus	>95
Scleroderma	50–90
Chronic active hepatitis	50–90
Heart disease with long-term procainamide (Pronestyl) therapy	50–90
Rheumatoid arthritis	<50
Rheumatic fever	<50
Juvenile rheumatoid arthritis	<50
Drug-induced states	
Anticonvulsants	<50
Hydralazine (Apresoline)	<50
Asbestosis	<50
Burns	<50
Myasthenia gravis	<50
Dermatomyositis	<50
Advanced age	5–20
Reference range	<5

agnostic tool, positive results must be confirmed by other means because they can be reported for patients who are free of autoimmune disease but who have other conditions (Table 19–6).

Osmolality

Osmolality is closely associated with electrolyte balance and the maintenance of homeostasis. *Osmolality* is a measure of the number of dissolved particles in a solution. Osmolality differs from specific gravity in that

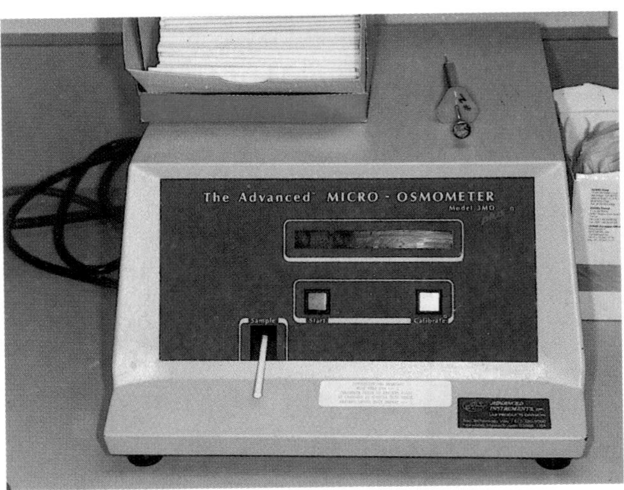

Figure 19–3. *Osmolality analyzer.*

the latter depends on the number and nature of the dissolved particles, whereas osmolality depends only on the number of dissolved particles. The number of dissolved particles in a solution can change important physical properties of the solution, which can have physiologic effects. Changes in osmolality affect a solution's boiling point, freezing point, vapor pressure, and osmotic pressure. Generally, whatever physiologic changes affect sodium will also affect osmolality. Osmolality testing can be performed on urine or serum, but is generally performed on both.

Hyperosmolality, or increased osmolality, is often associated with dehydration, diabetes mellitus, diabetes insipidus, and any other condition that affects **antidiuretic hormone (ADH)** levels. Hypo-osmolality, or decreased osmolality, is often associated with overhydration, loss of sodium, and any other condition that causes oversecretion of ADH (Fig 19–3).

PROCEDURE 19–1

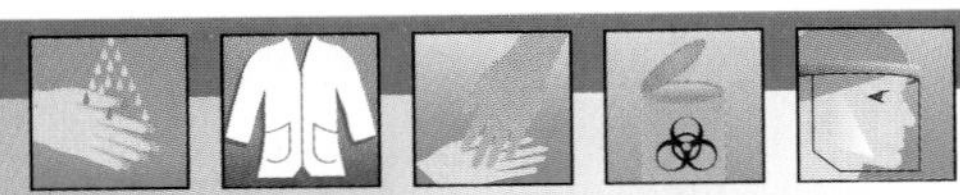

Assisting With Osmolality Testing

Principle

To perform and achieve proficiency in assisting with osmolality testing procedures

Equipment and Supplies

50 mOsm/kg standard
290 mOsm/kg standard
850 mOsm/kg standard
micro-osmometer
micropipette
distilled or deionized water
sample port cleaning probes
clean-catch urine specimen
1–3 mL of serum

Procedural Notes

When a solute is dissolved in a solvent, four of the properties of the solution are changed, in a roughly linear response to the amount of solute added:

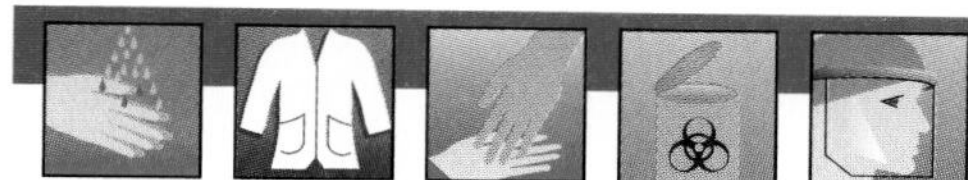

PROCEDURE 19–1

Assisting With Osmolality Testing (Continued)

1. The freezing point is lowered.
2. The boiling point is raised.
3. The osmotic pressure is lowered.
4. The vapor pressure is lowered.

The osmometer utilizes a thermostor probe to sense the sample temperature, to control the degree of supercooling and freeze induction, and to measure the freezing point of the sample.

Patient Preparation

No special preparation of the patient is required. Any questions that the patient has concerning the testing procedure should be reported to the technologist or the physician.

Specimen Requirements

Whole blood, serum, heparinized plasma, or urine may be used. **Check the requisition form to ascertain the type of specimen required.** Urine should be collected without preservatives and centrifuged to remove all gross particulate matter. If the analysis cannot be carried out soon after centrifugation, the specimen should be refrigerated or frozen. Before analysis, the refrigerated specimen should be warmed to facilitate the complete solution of any precipitated substances.

Interpretation of Results

Normal values:	Serum	278–308 mOsm/kg
	Urine	390–1090 mOsm/kg

Problem Solving

A patient reports to the laboratory for an osmolality test and asks you, "What is osmolality and why was this test ordered?" Your supervisor has given you permission to answer the patient's question. What are you going to tell the patient?

Radioimmunoassay

Radioimmunoassay (RIA) studies are useful because they have a high degree of specificity and sensitivity. RIA tests allow measurement of minute quantities of substances, such as immunoglobulins, vitamins, hormones, drugs, antibiotics, and carcinogens. In addition to RIA's specificity and sensitivity, the low cost of this diagnostic test contributes to its wide use. RIA testing involves three components:

1. The specific compound being tested—the patient's antigen (ligand)
2. A radioactive label attached to the specific compound being tested—labeled antigen
3. An antibody specific to the antigen being tested

To perform RIA, the patient antigen (ligand) and a known amount of the labeled antigen are mixed with the specific antibody. The antigens compete for binding sites on the antibody. Bound and free substances are then separated by charcoal absorption, salt or solvent precipitation, or solid-phase antibody or double-antibody techniques. The amount of patient antigen is based on a determination of either the free or the bound labeled antigen. A standard curve is used to quantify the patient's antigen.

Prostatic Acid Phosphatase

Acid phosphatases are enzymes that can be found in the kidney, spleen, liver, bone, red blood cells and platelets. In the male prostate gland, the activity of these enzymes is increased by 100 times. This finding makes prostatic acid phosphatase (PAP) a valuable test for diagnosing metastatic cancer and for determining prognosis. Acid phosphatase is also present in high concentrations in seminal fluid; therefore, testing for this enzyme may be useful in the investigation of rape cases.

Significantly elevated PAP levels usually indicate metastatic cancer of the prostate. Once the tumor is successfully treated, the enzyme level will drop, usually within 3 to 4 days. Moderately elevated PAP values can also occur in Paget's disease, hyperthyroidism, myeloma, and any bone cancer that has metastasized to bone tissue.

Palpation of the prostatic gland or prostatic biopsy procedures can cause elevated testing results. Therefore, when this test is ordered, the patient must be advised to refrain from palpation of the prostate gland for 2 to 3 days prior to testing. It may also be advisable to remind the physician of pretest protocols relating to palpation and biopsy. Drug use may also cause abnor-

Table 19–7
Significance of PSA Values

Category	*Range*
Normal	0–4 ng/mL or µg/L
Benign hypertrophy	4.0–8.0 µg/L
Prostatic cancer	>8.0 µg/L

Note: When test results exceed 4.0 µg/L, the test should be repeated to confirm results.

mal increases or decreases in PAP values. Either venous blood or seminal fluid may be used for this test.

Test Results. Normal values for PAP are 0 to 3.1 ng/mL. Elevated results should be reported immediately to the physician.

Prostate-Specific Antigen

Prostate-specific antigen (PSA) differs from PAP in that the former is found in both normal prostatic epithelial cells and prostatic cancer cells. Because of this factor, the PSA test is thought to be the most reliable for monitoring recurrent prostatic carcinomas. The American Cancer Society recommends that PSA testing by performed in conjunction with a digital rectal examination to screen patients for prostatic cancer. PSA is also a valuable test in establishing prognosis for patients at high risk for prostatic cancer. A venous blood sample is used for PSA testing (Table 19–7). It is important to note the patient's age on the collection tube label and on the laboratory request forms.

Paternity Tests/Genetic Studies

Paternity testing has become an important area of clinical laboratory testing. At one time, paternity was chiefly a factual legal issue; today, clinical laboratory tests play a valuable role in establishing paternity. Early paternity testing involved determining the blood groups of the mother, child, and suspected father. The ABO blood group type was then determined for each, and the inheritance patterns for the ABO blood group system were used generally to exclude paternity. Later, the **MN blood group** system and the Rh system were used,

Table 19–8
Rules of Inheritance and Exclusion of Paternity

Rule	*Description*
Rule 1	A child cannot have a genetic marker that is absent in both parents.
Rule 2	A child must inherit one pair of genetic markers from each parent.
Rule 3	A child cannot have a pair of identical markers (aa or bb) unless both parents have the marker (a or b).
Rule 4	A child must have the genetic marker (a or b) that is present as an identical pair in one parent (aa or bb).
Exclusion Type 1	The child is positive for a genetic marker that is absent in the mother and cannot be demonstrated in the alleged father.
Exclusion Type 2	In a system with more than two genetic markers, the child lacks both genetic markers that are demonstrated in the alleged father.
Exclusion Type 3	A child is homozygous for a genetic marker that is not present in both parents.
Exclusion Type 4	A child lacks a genetic marker and the alleged father is homozygous for the marker.

Example of exclusion type 2: The child lacks both the A and the B antigens from the father.

Phenotypes		
Mother	Child	Alleged Father
0	0	AB

Alert: Care must always be observed in exclusion of paternity owing to the variants that occur in all genetic systems used for paternity testing.

again to exclude paternity. Each of the parties tested—mother, child, and suspected father—was grouped in each system and the inheritance characteristics of each system were then compared. Although blood groups were the most familiar genetic tests, they were often insufficient by themselves.

Subsequent advances in technology led to advances in human genetics. The next major development involved human leukocyte antigen (HLA). The HLA system has become significant in paternity testing because the antigens present are controlled by several closely linked genetic factors (Table 19–8). The HLA system is also used to determine tissue compatibility for transplant candidates. Perfect tissue compatibility exists only between identical twins. A person's HLA type is determined by comparing the patient's lymphocytes against a panel of known HLA antiserums. HLA testing has also become important as a diagnostic tool for diseases such as **ankylosing spondylitis, multiple sclerosis,** and **myasthenia gravis,** among others.

As clinical medical technology continued to advance, tests designed to type, or "fingerprint," DNA became available. Until DNA typing was developed, the traditional method or paternity testing relied on the interpretation of chemical genetic markers, which are an expression of genetic material. In contrast, DNA typing involved direct testing of genetic material, rather than cellular expressions of genetic material. DNA typing has become an important tool for paternity testing, in addition to being used by law enforcement officials in the investigation, arrest, and prosecution of criminals.

Advances in DNA typing have led to advancements in the diagnosis and treatment of diseases with hereditary components. DNA testing, RNA testing, and chromosomal studies have emerged as important tools for genetic counseling, prenatal care, and the diagnosis and study of hereditary disorders.

Summary

Continued advances in clinical medical technology have led to an increased number of special procedures. Some of these procedures have replaced older technology, and have become routinely performed clinical laboratory procedures. Others have been used to provide additional information, but only under unusual circumstances; these tests continue to be performed in highly selective, specialized laboratories. Because of their specificity, sensitivity, and cost, a number of these tests are performed only in large laboratories.

Chapter Review

True or False

Circle T or F to indicate the correct answers to the following:

T F 1. The technique used to isolate and identify serum protein is called electrophoresis.

T F 2. ABG is an abbreviation for arterial blood gas.

T F 3. Hormones produced in a specific organ help to regulate that organ only.

Fill in the Blanks

Complete the following statements:

4. The fluorescent antibody study is most helpful in diagnosing ____________ .
5. ____________ is the measurement of the number of dissolved particles in a solution.
6. Osmolality tests can be performed on either ____________ or ____________ .
7. Radioimmunoassays are very useful because they are ____________ and ____________ .
8. Two tests that are used in diagnosing prostatic cancer are ____________ and ____________ .
9. There are ____________ types of viral hepatitis.
10. Tests that are usually part of a thyroid panel are: ____________ , ____________ , ____________ , and sometimes, ____________ .

Multiple Choice

Circle the letter that represents the single best answer:

11. A hepatitis profile includes:
    a. BUN and AFB
    b. RIA and ELISA
    c. CPK and LDL
    d. ELISA and BUN
12. Osmolality is closely associated with electrolyte balance and:
    a. Hemolysis
    b. Hemostasis
    c. Hematophoresis
    d. Homeostasis

Unit V

Serology and Immunohematology

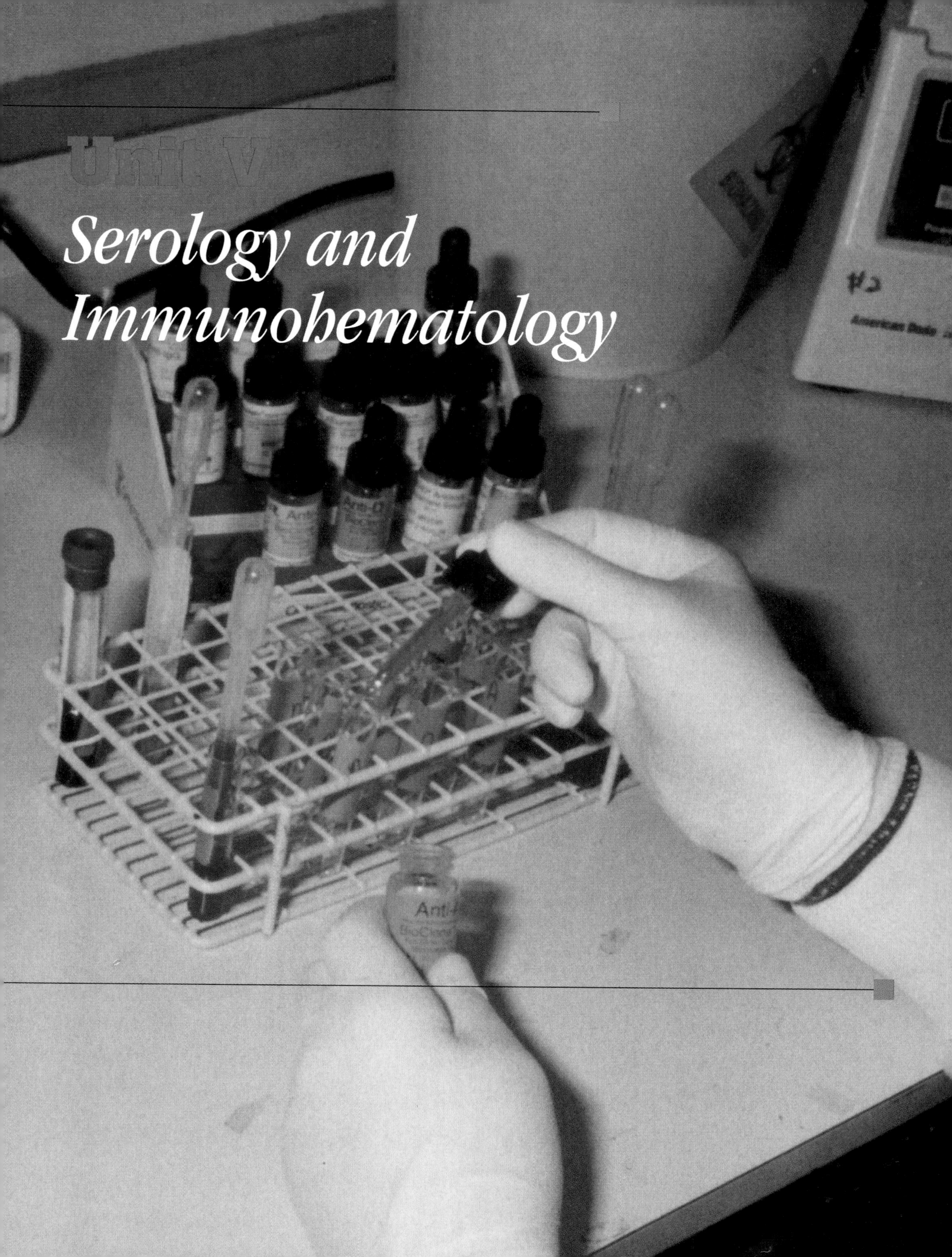

Vocabulary

antibodies: protein substances manufactured by lymphocytes when there is an antigen invasion
antigen: a foreign or natural material in the body that causes antibodies to be produced
B cells: lymphocytes that change into plasma cells and secrete antibodies
complement: blood protein that aids antibodies in destroying antigens
cytotoxin: a substance produced by the killer cells that destroys invading foreign cells
forensic: pertaining to the legal aspects of health care
immunoglobulins: major components of the humoral immune response
interferon: an antiviral protein secreted by the T cells that can stimulate macrophages to engulf bacteria
interleukins: proteins that activate immune responses and stimulate the growth of T-cell lymphocytes
lymphocytes: white blood cells that control the immune system response and produce antibodies to destroy antigens
lymphokines: chemicals produced by T-cell lymphocytes
lysis: destruction of a cell
macrophages: large phagocytes that destroy worn-out red blood cells
phagocytes: cells that can surround, engulf, and digest microorganisms and cellular debris
plasma cell: a cell originating from B-cell lymphocytes that secretes antibodies
sensitivity: the ability of a test to identify the condition or disease being tested for
serum: the liquid portion of blood that remains after clotting proteins and cells have been removed
specificity: the ability of a test to distinguish between a specific antibody or antigen being tested for from others not being tested for
T cells: lymphocytes that act directly on antigens to destroy them
typing of blood: laboratory testing to determine ABO grouping

Chapter Objectives

After reading this chapter, you should be able to:

1. Explain the immune response.
2. Identify two types of immunity.
3. Explain the antigen-antibody reaction in your body.
4. Describe the function of the B lymphocytes and the T cells.

Chapter 20
Introduction to Serology and Immunohematology

The immune system provides the body with special defensive responses against invading organisms. When bacteria enter the body, neutrophils travel to the invasion site to ingest the invading organisms. The inflammatory response begins as these **phagocytes** release proteins that attract other cells. **Macrophages** from local tissue and from the blood move in to clear away the dead cells and debris as the infection begins to subside.

This antibody-antigen reaction is an important process of the immune system. The body produces two specialized cells involved in the immune response. These cells are the T lymphocytes and B lymphocytes. When these special cells are exposed to an antigen, they become sensitized and an immune response specific to that particular antigen begins. An important component of the immune response is the ability of the immune system to produce an immune response to the same antigens at a later time. The ability of these sensitized cells to remember a specific antigen allows an immediate immune response any time exposure to that same antigen occurs in the future. This function of the immune system provides immunity that may last many years.

Scientists used blood **serum** for their investigations of antigen-antibody reactions. Today, these studies may be done on serum, plasma, whole blood, or urine samples. Such laboratory antigen-antibody studies are collectively called serology.

Immunohematology or Blood Bank

Immunohematology is another specialized area of immunology. In the clinical medical laboratory, immunohematology is commonly called the blood bank (Fig. 20–1). The blood bank is primarily concerned with supplying patients with compatible blood and blood products. To do this, the blood bank uses serologic techniques. Identification of blood groups and compatibility testing are necessary to ensure that blood that is transfused is com-

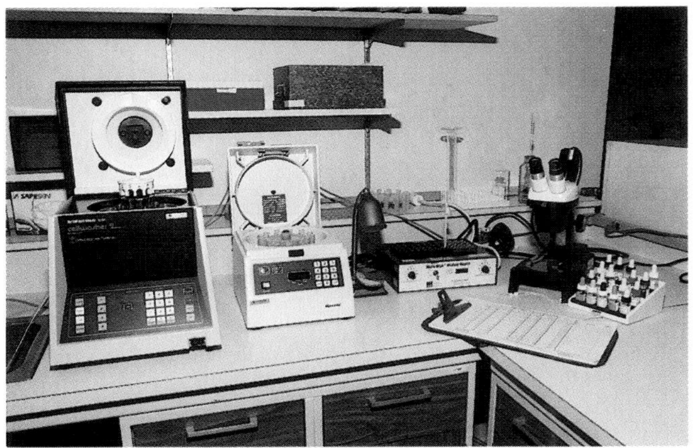

Figure 20–1. *Laboratory blood bank.*

patible with the patient's blood. Basic blood bank tests involve the ABO and Rh **typing of blood,** antibody screening, and compatibility testing (Fig. 20–2). The ABO blood group system and the Rh system provide the most common blood group antigens. When someone requires a transfusion, it is vitally important that both the recipient and the donor undergo blood typing to determine blood grouping compatibility. Generally, when the ABO type and Rh type of the patient and donor match, the blood is considered to be compatible and can be transfused.

Because blood groups are passed on from parents to offspring, blood group identification is also important in organ transplants, **forensic** testing, and determination of paternity.

Immune Response

Immunity is the state in which the body is unaffected by or protected from a pathogenic organism or foreign substance. Immunity may be active or passive. *Active immunity* is immunity that is acquired over a long period of time. Active immunity protects the body against new infections as a result of antibodies that have developed either naturally, after a previous infection, or artificially, after a vaccination. *Passive immunity* is immunity that is acquired from antibodies that are transferred either naturally through the placenta to the fetus or through the colostrum to an infant or artificially as a result of the injection of an antiserum or prophylactic therapy. Passive immunity is neither as permanent nor as long-lasting as active immunity.

Specific Immunity

Specific immunity is the classic immune response. Specific immunity involves major complex defense mechanisms of the immune system. The lack of a properly functioning immune system is incompatible with life (Fig. 20–3).

A properly functioning immune system requires that the body be capable of recognizing what belongs in the body and what is foreign. When a foreign substance is encountered, the substance initiates an immune system response. A foreign substance capable of initiating a response from the immune system is called an **antigen.** In addition to the property of recognition, the immune system response to an antigen is specific.

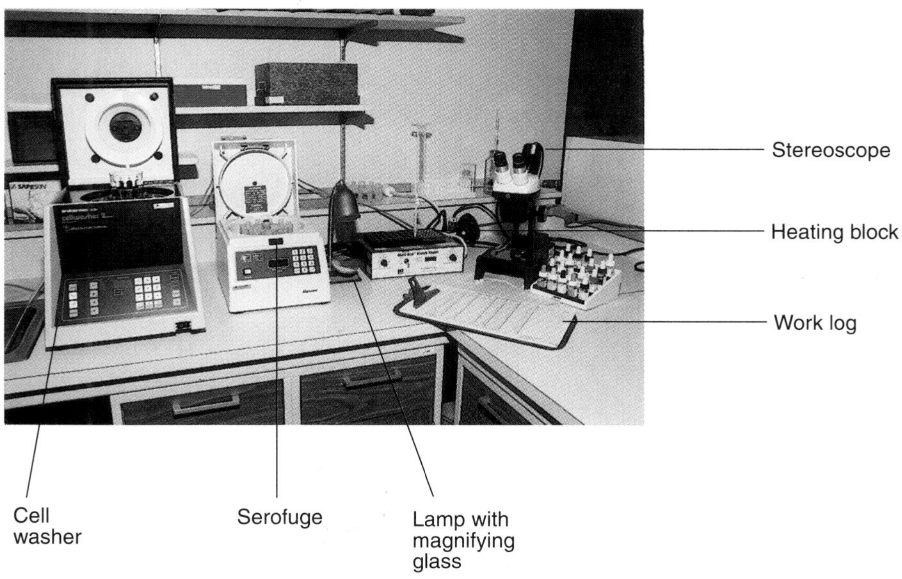

Figure 20–2. *Typical equipment in a blood bank work station.*

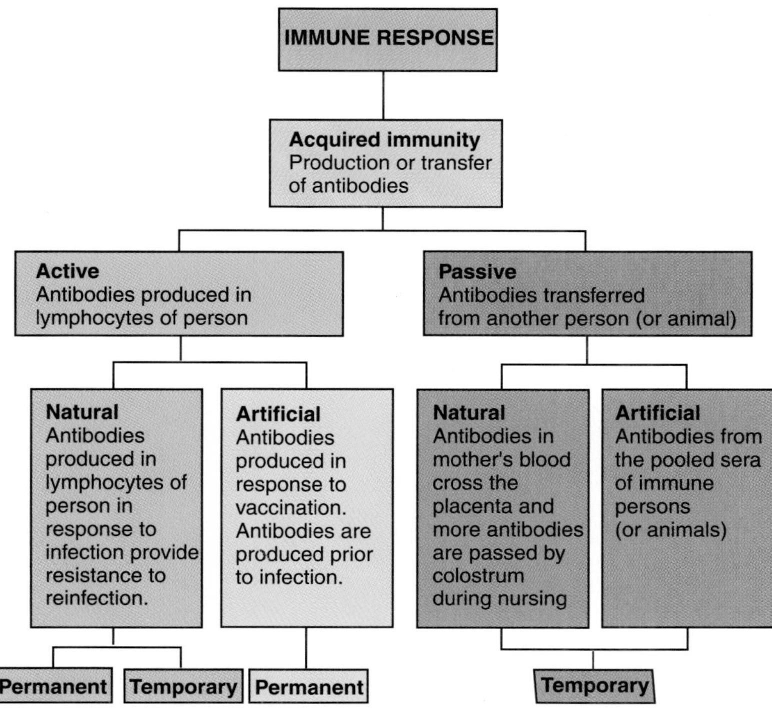

Figure 20–3. *Acquired immunity.*

In response to an antigen, the body produces antibodies. **Antibodies** are **immunoglobulins** produced in response to bacteria, viruses, or other foreign or antigenic substances. These antibodies are specific to the antigen that initiates the antibody's production.

When bacteria or viruses enter the body in significant numbers, the phagocytes are assisted by the body's next line of defense, the **lymphocytes.** There are two major types of lymphocytes: **B cells** and **T cells.** B cells originate in the bone marrow and migrate to lymphatic tissue. When a B cell is confronted with a specific antigen, it transforms into an antibody-producing cell called a **plasma cell.** The antibodies that are made by plasma cells are known as immunoglobulins, which are further classified as IgM, IgG, IgD, IgE, and IgA (Table 20–1). Immunoglobulins are found in plasma. They travel in the blood to a site of infection and react with and neutralize antigens. These antibodies can bind to the antigen in a bacterial wall and causes **lysis** of the bacterium. Sometimes, the antibody will coat the bacterium, thus helping a macrophage to ingest it. If the antigen is a toxin, the antibodies bind to and inactivate the toxin.

Nonspecific Immunity

The immune system consists of nonspecific immunity and specific immunity. *Nonspecific immunity* includes the anatomic mechanisms of immunity, such as the skin, mucous membranes, and body secretions. There is also a microbiologic mechanism, which comprises the normal flora or harmless microorganisms found throughout the body. This normal flora helps to prevent colonization of the body by pathogenic microorganisms. The phagocytic mechanism of immunity includes the body's phagocytic cells, such as macrophages, neutrophils, and monocytes. Additionally, there is also the mechanism of inflammation, which is the body's response to inhibit the spread of infection and promote healing. The pain, swelling, redness, and heat associated with injury or infection are a result of the body's inflammation mechanism. The body also has other mechanisms, most of which are biochemical or physiological (e.g., the complement system, **interferon,** and the pH of different body fluids).

Types of Immunity

Humoral Immunity

One type of immune response in which antibodies are produced is called humoral immunity. In addition to destroying antigens, the B cells transform into plasma cells and secrete antibodies called immunoglobulins. These immunoglobulins can activate a complex series of proteins in the blood called **complement.** Complement aids the antibody in destroying antigens, such as

Table 20–1
Immunoglobulins

	IgG	*IgA*	*IgM*	*IgD*	*IgE*
Location	Interstitial fluid Plasma Placenta	Tears Saliva Colostrum Gastrointestinal system Genitourinary system		Cord blood Serum	Interstitial fluid Serum
Activity	Forms antibodies Protects neonates Activates complement	Protects mucous membranes Aids antitoxins Assists in allergy responses	Responds to antigens Creates rheumatoid antibody Activates complement	Neutralizes toxic substances Assists in phagocytosis	Anaphylaxis Parasitic protection Allergic reactions
Normal values for adults ≥ 18 yrs of age	700–1500 mg/dL	60–400 mg/dL	60–300 mg/dL	Trace	Trace

bacteria or unwanted cells, by entering the blood and the lymphatic system and traveling to every part of the body, destroying the antigen (Fig. 20–4).

Humoral immunity involves the B lymphocytes, which originate in the bone marrow. B lymphocytes migrate to lymphoid tissue where they mature. When a B lymphocyte is exposed to an antigen, the B cells produce short-lived antibodies that seek out and destroy the antigens. The antibodies produced by the B cells are found in body fluids, particularly blood and lymph fluid. These antibodies then circulate throughout the body, which enables them to destroy the antigens wherever they are encountered. B lymphocytes have specialized memory cells that allow for an immediate response in the event of future exposure to the same antigen (Fig. 20–5).

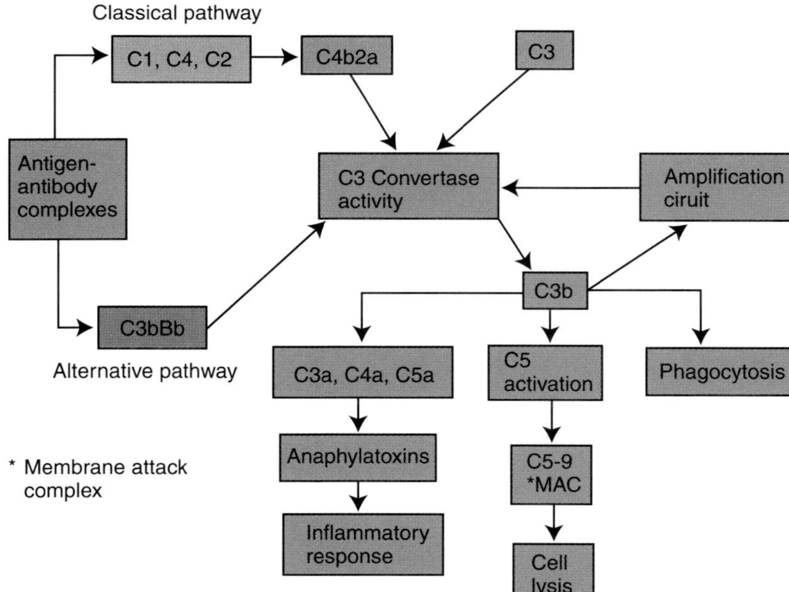

Figure 20–4. *Complement response.*

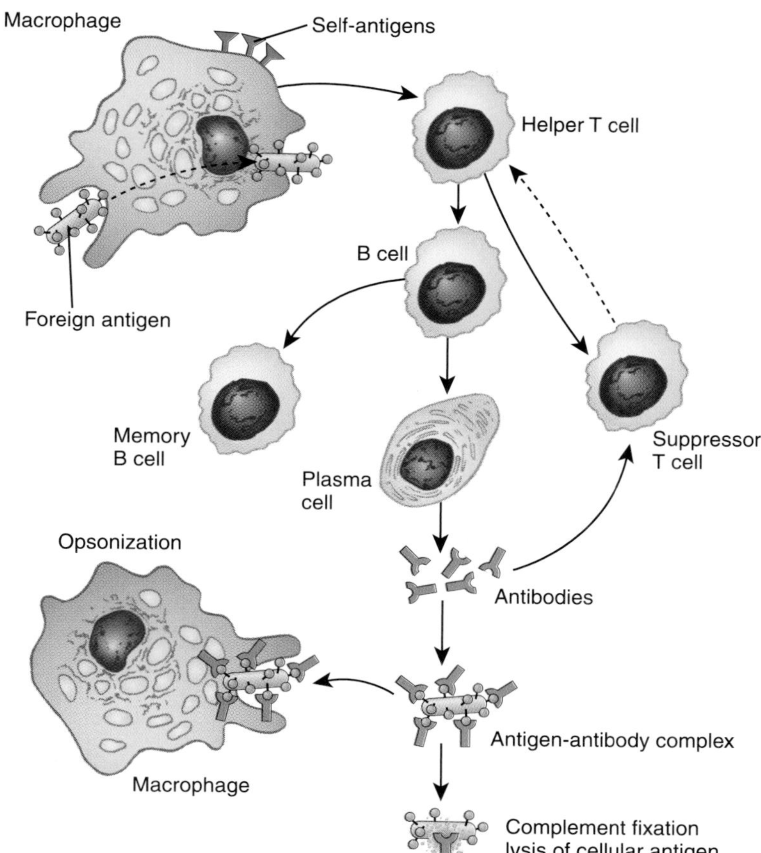

Figure 20–5. *Humoral immunity.*

Cell-Mediated Immunity

The immune response consists of two basic types of immunity: cellular immunity and humoral immunity. Cellular immunity is determined by the T lymphocytes or T cells. T lymphocytes originate in the bone marrow and migrate to the thymus where they mature and become available to respond to foreign substances or antigens. The T cells are released into the circulatory system and migrate to the spleen and lymph nodes. Once the T cells are exposed to a specific antigen, they divide and multiply in response to that specific antigenic stimulation. As a result of the exposure to the antigen, different types of T cells are produced. Killer T cells produce **cytotoxins** that are released when they bind with cancer cells, viruses, or foreign cells. Helper T cells assist the B lymphocytes in attacking the antigens. A third type of T lymphocytes, suppressor T cells, shut down the immune response when the antigen has been destroyed. Memory T cells provide an immunologic memory of the antigen so that the body will be able to respond immediately to future invasion by the same antigen.

Cell-mediated immunity is dependent on T-cell lymphocytes. T cells originate in the bone marrow and are processed in the thymus gland where they are acted upon by thymic hormones. They then migrate to all the lymph-containing organs. If an antigen encounters a T cell, the T cell can multiply very rapidly. These activated T cells engulf and digest the antigen (e.g., the cancer cell, virus, fungus, or bacterium). T cells also react to foreign tissues, such as skin grafts and organ transplants.

Some T cells are cytotoxic or killer cells. They can act directly on cells bearing antigens (tumor cells and tissue transplanted from an organ donor). Other T cells produce chemicals called **lymphokines,** such as interferon and **interleukins,** which have a toxic effect upon cells or bacteria. Interferon inhibits the ability of viruses to infect uninfected cells and stimulates macrophages to ingest bacteria. Interleukins activate T cells and are cytotoxic for some tumor cells, among other functions.

A special class of T cells, called helper cells, stimulate antibody production. Others regulate the amount of antibody produced by functioning as suppressor

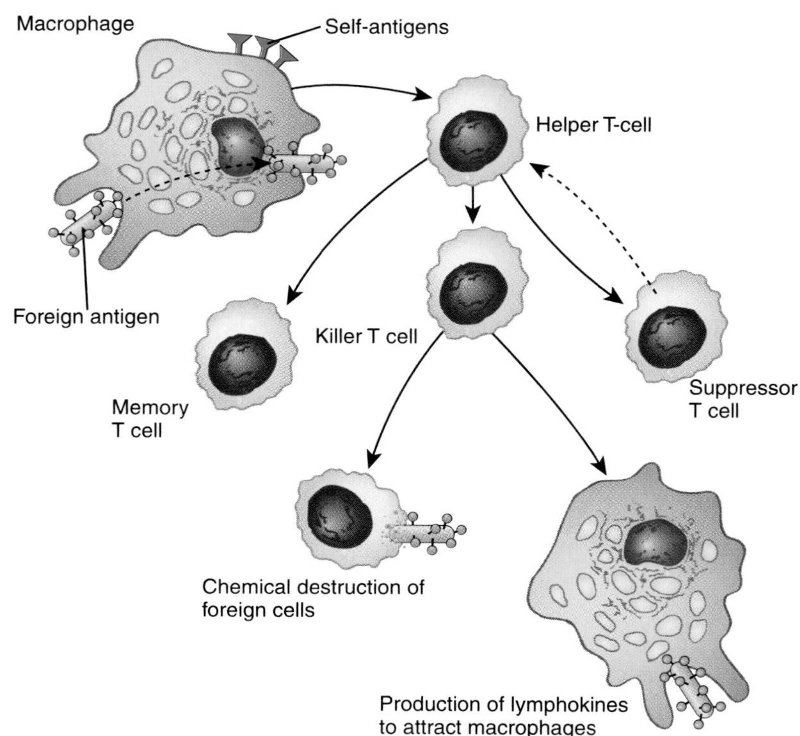

Figure 20–6. *Cellular immunity.*

cells that inhibit the activity of B-cell lymphocytes (Fig. 20–6).

Approximately 70% to 80% of the circulating lymphocytes are T cells. They are especially effective in the destruction of viruses, fungal infections, chronic bacterial infections, and foreign tissue (tumors).

Summary

Serologic testing can provide information that is useful in the diagnosis of many infectious diseases. Most of these tests are extremely valuable because they can be performed quickly and easily with a high degree of **specificity** and **sensitivity.** The immune system responds to invading organisms and produces the antibody antigen reaction. In this chapter you learned the importance of this system and how changes in the body in wellness and disease can be detected through analyzing the immune reaction. As diseases become more sophisticated, testing will also need to change to accommodate the needs of the medical profession and the people relying on these diagnostic procedures. The role the serology and immunohematology departments play will also continue to advance and aid in the determination of illness and evaluation of treatment.

PROCEDURE 20–1

Diagnostic Immunologic Testing

Principle

To obtain additional knowledge regarding immunologic disorders, thereby enhancing testing accuracy and patient education

Using library or department reference books, research the tests used in diagnosing immunologic diseases or disorders. Choose one test that interests you and write a report on the test. If you are unfamiliar with the references available, ask your instructor for suggestions of reference materials you might use.

Procedural Steps

Your report should include the following major points:

1. Purpose of the test
2. What the test consists of

PROCEDURE 20–1

Diagnostic Immunologic Testing (Continued)

3. Testing method
4. Test analyses
5. Test controls
6. Patient preparation (before and after the test)
7. Specimen collection requirements
8. Quality assurance and quality control
9. Your responsibilities and concerns throughout the procedure

Chapter Review

True or False

Circle T or F to indicate the correct answers to the following:

T F 1. Immunity is the state in which the body is affected by a pathogenic organism.

T F 2. Normal flora are harmful microorganisms found throughout the body.

T F 3. T cells and B cells are solely responsible for the immune response.

T F 4. Passive immunity is acquired over a long period of time.

Fill in the Blank

Complete the following statements:

5. Passive immunity is not as ______________ or ______________ as active immunity.

6. A foreign substance capable of initiating the immune system response is called an ______________.

7. ______________ are produced in response to an antigen.

8. B cells originate in the ______________ ______________.

Multiple Choice

Circle the letter that represents the single best answer:

9. The type of immunity in which antibodies are produced is:
   a. Humoral
   b. Cellular
   c. Active
   d. Passive
   e. Inborn

10. Cell-mediated immunity consists of:
    a. Killer T cells
    b. Helper T cells
    c. Suppressor T cells
    d. Memory T cells
    e. All of the above

Vocabulary

agglutination: the clumping together of blood cells caused by an antigen/antibody reaction
bioluminescence: a reaction, found in nature, between an enzyme and oxygen, producing cold light
brucellosis: a disease (also known as undulant fever) caused by coccal bacteria (brucella)
chemiluminescence: light generated as a result of a chemical reaction
cold light: light produced in the absence of heat
convalescent: pertaining to the period of recovery after an illness
exotoxins: poisonous substances secreted externally
flocculus: a small tuft or mass of fibrous material containing downy or flaky sheds
heterophil: an antibody that reacts with antigens other than the one it is expected to react with
infectious mononucleosis: an acute infection caused by the Epstein-Barr virus
in vitro: a biological reaction that occurs in an artificial environment
in vivo: a biological reaction occurring within the living body
luminol: organic compound with luminescent qualities
lysis: destruction of a cell by a lysin
salmonellosis: a disease caused by rod-shaped bacteria (salmonellae)
titer: the highest dilution of a serum required to cause clumping of particulate antigens
toxins: poisons, usually proteins, that cause antitoxins to form in the body, thus establishing immunity to a disease
VDRL: a serologic flocculation test for syphilis

Chapter Objectives

After reading this chapter, you should be able to:

1. Identify the body fluids that are used in serology.
2. Explain the sensitivity and specificity of serologic tests.
3. List and explain the categories into which serologic tests are classified.
4. Describe the methods used in testing for pregnancy, infectious mononucleosis, and rheumatoid arthritis.

Chapter 21
Serologic Testing and Procedures

The immune system involves a complex system of biochemical and physiological reactions that work as a team to protect the body against pathologic organisms and other foreign substances. These pathogenic organisms and foreign substances commonly include bacteria, viruses, **toxins,** cancer cells, allergens, and other foreign cells and tissues.

The serologic testing performed in the clinical medical laboratory generally involves the antigen-antibody reaction. When these reactions occur in the patient, they are termed **in vivo** reactions. When these reactions occur in a laboratory setting, they are said to be **in vitro** reactions. As a result of scientific and technologic advances, the in vitro study of the antibody-antigen reaction has become a very important diagnostic tool.

Immunologic or serologic methods of testing provide information about past or present infections by demonstrating antibodies against a particular organism, and by detecting components of causative organisms. In addition, the antibody titer can be monitored from its onset in the acute phase of disease to the **convalescent** phase of the disease by observing the titer elevation and its gradual decrease.

Serologic testing is also used to detect antibodies against organisms. The choice of test usually depends on the ordering physician and the practicality of the tests.

Test Preparation

As with all clinical medical laboratory testing, the collection, handling, and processing of specimens for serologic testing is very important. As the name denotes, most serologic testing is performed on serum. However, advances in technology have allowed testing of whole blood, urine, and other body fluids, as well.

Before specimen collection and processing or performance of any serologic testing, it is very important that the laboratory worker become familiar with the proper procedure for each test. This should include reviewing the package inserts provided by the test manufacturer. Such a review of the package insert will provide valuable information about the test, the principle on which the test is based, the reagents and equipment required, proper specimen collection procedures, preparation requirements, test procedures, and any precautions or warnings that pertain to the procedure. In addition, the inserts provide information on quality control, the interpretation of results, limitations of the procedure, performance characteristics, and references.

The sensitivity and specificity of serologic tests vary from procedure to procedure. As explained in Chapter 20, *sensitivity* is the ability of the test in question to identify those individuals having the condition or disease for which the test is being performed. *Specificity* is the ability of the test in question to distinguish the specific antibody or antigen being tested for from other similar antibodies or antigens. When performing serologic tests, sensitivity is important for determining false-positive and false-negative results. A *false-positive test result* indicates a test reaction that identifies a patient who does not have the condition or disease in question, but who nevertheless tests positive for that condition. Most serologic tests are qualitative. *Qualitative tests* indicate the presence or absence of the antigen or antibody for which the test is being performed. To properly diagnose and manage a specific disease, it is sometimes important for the physician to know the quantity of the antigen or antibody present. Quantitative tests involving antigens and antibodies are reported as titers. A **titer** is the lowest concentration or highest dilution of the specimen being tested that will produce an observable reaction. Determination of the titer is accomplished by diluting the specimen being tested and performing the serologic test in question on each dilution. Quantitative testing is routinely done on patients with rheumatoid arthritis or infectious mononucleosis, or in those who have tested positive on a qualitative pregnancy test. All serologic tests must be evaluated in conjunction with all other data available to the physician.

Testing Methods

Serologic tests can usually be classified into one of the following categories.

Bioluminescence/Chemiluminescence

Ongoing research and advances in immunoassay technology have identified new methods for quantitating substances that are present in the body in miniscule amounts. Among these advances are **bioluminescence** and **chemiluminescence.** These phenomena appear to have widespread applications in detecting extremely low levels of substances, such as hormones.

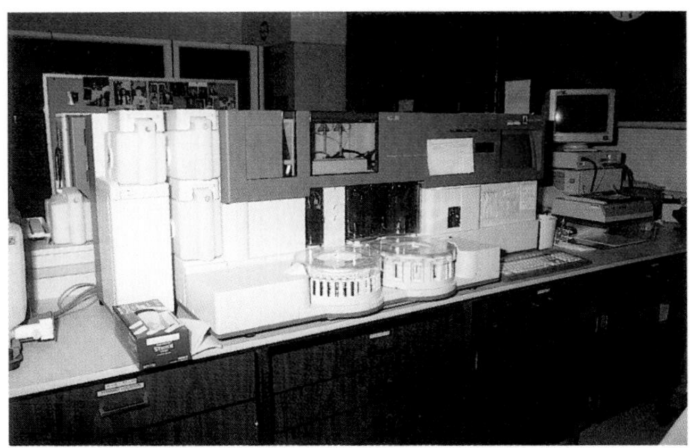

Figure 21–1. *Beckman ACS 180 Automated Chemiluminescence System.*

Bioluminescence is found in nature in the firefly and certain species of bacteria. **Cold light** is generated as a product of specific enzymatic reactions. Bioluminescence occurs when an enzyme-activated compound is combined with oxygen to create a new compound. This combination with oxygen causes a flash of light.

Chemiluminescence is light produced by a chemical reaction. These light-producing reactions occur at room temperature and require no energy source. Chemiluminescence involves a reaction between an organic compound, such as **luminol,** and oxygen (Fig. 21–1).

Any enzymatic or chemical reaction that produces oxygen or an oxygen compound can be joined with a luminescent reaction to generate light. The amount of light produced can then be correlated to the amount of enzyme or chemical present (Fig. 21–2).

Enzyme-Linked Immunosorbent Assay

The enzyme-linked immunosorbent assay (ELISA) is a sensitive technique that uses an enzyme-antibody-antigen combination absorbed onto the sides of a test wall. If the patient has antibodies or antigens for the disease agent, the linkage is formed and the antibody or antigen binds to an enzyme to produce a colored reaction, indicating a positive test result. If the patient does not have the serum antigen or the antibody sought, the enzyme is not linked and no color is visible. Enzyme-linked immunosorbent assays are simple to perform and are available in kit form. They are commonly used to test for acquired immunodeficiency syndrome (AIDS), hepatitis A, hepatitis B, and rubella (German measles), as well as certain toxic chemicals and drugs present in the serum (Fig. 21–3).

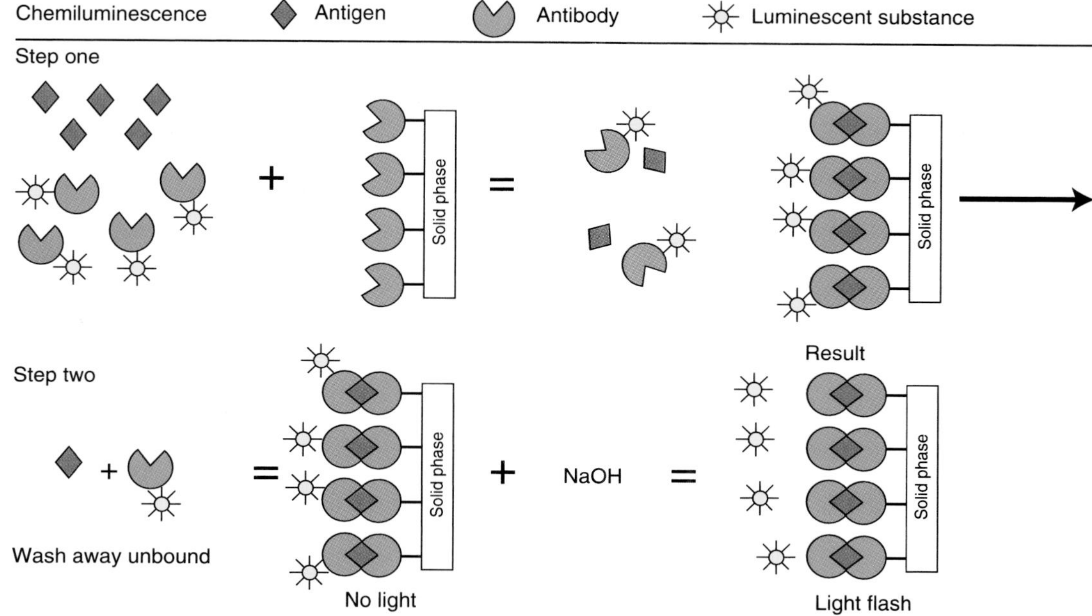

Figure 21–2. *Process of chemiluminescence.*

Agglutination Test

In agglutination testing, the antibody-antigen reaction involves attachment to a substance, such as latex beads or blood cells. Antibodies are capable of clumping together antigen molecules and bacteria. This process is called **agglutination.** Agglutination reactions can be performed on a slide or in a test tube by mixing the patient's serum with a specific antigen. The presence or absence of agglutination or clumping is then observed. When the antibody-antigen reaction takes place, it produces a result that is visible to the naked eye. These tests may be used, for example, to identify the ABO blood group and to diagnose **Brucellosis** and **salmonellosis.** In addition, **heterophil** agglutination tests are used to diagnose **infectious mononucleosis** (Fig. 21–4).

Radioimmunoassay

In radioimmunoassay (RIA), an antigen is labeled with a radioactive isotope. Using an antibody-antigen reaction with the labeled antigen, the quantity of the substance being measured can be determined (Fig. 21–5). Refer to the discussion on RIA in Chapter 19 for further details.

Precipitation Test

Tests involving precipitation are not as popular as ELISA or agglutination tests. Precipitation involves the formation of insoluble complexes too large to remain suspended in solutions. These complexes precipitate in a mass or **flocculus** that is visible to the naked eye. Precipitates will form when soluble antigens are com-

Figure 21–3. *Process of enzyme-linked immunosorbent assay (ELISA).*

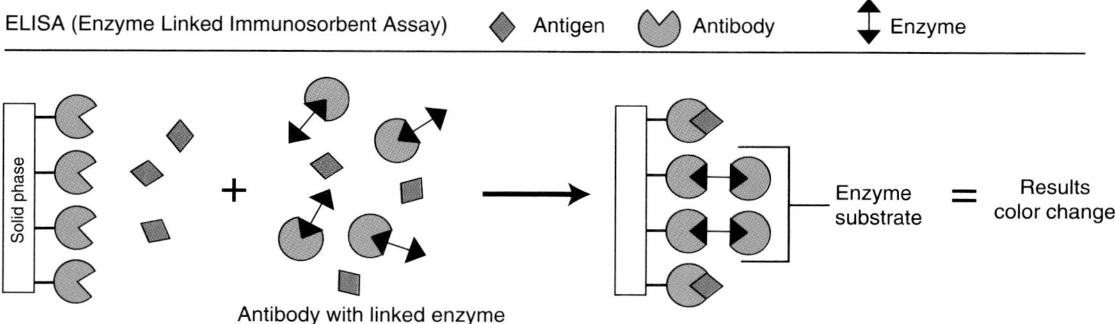

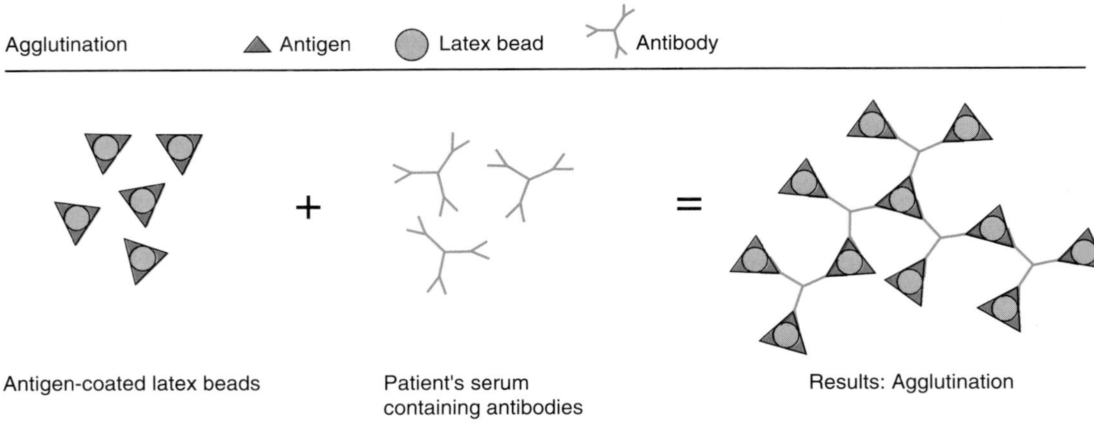

Agglutination ▲ Antigen ● Latex bead Antibody

Antigen-coated latex beads + Patient's serum containing antibodies = Results: Agglutination

Figure 21–4. *Process of agglutination.*

bined with antiserum containing a specific antibody. These tests are used mainly in the identification of bacterial **exotoxins** and antibodies of certain fungi (Fig. 21–6).

Complement Fixation Test

The complement fixation test involves a more tedious procedure. Complement is a substance found in normal serum that produces **lysis** when it is combined with antigen-antibody complexes. The patient's serum is first incubated with the antigen to be tested and a specific amount of complement. If an antigen-antibody reaction takes place, the complement will "fix" to these complexes. Erythrocytes coated with antibodies are then added to the combination and lysis occurs if there is any free complement left in the serum. The failure of lysis to occur implies that all of the complement was used up in the first phase of the test, indicating the presence of the particular antibody for which the test was performed. An example of a complement fixation test is the **VDRL** test (Fig. 21–7).

Neutralization Test

An antigen is said to be neutralized when it loses the ability to produce an injurious effect. An antigen-antibody combination causes such an effect. These tests are usually used in viral identification. The incubated known virus and test serum are inoculated into the tissue culture and the effects are noted. Animals may be used for this test. The test serum is given, and the animal is then challenged with the microorganism. If the antibody is present in the test serum, the animal is protected against the infection.

Fluorescent Antibody Test

In the fluorescent antibody test, an antibody's attachment to an antigen is identified under the fluorescent microscope through the use of a fluorescent dye. The test involves using a microscope slide upon which the clinical material has been fixed and overlaid with a specific preparation of antibody conjugated to dye. An antigen-antibody reaction is noted if fluorescent microorganisms are seen. The fluorescent treponemal antibody absorption (FTA-ABS) test for the diagnosis of syphilis is an example of a fluorescent antibody test (Fig. 21–8).

Testing Procedures

Pregnancy Testing

Serologic tests for pregnancy involve the detection of human chorionic gonadotropin (hCG), a hormone pro-

Figure 21–5. *Process of radioimmunoassay (RIA).*

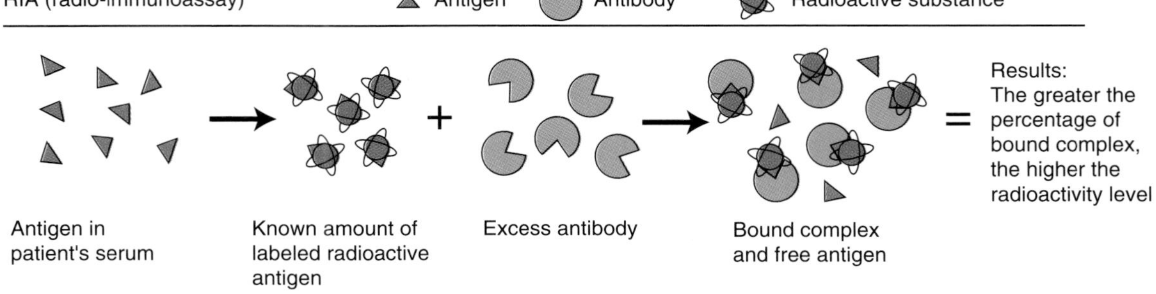

RIA (radio-immunoassay) ▲ Antigen Antibody Radioactive substance

Antigen in patient's serum → Known amount of labeled radioactive antigen + Excess antibody → Bound complex and free antigen = Results: The greater the percentage of bound complex, the higher the radioactivity level

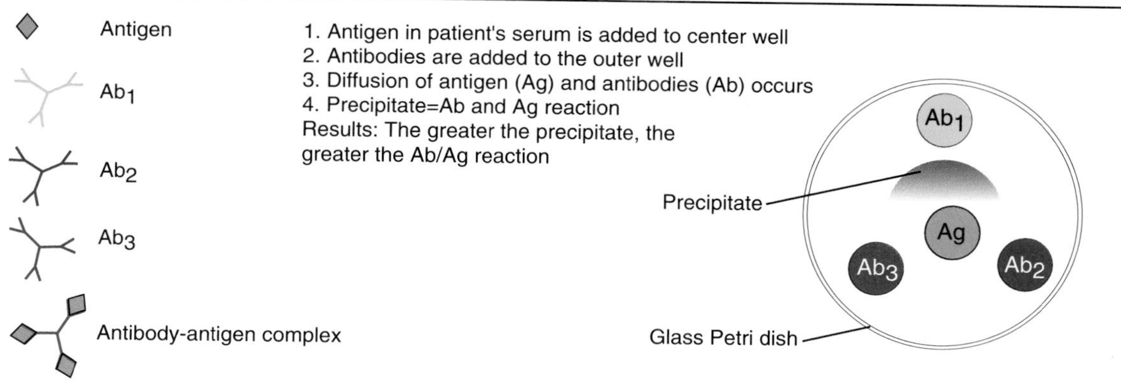

Figure 21–6. *Process of precipitation.*

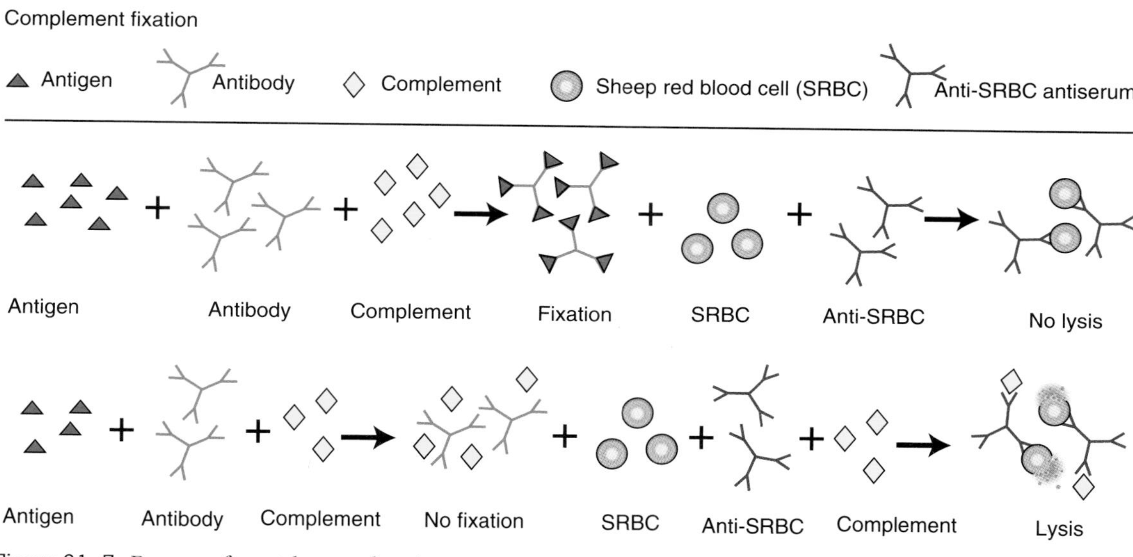

Figure 21–7. *Process of complement fixation.*

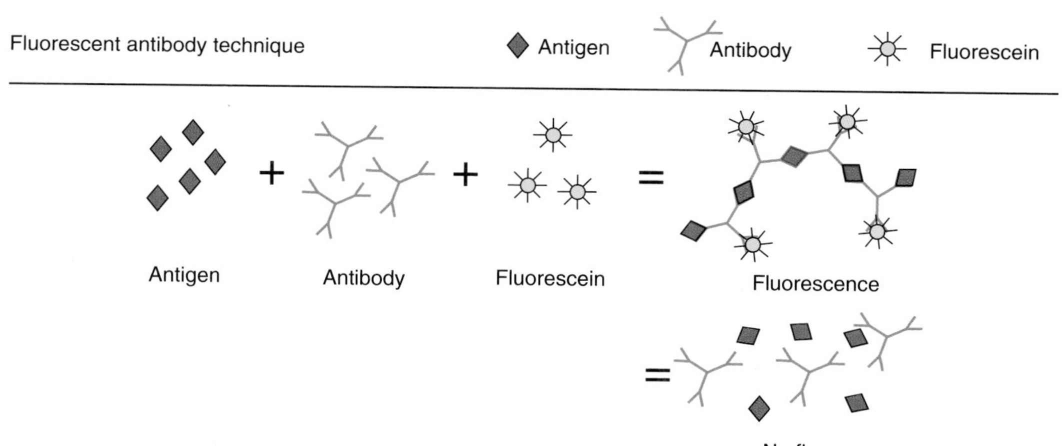

Figure 21–8. *Fluorescent antibody test.*

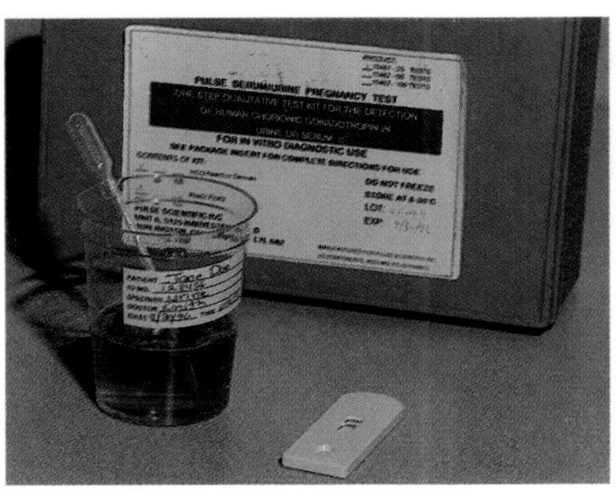

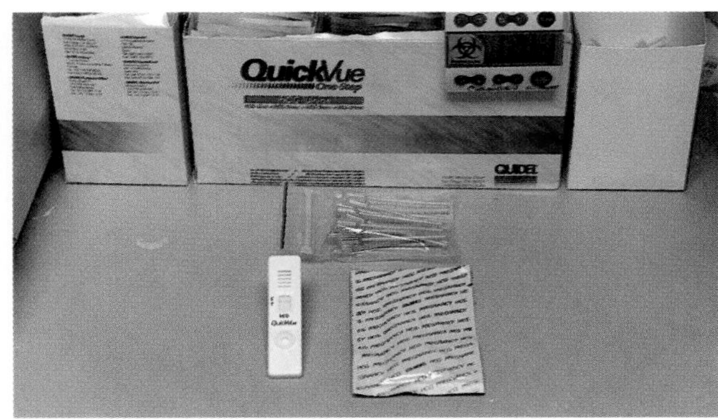

A B

Figure 21–9. A, *Pulse serum/urine pregnancy test*. B, *Quick Vue pregnancy test (hCG urine)*.

duced in the chorionic villi of the placenta and found in the urine and serum of pregnant women. Levels of hCG may be detected as early as 8 to 10 days after conception. In late pregnancy, hCG levels begin to decline, and pregnancy tests should be negative 3 to 4 days postpartum. Quantitative analysis of hCG is valuable in making a differential diagnosis of a viable pregnancy versus a nonviable pregnancy, in cases of multiple gestations, or in other conditions related to female reproduction.

Pregnancy testing can be performed on either serum or urine (Fig. 21–9*A* and *B*). A first-morning collection of urine generally contains the highest concentrations of hCG, however, and so is the specimen of choice for qualitative pregnancy testing. The first-morning urine is particularly valuable in detecting pregnancy in the early stages. However, any urine sample is suitable for testing. Pregnancy testing on a urine specimen should be performed as soon as possible, as hCG can be lost without proper storage. Specimens that will not be tested promptly should be refrigerated. Urine specimens that are grossly bloody, are contaminated by bacteria, contain excessive protein, or have a specific gravity of less than 1.005 are not acceptable for pregnancy tests.

False-negative tests commonly occur as a result of too low a specific gravity or testing too early in the pregnancy. False-positive tests are commonly associated with proteinuria and hematuria. If the physician is concerned that the patient may be in the early stages of pregnancy and the pregnancy test yields a negative result, the test should be repeated in 1 week. Pregnancy tests are generally done by agglutination inhibition or ELISA. The ELISA tests are popular because they are accurate and may be performed in one or two steps. In the agglutination inhibition test for pregnancy, agglutination occurs when anti-hCG antibodies combine with a latex bead coated with hCG (antigen). The agglutination inhibition test is designed in such a way that, when hCG is present in the urine of the patient being tested, no agglutination occurs. The anti-hCG binds with the hCG in the patient's urine, preventing the anti-hCG from binding with the hCG-coated latex beads. When the patient is not pregnant, there is no hCG in the patient's urine. Therefore, the anti-hCG is not inhibited and is free to bind with the hCG-coated latex beads. When this antibody-antigen reaction occurs, it forms a visible clumping and results in a negative test result.

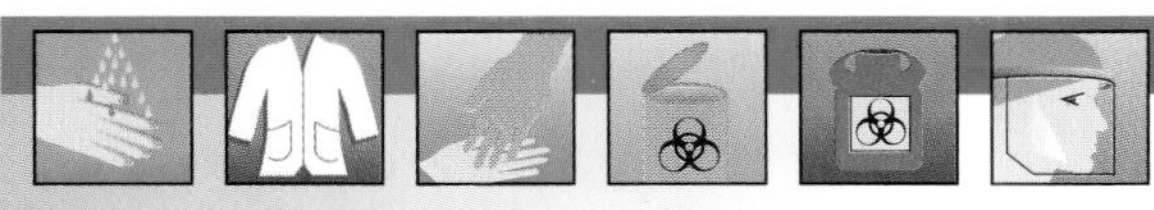

PROCEDURE 21–1

Performing a Pregnancy Test (ELISA Test)

Principle

To collect an appropriate sample and perform a pregnancy test with accuracy

Equipment and Supplies

QuickVue One-Step hCG Combo Test Kit or other slide test kit
watch or clock

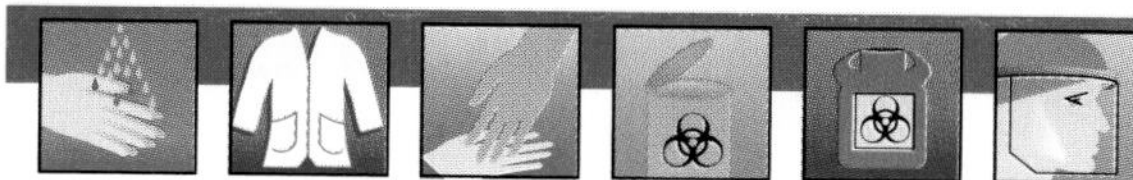

PROCEDURE 21–1

Performing a Pregnancy Test (ELISA Test) (Continued)

disposable pipette
specimen collection equipment and supplies

Procedural Steps

Obtaining a Specimen

Serum

1. Wash hands with disinfectant and dry them thoroughly. Don gloves and other protective gear, and follow universal precautions.
2. Assemble necessary equipment.
3. Explain the specimen collection procedure to the patient. No other special patient preparation is needed.
4. Collect a blood specimen by aseptic venipuncture using a tube that contains no anticoagulant agent.
5. Remove the serum from the clot as soon as possible.* Do not chemically modify the serum in any way.
6. Label the specimen with the appropriate patient information.

   ***If a serum separator was used, pour serum off into appropriate container. If a serum separator was not used, carefully remove the serum from the clot using a beral pipette, without disturbing the clot.**

Urine

1. Wash hands with disinfectant and dry them thoroughly. Don gloves and other protective gear, and follow universal precautions.
2. Assemble necessary equipment.
3. Instruct the patient in the proper technique for collecting a urine specimen in a clean container. First-morning specimens generally contain the highest concentrations of hCG and are recommended for early detection of pregnancy, but any urine sample may be successfully used for this test.
4. Label the specimen with the appropriate patient information.

Performing the Pregnancy Test

1. Wash hands with disinfectant. Put on gloves and other protective wear, and follow universal precautions. (Not necessary if done in previous steps.)
2. Assemble the necessary materials.
3. Review the manufacturer's procedural guidelines and follow them exactly.
4. Verify the patient's identification by checking the label on the patient's blood or urine specimen sample.
5. Remove the pregnancy test cassette from its container. Place on a clean, dry, and level surface.
6. Using a disposable pipette, add 3 drops of the patient's serum or urine to the sample well of the test cassette.
7. *When testing urine,* read the results in 3 minutes. *When testing serum,* read the results in 5 minutes.
8. After the appropriate interval, read the test result window. A blue control line next to the letter **C** *and* a pink-purple line next to the letter **T** is a positive test. If only a blue control line next to the letter **C** appears, this indicates a negative test. (NOTE: A blue control line should always appear in the window next to the letter **C**. If no visual control line appears, the test is invalid and must be repeated.)
9. If testing a urine specimen, repeat steps 5 through 8 on the positive urine control sample and the negative urine control sample.
10. Complete the necessary information on the report form.
11. Properly dispose of the patient's specimen and any disposable equipment according to biohazardous waste disposal guidelines.
12. Clean the work area and disinfect any reusable equipment.
13. Remove disposable protective clothing and gloves.
14. Wash hands with disinfectant.
15. Report the test results and enter the test performed in the laboratory log.

Interpreting Test Results

Positive Result: The appearance of any pink to purple line next to the letter **T** in the Result Window, along with a blue procedural Control Line next to the letter **C**, indicates a positive test result.

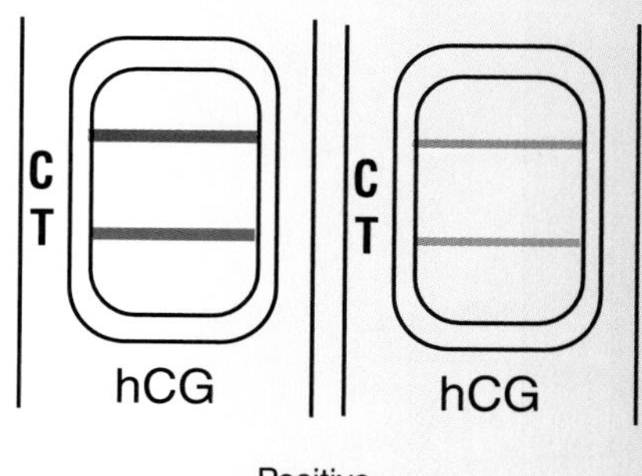

Positive

(continued)

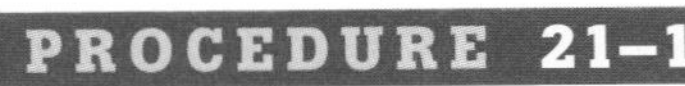

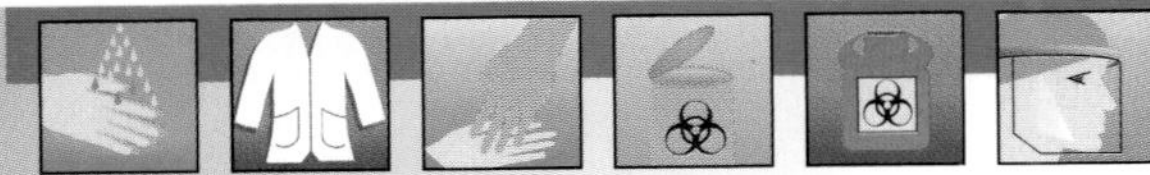

Performing a Pregnancy Test (ELISA Test) *(Continued)*

Negative Result: The appearance of the blue procedural Control Line next to the letter **C** only, and no pink to purple line next to the letter **T** after a 3-minute interval for urine and a 5-minute interval for serum indicates that the test result is negative.

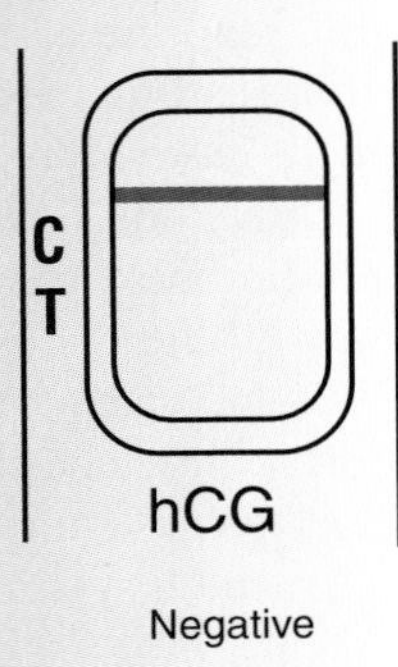

Negative

Invalid Result: A blue procedural Control Line should ALWAYS appear next to the letter **C** in the Result Window. If no blue procedural Control Line appears, the test is invalid.

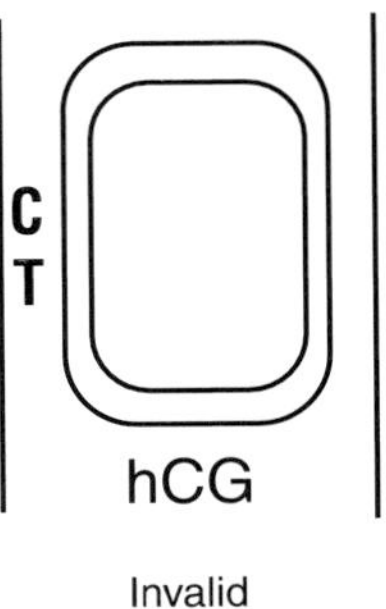

Invalid

Infectious Mononucleosis

Infectious mononucleosis is an acute viral infection caused by the Epstein-Barr virus (EBV). It is also called "mono" and is sometimes abbreviated "IM." Infectious mononucleosis is a disease commonly found in adolescents and young adults. Because it is believed to be transmitted orally, it is sometimes called the "kissing disease." Because of the vague, flu-like symptoms associated with infectious mononucleosis, diagnosis is usually based on the evaluation of clinical symptoms, hematologic testing, and serologic testing (Table 21–1). Infectious mononucleosis is characterized by fever, pharyngitis, swollen lymph glands, atypical lymphocytes, splenomegaly, hepatomegaly, fatigue, weakness, and headache. Infection typically confers permanent

Table 21–1
Differential Diagnosis of Infectious Mononucleosis

Clinical Findings	*Hematologic Findings*	*Serologic Findings*
Adolescents and young adults	Leukocytosis (12–25 $\times 10^9$/L)	Heterophil antibody
Vague onset	Lymphocytosis (60–90%)	EBV* antibody
Fever	Atypical lymphocytes	Cold agglutinins
Sore throat		
Lymphadenopathy (initially cervical)		
Splenomegaly		
	Slight monocytosis†	Positive monotest
	Neutropenia	

*Epstein-Barr virus.
†Refers to lymphocytes not monocytes.

immunity. Treatment is primarily symptomatic and usually includes bed rest.

Hematologic testing for infectious mononucleosis involves a complete blood count (CBC). Particular attention is paid to the patient's total white blood cell (WBC) count and the appearance of the patient's lymphocytes. In infectious mononucleosis, the lymphocytes may have an unusual or atypical appearance, and the patient may have an increased number of lymphocytes, termed *lymphocytosis*. Most patients exposed to EPV develop a heterophil antibody response. Heterophil antibodies are part of the widespread group of antibodies that are characterized by the ability to react with the surface antigens present on the red blood cells (RBCs) of different mammalian species. Most qualitative mononucleosis tests are slide tests. Slide tests yield rapid, reliable results, and are easy to perform. Specialized tests to detect the presence of EPV are available in reference laboratories and government-run public health laboratories.

Serologic test kits for infectious mononucleosis provide all the necessary reagents, materials, and controls. All that is needed is a small amount of the patient's plasma or serum. Some kits even allow testing of whole blood. Traditional tests for infectious mononucleosis, such as the Mono-Test (Wampole Laboratories) (Fig. 21–10*A*), are based on the agglutination of horse erythrocytes by the heterophil antibody present in patients with infectious mononucleosis. Because there are other antibodies present that will also react with horse erythrocytes, the serum is treated to remove these interfering antibodies before it is combined with the horse erythrocytes. Numerous commercial kits for testing for infectious mononucleosis are available, including the Pulse test (Pulse Scientific, Inc.) (Fig. 21–10*B*), Monoslide (Bectin Dickinson), Monospot (Meridian Diagnostics), and the Color Slide II (Seradyn).

Developments in solid-phase immunoassay technology have resulted in the capability for qualitative detection of infectious mononucleosis using easy-to-use test cassettes. Examples of this solid-phase immunoassay technology are Mono-Plus (Wampole Laboratories) and Concise Plus test for infectious mononucleosis (Rapid Diagnostic Technology) (Fig. 21–10*C*). In patients with hematologic and clinical evidence of infectious mononucleosis, a positive infectious mononucleosis test is usually diagnostic. However, caution must be exercised, as patients with infectious mononucleosis may test positive for long periods of time without any hematologic or clinical evidence of the disease. Conversely, serologic testing for infectious mononucleosis may yield negative results even though the patient has hematologic and clinical evidence of infectious mononucleosis.

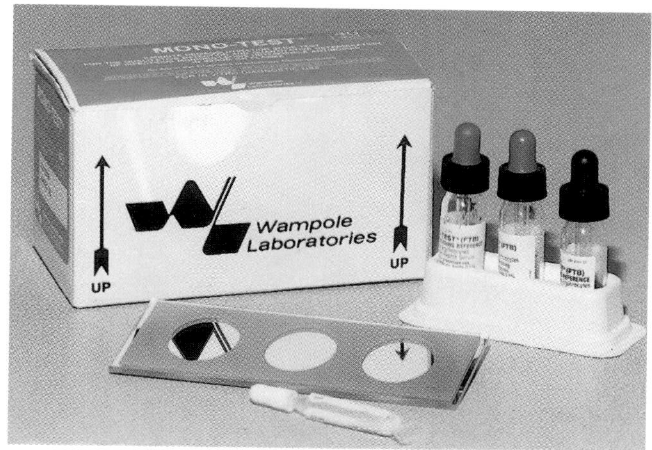

A

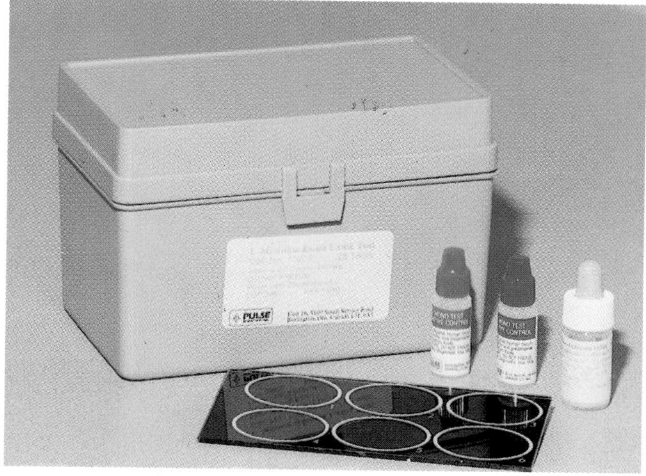

B

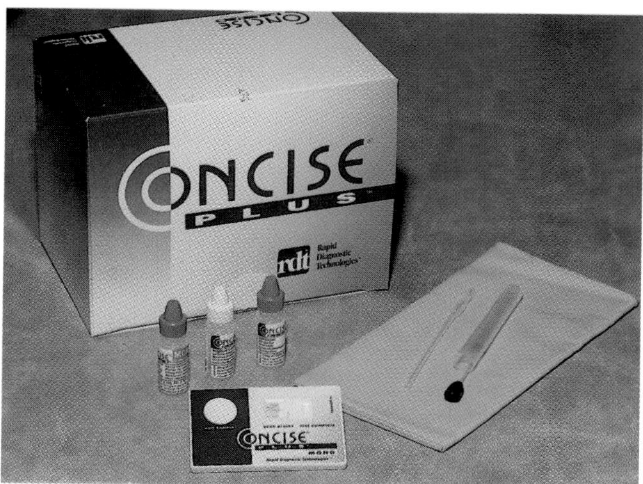

C

Figure 21–10. A, *Mono-Test (Wampole Laboratories)*. B, *Pulse test for infectious mononucleosis (Pulse Scientific Inc.)*. C, *Concise Plus test for infectious mononucleosis (Pulse Scientific, Inc.)*.

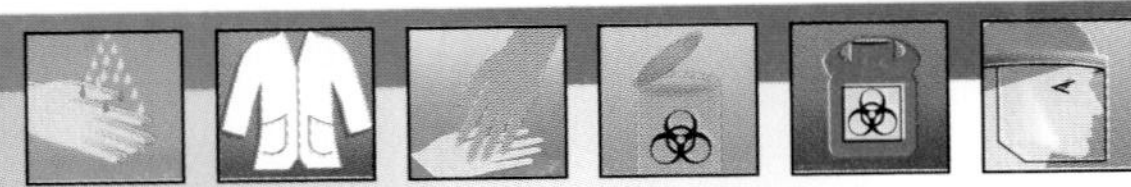

PROCEDURE 21–2

Testing for Infectious Mononucleosis (Solid-Phase Immunoassay)

Principle

To obtain the designated specimen, prepare it for infectious mononucleosis testing, perform an analysis, and report the results of the test following proper testing protocols

Equipment and Supplies

Mono-Plus Test Kit
centrifuge
micropipettor
positive control
negative control
watch or clock

Procedural Steps

Obtaining a Specimen

Serum

1. Wash hands, dry them thoroughly, and don gloves and protective apparel.
2. Assemble the necessary equipment.
3. Explain the specimen collection procedure to the patient.
4. Collect a serum sample by obtaining blood by aseptic venipuncture using a Vacutainer tube containing no anticoagulant.
5. Allow the blood to clot at room temperature (18° –24°C) and then centrifuge it at 1500 rpm for 10 minutes.
6. Separate the serum as soon as possible, after which it may be tested immediately.
7. Label the specimen with the appropriate patient information.

Plasma

1. Wash hands, dry them thoroughly, and don gloves and protective apparel.
2. Assemble the necessary equipment.
3. Explain the specimen collection procedure to the patient.
4. Collect the whole blood specimen into a tube containing anticoagulant (e.g., EDTA).
5. Remove the plasma from the clot or red cells as soon as possible to avoid hemolysis. Clear, nonhemolyzed specimens should be used for best testing results.
6. Label the specimen with the appropriate patient information.

Performing the Solid-Phase Immunoassay

1. Wash hands with disinfectant. Put on gloves and other protective gear and follow universal precautions. (Not necessary if done in previous steps.)
2. Assemble the necessary materials.
3. Review the manufacturer's procedural guidelines and follow them exactly.
4. Identify the patient's specimen by checking the label.
5. Allow the patient's sample, control samples, and test kit materials to come to room temperature.
6. Remove the Mono-Plus test cassette from the sealed pouch.
7. Label the test cassette with the patient's name.
8. Using the disposable micropipette, dispense 10 μL of the specimen into the sample well labeled **S**.

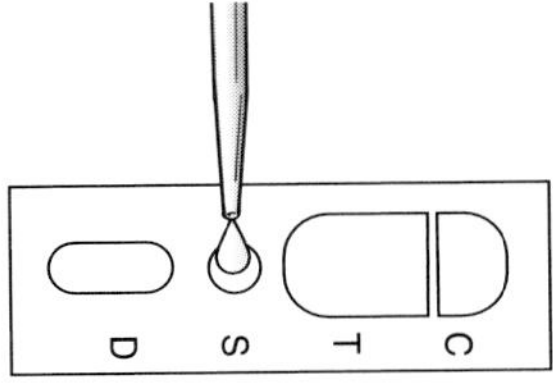

Specimen

9. Add 3 to 4 drops of developer solution to the solution well labeled **D**. Use caution not to touch the micropipette or the developer solution dropper to any surface or to the Mono-Plus (registered) test chamber.

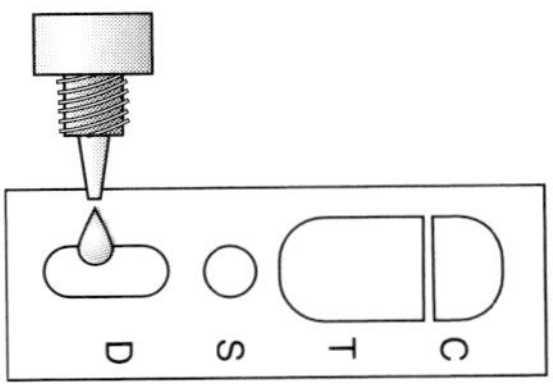

Developer

10. Results should be read in 8 minutes. Positive results may be reported sooner. However, an interval of 8 minutes is required to report a negative result.
11. Record the results.
12. Properly dispose of all test equipment according to biohazardous waste disposal guidelines.
13. Clean the work area and disinfect and store all reusable equipment.

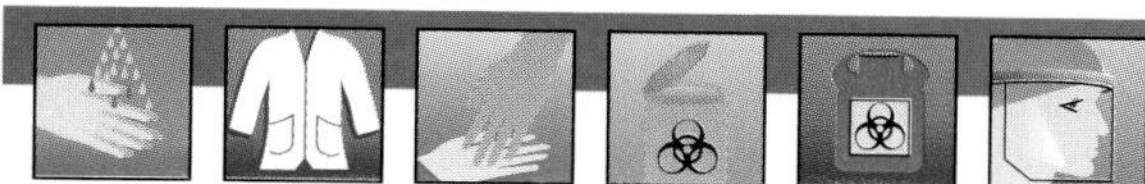

PROCEDURE 21–2

Testing for Infectious Mononucleosis (Solid-Phase Immunoassay) (Continued)

14. Remove gloves and other protective clothing.
15. Wash and disinfect hands.

Interpreting Test Results

Positive Result: The appearance of one pink-purple colored band in the Test Window (**T**) and in the Control Window (**C**) indicates that infectious mononucleosis–specific heterophil antibodies have been detected.

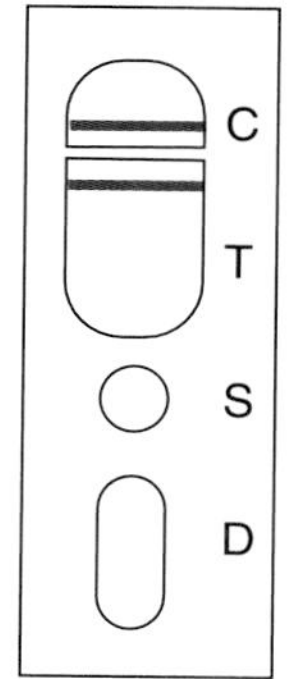

Positive

Negative Result: One pink-purple colored band in the Control Window (**C**), with NO distinct colored band appearing in the Test Window (**T**) (other than the normal faint background color), indicates that infectious mononucleosis–specific heterophil antibodies have not been detected.

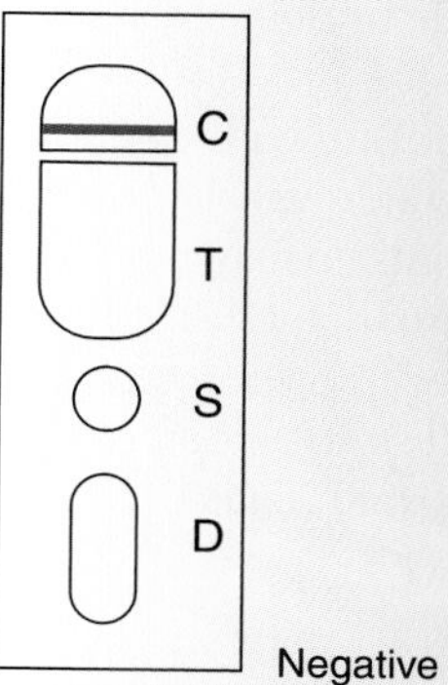

Negative

Invalid Result: A distinctive colored band should ALWAYS appear in the Control Window (**C**). The test is invalid if no band forms in the Control Window (**C**).

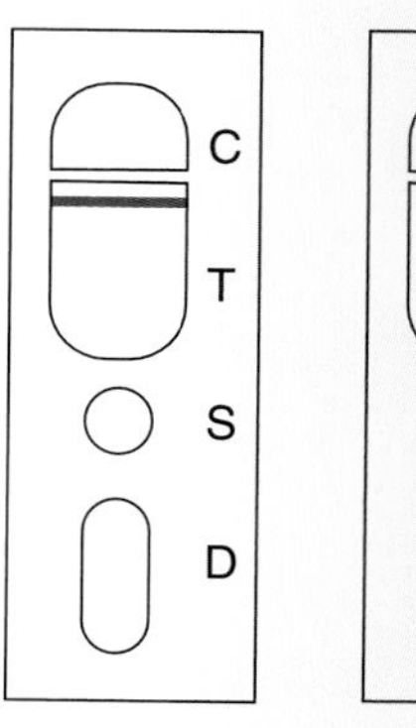

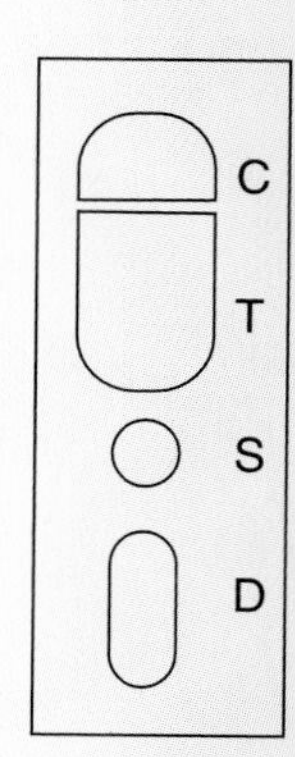

Invalid

Rheumatoid Arthritis

Rheumatoid arthritis is a chronic destructive and deforming systemic collagen disease that has an autoimmune factor. Rheumatoid arthritis is characterized by inflammation of the body's joints and related tissue (connective tissue).

The specific cause of rheumatoid arthritis is unknown. It is generally believed that the pathologic changes in the connective tissue are related to antigen-antibody reactions that are autoimmune in origin.

The diagnosis and treatment of rheumatoid arthritis is based on clinical symptoms, laboratory test results, radiologic studies and physical examination. Rheumatoid arthritis usually first appears in early middle age, and it affects women more frequently than men. Early symptoms of rheumatoid arthritis may include fatigue, weakness, loss of appetite, low-grade fever, anemia, and an increased erythrocyte sedimentation rate. Symptoms associated with the joints and related tissues include morning stiffness, joint pain or tenderness, swelling of joints, arthritic nodules, structural changes in the joints, and a positive serologic test for rheumatoid factor.

The serologic test for rheumatoid arthritis involves detection of the presence of rheumatoid factor (RF). RF is an immunoglobulin found in the serum of patients with rheumatoid arthritis. Immunoglobulins are formed in the bone marrow, spleen, and all lymphoid tissue, except the thymus. Immunoglobulins are structurally and antigenically distinct antibodies that are present in the serum and other body fluids. They are formed in response to specific antigens. The five classifications of immunoglobulins are IgA, IgD, IgE, IgG, and IgM. Of the patients diagnosed with rheumatoid arthritis, 75% to 85% have detectable levels of RF in their serum. RFs are immunoglobulins, usually IgMs, that are produced in response to human IgG (Table 21–2). RF levels are not usually elevated in other types of arthritis. Because of this, serologic tests that detect RF are valuable tools in the diagnosis of rheumatoid arthritis.

Treatment for rheumatoid arthritis varies. Bed rest, salicylate therapy, anti-inflammatory medications, physical therapy, and surgical procedures are among the treatments used.

The appropriate specimen for rheumatoid arthritis serologic testing is usually serum or synovial fluid. Synovial fluid is the lubricating fluid secreted by the synovial membranes of the joints.

Most serologic tests for rheumatoid factor use slide agglutination techniques, such as Seratest RF Latex Kit (Seradyn) and the RF Latex Test (Pulse Scientific, Inc.) (Fig. 21–11, *A* and *B*). The slide agglutination tests for rheumatoid factor are simple, rapid, qualitative methods for detecting rheumatoid factor. Special latex particles are coated with human immunoglobulin (IgG). If rheumatoid factors are present in the patient's serum or synovial fluid, the RFs, which are autoantibodies, will bind with the IgG and cause agglutination. The latex particles allow the agglutination to be visible to the

Table 21–2
Classification of Immunoglobulins

Type	*Location*	*Function(s)*
IgA	External secretions (tears, saliva, colostrum)	Primary antibody in the mucous membranes Conveys passive immunity to breast-fed infants Defends the body surfaces against invading microorganisms
IgD	B lymphocytes	Antigen receptor; increases in some allergic reactions (e.g., to milk and penicillin)
IgE	Lungs, skin, mucous membranes; basophils or mast cells	Defends against environmental antigens Important in allergic reactions Causes histamine release
IgG	Blood, extracellular fluid	Primary immunoglobulin present in human serum Crosses the placenta, producing prenatal immunity Important in defending against invasion by microorganisms Activates complement Major factor in conveying long-term immunity
IgM	Blood, circulating fluids	First immunoglobulin produced in immune response Controls ABO blood group Stimulates antibody activity Stimulates complement Significant factor in early immune response Defends against infection

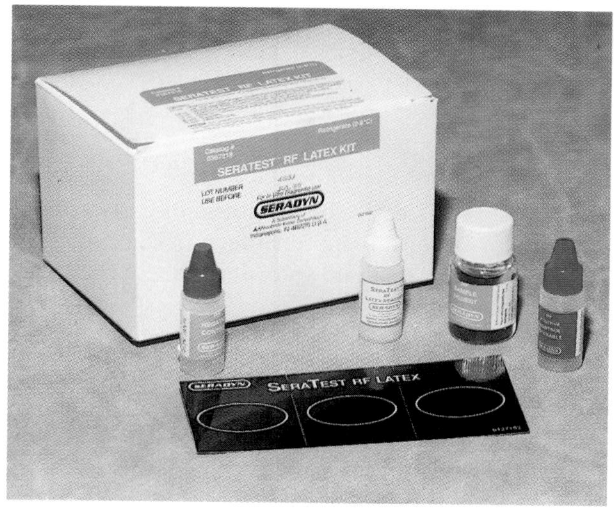

A

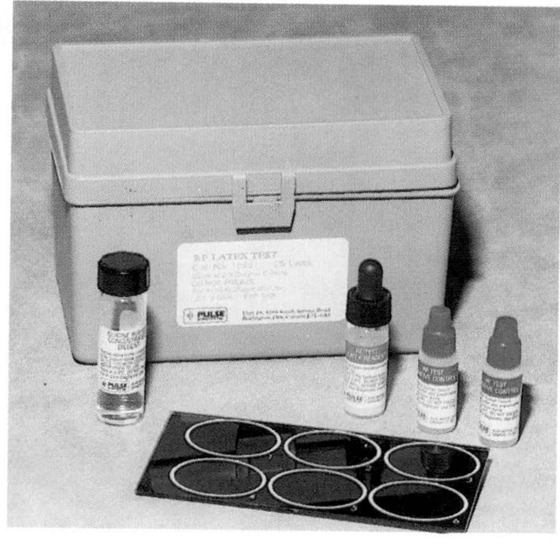

B

Figure 21–11. A, *Seratest RA Latex Kit (Sereadyn).* B, *RF Latex Test (Pulse Scientific, Inc.).*

naked eye. Quantitative testing for RF is accomplished by diluting the patient's serum or synovial fluid and testing the diluted samples. Specimens positive for RF exhibit agglutination, whereas specimens negative for RF show no agglutination. Because most normal individuals have low levels of RF in their serum, the patient's serum is diluted 1:20 before testing, using a glycine buffer. The dilution allows only significant levels of RF to be detected.

Diagnosis of rheumatoid arthritis should not be made solely on the basis of serologic testing for RF. Other inflammatory diseases may also cause a positive test result. In addition, only 75% to 85% of patients with rheumatoid arthritis have increased levels of RF. Therefore, a negative test does not rule out a diagnosis of rheumatoid arthritis. RFs can be used to monitor the course of rheumatoid arthritis, as RF levels will parallel the patient's condition.

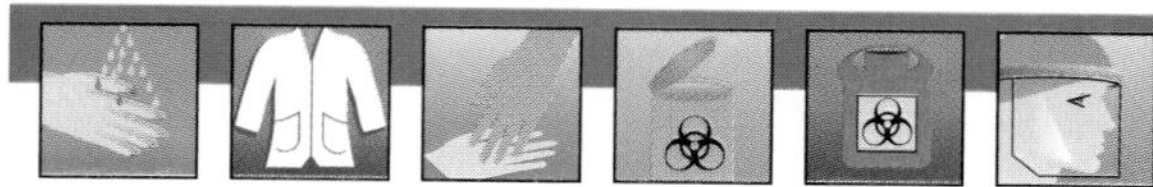

PROCEDURE 21–3

Performing a Slide Test for Rheumatoid Factor

Principle

To perform and report rheumatoid factor test results precisely following the manufacturer's instructions

Equipment and Supplies

timer
75-mm test tubes
test tube rack
specimen for testing
pipettes
rheumatoid slide test kit
applicator sticks

Procedural Steps

1. Wash hands with disinfectant. Put on gloves and other protective equipment and follow universal precautions.
2. Assemble the necessary materials.
3. Read the manufacturer's instructions, check the kit's expiration date, and check to be sure the kit is complete.

(continued)

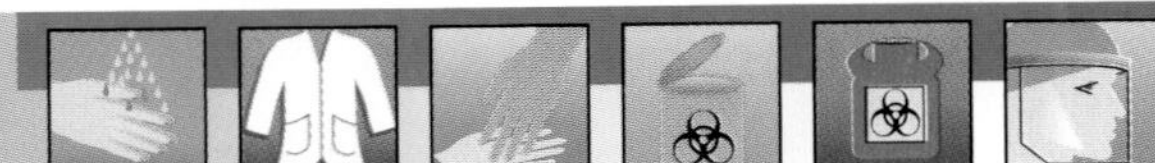

PROCEDURE 21–3

Performing a Slide Test for Rheumatoid Factor (Continued)

4. Allow the reagents to come to room temperature before performing the test.
5. Prepare a 1:20 dilution of the patient's serum using a glycine buffer (0.05 mL of serum in 0.95 mL of glycine buffer), as learned in Chapter 5, Procedure 5–1.
6. Dispense 1 drop of positive control serum onto the positive control ring on the slide.
7. Dispense 1 drop of negative control serum onto the negative control ring on the slide.
8. Dispense 1 drop of the patient's diluted serum onto the test ring on the test slide, using the dispenser spreader included in the test kit.
9. Gently mix the rheumatoid factor latex reagent.
10. Dispense 1 drop of the well-mixed rheumatoid factor latex reagent onto each of the control and test rings.
11. Use the spreader included in the test kit to mix the serum and the latex reagent thoroughly, spreading the mixture over the entire surface of the ring. **CAUTION: Use a separate spreader for each control or patient sample.**
12. Gently rock the slide using a figure-of-eight motion for 2 minutes.
13. Observe the rings on the slide for agglutination.
14. Report the results and record the test performed and the results in the laboratory log.
15. Properly dispose of all test materials according to hazardous waste disposal guidelines.
16. Disinfect and store all reusable equipment and reagents.
17. Clean and disinfect the work area.
18. Remove gloves and disposable protective equipment and discard appropriately.
19. Wash and disinfect hands.

Summary

Most serologic tests are available in kit form and are extremely sensitive in terms of negative and positive determinations. Whether you work in a physician's office laboratory or a hospital laboratory, it is critical that you become familiar with the sensitivity and specificity of every test you are responsible for performing. The results that you report will likely be used to diagnose or manage a patient with a specific disease or condition. You must assume responsibility for knowing the proper procedure for each test, which should include reviewing the package insert to be absolutely certain that the information provided by the manufacturer is followed for every test done. When you are entrusted with processing or performing serologic tests, you must follow the instructions provided by the manufacturer exactly as outlined.

Chapter Review

True or False

Circle T or F to indicate the correct answers to the following:

T F 1. An in vivo reaction occurs in the laboratory.

T F 2. Immunologic testing provides information about past and/or present infections.

T F 3. A false-positive reaction is one in which the patient tests negative but the disease or condition being tested for is really present.

T F 4. To determine a titer, the specimen must be diluted.

Fill in the Blanks

Complete the following statements:

5. The ______________ test is commonly used to detect AIDS.
6. The clumping of antigen molecules and bacteria together is called ______________ .
7. An example of a complement fixation test is the ______________ test.
8. Infectious mononucleosis is caused by the ______________ ______________ virus.

Multiple Choice

Circle the letter that represents the single best answer:

9. What hormone are you looking for in a pregnancy test?
   a. IgG
   b. hCG
   c. IgM
   d. Estrogen
   e. Testosterone

10. Most serologic tests for rheumatoid arthritis involve:
    a. Complement fixation
    b. Precipitation
    c. RIA
    d. Slide agglutination
    e. ELISA

Vocabulary

autologous: related to or belonging to self
forensic: pertaining to the legal aspects of a given test or procedure
genetically: pertaining to inheritance; relating to birth or origin
hemolytic: pertaining to the rupture of red blood cells (RBCs) and release of hemoglobin into the plasma
isoimmunization: development of antibodies in response to an antigen existing in alternative forms within the body and transferred to other humans who lack it
jaundice: yellowish color of the skin and mucous membranes secondary to hyperbilirubinemia
nomenclature: a classified system of technical names, such as for organisms or structures
prenatal: pertaining to the gestational time preceding birth
rouleaux: a roll of RBCs resembling a pile of coins

Chapter Objectives

After reading this chapter, you should be able to:

1. Discuss the ABO blood group system.
2. Describe how blood antibodies influence the system.
3. Discuss the research that led to the discovery of Rh.
4. List the signs and symptoms of hemolytic disease of the newborn.
5. Explain weak expression of D antigen.
6. Discuss your role in blood typing and crossmatching.
7. List the steps involved in determining blood type and Rh.

Chapter 22
Immunohematologic Testing and Procedures

In the clinical medical laboratory, the study of human blood groups, or immunohematology, is routinely performed in the blood bank department. Hence, the use of the term "blood banking" as an alternative to immunohematology. Immunohematologic tests are performed to prevent transfusion and transplant reactions, to identify the potential for hemolytic disease of the newborn, to determine parentage, and for **forensic** purposes.

The major clinical reason for performing immunohematologic tests, or blood banking, is to prevent problems caused by incompatibility of blood types. Crossmatching, or compatibility testing, is performed to prevent transfusion reactions in patients who are receiving blood transfusions. The second reason is to identify potential Rh incompatibility problems in expectant mothers. Rh incompatibility between expectant mothers and firstborn children may result in **hemolytic** disease of the newborn in second and succeeding pregnancies.

Although there are more than 300 different blood antigens, the two blood group systems of major clinical importance are the ABO system and the Rh system (Table 22–1).

Blood Group Systems

ABO System

Experiments performed by Karl Landsteiner in 1900 led to the discovery of the ABO blood group system and to the development of routine blood grouping procedures. Landsteiner discovered that human bloods could be classified into three groups, now named A, B, and O. The AB group was discovered a few years later. The letters A, B, O, and AB identify the type of antigen that each red blood cell (RBC), or erythrocyte, has on its surface. Type A has A antigen, type B has B antigen, type AB has an equal number of A and B antigens, and type O has neither A nor B antigens (Table 22–2).

Table 22–1
Major Blood Group Systems

System	***Significant Antigen(s)****
ABO	A, B
H	H
Lewis	Le^a, Le^b
I	I, i
P	P
Rh	D, C, c, E, e >50 antigens
MNS	M, N, S, s >37 antigens
Kell	K, k
Duffy	Fy^a, Fy^b
Kidd	Jk^a, Jk^b
Lutheran	Lu^a, Lu^b

*Collectively, there are more than 200 antigens.

Approximately 45% of the population of the United States has type O blood, 41% has type A blood, 10% has type B blood, and 4% has type AB blood. Blood group antigens are inherited (Table 22–3).

Blood Antibodies

In addition to discovering blood group antigens, Landsteiner also discovered that there were corresponding antibodies directed against the antigen absent from the person's RBCs. Blood group antibodies found in the serum or plasma are natural antibodies. The blood group antibodies are immunoglobulins of the IgM class.

In the ABO blood group system, the natural antibodies are of two types, classified as anti-A and anti-B. These antibodies are found in the plasma of persons who do not have the antigen present on their RBCs. For example, a person with blood group A antigens on the surface of his/her RBCs would have anti-B antibodies in his/her plasma. A person with blood group B antigens on the surface of his/her RBCs would have anti-A antibodies in his/her plasma. A patient with blood group A and B antigens on the surface of his/her RBCs would have neither anti-A nor anti-B antibodies in his/her plasma. A patient with type O blood lacks the blood group antigens A and B on the surface of his/her RBCs; therefore, both anti-A and anti-B antibodies are found in the plasma of persons with type O blood.

Rh System

The Rh system is the second major blood group system of concern in the clinical medical laboratory. However, unlike the ABO system, aspects of the genetics, nomenclature, and antigenic reactions of the Rh system remain unresolved, adding to its complexity.

The descriptive terms Rh-positive (Rh+) and Rh-negative (RH–) refer to the presence or absence of the RBC antigen D. There has been some confusion in the terminology of the Rh system owing to the different **nomenclatures** that have been applied to the Rh system. The Wiener nomenclature refers to the antigen as Rh (subset o) and the antibody as anti-Rh (subset o). This terminology has essentially been replaced by the Fisher-Race nomenclature, which refers to the Rh antigen as D and the antibody as anti-D (Table 22–4).

In 1940, Landsteiner and Wiener, after immunizing guinea pigs and rabbits with the RBCs of Rhesus monkeys, identified an antibody that agglutinated the RBCs in approximately 85% of the humans tested. They named this antigen the Rh factor. In modern usage, this is now called the D antigen. The Rh system was later expanded to include the C, c, E, and e antigens. However, the D antigen is the most clinically significant. Like the ABO system, the D antigen is **genetically** determined. However, unlike the ABO system, the Rh system has no naturally occurring antibodies. Anti-Rh

Table 22–2
Blood Compatibility

Recipient Blood*		***Compatible With***
RBC Antigen	***Plasma antibodies***	***Donor Types***†
Type O (no antigens)	Anti-A and anti-B	O
Type A (type A antigen)	Anti-B	O and A
Type B (type B antigen)	Anti-A	O and B
Type AB (type AB antigen)	None	O, A, B, and AB

*Patients with type AB blood are considered to be *universal recipients.*
†Patients with type O blood are considered to be *universal donors.*

Table 22–3
Frequency of Inherited ABO Blood Types

Ethnic Group	*O*	*A*	*B*	*AB*
Whites (%)	45	40	11	4
Blacks (%)	49	27	16	28
Native American Indians (%)	79	16	4	1
Asians (%)	40	28	27	5

antibodies, such as anti-D are formed only when Rh– patients are transfused with blood from an Rh+ donor, or when the blood of an Rh+ fetus passes through the placenta and enters the circulatory system of an Rh– mother.

Table 22–4
Rh Nomenclature for the Most Common Rh Antigens

*Rh-Hr**	*CDE*†	*Numerical*‡
Rh_0	D	Rh1
rh′	C	Rh2
rh″	E	Rh3
hr′	c	Rh4
hr″	e	Rh5

*Weiner
†Fisher and Race
‡Rosenfield

Hemolytic Disease of the Newborn

Hemolytic disease of the newborn (HDN), or *erythroblastosis fetalis,* causes severe **jaundice** in neonates and may result in mental retardation, stunted growth, or even death. The cause of HDN was unknown until the discovery of the Rh blood group system (Fig. 22–1).

HDN is a type of hemolytic anemia that occurs in neonates as a result of a fetal-maternal blood group incompatibility. The major cause of HDN is a blood group incompatibility involving the Rh system. However, ABO blood group system incompatibility can cause similar problems. HDN is caused by an antigen-antibody reaction in the blood of the newborn infant, resulting from the placental transmission of maternally formed antibodies against the incompatible antigens of the fetal blood. In Rh incompatibility, the hemolytic reaction occurs only when the mother is Rh– and the newborn is Rh+. This **isoimmunization** process rarely

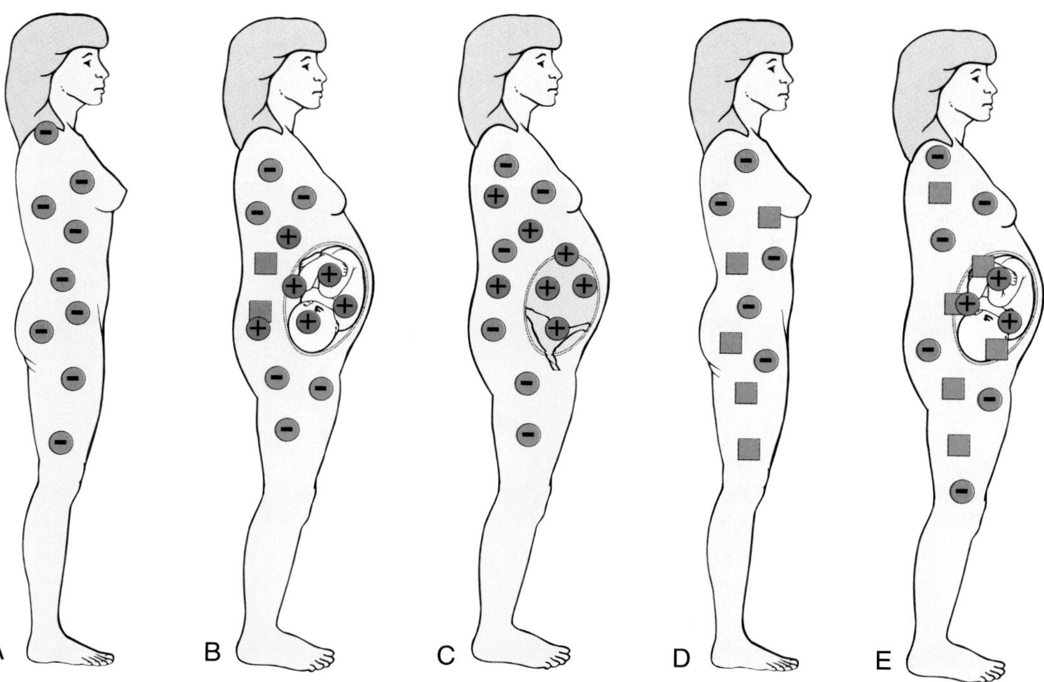

Figure 22–1. *Hemolytic disease of the newborn.* A, *Rh– female before pregnancy.* B, *Pregnancy with Rh+ fetus.* C, *Upon separation of placenta, a massive inoculation of mother occurs by Rh+ red blood cells.* D, *Mother becomes sensitized to Rh– blood and develops anti-Rh+ antibodies.* E, *Mother possesses positive Coombs test or has titer.*

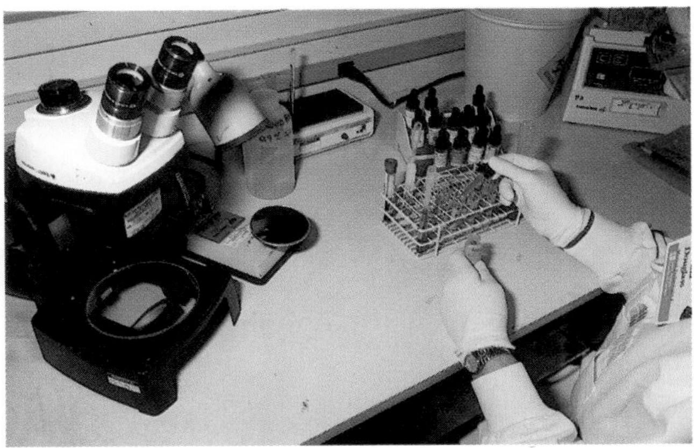

Figure 22–2. *In blood crossmatching, a patient's serum is checked against donor cells for compatibility.*

occurs with a first pregnancy, but there is an increased risk with each succeeding pregnancy. Maternal sensitization to the Rh factor can be prevented by the injection of a high-titer anti-Rh gammaglobulin preparation after the delivery or abortion of an Rh+ fetus. No sensitization occurs unless there is a transfer of fetal blood through the placental barrier and into the maternal circulatory system. Typical clinical symptoms of HDN include jaundice, severe anemia, and enlargement of both the liver and the spleen. The complications of HDN are serious and may even result in death. Prenatal blood group typing identifies mothers at risk of having infants with HDN. With proper prenatal testing and treatment, the complications of HDN can be avoided.

Weak Expression of D Antigen

Some individuals have a type of D antigen is expressed weakly. Because of this weak expression, additional testing must be performed to confirm whether a patient is Rh– or simply has a weakly expressed D antigen and is, instead, Rh+. This weak expression of the D antigen has been referred to as D (superset u). Current nomenclature classifies this as weak D blood, which is often designated as D+w.

Blood Grouping and Typing

Blood grouping and typing is routinely performed in hospital laboratories or in the physician's office laboratory (POL) prior to hospital admission, when patients may be receiving blood transfusions. Extreme caution should be taken when collecting and processing the specimens to ensure that the patient will receive compatible blood. Special caution is exercised in identifying transfusion patients and specimens to be used for blood grouping, typing, and compatibility testing. **Prenatal** grouping and typing is sometimes performed in the physician's office or in nonhospital laboratories.

Compatibility Testing/Crossmatching

Compatibility testing, or crossmatching, involves determination of the blood type of both the donor and recipient. Once the patient's blood group and type have been determined, donor blood units of the same group and type can then be selected from the blood bank for compatibility testing. Compatibility testing requires that the recipient's serum be reacted with the donor's RBCs. The presence of hemolysis and/or agglutination indicates incompatibility, in which case the donor blood is not suitable for transfusion into the patient (recipient). However, the absence of hemolysis and agglutination indicates that the donor blood is compatible and would be suitable for transfusion (Fig. 22–2).

When a patient receives incompatible blood, serious problems can develop as a result of a transfusion reaction. In a transfusion reaction, patients experience chills, fever, headache, hives, and burning sensations. Symptoms can become quite severe and can lead to renal failure and shock.

Because of the concern over the transmission of disease through blood transfusion, particularly human immunodeficiency virus (HIV) and hepatitis, there has been an increase in alternative sources of transfusion blood. Blood for transfusion comes from donors within a community. All donated blood is grouped, typed, and screened for HIV and hepatitis, in addition to a number of other diseases. There is also a detailed screening of donors before they are accepted as blood donors. The blood supply in the United States is extremely safe, and cases of disease transmission occurring as a result of blood transfusions are rare (Fig. 22–3).

Figure 22–3. *Unit of blood.*

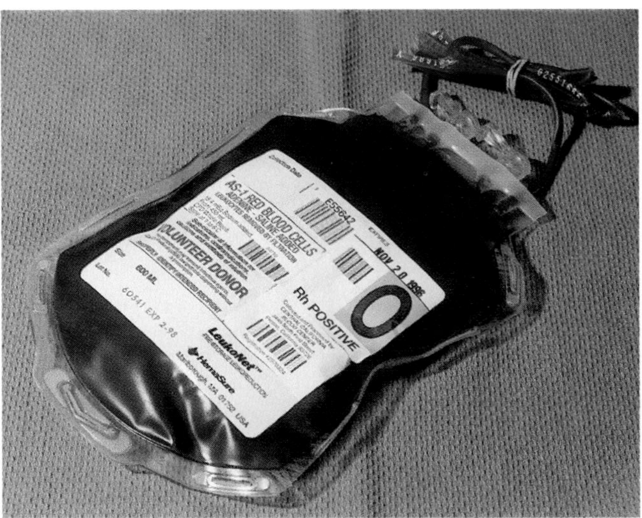

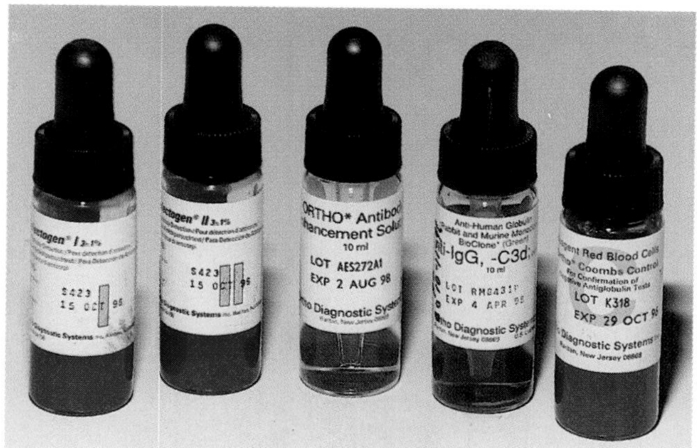

Figure 22–4. *Antibody screening cells.*

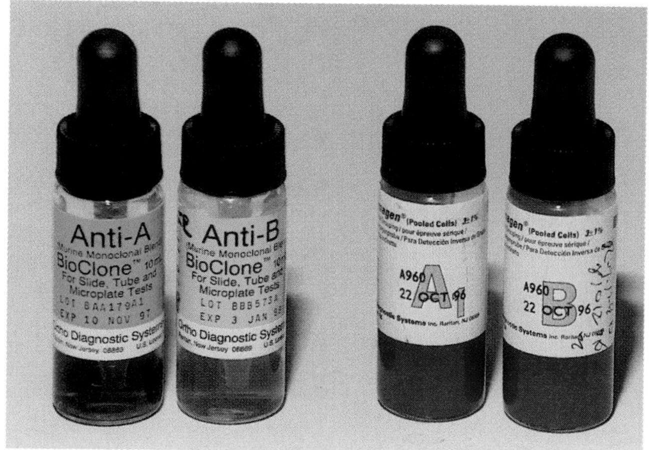

Figure 22–5. *ABO antiserum and cells.*

There has been an increase in **autologous** transfusions in recent years. An autologous transfusion is one in which the patient donates his or her own blood for transfusion at a later date. Similarly, family members and friends of patients may donate specifically for a particular patient, if they have blood of the same group and type as the patient.

In addition to blood grouping, typing, and compatibility testing, crossmatching involves an antibody screen (Fig. 22–4). The antibody screen serves to detect antibodies present in the patient's blood that are a result of previous sensitization to an antigen, usually from a previous blood transfusion. The antibody screen is performed on the recipient's serum to determine whether there are any clinically significant antibodies other than the ABO system antibodies. It is common for patients with a history of multiple blood transfusions to develop acquired blood group antibodies. Once it is determined that the patient has a blood group antibody, further testing can identify the antibody. Once the antibody is identified, donor blood can be screened to eliminate blood with the antibody in question and to locate suitable blood that will be compatible with the patient's blood.

Immunohematology, or blood bank testing, is very complex and serious work and should only be attempted by qualified and highly skilled laboratory personnel. When working in the POL, knowledge of how blood is typed and crossmatched will enable you to answer questions frequently asked by patients. In addition, when drawing blood that will be sent to a hospital laboratory for testing, such knowledge will ensure accuracy and precision (Table 22–5).

Testing Procedures

Determination of ABO Group

Determination of ABO blood groups is a simple test that can easily be performed. The test detects the presence of A or B antigens on RBCs based on the presence or absence of agglutination with a known antiserum (Fig. 22–5). When the antigen on the patient's

Table 22–5
Minimum Draw Volumes for Blood Banking*

Assay	*Minimum Whole Blood Volume (mL)*	*No. of Full Pink-Top Microtainers*[†]
Antibody identification	5–6	Amount too great for Microtainer use
Crossmatch	2.5	3–4
Direct Coombs test	0.5	3–4
Elution	3–4	4–5
Type and screen	1.5	2

*The blood bank should be consulted to verify the necessity of the draw and the amount of blood required.
[†]A full Microtainer tube holds 0.75 mL. Microtainer tubes are color-coded, denoting specific additives.

REACTION GRADING

The degree of red cell agglutination observed in any blood bank test procedure is significant and should be recorded. A system of grading is illustrated.

Description	Reaction*	Grade	
Button of cells remains in one clump after being dislodged from wall of test tube. Background is clear.		++++	4+^s
Button breaks into two or three clumps after being dislodged. Background is clear.		++++	4+
Button breaks into four to six large clumps. Background is clear.		+++±	3+^s
Button breaks into many large clumps. Background is clear.	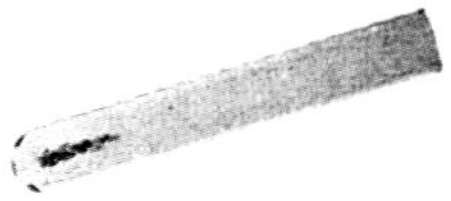	+++	3+
Button breaks into many medium-sized clumps. Background may become slightly cloudly.		++±	2+^s
Button breaks into many small clumps. Background becomes more cloudy.	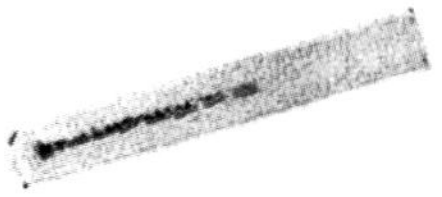	++	2+
Button breaks into numerous tiny clumps. Background becomes very cloudy.	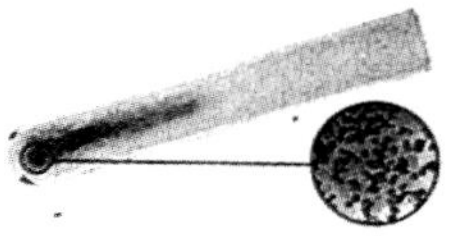	+	1+
Very fine agglutinates in a sea of free cells.	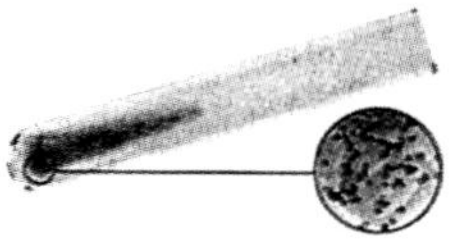	±	±
No visible agglutinates.	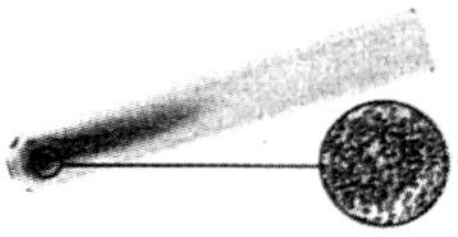	0	Neg.

Bibliography:
Technical Methods and Procedures
of the American Association of Blood Banks
Sixth Edition 1974

*Utilizing 5% cell suspension.

ORTHO DIAGNOSTICS INC.
Raritan, New Jersey 08869

Figure 22–6. *Agglutination reactions. (Courtesy of Ortho Diagnostics, Inc., Raritan, NJ.)*

RBCs corresponds to the antibody, agglutination occurs. If the corresponding antigen is not present on the RBCs, no agglutination will occur. For example, Type A blood will agglutinate in the presence of anti-A antiserum, but not in the presence of anti-B antiserum. Type B blood will agglutinate in the presence of anti-B antiserum, but not in the presence of anti-A antiserum. Type O blood will not agglutinate in the presence of anti-A antiserum or anti-B serum, whereas Type AB blood will agglutinate in the presence of both anti-A antiserum and anti-B antiserum. The test can be performed by using either a slide test or a tube test (Fig. 22–6).

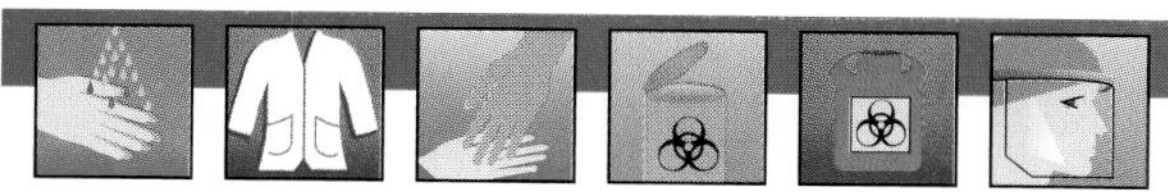

PROCEDURE 22–1

Determining ABO Group Using a Slide Test

Principle

To ensure that the patient will receive compatible blood by determining ABO group using a slide test. **CAUTION: Special caution is exercised in identifying transfusion patients and specimens to be used for blood grouping, typing, and compatibility.**

Equipment and Supplies

glass slides with frosted ends
anti-A and anti-B serum
applicator sticks
loaded Autolet
alcohol prep pads
sterile gauze flats (1 × 1 inch)
laboratory marker or pencil

Procedural Steps

1. Wash hands thoroughly and dry them, observing universal precautions. Don gloves.
2. Assemble and prepare the necessary equipment and supplies.
3. Place 1 drop of anti-A serum on a clean, labeled, glass slide.
4. Place 1 drop of anti-B serum on a second, clean, labeled, glass slide.
5. Place 1 drop of anti-A, anti-B serum on a third, clean, labeled, glass slide, if parallel tests are to be performed with this reagent.
6. Explain the procedure to the patient.
7. Select the puncture site (see Chapter 11).
8. Very gently rub the patients' selected finger along the sides.
9. Clean the site with an alcohol prep pad and dry it with sterile gauze.
10. Firmly grasp the patient's finger on the sides, near the site to be punctured.
11. Hold the Autolet at a right angle to the site and puncture the finger.
12. Wipe away the first drop of blood with sterile gauze.
13. Apply gentle pressure to cause the blood to flow freely.
14. Place 1 large drop of blood on each of the three prepared slides.
15. Cover the puncture site with sterile gauze and instruct the patient to apply pressure to the site.
16. Mix the antiserum and RBCs thoroughly, using a clean applicator stick for each slide. The mixture should be spread over an area measuring approximately 20 mm × 40 mm.
17. Gently tilt the slide continuously for up to 2 minutes. **CAUTION: Do not place the slide over heated surfaces, such as an Rh viewbox, during this time.**
18. Read, interpret, and record the results of the reaction for all slides.

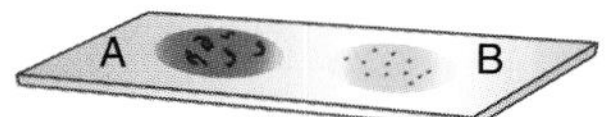

TYPE A
A = Agglutination
B = No agglutination

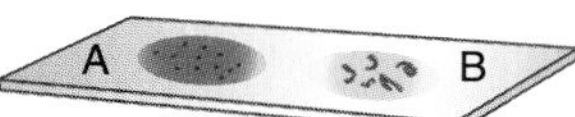

TYPE B
A = No agglutination
B = Agglutination

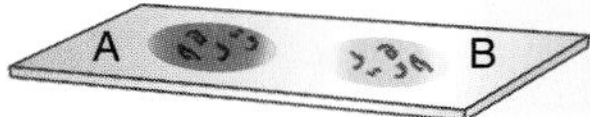

TYPE AB
A = Agglutination
B = Agglutination

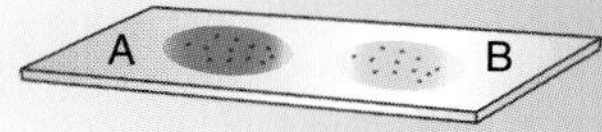

TYPE O
A = No agglutination
B = No agglutination

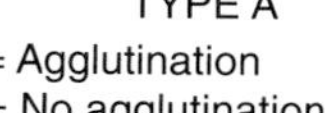

ABO group slide test reactions

(continued)

PROCEDURE 22–1

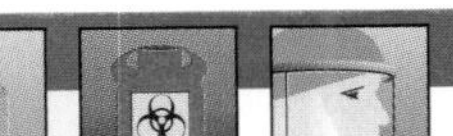

Determining ABO Group Using a Slide Test (Continued)

19. Discard all disposable equipment according to biohazardous waste disposal guidelines.
20. Clean the work surface and store all reusable equipment and reagents.
21. Remove all protective equipment and gloves.
22. Wash and disinfect hands.

Interpretation of Results

Positive Result: Strong agglutination of RBCs in the presence of any ABO grouping antiserum constitutes a positive result.

Negative Result: A smooth suspension of RBCs at the end of 2 minutes indicates a negative test result.

Indeterminate Result: Samples yielding weak or doubtful reactions should be retested using the tube test method.

PROCEDURE 22–2

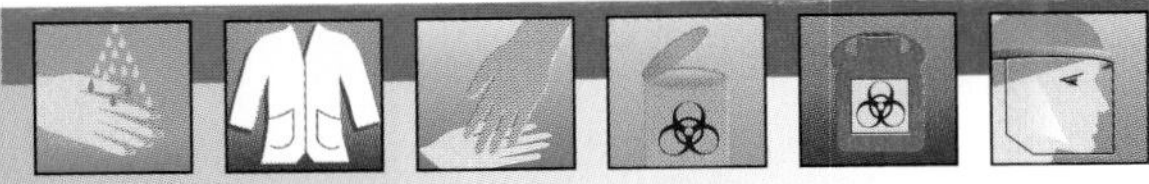

Determining ABO Grouping Using a Tube Test

Principle

To identify a patient's blood group using accurate specimen collection and processing methods

Equipment and Supplies

anti-A and anti-B antiserum
4 75-mm test tubes
label marker
disposable pipettes
centrifuge
tube rack
blood specimen for testing
physiological saline

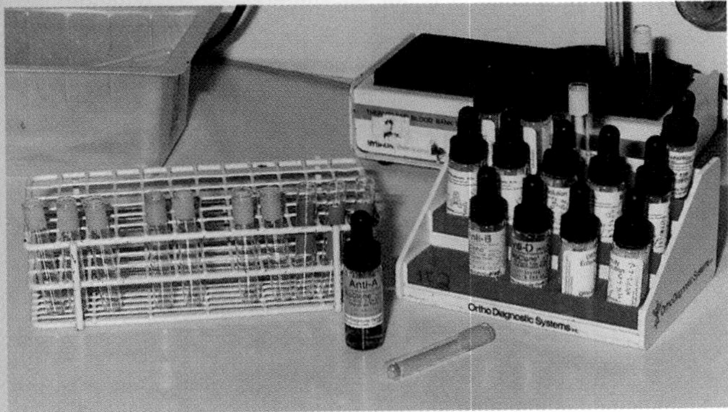

ABO test tube system

Procedural Steps

1. Wash hands thoroughly and dry them, observing universal precautions.
2. Assemble and prepare the necessary equipment and supplies.
3. Explain the procedure to the patient.
4. Put on gloves.
5. Perform venipuncture to obtain 75 mm of blood for testing.
6. Place 1 drop of well-mixed blood into a test tube and add 19 drops of saline. Mix by inversion. Label this tube "2%–5% cells."
7. Properly label two test tubes **A** and **B**.
8. Place 1 drop of anti-A antiserum in the test tube labeled **A**.
9. Place 1 drop of anti-B antiserum in the test tube labeled **B**.
10. Add to each tube 1 drop of a 2%–5% suspension of RBCs to be tested.
11. Mix the contents of each tube gently and centrifuge for 15 to 30 seconds at approximately 900–1000 rpm.
12. Resuspend the RBCs by gently tapping the

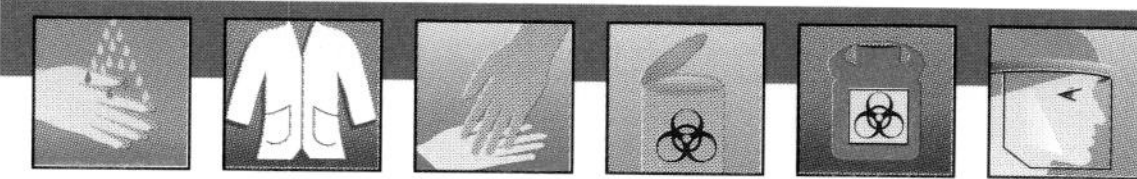

PROCEDURE 22–2

Determining ABO Grouping Using a Tube Test (Continued)

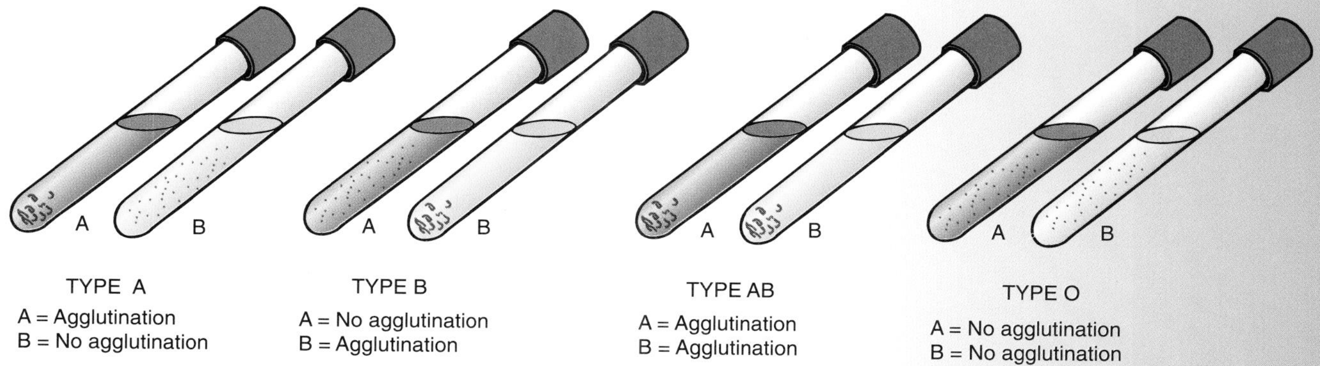

ABO group tube test reactions

side of the tube. Examine the cells for agglutination.

13. Read, interpret, and record the test results. Results can be confirmed by using ABO serum testing. ABO serum testing or indirect typing involves testing the patient's serum against RBCS with known antigens present.
14. Discard all disposable equipment according to biohazardous waste disposal guidelines.
15. Clean the work surfaces and store all reusable equipment after disinfecting them in a 10% bleach solution.
16. Remove all protective equipment and gloves.
17. Wash and disinfect hands.

Interpretation of Results

Positive Result: Agglutination and/or hemolysis in any tube indicates a positive test result.

Negative Result: The absence of agglutination and/or hemolysis and the presence of a smooth suspension of RBCs indicates a negative test result.

Indeterminate Result: Any discrepancies in reaction should be resolved by further testing.

Figure 22–7. *Determination of Rh type using anti-D antiserum and Rh control.*

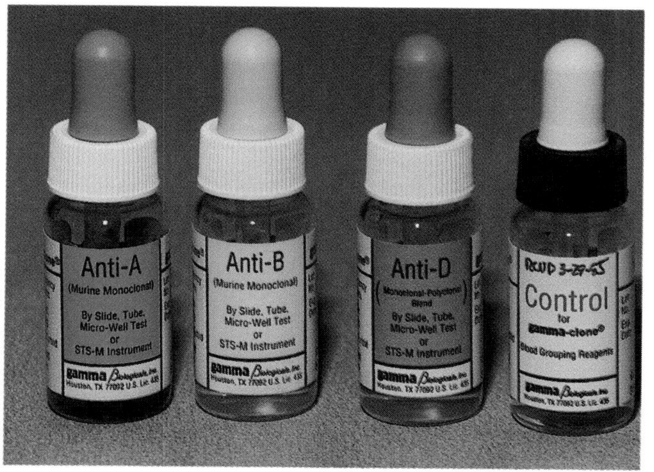

Determination of Rh Type

The determination of Rh type is a simple test that can be performed with a minimum amount of equipment. The test detects the presence of D antigens on the surface of RBCs based on the presence or absence of agglutination with anti-D antiserum. When the D antigen is present, agglutination occurs when the anti-D antiserum is reacted with the RBCs. If the D antigen is not present, no agglutination will occur. Rh+ (D+) blood will agglutinate in the presence of anti-D antiserum, but not in the presence of the Rh control (Fig. 22–7). Rh– (D–) blood will *not* agglutinate in the presence of anti-D antiserum, nor will it agglutinate in the presence of the Rh control. The determination of Rh type can be accomplished by either a slide test or a tube test.

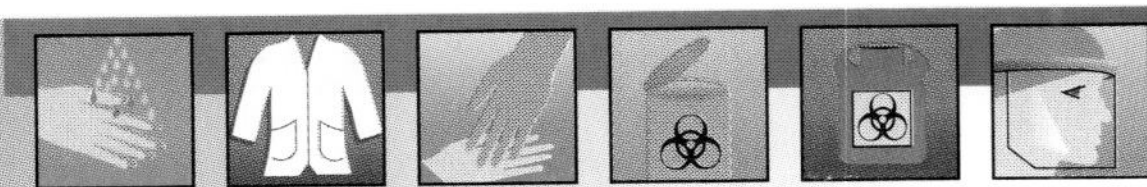

PROCEDURE 22–3

Determining Rh Group Using a Slide Test

Principle

To detect the presence of D antigens on the surface of RBCs based on the presence or absence of agglutination with anti-D antiserum

Equipment

glass slides with frosted ends
anti-D serum
applicator sticks
loaded Autolet
alcohol prep pads
sterile gauze flats (1 × 1 inch)
laboratory marker or wax pencil
lighted viewbox

Procedural Steps

1. Wash and disinfect hands. Put on gloves and other protective equipment.
2. Follow universal precautions.
3. Assemble and prepare the necessary equipment.
4. Label one slide **D** and the other **C**.
5. Place 1 drop of anti-D serum on the glass slide labeled **D**.
6. Place 1 drop of the appropriate control reagent on the slide labeled **C**.
7. Perform a capillary puncture to secure a blood specimen.
8. To each slide, add 2 drops of the patient's whole blood.
9. Thoroughly mix the RBC suspension with the anti-D serum, using a clean applicator stick for each slide, and spread the reaction mixture over an area measuring approximately 20 mm × 40 mm on each slide.
10. Simultaneously place the slides on the viewbox and tilt them gently and continuously to observe for agglutination. **NOTE: Most manufacturers require that the test be read within 2 minutes because drying of the reaction mixture may cause the formation of rouleaux, which may be mistaken for agglutination.** **CAUTION: Drying around the edges of the reaction mixture must not be confused with agglutination.**

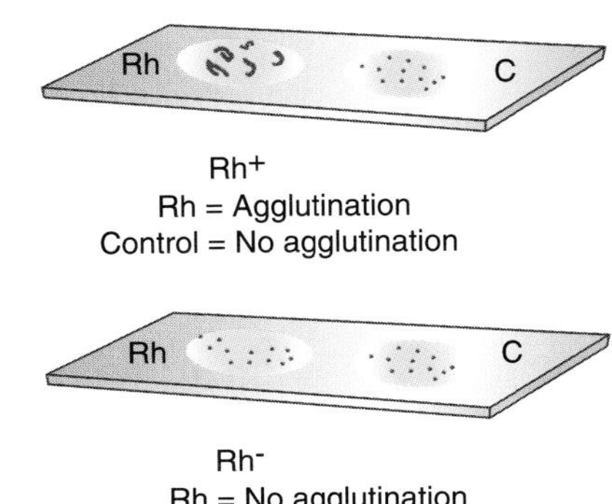

11. Interpret and record the results of the reactions on both slides.
12. Discard all disposable equipment according to biohazardous waste disposal guidelines.
13. Clean and store all reusable equipment and reagents.
14. Clean all work surfaces.
15. Remove all protective equipment and gloves.
16. Wash and disinfect hands.

Interpretation of Results

Positive Result: Agglutination with the anti-D serum in a smooth suspension on the control slide constitutes a positive result and indicates that the RBCs being tested are Rh+ (D+).

Negative Result: No agglutination with anti-D serum and Rh control suggests that the RBCs are Rh– (D–). Further testing is required to determine whether the RBCs that type as Rh– (D–) carry a weak D antigen.

Indeterminate Result: If there is agglutination on the control slide, the anti-D serum test must not be interpreted as yielding a positive result without further testing.

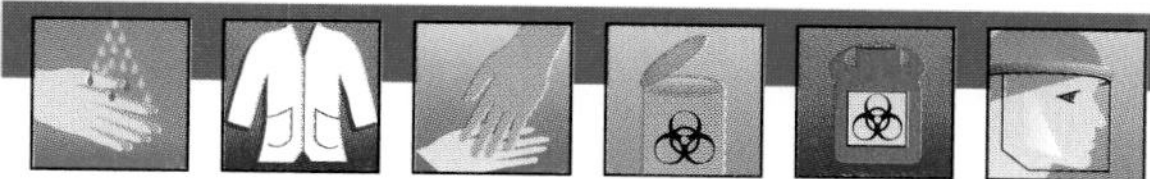

PROCEDURE 22–4

Determining Rh Using a Tube Test

Principle

To identify a patient's Rh through the detection of D antigens on the blood surface

Equipment and Supplies

two 75-mm test tubes
laboratory marker
disposable pipettes
tube rack
blood specimen for testing
anti-D serum
centrifuge

Procedural Steps

1. Wash and disinfect hands and don gloves and protective gear.
2. Follow universal precautions.
3. Assemble and prepare the necessary equipment.
4. Verify the identification of the patient by checking the specimen label. Properly label the containers **D** and **C**.
5. Place 1 drop of anti-D serum in the test tube labeled **D**.
6. Place 1 drop of the appropriate control reagent in the test tube labeled **C**.
7. To each test tube, add 1 drop of a 2%–5% suspension of the RBCs to be tested. NOTE: Blood prepared for ABO testing can be used if both tests are being done consecutively. If not, a blood specimen must be obtained and prepared as it was in Procedure 22–2.
8. Mix gently and centrifuge for 15 to 30 seconds at 900–1000 rpm.
9. Gently resuspend the RBCs by tapping the sides of the test tube. Examine the cells for agglutination. **NOTE:** Adding 1 drop of saline to each test tube before suspending the RBCs button will provide additional fluid to facilitate resuspension.
10. Grade the reactions and record the test and control results.

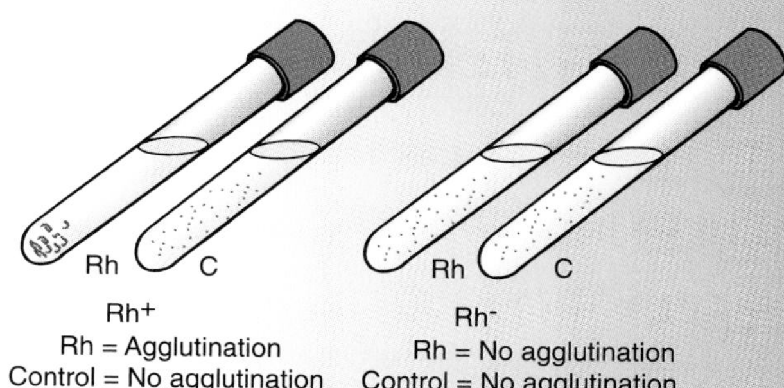

11. Discard all disposable equipment according to biohazardous waste disposal guidelines.
12. Clean all work surfaces and equipment with a 10% bleach solution. Return all reusable equipment and reagents to the proper storage area.
13. Remove all protective equipment and gloves.
14. Wash and disinfect hands.

Interpretation of Results

Positive Result: Agglutination equal to or greater than 2+ in the anti-D tube and a nonreactive control constitute a valid test and indicate that the RBCs being tested are Rh+ (D+).

Negative Result: A smooth suspension of RBCs in both the anti-D and the Rh control tubes constitutes a negative test result.

CAUTION: Although blood from patients may be classified as D- at this point, donor blood must be further tested for weakened forms of the D antigen.

Indeterminate Result: If there is agglutination in the control tube, or if the agglutination in the anti-D tube is less than 2+, the Rh type must not be interpreted as positive without further testing.

Summary

Immunohematology is a specialized field that usually involves tests performed in the hospital laboratory. If you work in a POL, you may never have occasion to assist with these procedures. However, you will likely be present when patients are advised that these tests are necessary, so you may be in a position to answer patients' questions about these procedures. By fully understanding the methods used and the testing process, you will be able to help the patient gain an understanding of the procedures and to offer reassurance. It is important to remember that through knowledge comes acceptance and understanding.

Chapter Review

True or False

Circle T or F to indicate the correct answers to the following:

T F 1. The two major blood grouping systems are the ABC and the Rh.

T F 2. If you have type AB blood, you carry B antigens.

T F 3. HDN is a type of hemolytic anemia.

T F 4. HDN is caused by an antigen-antibody reaction in the blood of the neonate.

Fill in the Blanks

Complete the following statements:

5. When testing blood for compatibility, the presence of ______________ and ______________ indicates incompatibility.

6. Receiving incompatible blood could lead to ______________ ______________ and ______________ .

7. Two diseases that are of concern when a blood transfusion is necessary are ______________ and ______________ .

8. An ______________ transfusion is one in which the recipient receives their own donated blood.

Multiple Choice

Circle the letter that represents the single best answer:

9. Compatibility testing requires that the:
   a. Recipient's RBCs be reacted with the donors' serum
   b. Recipient's serum be reacted with the donor's serum
   c. Recipient's RBCs be reacted with the donor's RBCs
   d. Recipient's serum be reacted with the donor's RBCs
   e. Recipient's RBCs and serum be reacted with the donor's RBCs and serum

10. A person's ABO group and Rh can be determined using:
    a. Tube or slide testing
    b. Tube testing only
    c. Slide testing only
    d. Microscopic analysis
    e. All of the above

Unit VI
Microbiology

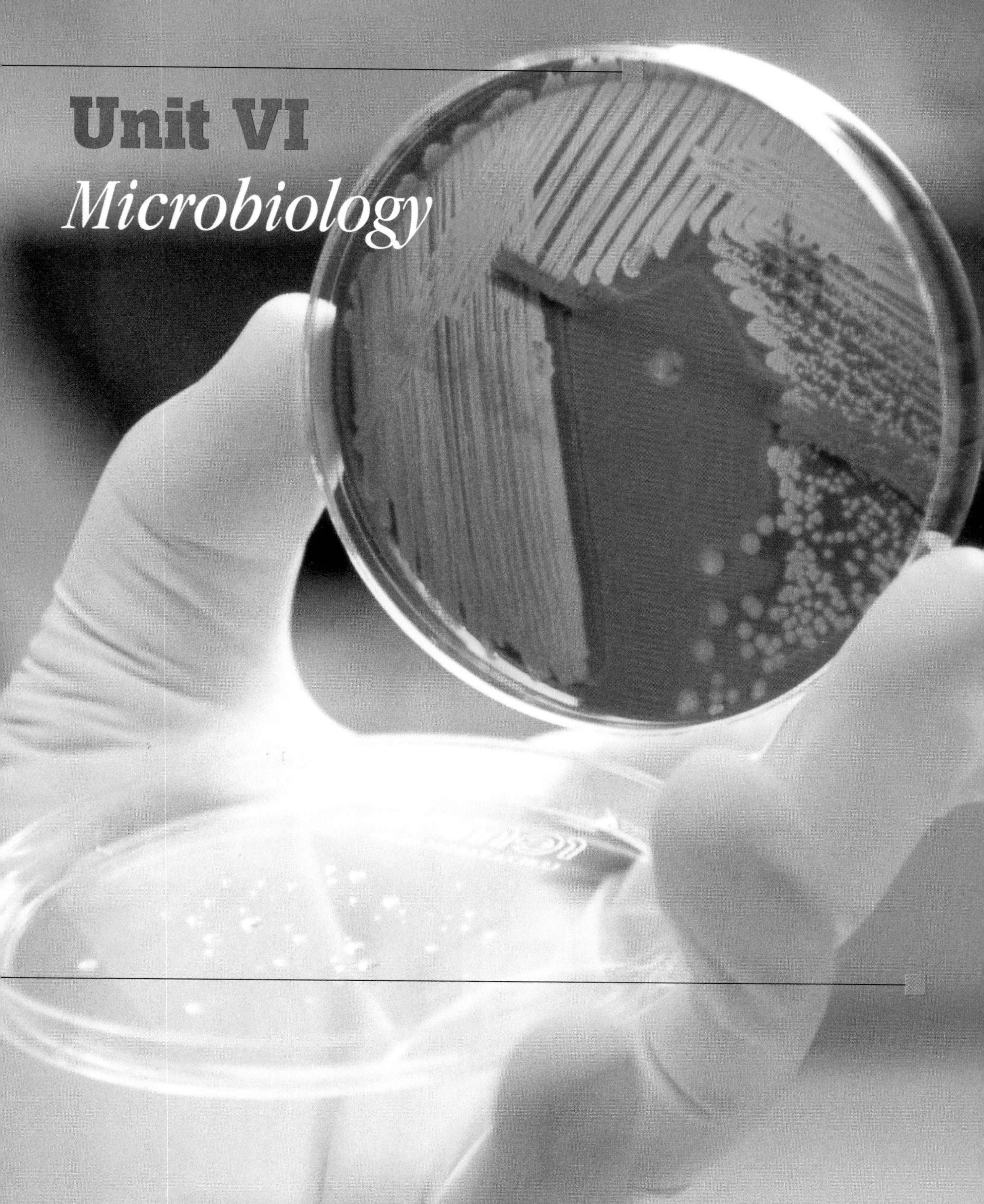

Vocabulary

autoclave: an instrument that uses steam, dry heat, or chemicals at high pressure to kill possible contagious or infectious agents

epidemic: rapid, widespread occurrence of disease among many people in a given region at the same time

morbidity: the ratio of sick to well people in a given community

mortality: the ratio of the total number of deaths occurring to the total or given population

nosocomial: pertaining to or beginning in a hospital; generally refers to the spread of infection among patients, staff, and visitors inside the hospital

Chapter Objectives

After reading this chapter, you should be able to:

1. Discuss the major role of the bacteriology department.
2. Explain elements that affect morbidity and mortality rates in the laboratory.
3. List the reasons why collection and transportation of specimens are critical to testing accuracy.
4. Describe the OSHA standards that are strictly followed when handling biohazardous materials.
5. Name the various methods for decontaminating infectious materials.

Chapter 23
Introduction to Microbiology

In the clinical laboratory, the microbiology or bacteriology department is an important area. Many tests ordered by the physician will be performed within this division of a large laboratory. The clinical microbiologist deals with the prevention, diagnosis, and management of infectious and/or contagious diseases. Without input from the bacteriology laboratory, many diseases could not be diagnosed and treated properly.

It is extremely important that specimens for bacteriology be collected carefully to avoid contamination so that the best possible results are obtained. The major role of the bacteriology department is to determine the agent(s) causing a disease and to provide information regarding the most effective treatment. In addition, responsibilities include preventing **nosocomial** infections, as well as assisting with infection control in the physician's office and in the community at large. Clinical microbiologists work closely with physicians, pharmacologists, and public health officers to identify infectious diseases and to prevent their spread. Early diagnosis and treatment of possible infectious diseases are significant in reducing the **morbidity** and **mortality** rates.

Specimen Collection and Transport

When we consider the consequences of a disease reaching **epidemic** proportions, the correct collection techniques and transport of specimens for bacteriology testing become critical. An improperly collected or transported specimen can severely limit the speed, dependability, and quality of the information that the bacteriology laboratory can provide to the physician. On the other hand, a correctly collected and transported specimen can speed to the physician accurate information that is necessary for the diagnosis and treatment of possible epidemiologic disease. We like to think that, because of our excellent health care system, we are protected against disease outbreaks, such as Ebola virus and typhoid; this is true only if we, as members of a health care team, do all we can to ensure disease prevention.

The prime concern is to avoid introducing contaminating microorganisms into a specimen. Contamination can result from exposure to microor-

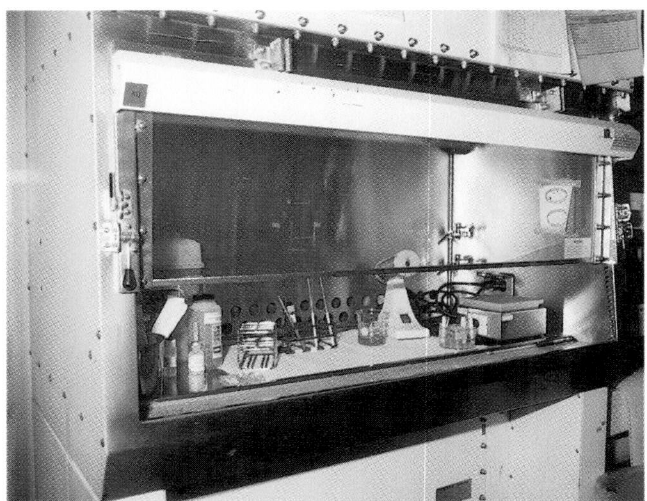

Figure 23–1. *Biohazard cabinet.*

ganisms originating from the patient, the person collecting the specimen, or the environment, or from introducing the unwanted organism into a specimen. When a specimen is contaminated by extraneous microorganisms, significant difficulty is encountered in interpreting the information provided by the specimen.

All persons responsible for the collection and transportation of specimens for bacteriologic testing should be familiar with each laboratory's procedures in this area. Most laboratories provide all laboratory personnel with manuals and/or hands-on training in the proper techniques. Additionally, most laboratories will provide the proper specimen collection apparatus and

Figure 23–2. *Standard laboratory apparel.*

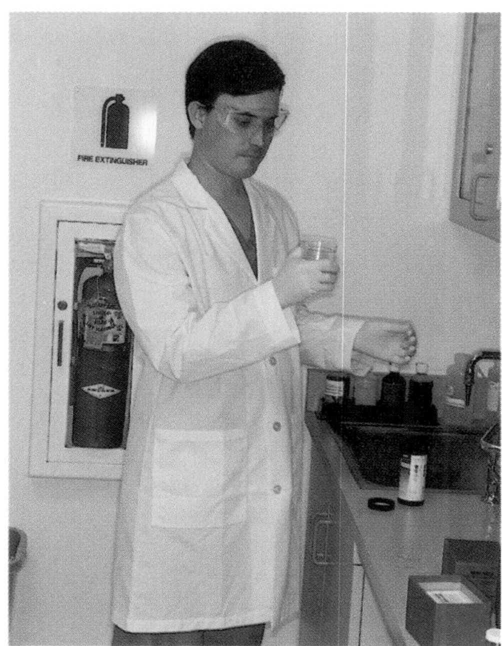

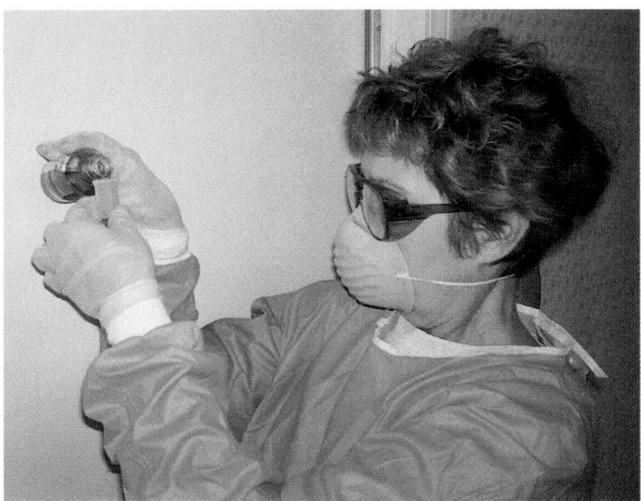

Figure 23–3. *Special safety apparel: gloves, barrier gown with knit cuffs, mask, safety goggles.*

instructions to a physician's office laboratory (POL) upon request without charge.

Specimens that are improperly collected or transported will be rejected by the clinical laboratory. (Refer to Appendix A for specimen rejection policy and procedure.) A specimen that has been improperly collected and/or transported may be the only specimen available for testing. In this situation, the clinical microbiologist will need to work closely with the staff involved in specimen collection and transport in order to avoid similar problems in the future and still provide helpful information to the physician or public health officer.

Safety Considerations

Infectious and contagious diseases can be transmitted easily from person to person by direct or indirect contact. For this reason, it is important that the OSHA stan-

Figure 23–4. *Decontaminating a work area.*

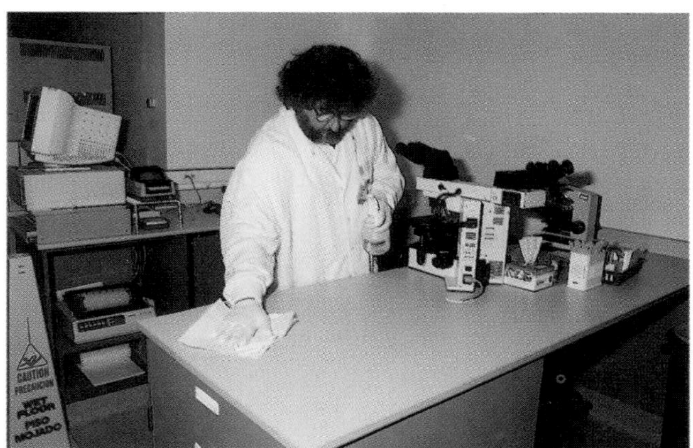

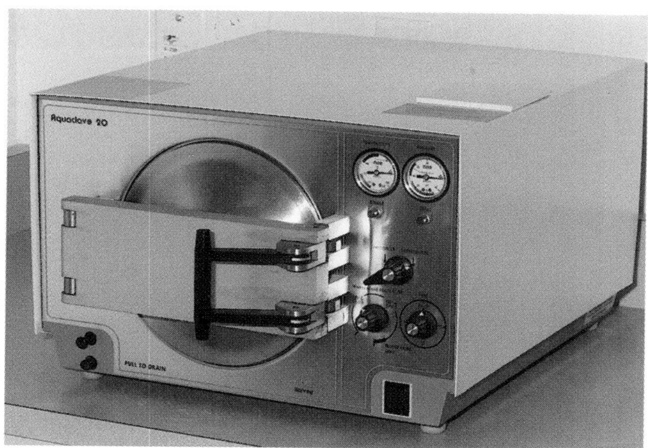

Figure 23–5. *Steam/gas autoclave.*

dards pertaining to biohazardous materials be strictly adhered to by health care personnel. Health care workers, both inside and outside the laboratory, can become exposed to agents capable of causing infectious disease on a daily basis. Agents, such as bacteria, fungi, parasites, and viruses, are capable of causing serious disease, so strict adherence to safety rules is required to prevent disease transmission.

Microbiology laboratories contain appropriate safety equipment. Biological safety cabinets and biohazard devices that encase a work area help to protect laboratory personnel from accidental exposure to infectious diseases (Fig. 23–1). Air that contains infectious materials can be decontaminated by passing it through a high-efficiency particulate air (HEPA) filter or by exposure to ultraviolet light or heat. In addition to gloves, laboratory coats and other protective clothing should be worn over conventional street apparel (Fig. 23–2). Moreover, certain activities in the laboratory may require additional protective clothing (Fig. 23–3). Strict decontamination procedures must always be followed.

All materials containing potentially infectious agents must be decontaminated and/or disposed of according to OSHA standards. Biohazard containers should be used.* Work benches and other surface areas are cleaned with liquid antiseptic agents (Fig. 23–4). A 10% solution of sodium hypochlorite (household bleach in water) is an effective agent against viral contamination. If a prepared antiseptic solution is used, a new mixture should be prepared every 7 days to maintain effectiveness. When using commercial antiseptics, always check the expiration date. Reusable materials must be sterilized in an **autoclave** (Fig. 23–5) according to the manufacturer's specifications.

*The Centers for Disease Control (CDC) provide etiologic agent labels with the biohazard symbols. The telephone number of the local Haz-Mat agency is listed in the phone book, or you may write to the CDC, Atlanta, Georgia.

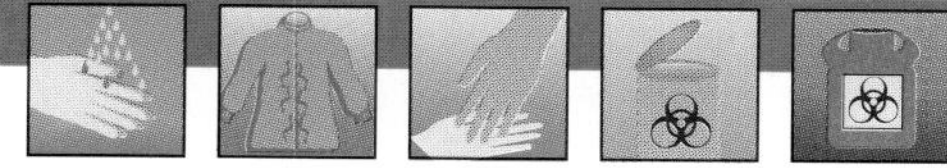

PROCEDURE 23–1

Decontaminating a Laboratory Area

Principle

To clean laboratory work stations, equipment, and other surface areas with liquid antiseptic agents

Equipment and Supplies

cleaning cloths
antiseptic cleaning solution or 10% bleach solution
microscope cleaner
basin or small pail to hold cleaning solution

Procedural Steps

1. Remove all jewelry and put in a safe, secure place.
2. Wash hands and dry them thoroughly.
3. Put on a barrier gown, gloves, and goggles.
4. Collect all the decontamination supplies you will need.
5. Using special microscope cleaner, thoroughly wipe off all microscopes, paying particular attention to the areas that come in contact with the user and with the sample. Dry any wet areas with a clean cloth.

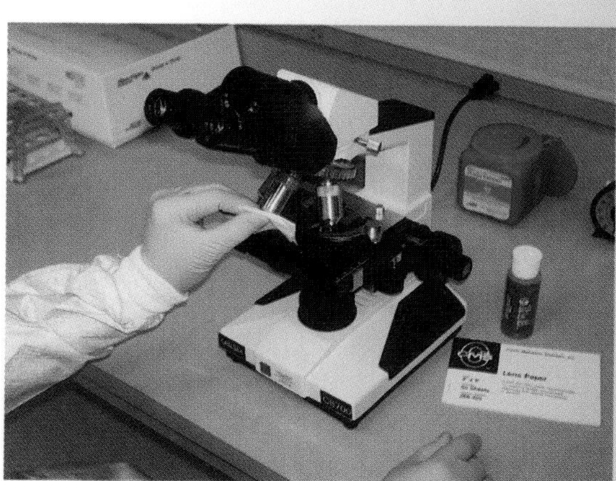

Clean specimen contact areas.

(continued)

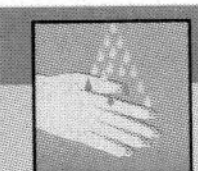 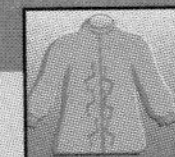 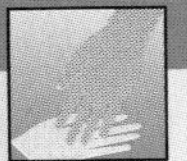 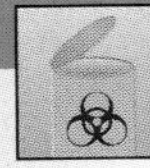 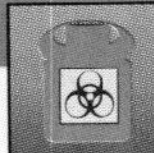

PROCEDURE 23–1

Decontaminating a Laboratory Area (Continued)

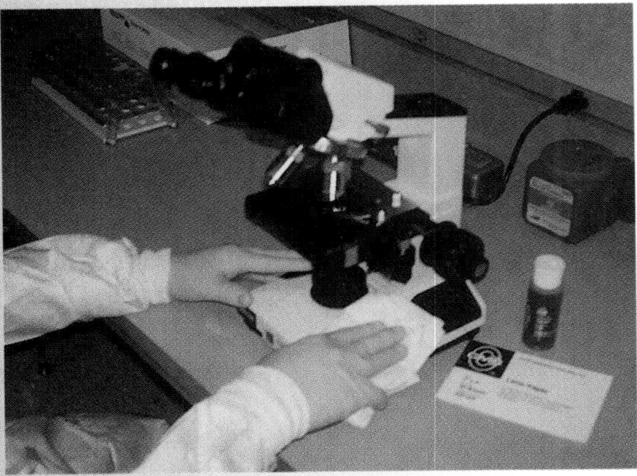

Use a soft clean towel to dry any wet areas.

6. Using a cleaning cloth soaked in 10% bleach solution or the designated commercial antiseptic, wipe the remaining equipment following the same technique as used on the microscopes.

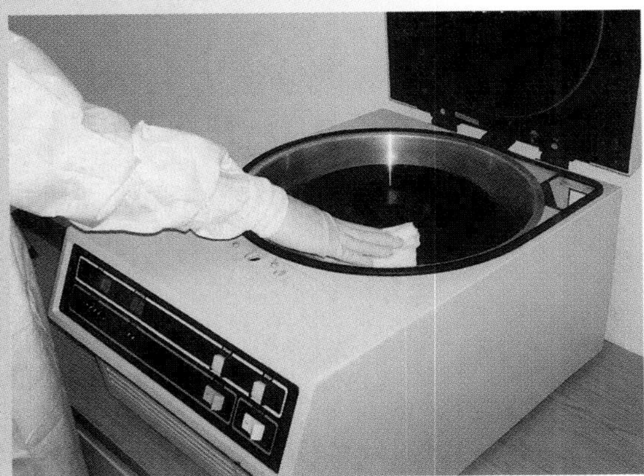

Clean the centrifuge.

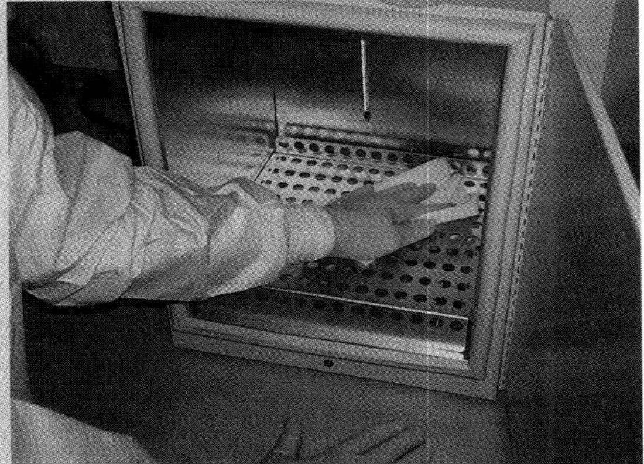

Clean the incubator.

7. Rinse the cleaning cloth in the cleaning solution and use it to wash off all countertops/work areas. Dry the areas with a clean cloth.

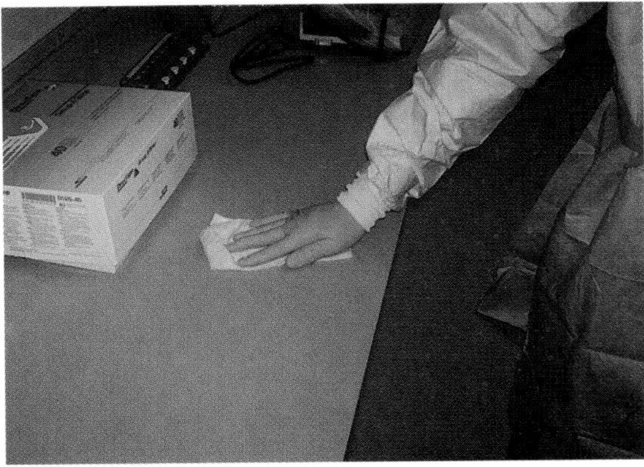

Clean counter tops.

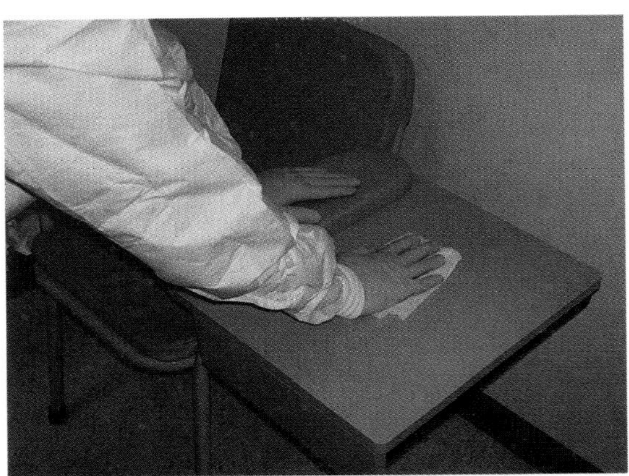

Clean work top areas.

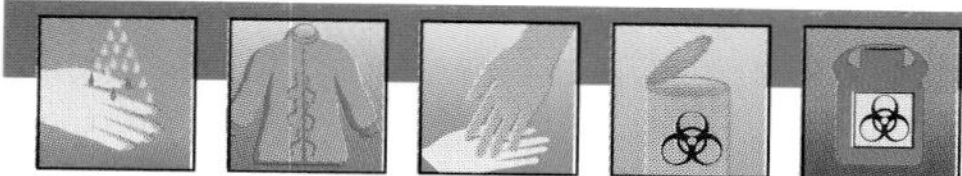

PROCEDURE 23–1

Decontaminating a Laboratory Area (Continued)

8. Rinse the cleaning cloth and wash all storage cabinet doors, paying extra attention to the knobs and edges used to open and close doors. Dry these areas with a clean cloth.

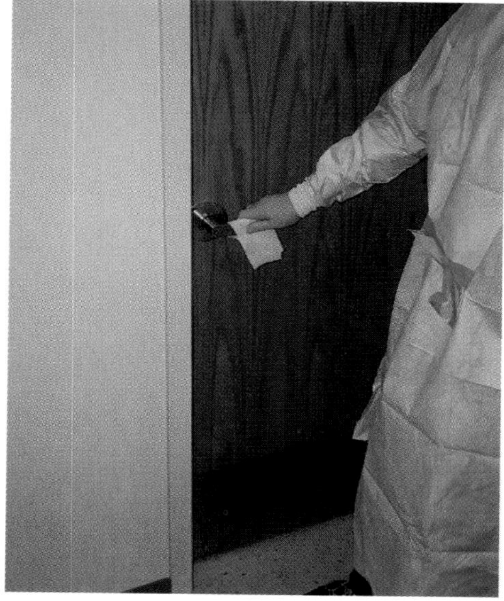

Clean door knobs.

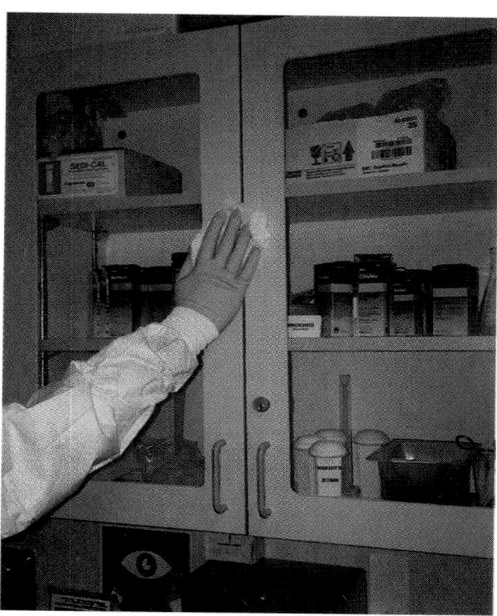

Clean cabinet doors.

9. Rinse the cleaning cloth again in the solution and complete the cleaning by washing any knob, door edge, or other surface that has been contaminated. Dry these surfaces with a clean cloth.

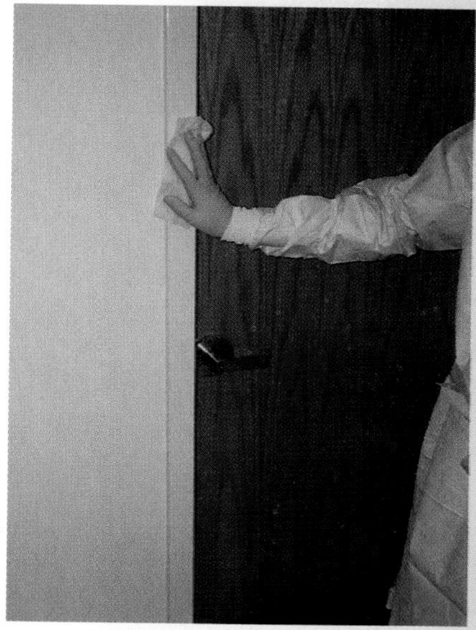

Clean door frames.

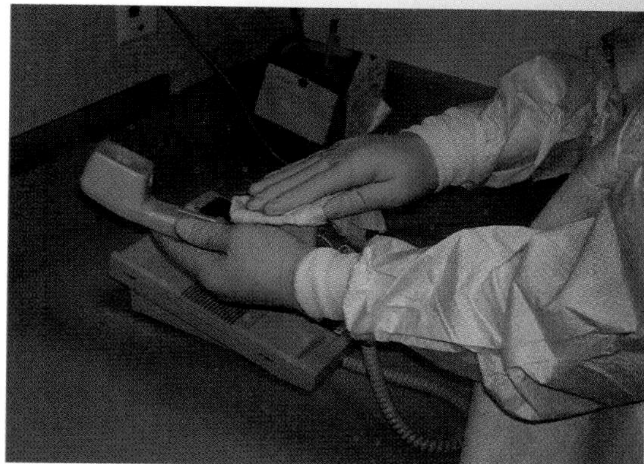

Clean the telephone.

NOTE: It is always better to wash an area that really did not need to be washed than to skip an area that was contaminated.

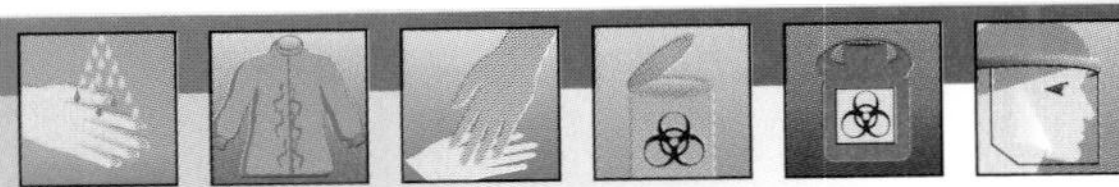

PROCEDURE 23–2

Decontaminating a Biohazardous Spill

Principle

To decontaminate and dispose of materials containing potentially infectious producing agents according to OSHA standards

Equipment and Supplies

1 clear Zip-Loc bag
1 oz emergency sanitation (ESP) liquid-congealing powder
1 pick-up disposable spatula
3–5 paper towels
1 germicidal cloth
1 biohazard bag with tie

Procedural Steps

1. Wash hands and dry them thoroughly.
2. Assemble necessary supplies.

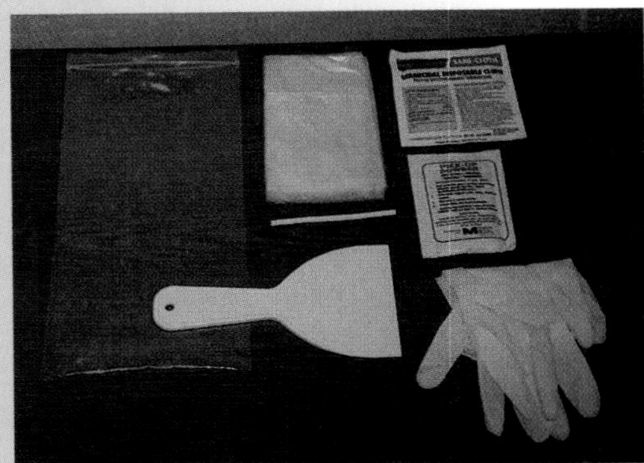

Collect supplies.

3. Put on all biohazard apparel
4. Sprinkle ESP congealing powder uniformly over the spill until thoroughly covered.

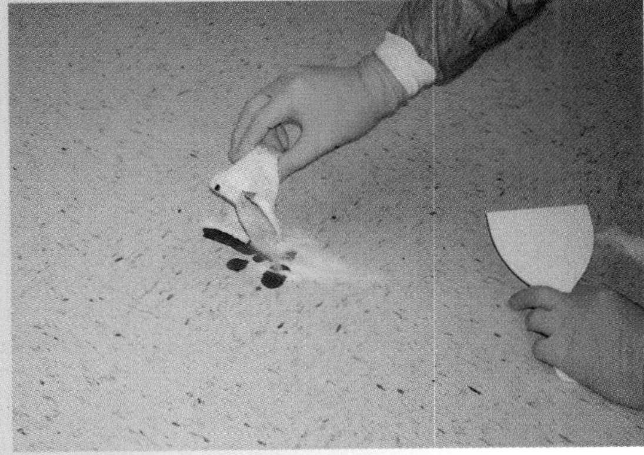

Sprinkle ESP congealing powder over the spill.

5. Using the spatula, stir the spilled material to speed the congealing process.

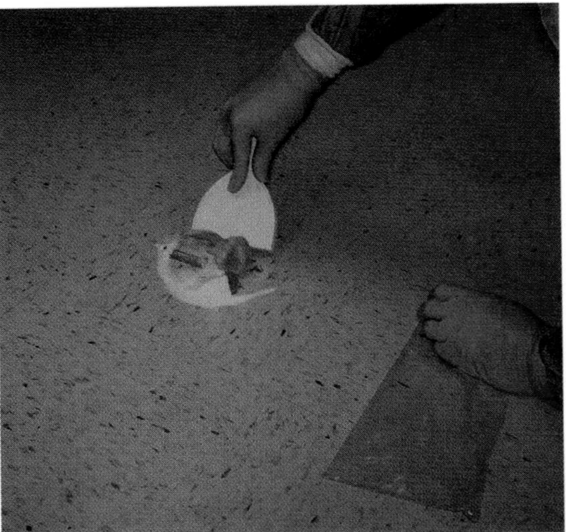

Mix with a spatula.

6. When the liquid is sufficiently congealed, use the spatula to scoop up the spill.
7. Place the spill into the Zip-Loc bag.

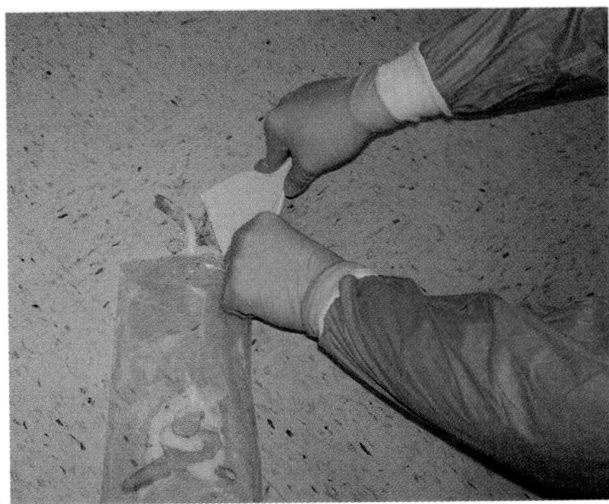

Scoop up spill and place in bag.

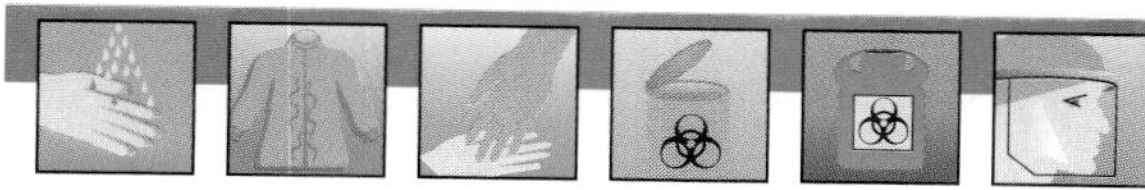

PROCEDURE 23–2

Decontaminating a Biohazardous Spill (Continued)

8. Place the spatula into the Zip-Loc bag and seal the bag.

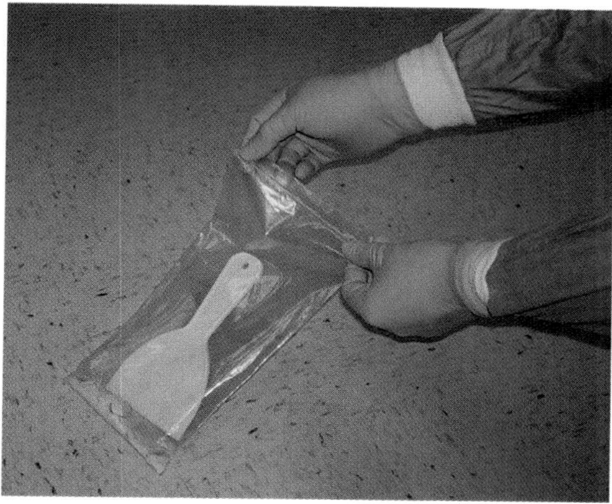

Place spatula in bag.

9. Wipe the area thoroughly with the germicidal cloth.

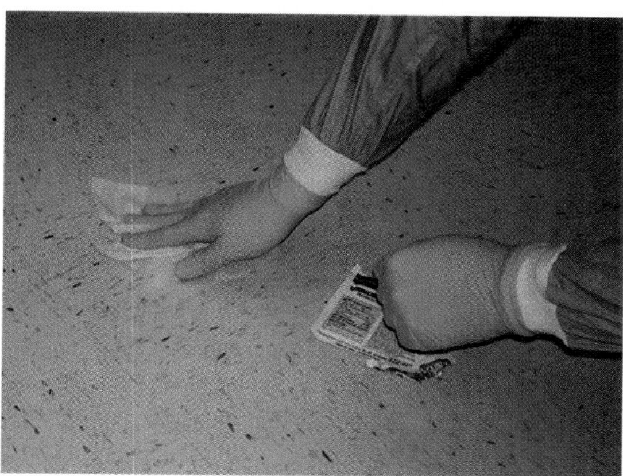

Clean area thoroughly with germicidal cloth.

10. Dry the area using paper towels.

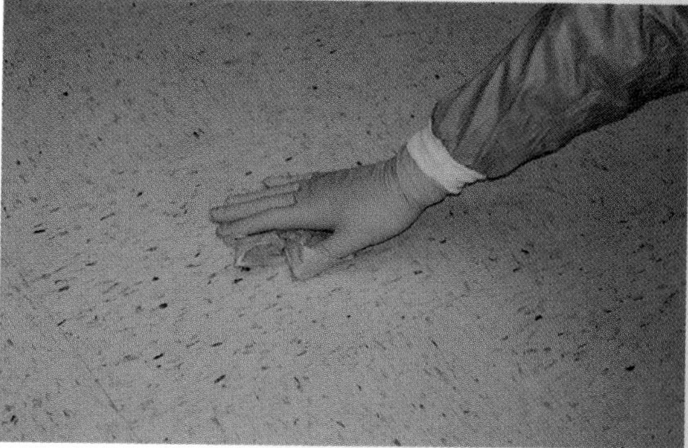

Dry area with paper towels.

11. Place the sealed bag, germicidal cloth, and paper towels into the biohazard bag and seal it securely with the tie provided.

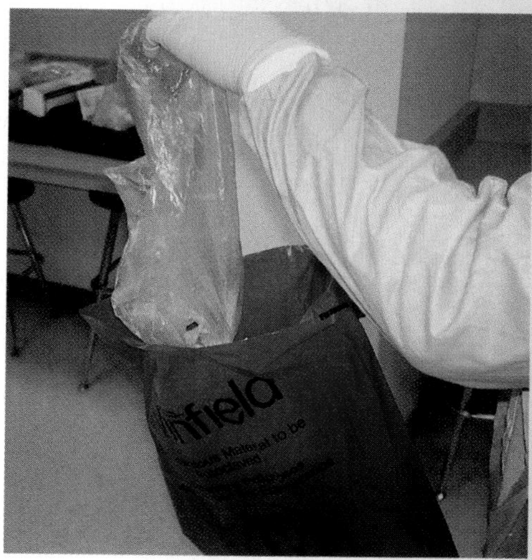

Place contaminated items in biohazard bag.

12. Dispose of the bag in an approved container.
13. Remove gloves, goggles, mask, and barrier gown and deposit these items in the designated container.
14. Wash hands and dry them thoroughly.
15. Report and record the incident and the procedure used to clean up and decontaminate the spill.

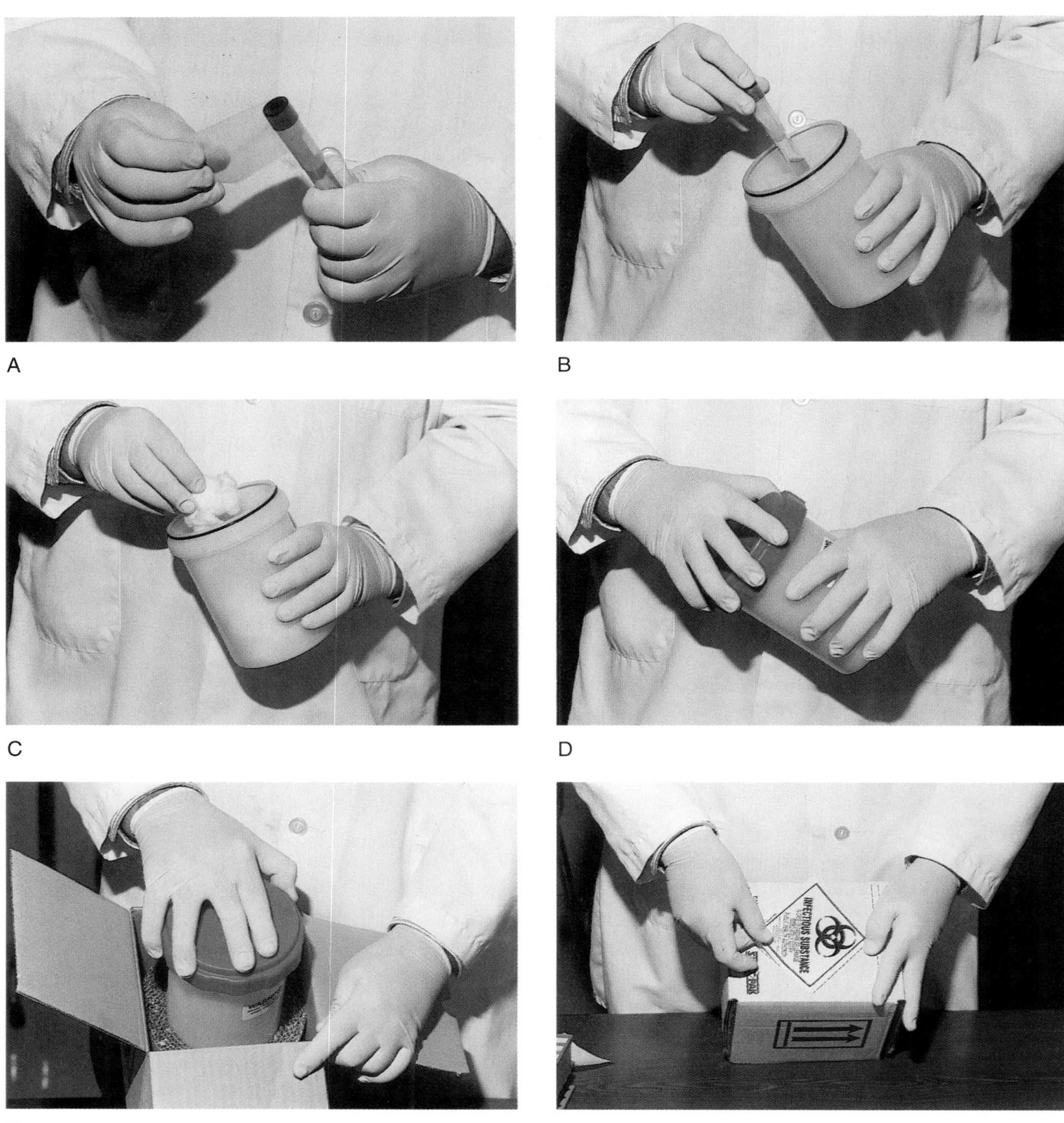

Figure 23–6. *Preparing a specimen for mailing.* A, *Special tube is sealed with leakproof tape.* B, *Sealed tube is placed in container.* C, *Container is packed with an absorbent material.* D, *Container holding tube is placed in cardboard outer container with screw-top lid.* E, *Container is placed into special cardboard mailing carton.* F, *Medical specimen label is placed on mailing container.*

Mailing and Shipping Specimens

Special testing may require that specimens be transported to laboratories outside of your area. This will require use of the U.S. Postal Service or transport by private carrier. Specimen mailing or shipping containers must be obtained and used. It is wise to have these mailing containers on hand for use within the laboratory. Most large laboratories provide these materials, at no cost, and many also have a courier pick-up service. Generally, the specimen is collected in a special vial or tube, preferably with an unbreakable plastic or glass inner core. This vial or tube is sealed with special tape to prevent leakage (Fig. 23–6*A*) and is then placed in a larger, outer container (Fig. 23–6*B*) that is packed with absorbent material (Fig. 23–6*C*). This outer container is usually metal or plastic with a leakproof, screw-top lid (Fig. 23–6*D*). This container should hold enough absorbent material to absorb the entire contents of the inner vial or tube, should it break. The metal or plastic container is then inserted into a special cardboard mailing carton (Fig. 23–6*E*). The mailing label is attached to the cardboard mailing carton, along with any warning labels that are required. If you are using U.S. Postal Service, the label must specify the contents as medical specimens (Fig. 23–6*F*),

Summary

The most important factor influencing the accuracy of laboratory test results is the method used for specimen collection and processing. When working in the laboratory collecting area, you must be familiar with specimen collection protocols and appropriate methods for specimen transport. Each laboratory receiving specimens for testing generally has specific rules to follow for preparing specimens for transport. The laboratory worker's ability to meet these specimen collection standards directly influences the quality of the specimens submitted. Careful preparation of the patient, meticulous equipment preparation and maintenance, and frequent checking of pertinent protocols to ensure correct and accurate specimen handling and processing are among the most important services you can provide.

Chapter Review

True or False

Circle T or F to indicate the correct answers to the following:

T F 1. When collecting specimens, a primary concern is avoiding specimen contamination.

T F 2. Infectious diseases are always transmitted by direct contact.

T F 3. Laboratory coats are routinely worn in the laboratory area.

T F 4. A nosocomial infection refers to an infection spread through nasal secretions.

T F 5. The major role of bacteriology is to identify bacteria.

Fill in the Blanks

Complete the following statements:

6. When decontaminating reusable materials, you sterilize them in an ______________ .
7. CDC is an abbreviation for ______________ ______ ______________ ______________ .
8. The standards set by OSHA are designed to protect ______________ .

Multiple Choice

Circle the letter that represents the single best answer:

9. The term *morbidity* refers to the ratio of:
   a. Deaths to the total population
   b. People hospitalized to the number of hospital beds available
   c. Sick to well persons in a community
   d. World epidemics to regional epidemics
   e. Accidental deaths to natural deaths
10. A _____ solution of household bleach and water is an effective agent against viral contamination.
    a. 10%
    b. 20%
    c. 30%
    d. 40%
    e. 50%

Vocabulary

asymmetric: characterized by a lack of similarity of size, shape, or position
bacteriostatic: substance that inhibits or retards bacterial growth
bilayered: split, or with two distinct layers present
flagellate: any microorganism having a long, whiplike, mobile appendage
hyphae: filaments or threads composing the mycelium of a fungus
medium: a nutritive substance upon which bacteria are placed for growth
mordant: a substance that fixes or intensifies a stain or dye
morphology: the study of the form and structure of organisms, organs, tissues, or cells
peptidoglycan: a polysaccharide attached to short, cross-linked peptides found in bacterial cell walls
phagocytosis: the engulfing of microorganisms or other cells and foreign particles by phagocytes
proteinaceous: pertaining to any protein that is a large organic compound made up of one or more chains of amino acids
spores: refractile, oval bodies formed within bacteria; regarded as a resting stage during the life cycle of a cell
vibrio: an organism of the genus *Vibrio,* or other motile spirillum organism

Chapter Objectives

After reading this chapter, you should be able to:

1. Identify the factors that can affect the Gram stain.
2. Explain why glass slides with frosted ends are desirable.
3. Describe the technique used for smearing three types of specimens.
4. State the reasons why methanol fixation is replacing the old standard of heat fixation of smears.
5. List the steps involved in obtaining an organism colony from a Petri dish.
6. Identify the universal technique used to stain bacteria.
7. Explain the function of a mordant.
8. Compare the Wescor stainer with manual staining.
9. Explain the value of a control slide when performing an in-house slide preparation.
10. Describe the uses of a direct saline mount.
11. Identify the wet mount examination used to diagnose fungus.
12. List fluids that may be used for direct visualization using India ink preparation.

Chapter 24

Smear Preparation, Staining Techniques, and Wet Mounts

Since the work of van Leewenhoek in the 17th century, microscopic methods for the diagnosis of infectious diseases have been the fastest way to determine the presence of disease-producing microorganisms. Direct visualization by wet preparations and/or staining techniques is an important tool in the clinical laboratory's arsenal. A microscope and a Gram stain are the first elements required to identify an unknown organism.

The Gram Stain

The Gram stain is used to classify bacteria on the basis of their form, size, cellular **morphology,** and Gram stain reaction. It is a critical test for the rapid presumptive identification of infectious agents, and it also is a means by which the quality of a clinical specimen can be evaluated. The test was originally developed in 1884 by Hans Christian Gram. In 1921, it was modified by Hucker to the test we use today.

When exposed to the Gram stain, bacteria stain either gram-positive (deep violet) or gram-negative (light to dark red) on the basis of differences in cell wall composition and structure (Fig. 24–1). Gram-positive bacteria have a thick **peptidoglycan** layer and large amounts of teichoic acids. This combination prevents them from being affected by alcohol decolorization; therefore, they retain the initial stain of crystal violet, which imparts a deep violet color. Gram-negative cell walls have a single peptidoglycan layer attached to an **asymmetric,** lipopolysaccharide, phospholipid, **bilayered,** outer membrane interspersed with protein. The outer membrane is damaged by the alcohol decolorizer, allowing the crystal violet iodine complex to leak out and be replaced by the Safranin counterstain (red). The Gram stain can be affected by many factors, including culturing, age, antibiotics, the **medium** in which the bacteria is growing, incubation atmosphere, **phagocytosis,** and staining technique.

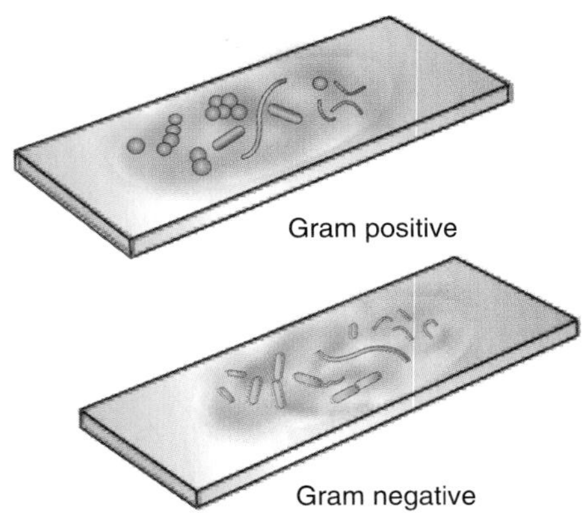

Figure 24–1. *Gram-positive and gram-negative stained bacteria.*

Smear Preparation

Proper smear preparation will produce a thin monolayer of organisms for easy visualization but will be thick enough to reveal characteristic arrangements of the bacteria. **Always wear latex gloves and a laboratory coat and follow all other universal precautions when handling clinical specimens.**

Precleaned, glass slides with frosted ends should be used for the smear. The frosted ends are desirable, as they allow accurate labeling and convenient handling. Frequently, a direct smear is prepared from the swab used to obtain the sample. A smear can be from any body opening, including the genitals or wounds (such as surgical sites, bites, cuts, or body ulcers). The best process is to obtain two swabs, one for the culture and one for the smear. However, often, this is not possible, so one swab must be used for both the culture and the smear. If this is the case, the specimen is cultured first. Then, before the thioglycolate tube is inoculated, the smear is prepared. The danger in using one swab is that the target area may be missed, thus invalidating the entire testing process. You will want to check laboratory protocols for smear preparation to determine the exact procedure for obtaining a smear specimen.

Smearing and Fixation Technique

To prepare the smear, gently roll the swab across the slide, in one direction, leaving a thin film of the specimen material on the slide. Specimens not received on swabs can be spread over a large area by using sterile swabs or a heat-sterilized wire loop to form a thin film on the slide (Fig. 24–2). Extremely thick specimens can

Figure 24–2. *Procedure for smear preparation using a swab.*

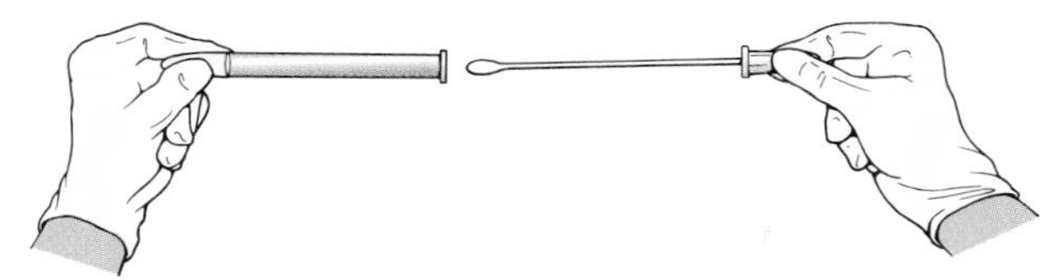

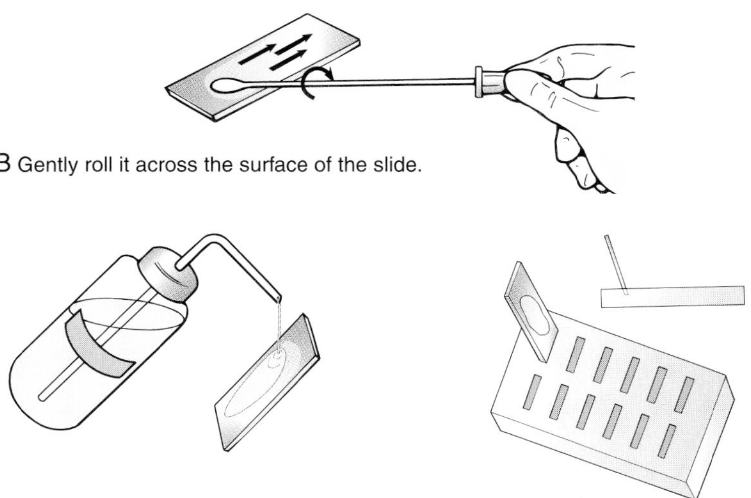

B Gently roll it across the surface of the slide.
C Flood slide with methanol for one minute.
D Drain slide and allow it to dry.

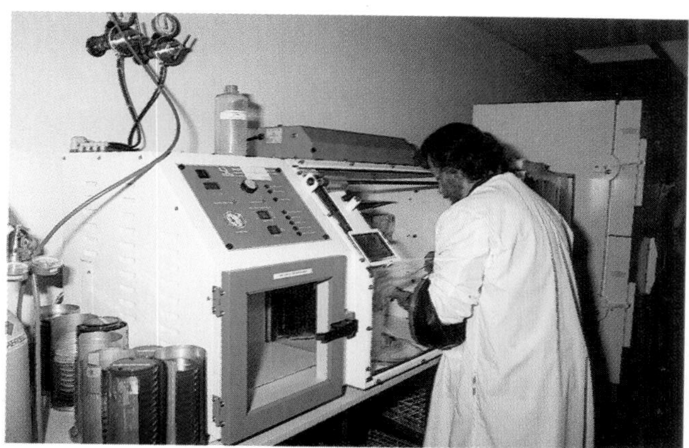

Figure 24–3. *Anaerobic chamber.*

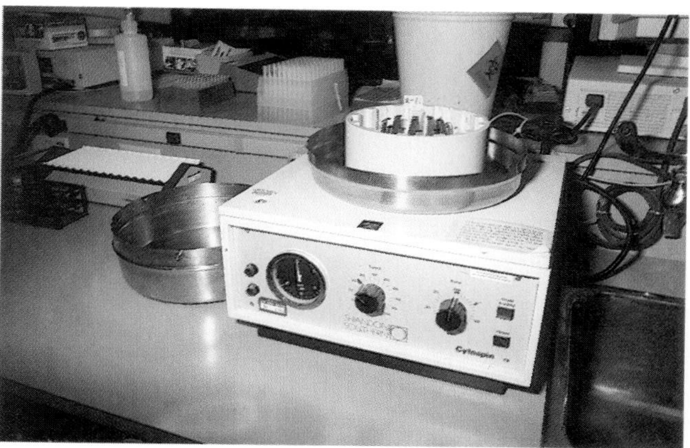

Figure 24–4. *Cytospin slide centrifuge.*

be placed on one slide, covered with a second slide, and pulled apart. The excess on the edge of the slide can then be removed using a disinfectant-soaked paper towel. **The smearing and fixation technique must be done in a biosafety cabinet (Fig. 24–3).**

A more commonly used technique for thick specimens is to place a drop of saline on the slide to facilitate smear preparation. Smears of cerebro spinal fluid or other body fluids requiring centrifugation may be prepared by using a Cytospin slide centrifuge to concentrate the fluids (Fig. 24–4). This method is used to increase the likelihood of visualizing bacteria and to decrease examination time for more rapid results. Using slides with etched rings helps to locate the inoculated area (Fig. 24–5).

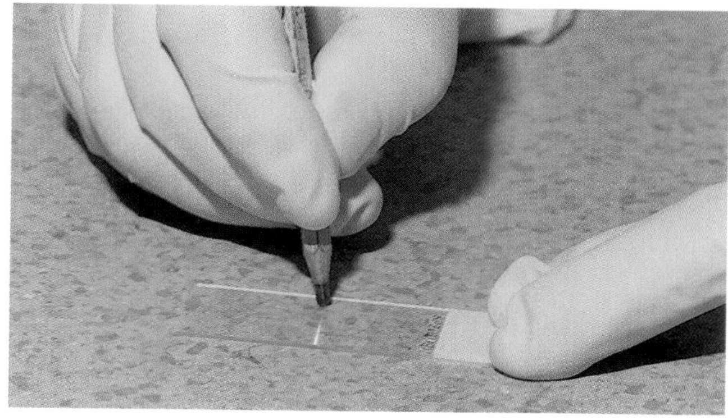

Figure 24–5. *Etching a slide.*

Smears should be air-dried on a flat surface or on an electric slide warmer heated to 60°C. The slide is placed on the supporting rods of the stain rack and then fixed by covering the slide with methanol for 1 minute. The residual methanol is then drained off without rinsing and is allowed to air-dry again. The slide is then ready to stain. Do not heat-fix the slide before staining. Methanol fixation is preferred over the old standard of heat-fixing smears because it prevents lysis of red blood cells (RBCs), gives a cleaner background, does not affect bacterial morphology, and is safer.

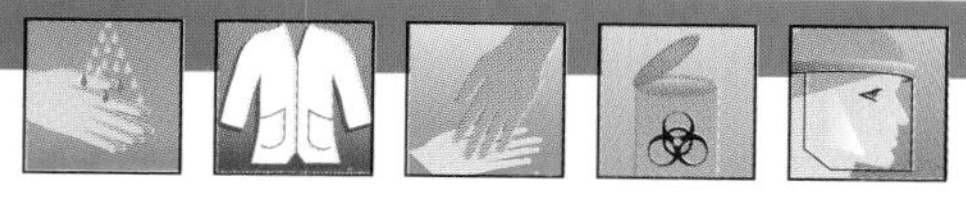

PROCEDURE 24–1

Preparing a Direct Smear

Principle

To prepare a slide using a direct smear of cultured bacteria as preparation for Gram staining and microscopic examination

Equipment and Supplies

frosted, precleaned slides
laboratory marker
swab containing the specimen
stain rack
methanol
watch or timing device

Procedural Steps

1. Wash hands and dry them thoroughly.
2. Label a slide with the patient's name.

(continued)

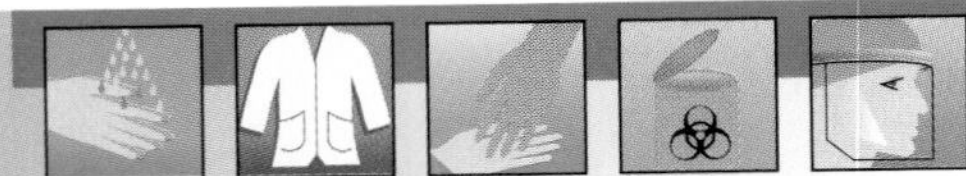

PROCEDURE 24–1

Preparing a Direct Smear (Continued)

3. Put on gloves and other protective gear.
4. Carefully remove the swab from its transport media and gently roll it across the surface of the slide

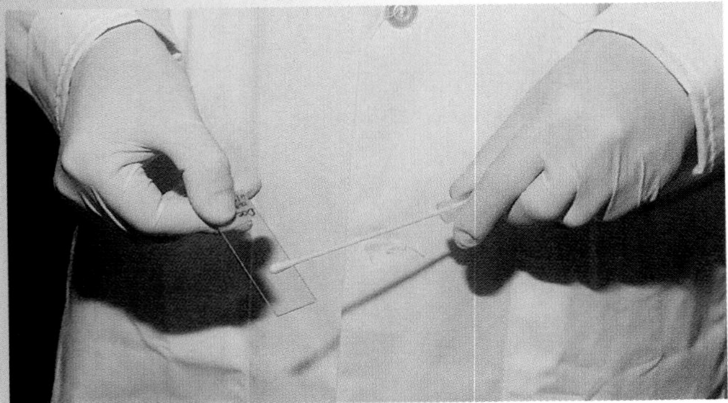

Gently roll the swab across the surface of the slide.

5. Place the slide on a flat surface to dry. Return the swab to the transport media.
6. Place the slide on the supporting rods of the stain rack.
7. Fix the slide by covering it with methanol for 1 minute.

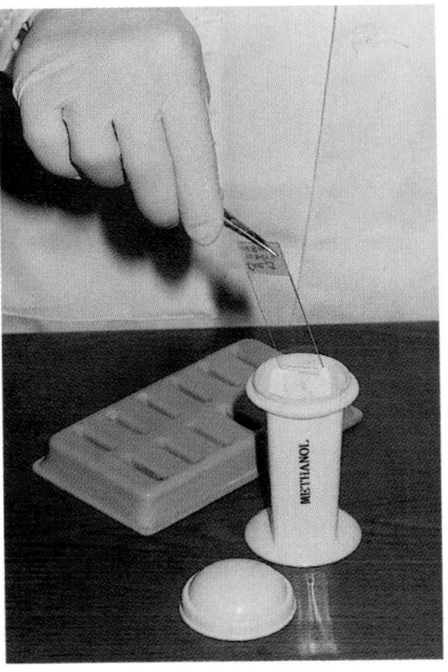

Fix the slide by dipping it into methanol and allow it to dry.

8. Drain off the remaining methanol and allow the slide to air-dry again.
   NOTE: Methanol fixation has replaced heat fixation as the preferred method.
9. The slide is now ready to stain.
10. If appropriate, proceed to staining the slide for viewing. Otherwise, clean the work area.
11. Discard all disposable waste according to laboratory protocols/OSHA standards.
12. Remove gloves and protective gear. Wash hands.

Bacterial Smears on Media

Smears from bacteria growing on media are made by putting a drop of **bacteriostatic** saline on the slide along with a small portion of one colony of the organism. The colony is obtained by lifting the lid of the Petri dish containing the media and using a sterile wire loop, sterile plastic disposable loop, or sterile applicator stick to pick up a small portion of a single pure colony (Fig 24–6). Smears from blood agar should only be made from colonies that are 24 hours old or less. In older colonies, the cell walls tend to break down, causing unreliable Gram stain results. The smear is then air-dried and methanol-fixed, after which the slide is ready to stain.

Staining Bacteria

Gram staining is routinely performed in the microbiology section of the clinical laboratory. Bacteria (or microorganisms, as they are sometimes called) are so tiny and virtually colorless that their morphology cannot be determined without first staining them. The Gram stain is the universal technique used to stain bacteria after they have been methanol-fixed.

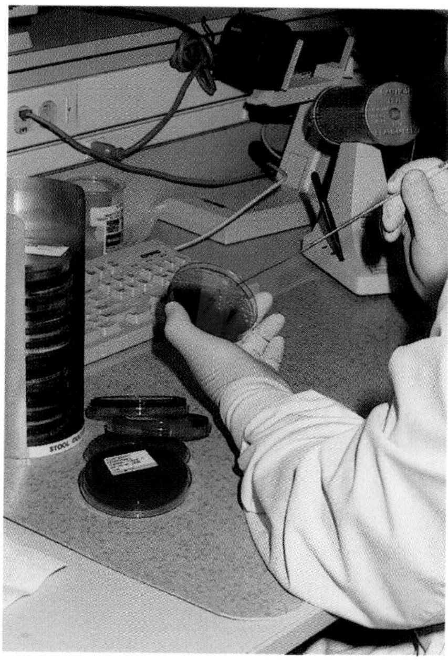

Figure 24–6. *A portion of single colony is picked up using a sterile loop.*

The staining procedure involves the sequential application of primary stain **mordant,** decolorizer, and counterstain to a bacterial smear. The stains are taken up differentially by the organisms according to the chemical composition of the cell walls. A fixed smear is placed on a staining rack and the primary stain crystal violet is poured onto one end of the smear until the whole slide is covered (Fig. 24–7*A*). The stain is allowed to remain in place for 30 seconds. The crystal violet is then decanted by lifting one end of the slide and rinsing the slide gently with distilled or deionized water (Fig. 24–7*B*). **CAUTION: Excessive rinsing in this step could cause the crystal violet to be washed from gram-positive cells.**

The Gram iodine solution, called a mordant, causes the dye to adhere to the object being stained. The slide is flooded with iodine solution and allowed to sit for 30 seconds (Fig. 24–7*C*), after which the slide is gently rinsed with distilled or deionized water. The slide is then decolorized, usually with an acetone alcohol mixture, by letting the solution flow over the smear with the slide held at an angle. Rinsing is discontinued when the runoff becomes clear (Fig. 24–7*D*). The de-

Figure 24–7. *Gram staining technique.*

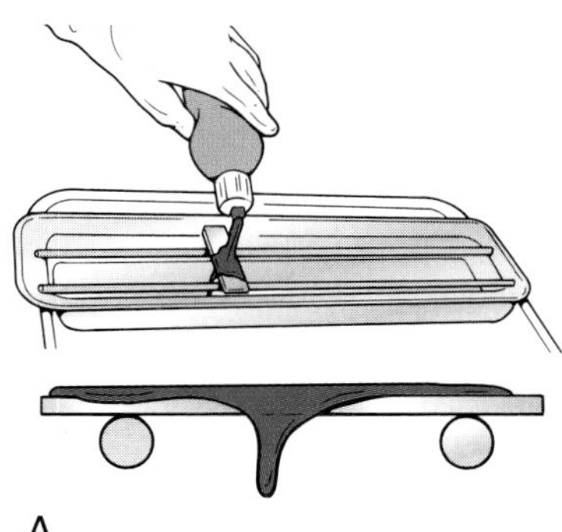

A
Pour crystal violet stain onto one end of the slide until the slide is covered.

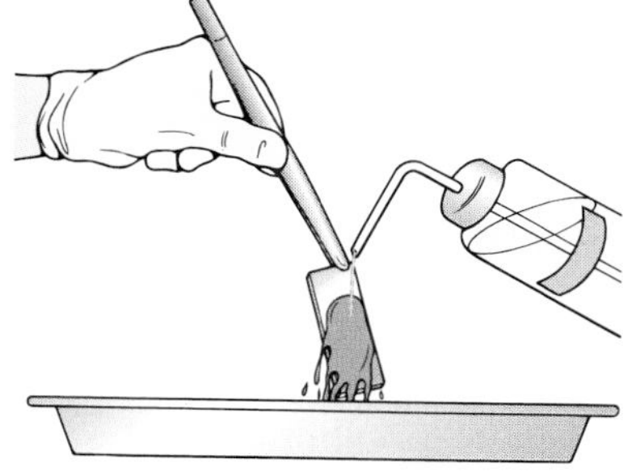

B
Lift one end of the slide and rinse gently with distilled or deionized water.

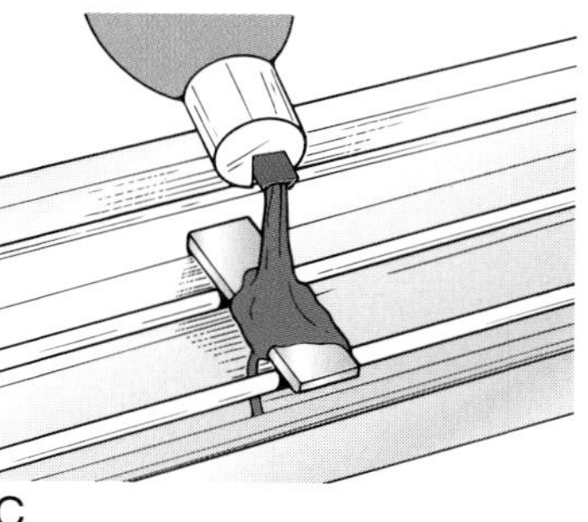

C
Flood the slide with iodine solution.

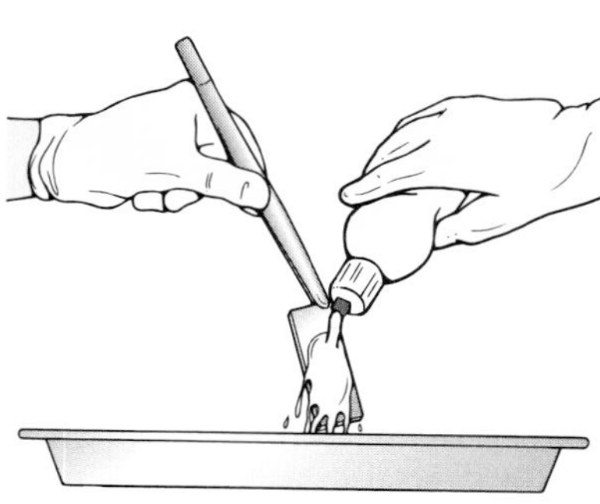

D
Hold the slide at an angle and decolorize with an acetone/alcohol mixture.

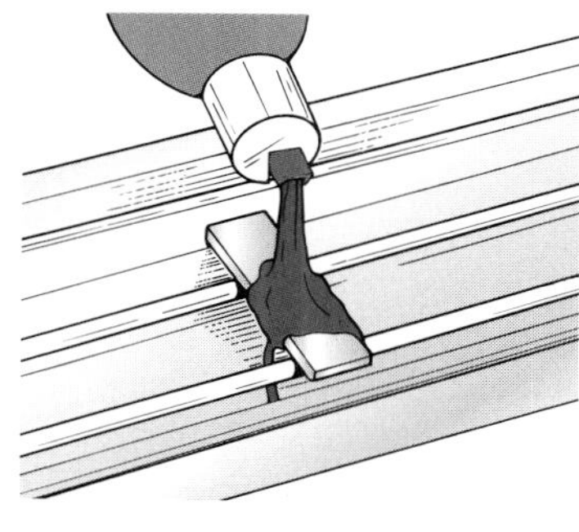

E
Flood the slide with safranin.

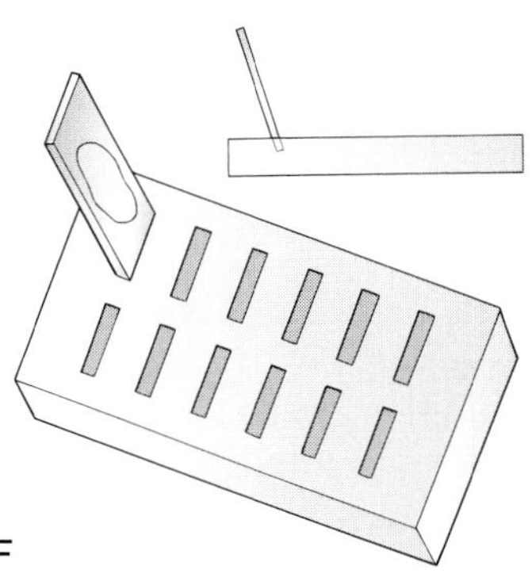

F
Drain the slide and air-dry it in a slide dryer.

colorization time is adjusted according to the thickness of the smear and the type of decolorizer used. Excessive rinsing with the decolorizer can cause the dye's iodine complex to be washed from gram-positive cells. Safranin is now the preferred counterstain. The slide is flooded with safranin, which is allowed to remain in place for 30 seconds (Fig. 24–7*E*). The safranin will have no effect on gram-positive cells (which stain violet), but the gram-negative cells will stain red. Excess counterstain is removed with a gentle flow of distilled or deionized water. The slide is then drained and allowed to air-dry in an upright position, or it may be dried by a commercial slide drier (Fig. 24–7*F*). Once the slide is dry, it is ready to be examined microscopically.

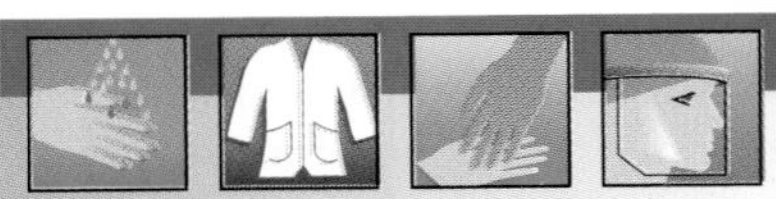

PROCEDURE 24–2

Gram Staining a Culture Slide

Principle

To stain bacteria in preparation for microscopic examination and categorization based on the reaction of the bacteria to the stain and their characteristics

Equipment and Supplies

a fixed slide (as prepared in Procedure 24–1)
crystal violet stain
Gram iodine stain
stain rack
deionized or distilled water
decolorizer (acetone/alcohol mixture)
safranin stain

Procedural Steps

1. Place the fixed slide on a staining rack.
2. Pour the primary stain, crystal violet, onto one end of the slide until the whole slide is covered. Allow the stain to remain in place for 30 seconds.
3. Decant by lifting one end of the slide and then gently rinse the slide with distilled or deionized water.
4. Flood the slide with iodine solution (mordant). Allow the mordant to remain in place for 30 seconds.
5. Repeat the water rinse.
6. Hold the slide at an angle and apply decolorizer (alcohol/acetone) by letting the solution run over the smear until the runoff becomes clear.
7. Return the slide to the stain rack. Flood the slide with safranin stain (counterstain). Allow the stain to remain on the slide for 30 seconds.
8. Gently rinse the slide with distilled or deionized water.
9. Place the slide in an upright position and allow it to air-dry.
10. Once the slide is dry, it is ready to be examined microscopically.
11. Clean the work area, discarding all waste according to laboratory protocol/OSHA standards. Return unused supplies to the proper storage area.
12. Remove gloves and wash hands.

Expected Results

Primary stain: Turns to purple all bacteria in the smear.
Mordant: Causes no change in the appearance of the bacteria.
Decolorizer: Gram-negative cells no longer appear purple.
Counterstain: Gram-negative cells turn pinkish red, whereas all the gram-positive cells remain purple.

Automatic Gram Staining

Some manufacturers recommend an interval of 1 minute, instead of the 30 seconds mentioned in the steps just outlined. Moreover, Wescor Manufacturing has developed an automatic Gram stainer. Resembling a desktop centrifuge, this device can methanol-fix and stain multiple slides simultaneously according to a preset cycle (Fig. 24–8). All the slides can be stained in about 3 minutes with no variation in staining technique. A smear slide for quality control can be purchased commercially or prepared in-house.

In-House Control Slide

A prepared in-house control slide contains one loopful of *Escherichia coli,* gram-negative rods that stain red, and *Staphylococcus aureus,* gram-positive cocci that

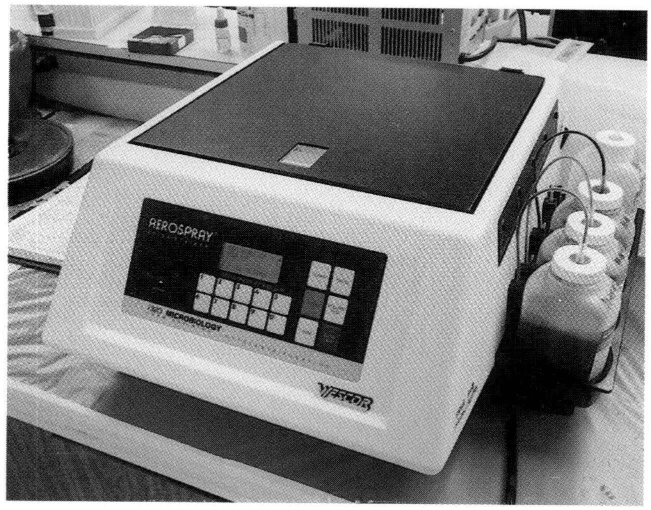

Figure 24–8. *Wescor stainer.*

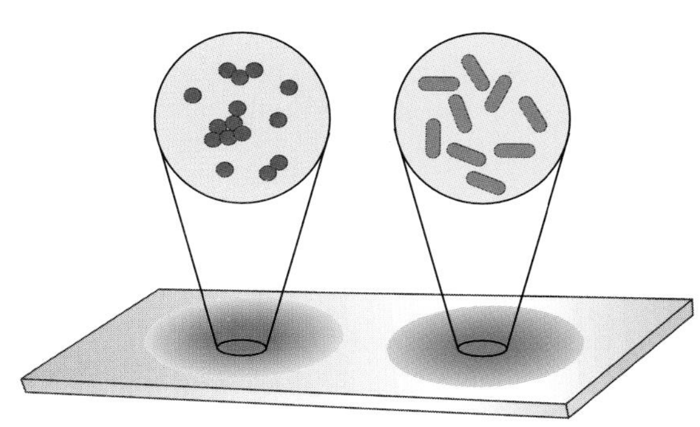

Figure 24–9. *The control slide shows violet cocci (gram-positive* Staphylococcus aureus*) and red rods (gram-negative* Escherichia coli*).*

Figure 24–10. *The three basic shapes of bacteria.*

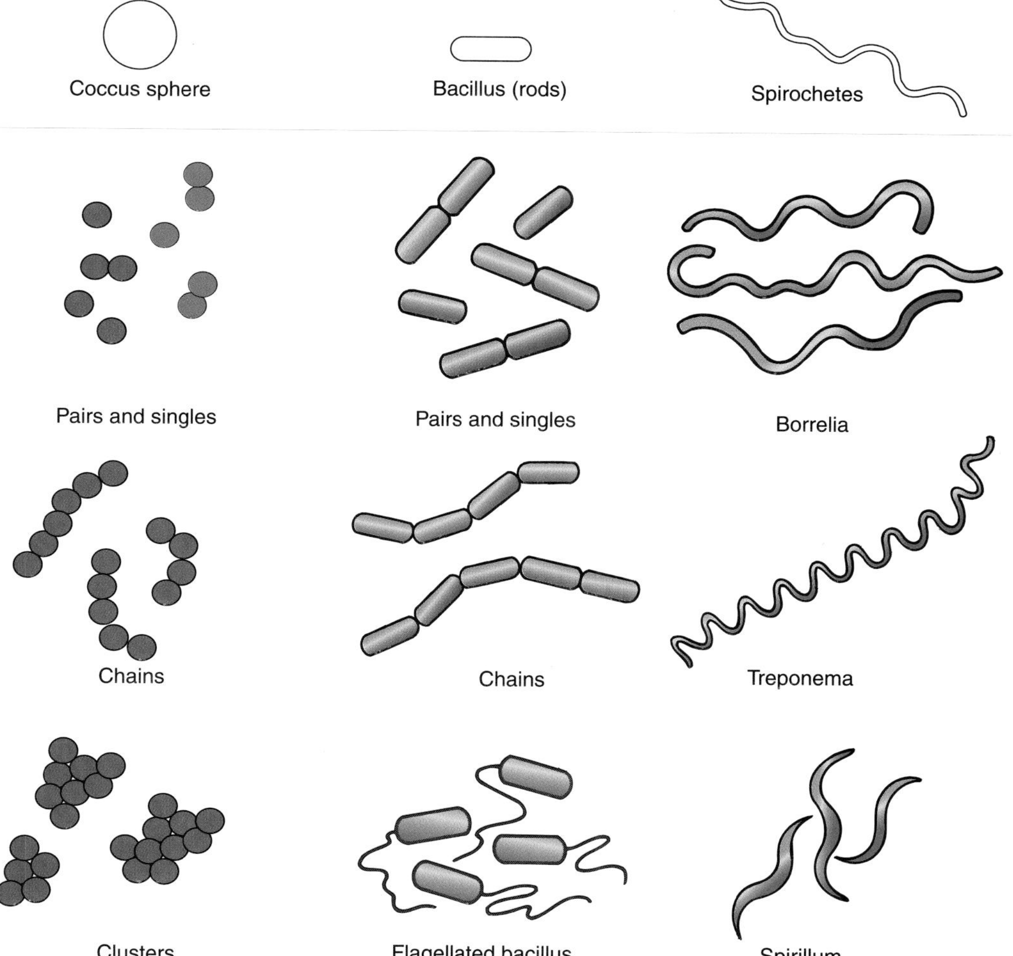

stain violet, which are mixed at each end of a single slide. The control slide is stained at the same time as the slides with the unknown organisms. If the control slide stains correctly, violet cocci and red rods should be visible when the slide is examined under the microscope (Fig. 24–9). If this is the case, the Gram staining procedure was performed correctly, and the reagents functioned properly.

Microscopic Analysis

Examine the stained smear first under the low-power lens (10×) and then under the high-power lens (40×). Swing this lens away and put a drop of oil on the smear. View the smear under the oil-immersion lens (100×). Individual bacterial cells have one of three general shapes: spheres, rods, or spirals (Fig. 24–10).

The spherical bacteria are known as cocci (singular form, coccus), meaning "berry" in Latin. Cocci are able to assume a variety of arrangements depending on how they divide during replication. The most common forms are irregular, grape-like clusters (usually indicative of staphylococci) or chains consisting of four or more cocci (usually indicative of streptococci) (Table 24–1).

Rod-shaped or oval bacteria are called bacilli (singular form, *Bacillus*) or rods. They appear either singly or in chains. Some bacilli, like some cocci, appear broad and rounded. These organisms are termed coccobacilli (see Table 24–1).

Spiral bacteria include two types of organisms: the **vibrio,** which resembles a curved rod or comma, and the spirillum, which resembles a rigid spiral or corkscrew (see Table 24–1).

Some bacteria, such as *Mycobacterium* or *Nocardia,* may not appear to be either gram-positive or gram-negative. This is because of their waxy outer coating, which does not stain easily using the Gram stain process (see Table 24–1).

PROCEDURE 24–3

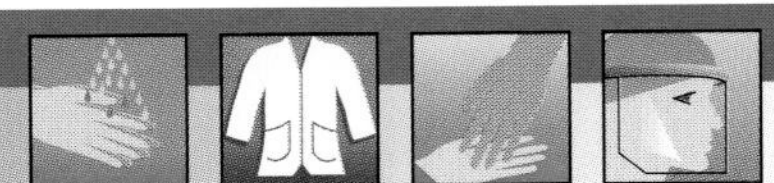

Recognizing Types of Bacteria

Principle

To gain familiarity with the morphology of different types of bacteria

Equipment and Supplies

text paper
colored pencils

Procedural Steps

1. Study the diagrams of bacteria that appear in the text of this chapter.
2. In the space provided, draw each of the following types of bacteria: cocci, rods, spirilla.
3. Compare your drawings to the text illustrations and correct any inaccuracies.

Cocci	**Rods**	**Spirilla**

Table 24–1
Important Pathogenic Bacteria

Genus/Species	Subtype	Gram Stain Reaction
Bacillus anthracis	Spore-forming rod	+
Bacteroides fragilis	Rod	–
Borrelia species	Spirochete	–
Campylobacter jejuni	Rod	–
Clostridium tetani	Spore-forming rod	+
Clostridium perfringens	Bacillus	+
Corynebacterium diphtheriae	Rod	+
Enterococcus species	Cocci	+
Escherichia coli	Rod	–
Haemophilus influenzae	Rod	–
Klebsiella pneumoniae	Rod	–
Legionella species	Rod	–
Leptospira species	Spirochete	–
Listeria species	Rod	+
Mycobacterium leprae	Beaded rod	AFB
Mycobacterium tuberculosis	Beaded rod	AFB
Neisseria gonorrhoeae	Diplococcus	–
Neisseria meningitidis	Diplococcus	–
Pasteurella species	Rod	–
Propionibacterium species	Bacilli	+
Proteus vulgaris	Rod	–
Pseudomonas aeruginosa	Rod	–
Shigella species	Rod	–
Salmonella species	Rod	–
Staphylococcus aureus	Coccus/clusters	+
Streptococcus pyogenes	Coccus/chains	+
Streptococcus pneumoniae	Diplococcus	+
Treponema pallidum	Spirochete	–
Vibrio cholerae	Curved rod	–
Yersinia pestis	Rod	–

+, Gram-positive stain; –, Gram-negative stain; AFB, Acid-fast bacillus; requires special stain.

Recording the Test Results

Once the staining process is complete, the relative number of observed bacteria is recorded. Two commonly used quantitation systems are numerical and descriptive (Table 24–2). For example, the results might be recorded as 1+ gram-negative streptococci, or moderate gram-negative bacilli (see Table 24–2).

Wet Mounts

Like the Gram stain, the direct visualization of a clinical specimen is an important diagnostic tool in the clinical microbiological laboratory. Using brightfield microscopy or phase-contrast microscopy, specimens can be applied directly to the surface of a slide for immediate examination. This technique is useful for liquid specimens, such as urine, urine sediment, vaginal discharge, cerebrospinal fluid, and other aspirated fluids. It is also useful for stool, sputum, and wound exudate. These specimens may be prepared in a number of ways.

Direct Saline Mount

Nonliquid specimens may be diluted using equal parts of sterile physiological (normal) saline (0.85%–0.9%). The specimen on the slide is then overlaid with a coverslip and is examined directly under the microscope. This type of wet slide preparation is known as a direct saline mount or direct wet mount. *Trichomonas vaginalis* is an example of an organism that is usually diagnosed using a direct saline mount (Fig. 24–11*A*).

Table 24–2
Quantitation Systems for Recording Observed Bacteria

Quantitation	*Significance*
NUMERICAL	
1+	<1 per oil-immersion field
2+	1 per oil-immersion field
3+	2–10 per oil-immersion field
4+	predominant, or >10 per oil-immersion field
DESCRIPTIVE	
Rare	<1 per oil-immersion field
Few	1–5 per oil-immersion field
Moderate	5–10 per oil-immersion field
Many	>10 per oil immersion field

Potassium Hydroxide (KOH) Mount

Some specimens contain **proteinaceous** material that makes direct examination difficult. A 10% potassium hydroxide (KOH) preparation is helpful when examination proteinaceous specimens for fungal elements, such as would be present in a yeast infection. A KOH preparation is useful when examining skin or nail scrapings because it digests the specimen, leaving the fungal elements intact. It is also useful in the diagnosis of vaginal yeast infections. The procedure is essentially the same as for the direct saline mount, with the exception that KOH is substituted for saline in the preparation. Fragments of skin scales, nails, or hair are suspended in a drop of 10% KOH. A coverslip is placed over the drop and the slide is allowed to sit at room temperature for about 30 minutes. Gentle heating may speed the digestion of the proteinaceous material in the specimen, although caution should be exercised so

Figure 24–11. A, *Direct mount slide preparation.* B, *India ink slide preparation.*

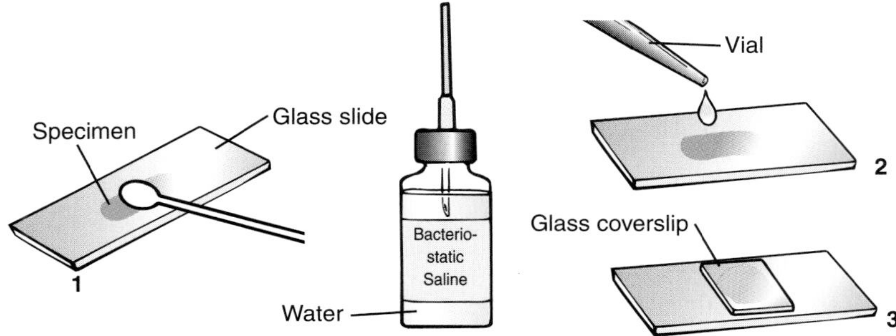
Specimen
Glass slide
1
Bacterio-static Saline
Water
Vial
2
Glass coverslip
3
Wet Mount (normal saline direct mount slide preparation)
1. Gently roll the specimen onto the slide.
2. Mix the specimen with one drop of saline.
3. Cover with coverslip and examine microscopically.
A

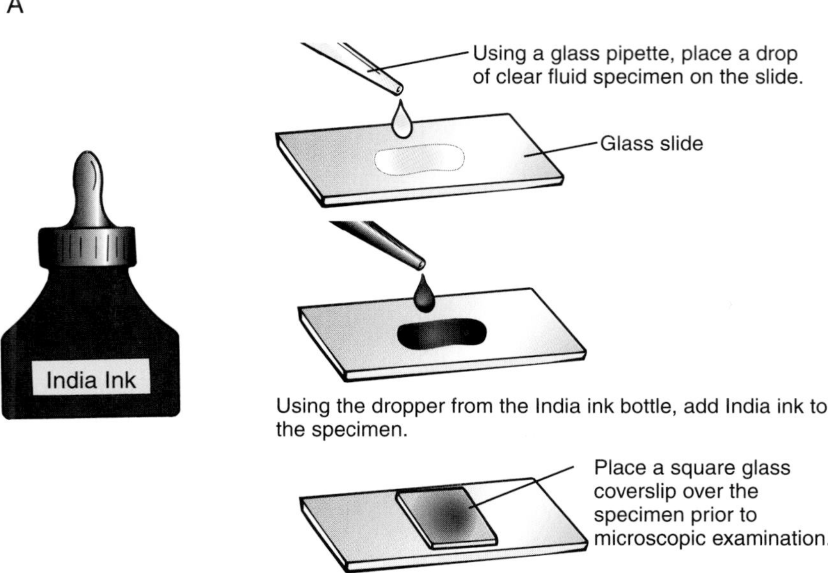
Using a glass pipette, place a drop of clear fluid specimen on the slide.
Glass slide
India Ink
Using the dropper from the India ink bottle, add India ink to the specimen.
Place a square glass coverslip over the specimen prior to microscopic examination.
B

as not to overheat and damage the fungal elements. The presence of fungal elements can be enhanced by the addition of commercially prepared stains, such as lactophenol cotton blue. The slide is then placed under the microscope and examined for fungal **hyphae** or **spores,** first at a magnification 10×, and then 40×. Microscopic findings are reported immediately for confirmation.

India Ink Preparation

The direct visualization of encapsulated yeast is enhanced by the use of India ink (Pelikan brand). This process is useful when the presence of *Cryptococcus neoformans* is suspected in cerebrospinal fluid and other body fluids. The clinical specimen is first centrifuged, after which equal parts of sediment and India ink are combined and examined under a brightfield microscope, using first the low-power (10×) and then the high-power (40×) objective. The encapsulated yeast will exclude the India ink, causing the capsule to appear as a clear halo around the organism (Fig. 24–11*B*).

Summary

The medical or laboratory assistant is seldom responsible for the microscopic analysis of prepared slides. In most laboratory settings, the assistant will prepare the slide, place it under the microscopic lens, and set the focus. Once this is completed, the physician or laboratory technologist will read the slide and record the results. It is the assistant's role to make sure that the slide is properly prepared and ready for viewing. To do this correctly, the assistant must be skilled in preparation techniques, be able to recognize microorganisms, and be able to determine whether a slide has been prepared correctly.

In direct wet mount slide preparation, time is a very important element, directly affecting the accuracy of results. The tiny organisms seen under the microscope die quickly when removed from their growing environment. Many wet mounts are of specimens taken from the genital area of a patient, which means that the patient submitted to a personal examination. When you receive such a specimen and perform the test, strive for both accuracy and speed, so as not to subject the patient to a repeat test. These types of procedures, when done correctly, will build your confidence as a valuable health team member.

Chapter Review

True or False

Circle T or F to indicate the correct answers to the following:

T F 1. Gram-positive bacteria will appear red when stained.

T F 2. Methanol replaced the heat fixation method in slide preparation.

T F 3. Specimens for a direct saline mount must be examined within 2 hours of collection.

T F 4. The KOH preparation is used when examining fungus.

T F 5. *Trichomonas vaginalis* is primarily diagnosed on the basis of a direct saline mount.

Fill in the Blanks

Complete the following statements:

6. India ink is a useful tool when examining

 ____________ .

7. India ink causes the capsule to appear as a

 ____________ .

8. Another name for Gram iodine solution is

 ____________ .

9. Morphology refers to the ____________ and

 ____________ of organisms, organs, tissues, or cells.

Multiple Choice

Circle the letter that represents the single best answer:

10. Potassium hydroxide preparation is a ____________ solution.
 a. 10%
 b. 20%
 c. 30%
 d. 40%
 e. 50%

11. Refractile oval bodies formed within bacteria are:
 a. Flagellates
 b. Hyphae
 c. Spores
 d. Cocci
 e. Fungus

12. A smear slide for quality control is used to:
 a. Identify gram-positive bacteria
 b. Identify gram-negative bacteria
 c. Determine whether the Gram stain was done correctly
 d. Confirm proper function of the reagents
 e. c and d

Vocabulary

anaerobic: capable of living or growing in the absence of molecular oxygen

bacitracin: an antibacterial substance, obtained from a strain of Bacillus, which is useful in the treatment of a wide range of infections

bacteriuria: bacteria in the urine

endocarditis: inflammation of the lining of the heart and heart valves

glomerulonephritis: inflammation of the glomerulus located in the nephron of the kidney

hemin: nutrients present in lysed red blood cells (RBCs)

hemolytic: pertaining to the rupture of erythrocytes and the release of hemoglobin into plasma

inoculum: serum or other substance introduced onto culture media

lysis: destruction or decomposition of cells or cell contents

nonfastidious: an organism that has no precise nutritional or environmental requirements for growth and survival

normal flora: microorganisms that live on or within the body and compete with disease-producing microorganisms, thereby providing a natural immunity against certain infections

pathogenic: pertaining to any disease-producing agent or microorganism

Petri dish: a round, shallow, flat-bottomed transparent glass or plastic dish with vertical sides and a cover that is similar and slightly larger

pyuria: pus in the urine

Chapter Objectives

After reading this chapter, you should be able to:

1. List the guidelines for collecting and transporting specimens for culture.
2. Identify five conditions that are important for the growth of microorganisms.
3. Name the areas of the body that normally contain bacteria.
4. Describe the temperature range needed to grow bacteria.
5. List the forms of culture media and identify the pathogens that will grow on each.
6. Explain the technique for streaking a Petri dish.
7. List the procedural steps for collecting a throat specimen for culture.
8. Outline the steps involved in performing a urine culture.
9. Describe the technique for using a sterile loop to prepare a urine culture.
10. Explain why a bacitracin disk is used in throat cultures.
11. Explain why timing of throat cultures is necessary to ensure optimal diagnostic accuracy.
12. Discuss the rationale for performing a rapid strep test on a throat swab.

Chapter 25
Culture Techniques

Specimens collected for microbiologic testing reflect that patient's condition or disease. A sufficient amount of specimen must be collected to ensure complete and accurate testing. Fluid from the source of the problem is the ideal specimen for microbiologic testing. However, purulent drainage or tissue is also frequently used. As the specimen can originate anywhere on or in the body, proper identification of the specimen to be tested is extremely important.

Specimen Collection and Transportation Procedures

Improperly collected or transported specimens often result in a failure to isolate the **pathogenic** or causative organism. The specimen must be identified properly, and any clinical information that may aid the microbiologist should be provided. Observing the appropriate steps for collecting and transporting specimens is critical to the integrity of the specimen and the accuracy of any testing.

GUIDELINES

Guidelines for Proper Collection and Transport of Biologic Specimens

- The specimen should be collected in the area most likely to produce the suspected microorganism, with as little contamination as possible.
- Specimen quantity should be sufficient to permit the required examinations.
- Specimens should be placed in designated sterile containers. These containers protect the specimen from contamination and also protect handlers from exposure to the microorganism.
- Whenever possible, the specimen should be collected soon after the onset of the disease, as the likelihood of isolating the causative microorganism is greatest at that time.
- Whenever possible, the specimens for microbiologic examination should be collected before the administration of antimicrobial agents.

- Once collected, the specimens should be transported promptly to the laboratory for testing. Some bacteria are susceptible to changes in temperature, and all bacteria are susceptible to drying.
- Specimens that are improperly collected or transported may be rejected. It is important that the facility's guidelines for rejection be scrupulously observed, and that all rejections be explained to the physician who ordered the examination.

Special care must be taken in the collection and handling of certain specimens. For example, **anaerobic** specimens, which are air-intolerant, must be transported in special transportation apparatus. Successful isolation and identification of anaerobes depends on the use of a proper anaerobic container. Anaerobic collection devices provide an oxygen-free environment in which to collect and transport the specimen.

Conditions for Bacterial Growth

Like all organisms, bacteria require a specific environment for life. Temperature, moisture, nutrients, pH, and salt concentration are all important for the growth of microorganisms. Bacteria may be pathogenic or nonpathogenic. The latter do not ordinarily cause disease or infections; however, they are opportunistic microorganisms which, under certain circumstances, may cause infection or disease. Many areas of the body normally contain bacteria, which population of bacteria is called **normal flora.** For example, the upper respiratory tract and the intestinal tract are full of bacteria that are non–disease-producing and are present in healthy individuals.

Aerobic bacteria grow best in an atmosphere containing oxygen. Some organisms that appear to be anaerobic are able to grow under either aerobic or anaerobic conditions. These are called facultatively anaerobic organisms. Microaerobic organisms grow best in atmospheres of reduced oxygen tension.

The growth of most bacteria is enhanced when the cultures are incubated at 35°C, which is close to the normal human body temperature. However, some bacteria may grow better at lower temperatures (e.g., 30°C) or at higher temperatures (e.g., 42°C). Typically, bacteria found on the surface of the body grow best at lower temperatures, whereas bacteria that originate internally grow best at 35°C.

Figure 25–1. *Enrichment, supportive, selective, and differential media.*

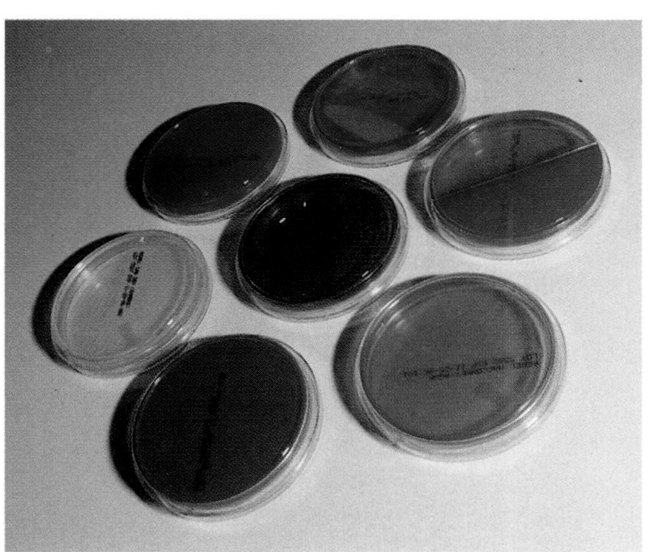

Culture Media

Before pathogens can be isolated and identified, they must first grow on artificial culture media. Culture media are generally agar-based, solid media in **Petri dishes.** Special-purpose media include enrichment, supportive, selective, and differential media (Fig. 25–1).

- *Enrichment media* is used to encourage the growth of a particular organism while suppressing the growth of unwanted organisms.
- *Supportive media* allow **nonfastidious** organisms to grow at their natural rates.
- *Selective media* are inhibitory to all organisms except the targeted organism to be grown. Selective media usually contain antibiotics or other chemical agents to inhibit unwanted microorganisms.
- *Differential media* allow for the cultural characteristics of different microorganisms to be morphologically identified from microorganisms with different characteristics (Table 25–1).

Frequently Used Artificial Culture Media

There are hundreds of different types of artificial culture media, which may be solid, liquid, or semi-solid. Media may come in plates, tubes, or in jars. The following are examples of some of the more commonly used culture media.

Many other types of culture media are used for anaerobic organisms, fungus, and Microbacterium species.

Blood Agar

Blood agar is the most commonly used media in the microbiology laboratory. It supports all but the most fastidious bacteria. This type of media consists of a

Table 25–1
Commonly Used Primary Plating Media

Medium	*Abbreviation*	*Form Media Used as*	*Type of Medium*	*Expected Isolates*	*Differential Reactions*	*Comments*
Anaerobic CDC Blood Agar (Brucella)	BRUC or BRU	Plate	Enriched	All types aerobic/anaerobic and gm(+) & gm(−)	Hemolysis	Supports growth of all strict anaerobic and facultatively anaerobic bacteria.
Anaerobic Colistin-Nalidixic Acid Agar	ANA-CNA or CNA	Plate & Biplate	Enriched, selective	Growth of most gm(+) & gm(−) anaerobes; inhibits facultative anaerobic gm(−) bacteria	*C. perfringens* double zone of hemolysis	
Anaerobic Kanamycin Bile Esculin Agar	KBE	Plate & Biplate	Differential, selective	*B. fragilis* group	BE (+): Brown/black pigment BE (−): No pigment formed	Provides presumptive ID of *B. fragilis* group.
Anaerobic Laked Blood w/Kanamycin & Vancomycin Agar	LKV	Plate	Selective	*Bacteroides* spp.; pigmented anaerobic gm(−) rods, or *F. mortiferum*	Enhances pigment production in pigmented anaerobic gm(−) organisms	Yeasts & kanamycin-resistant gm(-) bacilli may grow on this medium.
Blood Agar/MacConkey Agar	BAP/MAC	Biplate	BAP—Enriched, differential MAC—Differential, selective	BAP = gm(+) & gm(−) organisms MAC = gm(−) enteric bacilli	BAP = Hemolysis patterns MAC = Lac(+):pink Lac(−):colorless	MAC: gm(+) organisms inhibited by bile salts.
Chocolate/Modified Thayer-Martin Agar	CHOC/MTM	Biplate	CHOC—Enriched MTM—Selective	CHOC = *H. influenzae, N. gonorrhoeae & meningitidis* MTM = *N. gonorrhoeae & meningitidis*	NA	CHOC = see info under CHOC. MTM = Vancomycin inhibits gm(+) organisms. Colistin inhibits gm(−) organisms. Nystatin inhibits yeast.
Blood Agar	BAP	Plate	Enriched, differential	gm(+) & gm(−) organisms	Hemolysis patterns	
Brain Heart Infusion Agar w/Blood, Chloramphenicol & Gentamicin	BHI/BCG or BHI W/B.C.G.	Slant	Enriched, selective	Various fungi		Antibiotics inhibit growth of many gm(+) & gm(−) bacteria & allow fungi to grow.
Campylobacter-Cefoperazone-Vancomycin-Amphotericin Agar	CVA	Plate	Enriched, selective	Isolation of *Campylobacter* spp.	NA	
Chocolate Agar	CHOC	Plate	Enriched	*H. influenzae,* gonococcus *N. meningitidis*	NA	Low agar content provides increased moisture needed by some organisms.
Cooked Meat w/Glucose Broth	CMG	Tube	Enriched	Aerobic & anaerobic, gm(+) & gm(−)	NA	

(continued)

Table 25–1

Commonly Used Primary Plating Media *(Continued)*

Medium	***Abbreviation***	***Form Media Used as***	***Type of Medium***	***Expected Isolates***	***Differential Reactions***	***Comments***
Colistin-Nalidixic Acid Agar	CNA	Plate	Enriched, selective	Gm(+) organisms	Hemolysis patterns	Colistin inhibits gm(–) organisms; nalidixic acid inhibits *Proteus*. spp.
Dermatophyte Test Medium	DTM	Slant	Enriched, selective	Dermatophyte isolation	NA	
Hektoen Enteric Agar	HE	Plate	Differential, selective	*Salmonella* & *Shigella* spp.	*Salmonella* and *Shigella*: Blue, green Normal enterics: Orange, yellow	Has lactose, sucrose & salicin; most *Enterobacteriaceae* ferment one of these. Detects H_2S also.
Loeffler Agar	LAS	Slant	Enriched	*Corynebacterium* spp.	NA	Coryneforms grow in angular groups.
Lowenstein-Jensen Agar	LJ	Slant	Enriched	Isolation of AFB	NA	
Lowenstein-Jensen Gruft	LJG	Slant	Enriched, selective	Isolation of AFB	NA	
MacConkey Agar	MAC	Plate	Differential, selective	Gm(–) enteric bacilli	Lactose (+): pink Lactose(–): colorless	Gm(+) organisms are inhibited by bile salts.
MacConkey w/Sorbitol Agar	SMAC	Plate	Differential, selective	Isolation of *E. coli* 0157:H7	Sorbitol (+): pink Sorbitol(–): colorless	*E. coli* 0157:H7 does NOT ferment sorbitol.
Mannitol Salt Agar	MAS	Plate	Differential, selective	Isolation of staphylococci	Mannitol(+): yellow Mannitol(–): pink, colorless	*S. aureus* colonies are Mannitol (+).
Mycobiotic Agar (Mycosel)	MYCO	Slant	Selective	Various fungi & gm(+)	NA	
Sabouaud Dextrose Agar	SDA	Plate & Slant	Enriched	Various fungi & gm(+) &gm(–) bacteria		
Selenite Broth	SEL	Tube	Enriched, selective	Enrichment for *Salmonella & Shigella*	NA	
Streptococcus Selective Agar	SXT	Plate	Differential, selective	Isolation of β-hemolytic strep	Patterns of hemolysis	Most gm(–) organisms are inhibited.
Thiosulfate-Citrate-Bile Salts-Sucrose	TCBS	Pour Plate	Differential, selective	Isolation of *Vibrio* spp.	Sucrose(+): Yellow or orange Sucrose(–): Green	MAC most other gm(–) organisms: MAC not recommended for culture of *Vibrio*.
Xylose-Lysine Desoxycholate Agar	XLD	Plate	Differential, selective	Enteric pathogens (e.g., *Salmonella* & *Shigella*)	Normal enterics: Yellow Enteric pathogens: Pink to red	Contains xylose, lactose and sucrose; normal enteric flora usually ferment at least one of these. Detects H_2S, which shows as black pigment.

gm(+), gram-positive; gm(–), gram-negative; AFB, acid-fast bacilli.

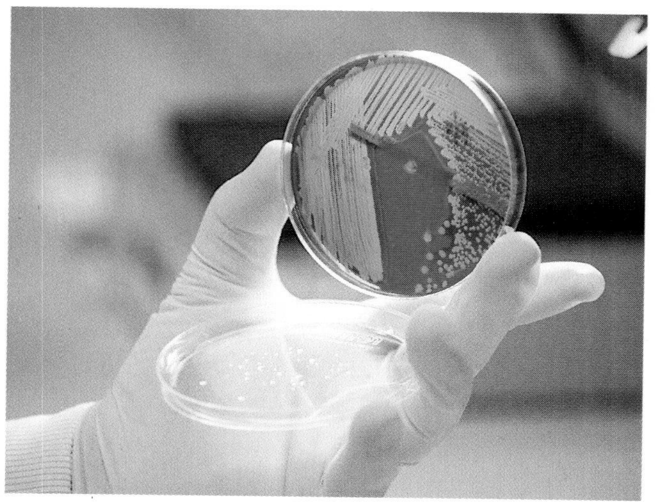

Figure 25–2. *Clear area around lysed red blood cells.*

chemical base and 5% sheep blood. Blood agar allows us to determine whether an organism is **hemolytic.** Beta-hemolytic bacteria cause complete **lysis** of red cells, producing a clear area around the colony of bacteria (Fig. 25–2). Alpha-hemolytic bacteria cause incomplete lysis, producing a greenish coloration around the colony (Fig. 25–3). Bacteria that have no hemolytic effect are sometimes called gamma-hemolytic bacteria (Fig. 25–4).

Chocolate Agar

Chocolate agar uses the same base as blood agar but is prepared differently. The temperature is raised during preparation, which results in partial lysis of the red blood cells (RBCs) and causes the media to turn a chocolate color (Fig. 25–5). Nutrients present in the lysed cells are released into the media. These nutrients, known as **hemin** (X factor), and a coenzyme called V factor, are added to supplement the agar, creating a nutrient-rich culture media. *Neisseria gonorrhea, Haemophilus* species, and other fastidious organisms grow best on chocolate agar.

Figure 25–3. *Incomplete hemolysis producing greenish coloration.*

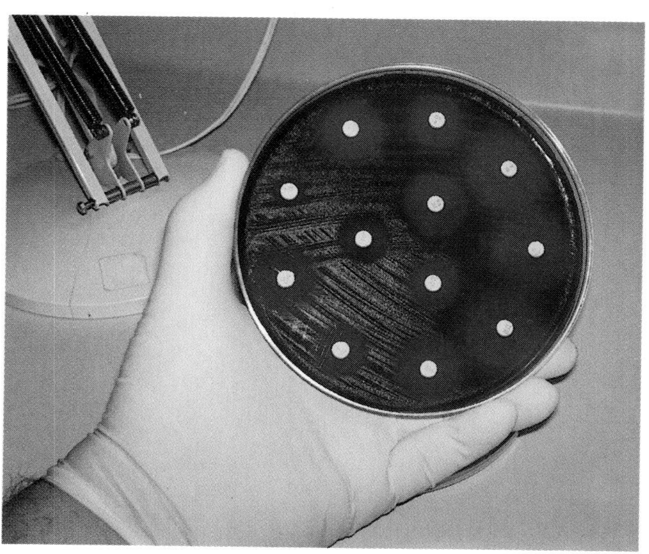

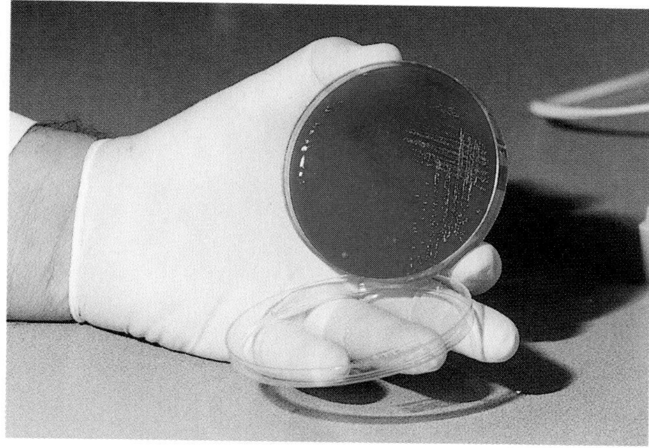

Figure 25–4. *Gamma hemolytic strep.*

MacConkey (MC) Agar

MacConkey (MC) agar is a selective and differential medium that inhibits the growth of gram-positive cocci while allowing gram-negative bacilli to grow easily. Lactose-fermenting, gram-negative bacteria produce colonies that range in color from pink to red (Fig. 25–6). Nonlactose fermenters remain colorless (Fig. 25–7). MacConkey agar is useful in the isolation of enteric bacilli.

Figure 25–5. *Chocolate agar.*

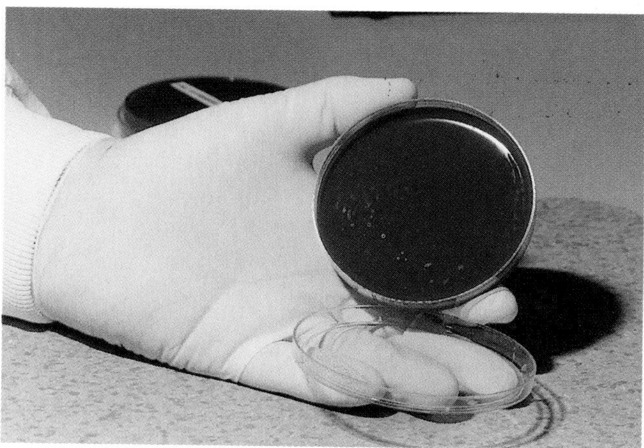

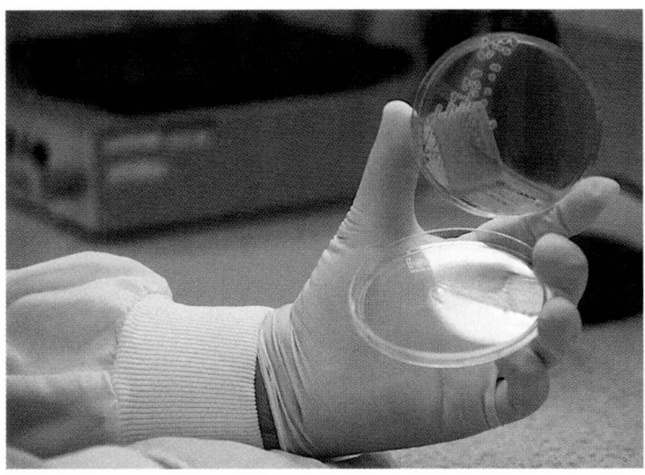

Figure 25–6. *Gram-negative bacilli, showing pink to red color range.*

Chopped Meat (CM) Broth

Chopped meat (CM) broth consists of ground meat in a nutrient broth (Fig. 25–8). It comes in a capped tube and promotes the growth of most bacteria, especially anaerobes.

Streptococcal Selective Agar (SSA)

Streptococcal selective agar (SSA) is modified sheep agar that inhibits most streptococci, except for *Streptococcus pyogenes* and *Streptococcus agalactiae*. These organisms are beta-hemolytic, and can be readily observed on SSA (Fig. 25–9). This type of media is used primarily for the detection of *Streptococcus pyogenes,* a group A streptococci obtained from throat swabs.

Thayer-Martin (TM) Agar

Modified Thayer-Martin (TM) agar is chocolate agar that has been enriched with vitamins and other supplements and to which has been added antibiotic inhibitors. It is primarily used to culture pathogenic *Neisseria* species.

Figure 25–7. *Colorless nonlactose fermenters.*

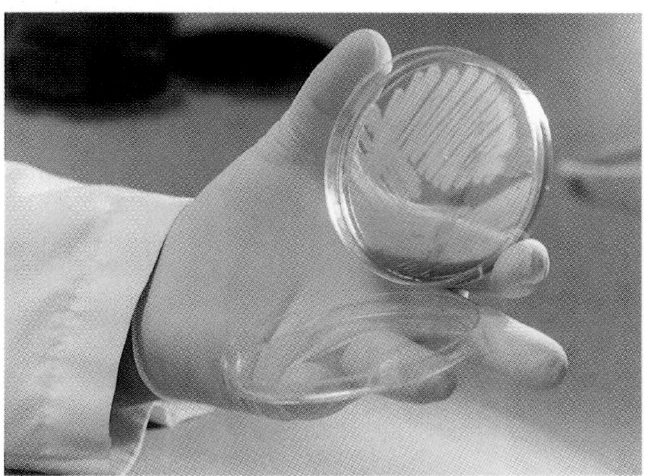

Hektoen Enteric (HE) Agar

Hektoen enteric (HE) agar is a selective and differential medium that inhibits normal fecal flora while allowing the growth of *Salmonella* and *Shigella* species. The colonies of lactose-fermenting bacteria are yellow (Fig. 25–10*A*). Hydrogen sulfide–producing bacteria, such as the *Salmonella* species, cause a black precipitation to form around the colonies (Fig. 25–10*B*).

Basic Culture Techniques

Specimens for bacterial culture are inoculated to media by spreading or streaking the specimen over the surface of the agar. A pattern is used to allow quantitation of bacterial growth, as well as the isolation of individual colonies of bacteria.

The basic streaking pattern is illustrated in Figure 25–11, *A* and *B*. The plates are divided into quadrants, with an initial streak placed in the first quadrant. The second streak goes into the second quadrant, thus spreading the colonies for isolation. The third and fourth streak areas continue on until the plate is filled. The streaking is accomplished by using a sterile microbiologic loop. These loops may be plastic and dispos-

Figure 25–8. *Chopped meat broth agar.*

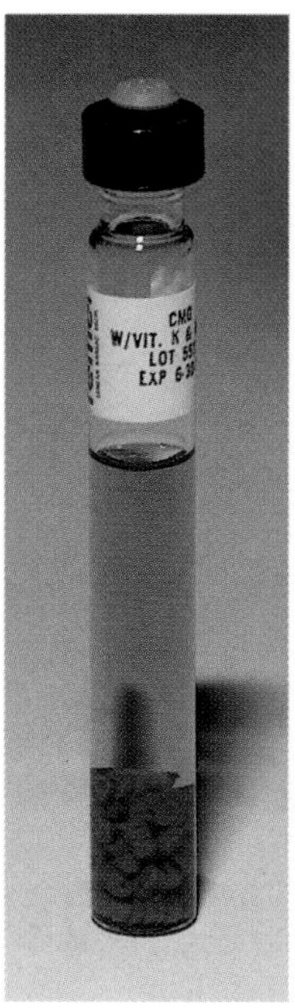

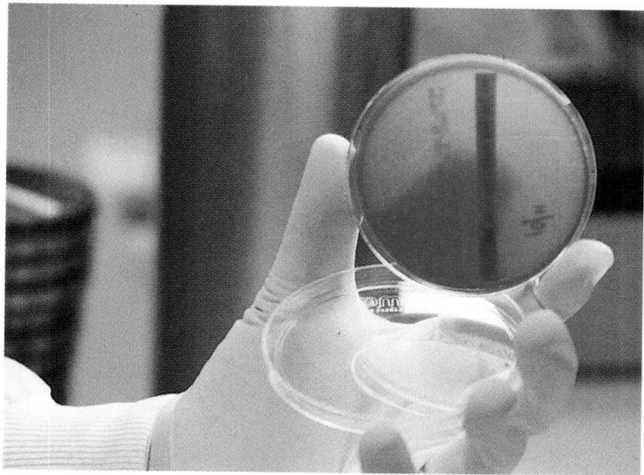

Figure 25–9. *Photo of hemolysis on SSA*

able, or they may be wire and reusable. The wire loops are sterilized between streaks using heat (Fig. 25–11*C*).

PRECAUTION: Bunsen burners or other open flames are hazardous and are not advised for use in sterilizing microbiologic loops. The preferred method is using a flameless heating element that eliminates aerosols, a totally self-contained cinerator unit, or disposable loops.

Urine Culture

Unlike the infectious agents of other specimen types, the etiologic agents of urinary tract infection are limited to a few rapidly growing microorganisms.

Pyuria, together with **bacteriuria,** is an important factor in establishing the presence of a urinary tract infection. Several guidelines for the interpretation of significant bacteriuria in a variety of patient populations have been suggested.

Urine specimens are submitted for culture from patients with symptoms of urinary tract infection and from asymptomatic patients with a high risk of infection. *Klebsiella-Enterobacter* species, *Proteus* species, and *Pseudomonas* species constitute a majority of the organisms isolated in such patients.

Specimen Collection

Urine is normally a sterile body fluid, but if collected improperly, it can become contaminated with microbiota from the perineum, prostate, urethra, or vagina. The assistant MUST provide detailed instructions to ensure proper specimen collection.

The best sample is a clean-voided midstream specimen collected in a sterile container. For detailed collection instructions, refer to Chapter 7. Obtain an early-morning specimen whenever possible because of the increased bacterial counts after overnight incubation in the bladder. Do not have the patient force fluids in order to void, as excessive fluid intake will decrease the colony count. If the patient has been asymptomatic, have him or her collect three consecutive early-morning specimens. If the urine specimen must be transported, collect at least 3 mL of urine into a transport tube containing a preservative to avoid an inhibiting or diluting effect on the microorganisms.

Semiquantitative Streaking

An inoculating loop, calibrated to retain 0.001 mL of urine, is immersed into an uncentrifuged urine sample and a streak is made across the center of an agar plate.

Figure 25–10. A, *Lactose-fermenting bacteria.* B, *Black precipitation around colonies.*

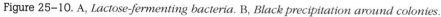

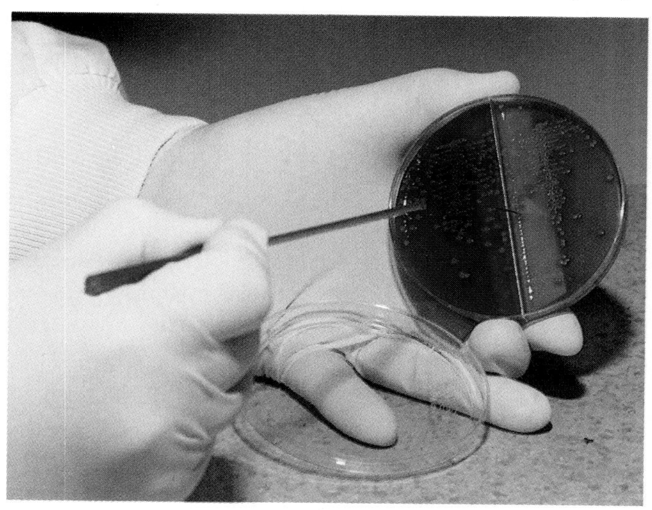

A

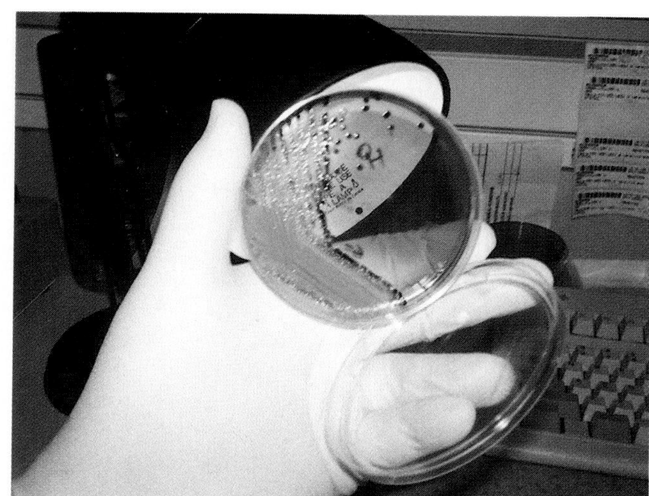

B

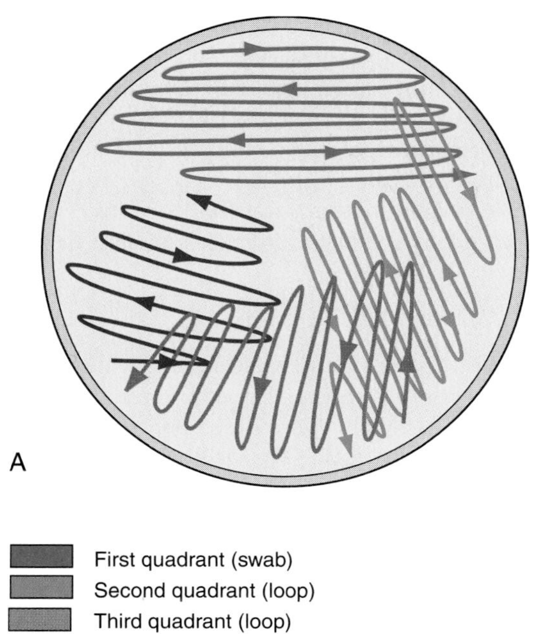

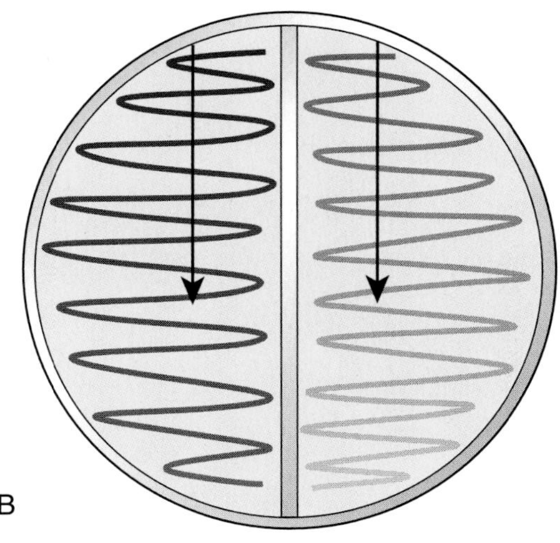

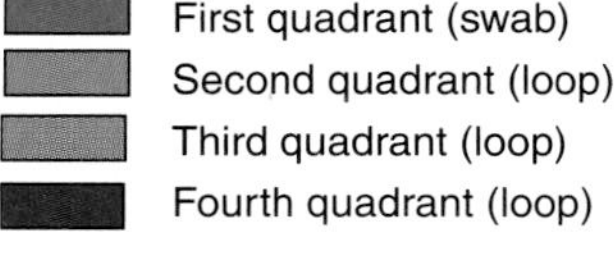

Pattern used to count the number of colonies of bacteria that appear on the surface of the original incubated inoculum

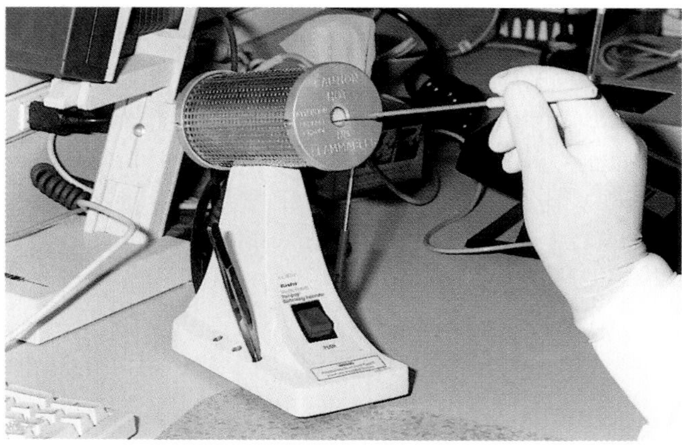

Figure 25–11. A, *Drawing of basic streaking pattern.* B, *Pattern for counting the number of colonies.* C, *Loop incinerator.*

The inoculum is then diluted by spreading it evenly at right angles to the primary streak (see Fig. 25–11*A*). Remember to resterilize your loop between each phase of the streaking procedure. Label the agar side of the Petri dish with the patient's name, the date and time, and the type of specimen used. Place the sample into the incubator, agar side up.

After 18 to 24 hours of incubation, the number of colonies of bacteria in the urine sample is estimated by counting the number of colonies that appear on the surface of the media. To count the colonies, lightly score a straight line from edge to edge, through the center of the agar. Using the wire loop, count the colonies on each side of the dish, following a zigzag pattern (Fig. 25–11*B*). If 50 colonies are counted using the 0.001 mL loop, the number of colonies should be multiplied by 1000 to yield a total of 50,000 colonies/mL in the urine sample.

Throat Culture for Group A Streptococcus

Although viruses cause some sore throats, the primary cause of bacterial pharyngitis in North America is *Streptococcus pyogenes* or group A streptococci ("strep"). Group A strep is important because infection can occasionally lead to bacterial **endocarditis,** rheumatic fever, or acute **glomerulonephritis.**

Collection Technique

A sufficient sample of organisms must be collected to grow a representative throat culture. This is accomplished by swabbing the throat with a sterile Dacron

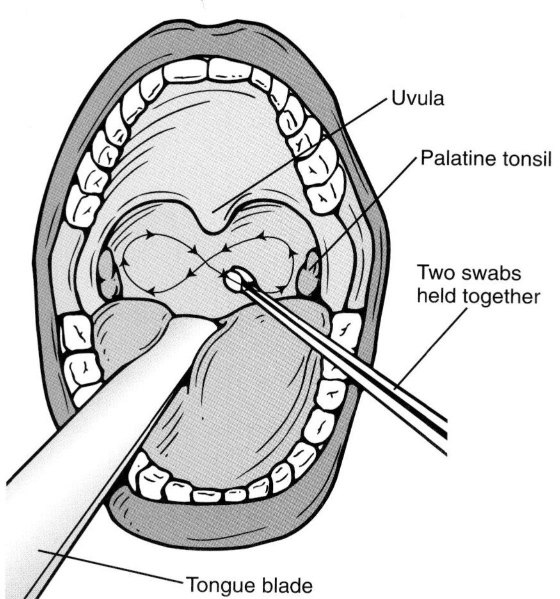

Figure 25–12. *Technique for obtaining a throat sample.*

swab. **Cotton swabs may inhibit Streptococcus and so should not be used.** While holding the patient's tongue down with a depressor, the specimen is taken directly from the back of the throat and tonsils (Fig. 25–12). Avoid touching the swab to the teeth or the inside of the mouth during collection of the specimen. The swab should be rubbed on the target areas in a horizontal, lazy-8, or large circular pattern. Two swabs can be done at the same time. One is then used for the enzyme test and, if it is negative, the second swab is used for the culture. The swab is placed in a sterile collection tube with media if a culture is to be done. The tube must be labeled with the patient's full name and any other necessary identification (e.g., patient number, date of birth, etc.) (Fig. 25–13, *A* and *B*).

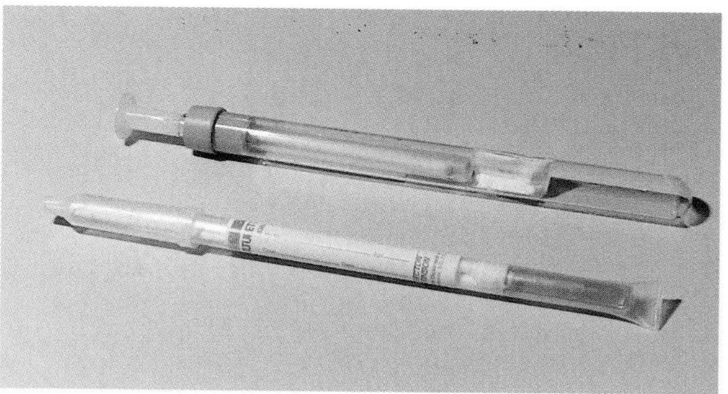

A

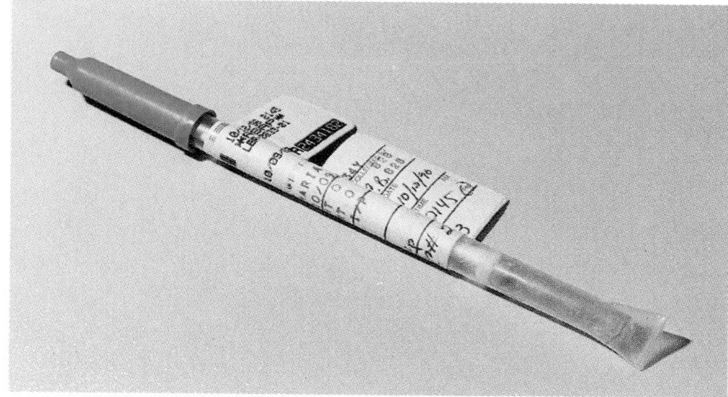

B

Figure 25–13. A, *Sterile collection tube.* B, *Labeled collection tube.*

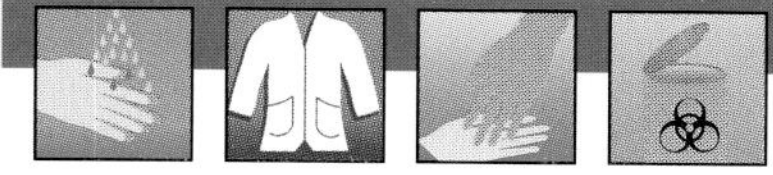

PROCEDURE 25–1

Obtaining a Throat Swab for Culture

Principle

To obtain an adequate, noncontaminated sample for culture and screening for group A beta-hemolytic Streptococcus

Equipment and Supplies

tongue depressor
2 sterile dacron swabs
sterile specimen container with transport media
laboratory marker

Procedural Steps

1. Wash hands and dry them thoroughly.
2. Assemble needed supplies and obtain a laboratory request form.
3. Explain the procedure to the patient.
4. Put on gloves.
5. Position the patient and adjust the light source to provide visualization of the pharyngeal area.
6. Carefully remove both swabs from the sterile wrapping.
7. Instruct the patient to open his or her mouth and say "ah."

(continued)

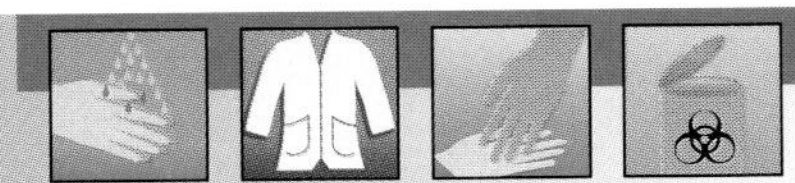

PROCEDURE 25–1

Obtaining a Throat Swab for Culture (Continued)

8. Depress the tongue with the tongue blade.
9. Holding both swabs together, firmly swab the tonsillar pillars and any area that appears to be infected using a figure-of-eight or circular pattern.
10. Place swabs containing the specimen in the media transport tube.
11. Label the container.
12. Dispose of all contaminated materials according to laboratory protocol and OSHA standards.
13. Remove gloves and wash your hands.
14. Record the procedure in the laboratory logbook.

Testing Technique

Routine throat cultures are grown on 5% sheep blood agar, MacConkey agar, chocolate agar, or SSA. Throat cultures for beta-hemolytic streptococci are inoculated to 5% sheep agar and SSA. To inoculate a throat culture, lift the lid on the properly labeled agar plate just enough to allow entrance of the swab. Gently roll the swab across the surface of one quadrant of the plate (Fig. 25–14). Then use a sterile loop to spread the **inoculum** across the area where the specimen was just placed. Spread the inoculum into the second quadrant with the loop, crossing the first quadrant two or three times. Use the loop to spread the specimen into the third quadrant by entering the second quadrant two or three times. When streaking the organism from the third quadrant to the fourth, the loop enters the previously streaked third quadrant two or three times (Fig. 25–11*A*). The agar plate is turned a quarter turn each time a quadrant is streaked. This technique is called *streaking for isolation,* as the number of organisms introduced to each quadrant is fewer than the number in the one before. Most laboratories place a disk of **bacitracin,** an antimicrobial, on the overlap between the first and second quadrants of the plate to give an early indication of the presence of group A streptococcal organisms (Fig. 25–15). Bacitracin inhibits the growth of this organism.

After streaking, the plate is incubated for 18 to 24 hours at 35°C in a candle jar or CO_2 incubator (Fig. 25–16). Growth of streptococci is enhanced by incubation in an environment of increased CO_2. Agar plates are incubated upside down to prevent condensation from dropping onto the agar surface.

Figure 25–14. *The lid of a Petri dish opened and the swab being rolled across one quadrant.*

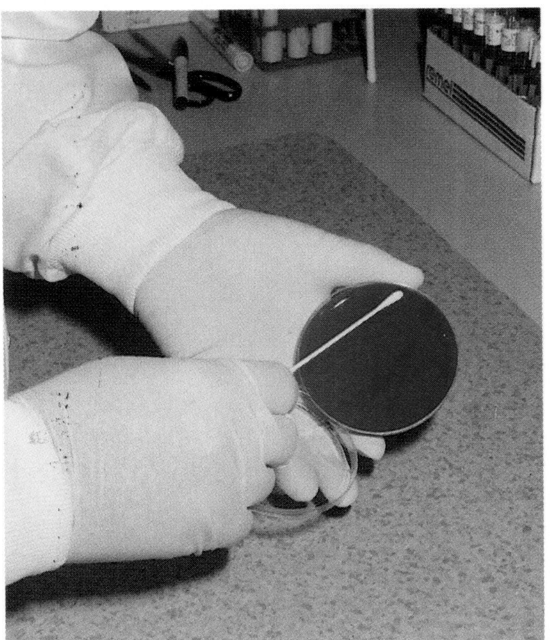

Figure 25–15. *Culture plate with placement of bacitracin disk in the first quadrant.*

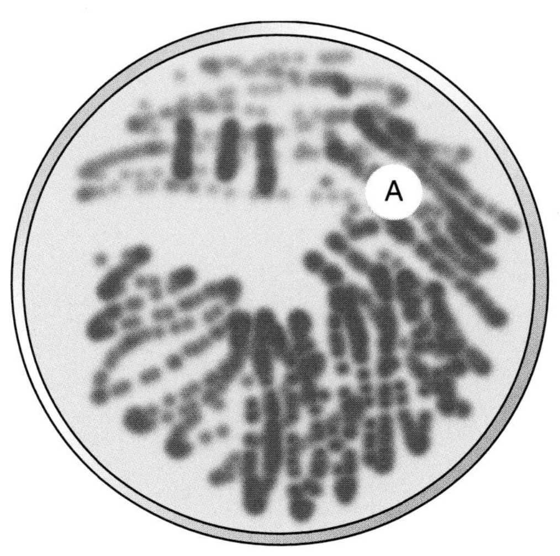

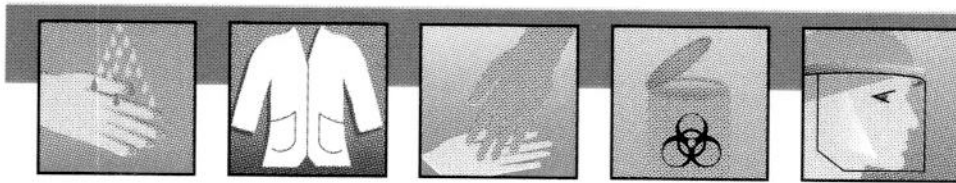

PROCEDURE 25–2

Preparing a Throat Swab Culture

Principle

To inoculate throat specimens and isolate streptococcal organisms using the proper technique and streaking pattern

Equipment and Supplies

thumb forceps
bacitracin disk
sterile specimen container containing swabs with bacteria
blood agar plate
wire inoculating loops
loop incinerator
incubator set at 35°–37°C
laboratory marker
loop holder

Procedural Steps

1. Wash hands and dry them thoroughly.
2. Assemble all equipment and supplies.
3. Turn on the loop incinerator.
4. Place the inoculating loop in a holder close to your work area.
5. Put on gloves and other protective gear.
6. Pick up the specimen container with your nondominant hand and remove the cap.
7. Remove one of the swabs.
8. Recap the container and set aside for later use.
9. Place a blood agar plate on the table, agar side down, and lift the lid.
10. Roll the swab through the first quadrant.
11. Place the swab in a biohazard waste container.
12. Sterlilize the loop in the loop incinerator and allow it to cool.
13. Using the loop, streak for isolation of colonies in the second, third, and fourth quadrants (see Fig. 25–11).
14. Use the loop to make three stabs in the agar in the first quadrant.
15. Resterilize the loop and sterilize the thumb forceps.
16. Using the sterile thumb forceps, remove one bacitracin disk from the disk vial.
17. Place the disk on the agar in the overlap between the first and second quadrant.
18. Resterilize the thumb forceps.
19. With the laboratory marker, label the agar side (bottom) of the plate with the patient's name and the date.
20. Place the agar plate in the incubator, agar side up.
21. Record the procedure in the laboratory logbook.
22. Dispose of all biohazardous waste according to laboratory protocols and OSHA standards. Clean and disinfect the work area.
23. Remove gloves and wash hands.

Interpreting Results

Identification of organisms is based on the presence of beta-hemolytic streptococci that are inhibited by bacitracin. The colonies themselves appear slightly opaque and are about the size of pinpoints. Additional identification may be based on biochemical and serologic testing. Unless the specimens test positive in the first 24 hours of incubation, throat cultures are finalized 48 hours after inoculation, although there is a trend toward finalizing negative cultures in less than 48 hours.

Rapid Strep Test

Frequently, in the physician's office, there is a need to establish a quick diagnosis for suspected streptococcal infection so that antibiotics may be started immediately. Rapid strep tests usually require 4 to 10 minutes to process. When using this type of testing, the physician is able to obtain the test results quickly, and can confirm the diagnosis in a very short period of time. The patient can then be started on antibiotics (if appropriate) and all can be accomplished in one office visit.

The most commonly used procedure is the direct antigen identification test, which confirms the presence of group A streptococcus through an antigen-antibody reaction (Fig. 25–17). If the group A streptococcus antigen is present in the specimen, it will combine with antibody-sensitized particles to produce agglutination or a color change that can easily be observed with the naked eye.

When performing a rapid strep test in the laboratory, it is always important to read the directions that are included with each commercially available antigen identification test. Once the directions are read, be sure to follow them exactly as written. Results will be inconclusive if shortcuts are taken.

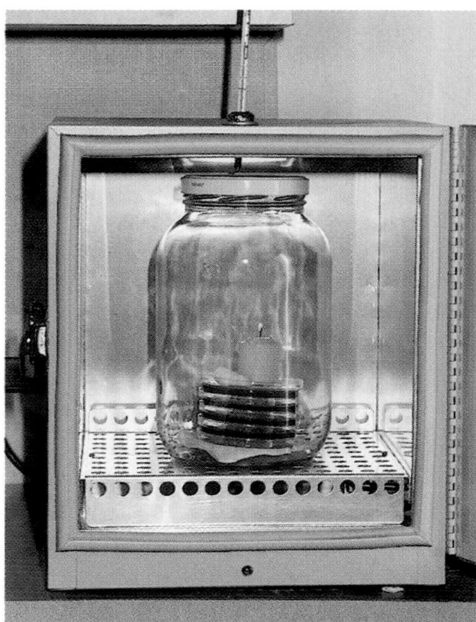

Figure 25–16. *The candle jar.*

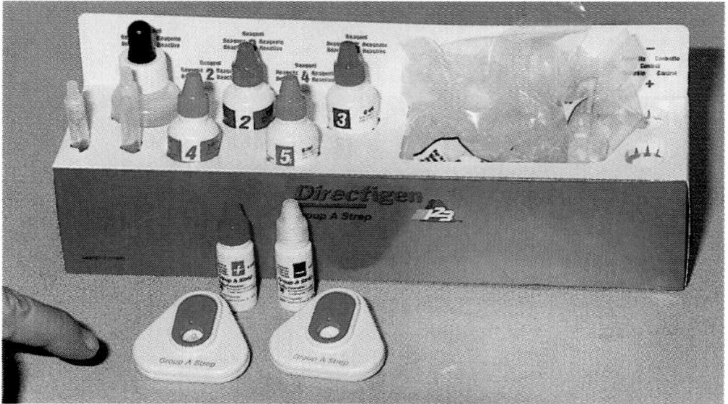

A

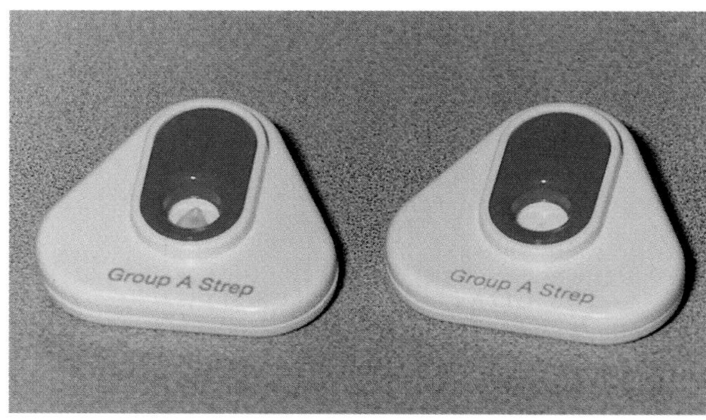

B

Figure 25–17. A, *Becton-Dickenson Directigen–Group A rapid strep test.* B, *Test results: left, positive; right, negative.*

TEST

Examples of Antigen Identification Tests

- Abbott Laboratories: *TestPack Strep A*
- Access Medical Systems, Inc.: *Access Icon Strep A*
- Becton Dickinson: *Directigen*
- Ventrex Laboratories: *Ventrescreen*

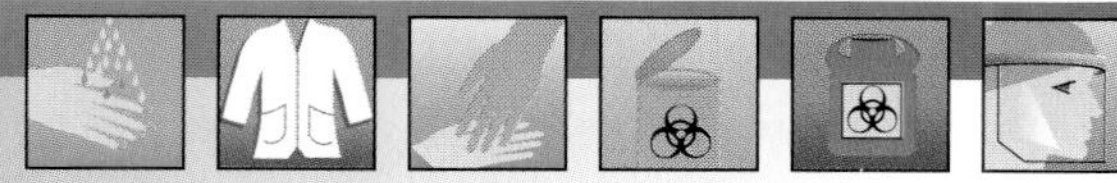

PROCEDURE 25–3

Performing a Rapid Strep Test

Principle

To prepare a slide for microscopic identification of group A beta-hemolytic streptococci

Equipment and Supplies

Abbott TestPack +Plus Strep A
clock or watch
throat swab obtained in Procedure 25–1

Procedural Steps

1. Before beginning the assay, bring all reagents and reaction disks to room temperature (minimum of 30 minutes).
2. Position all bottles vertically, and dispense reagents slowly as free-falling drops. Avoid reagent contact with eyes, as the reagent is an irritant.
3. Wash hands, dry them thoroughly, and put on gloves and other protective gear.
4. Add 3 drops of **reagent 1** to an extraction tube. This solution should be pink.
5. Add 3 drops of **reagent 2** to the same tube. This solution should turn yellow.
6. Place the specimen swab in the tube, twirling the swab to mix.
7. Let stand for exactly 1 minute.
8. Add 3 drops of **reagent 3** to the same tube, again twirling the swab in the tube to mix. This solution should be pink.
9. Express the liquid from the swab by squeezing the tube with the thumb and forefinger and rotating the swab as it is withdrawn. The liquid must be thoroughly removed from the swab. Best results are achieved when the liquid reaches or exceeds the line on the tube.

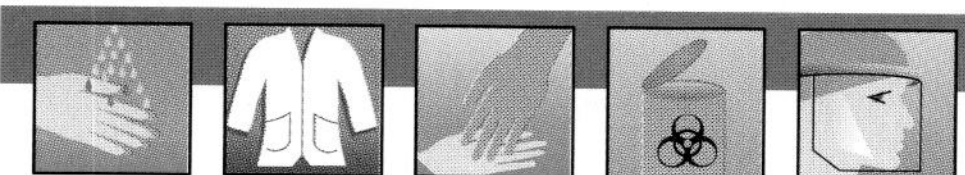

PROCEDURE 25–3

Performing a Rapid Strep Test (Continued)

10. Discard the swab in biohazard waste container.
11. Remove the **reaction disk** from the pouch and place it on a dry, flat surface.
12. Pour the entire contents of the tube into the **sample well.**
13. Read the test results when the entire **end of assay window** turns red (in approximately 5–10 min).
14. Properly dispose of all contaminated waste, including the specimen swab, gloves, extraction tube, and reaction disk, after use. Items contacting samples should be considered potentially infectious.
15. Record the test results and enter the test in the laboratory logbook.

Interpretation of Results

Positive Result: A **plus sign (+)** in the **result window** indicates a positive test result for group A streptococcal antigen. A pink or red color (darker than the background) on the **patient bar** is interpreted as a positive result even if it has less color than the **control bar.** In the presence of very low antigen levels, only a portion of the plus sign may develop.

Negative Result: A **minus sign (–)** in the **result window** indicates a negative test result for group A streptococcal antigen. If the test result is inconsistent with the patient's clinical presentation, a follow-up throat swab should be collected for repeat testing or culture.

Summary

When obtaining specimens that are likely to be of an infectious nature, it is important to remember the rules of basic asepsis. By practicing good techniques, you can prevent and control infection of yourself and fellow employees.

Infected individuals need treatment as quickly as possible. The method and technique used to obtain a specimen for culture and the accuracy of culture preparation will ensure early diagnosis and treatment of the patient.

Chapter Review

True or False

Circle T or F to indicate the correct answers to the following:

T F 1. Anaerobic microorganisms are air-tolerant.

T F 2. Rapid strep tests require 40 to 60 minutes before results can be obtained.

T F 3. Bacteria that are capable of producing disease are pathogenic.

T F 4. Most bacteria grow best in temperatures greater than 45°C.

Fill in the Blanks

Complete the following statements:

5. The most commonly used culture media is

_____________ _____________ .

6. Elements important for the growth of microorganisms are:

_____________ , _____________ , _____________ ,

_____________ , and _____________ .

7. MacConkey agar is a _____________ and

_____________ media.

Multiple Choice

Circle the letter that represents the single best answer:

8. Throat cultures are usually grown on:
   a. Mannitol salt agar
   b. Chocolate agar
   c. Thayer-Martin agar
   d. Chopped meat agar
   e. 5% sheep blood agar
9. Blood agar will determine whether an organism is:
   a. Aerobic
   b. Nonfastidious
   c. Hemolytic
   d. Fastidious
   e. Gram-negative
10. An organism that lives and grows in the absence of molecular oxygen is:
    a. Anaerobic
    b. Aerobic
    c. Hemolytic
    d. Spore
    e. Nonfastidious

Vocabulary

bacteremia: the presence of bacteria in the blood

cellulitis: a diffuse inflammatory process within solid tissues

coagulase: an enzyme that causes coagulation of citrated plasma

commensal: living on or within an organism without causing harm to the host; nonparasitic

exudate: a fluid with a high concentration of protein and cellular debris that has escaped the blood vessels, usually as the result of inflammation

fascia: a sheet of fibrous connective tissue deep in the body that supports and separates muscles

gonorrhea: a sexually transmitted infection characterized by inflammation of the mucous membranes of the reproductive and urinary tracts

mastoditis: inflammation of the air cells of the portion of the temporal bone lying behind the external opening of the ear

meningitis: an inflammation of the meninges causing edema of the brain's covering, which, in turn, causes pressure on brain tissue

necrosis: morphologic changes indicative of cell death caused by enzymatic degradation

nosocomial: pertaining to or acquired during hospitalization, as in an infection

opportunistic: denoting a normally harmless species of bacteria that becomes pathogenic under specific circumstances

otitis media: inflammation of the middle ear

paronychia: inflammation involving the folds of tissue surrounding the nail

pharyngitis: inflammation of the throat

phlegm: a viscid mucus excreted from the respiratory tract

polymorphs: leukocytes appearing in different forms in different developmental stages

sebaceous: an oil-secreting gland in the skin

subarachnoid: between the surface layer and the pia mater layer of the skull

sudoriferous: glands in the skin that produce sweat

suppuration: the formation or discharge of pus

tonsillitis: inflammation of the palatine tonsils in the throat

urethritis: inflammation of the canal that extends from the bladder to the outside of the body

Chapter Objectives

After reading this chapter, you should be able to:

1. Define and explain normal flora.
2. Distinguish between the genus and the species name of bacteria.
3. Describe the four standard factors used for identifying bacteria.
4. Identify the pyogenic species that are common bacterial pathogens, and give examples of diseases caused by each.
5. Identify the genus Enterobacteriaceae and the common species in this group.
6. Distinguish between commensal and nosocomial infections.
7. Identify the *Mycobacterium* species and the major infections they cause.
8. Explain why health care workers are susceptible to *Mycobacterium tuberculosis*.
9. Describe the purpose of rapid chemical tests.
10. Outline six types of rapid chemical testing procedures and the bacteria each will identify.
11. Compare manual, semi-automated, and automated testing systems.
12. List the most frequently diagnosed bacteria in each of the body systems.
13. Identify existing conditions that make a person susceptible to disease.

Chapter 26
Bacteriology

Bacteria are single-celled organisms that are found everywhere in our environment. Their natural habitats include fresh water, salt water, soil, and living organisms. Most bacteria are not harmful to us, and within their normal habitats, they play a vital role in aiding body functions. However, a small percentage of bacteria are responsible for a wide range of common infections.

Normal Flora

Living within every body is a group of microorganisms called normal flora. These bacteria live in specific locations where there is a favorable environment. As long as they remain in their resident environment, these bacteria remain beneficial to us and do not pose problems to healthy normal tissue and body functions. However, if these flora move out of their natural sites into areas within our bodies that do not recognize them, they may become pathogenic, (in which case they are said to cause **opportunistic** infections.

Bacterial Nomenclature

When referring to bacteria, we use two names. The first is the genus and the second is the species. The genus name is always capitalized, but the species is not. For example, let us consider *Streptococcus viridans* and *Streptococcus pyogenes*. Both of these bacteria come from the same bacterial family and the same genus. This tells you that the two bacteria are similar or are related. Now look at the species name. Each of these species is different enough to be given its own name. Think of your own name. You share your last name with your siblings, even some of your cousins perhaps, but each of you is an individual. Thus, you are given different first names to allow identification as individuals belonging to a family.

When looking at laboratory reports, you will notice that, frequently, the

Table 26–1
Bacterial Colony Morphology

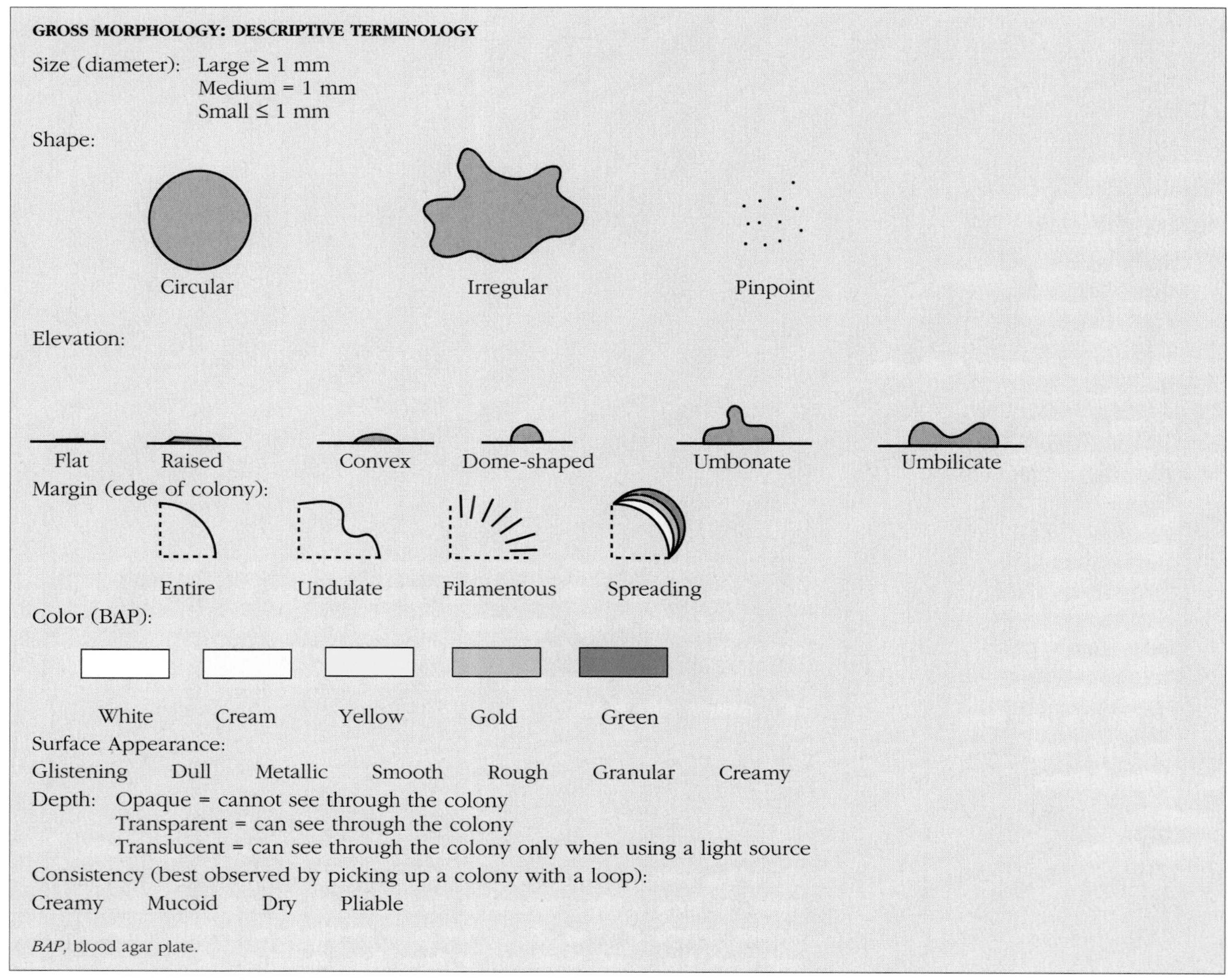

GROSS MORPHOLOGY: DESCRIPTIVE TERMINOLOGY

Size (diameter): Large ≥ 1 mm
Medium = 1 mm
Small ≤ 1 mm

Shape:

Circular Irregular Pinpoint

Elevation:

Flat Raised Convex Dome-shaped Umbonate Umbilicate

Margin (edge of colony):

Entire Undulate Filamentous Spreading

Color (BAP):

White Cream Yellow Gold Green

Surface Appearance:

Glistening Dull Metallic Smooth Rough Granular Creamy

Depth: Opaque = cannot see through the colony
Transparent = can see through the colony
Translucent = can see through the colony only when using a light source

Consistency (best observed by picking up a colony with a loop):

Creamy Mucoid Dry Pliable

BAP, blood agar plate.

genus name is shortened. For instance, *Escherichia coli* may be written *E. coli, Streptococcus pyogenes* may be abbreviated *S. pyogenes,* or *Staphylococcus aureus* may be written *S. aureus.* Thus, it is important that you learn both the genus and the species names of the common pathogens.

Bacterial Grouping

There are four standard factors used to identify bacteria in the laboratory. Identification is based on (1) cellular morphology, (2) colony morphology, (3) biochemical testing, and (4) antibiotic sensitivity testing (Tables 26–1 and 26–2).

In the laboratory, bacteria are usually divided into four basic groups: gram-positive cocci, gram-negative cocci, gram-positive bacilli, and gram-negative bacilli. Other, less commonly encountered morphologic shapes are curved rods and spirals. This grouping reflects the shape and color that the bacteria assume when they are stained (Fig. 26–1, *A* and *B*).

Gram staining of isolated colonies provides information on the cellular morphology of bacteria. Protocols for definitive identification and antibiotic sensitivities are based on bacterial cell morphology. Gram stain results are not always indicative of the bacteria's cellular morphology, however. Certain gram-positive bacteria lose some of their cell wall integrity and appear to

Table 26–2
Colony Morphology on Blood Agar Isolation Media

Organism	*Morphology*
GRAM-NEGATIVE	
Branhamella (Moraxella) species	Whitish, medium to large, raised or dome-shaped
Escherichia coli	Gray, mucoid, flat or dome-shaped; may be beta-hemolytic
Neisseria meningitidis	Medium to large, creamy and gray; alpha-hemolytic
Pseudomonas aeruginosa	Flat, gray, spreading
GRAM-POSITIVE	
Enterococcus species	Gray, medium; usually no hemolysis
Corynebacterium species	White, dry, may be sticky
Listeria monocytogenes	Whitish gray, similar to group B streptococcus; flat, narrow zones of beta-hemolysis
Staphylococcus aureus	Large, convex, white-yellow, creamy, opaque; may be beta-hemolytic
Staphylococcus epidermidis	White-gray, raised, creamy
Streptococcus pneumoniae	Umbilicate; alpha-hemolysis (greenish color); may be mucoid or teardrop-shaped
Streptococcus pyogenes	Pinpoint to medium; clear zone of beta-hemolysis; translucent, dull, gray
Streptococcus viridans	Pinpoint to medium; white-gray; caramel odor; alpha-hemolysis (greenish color) surrounding colony
YEAST	
Candida albicans	White, creamy; bread odor

stain like gram-negative organisms (see Tables 26–1 and 26–2).

Common Bacterial Pathogens

Pyogenic Organisms

One very common group of bacterial pathogens are labeled pyogenic (pus-producing). This group includes staphylococci, streptococci, pneumococci, gonococci, meningococci, and the coliform organisms. Whenever these organisms cause an infection within our bodies, we see an acute inflammatory response culminating in a massive infiltration by **polymorphs.** If our internal defenses are strong enough to destroy the invading organism, the infection will recede and disappear. If the invading organism persists, it will proceed on a mission of destruction, causing tissue **necrosis** and **suppuration.**

Staphylococci

Staphylococci are gram-positive cocci that usually grow in clusters. They are commonly found on the skin and are subdivided into two groups based on their ability to produce an enzyme called **coagulase.** The coagulase-positive organisms are generally the pathogens, whereas the coagulase-negative organisms are usually harmless, considered to be part of the indigenous flora (Fig. 26–2).

Staphylococcus aureus is a coagulase-positive organism. The nasal cavity is a pathogenic reservoir for this pathogen, and it can easily be spread to the skin. When the hands become contaminated, *S. aureus* can be transferred to other objects and people through touch. Skin lesions, including abscesses, postoperative wound infections, boils, carbuncles, **paronychia,** and impetigo, may be caused by *S. aureus.* A typical lesion is a circumscribed area of inflammation with suppuration. Other important staphylococcal infections include

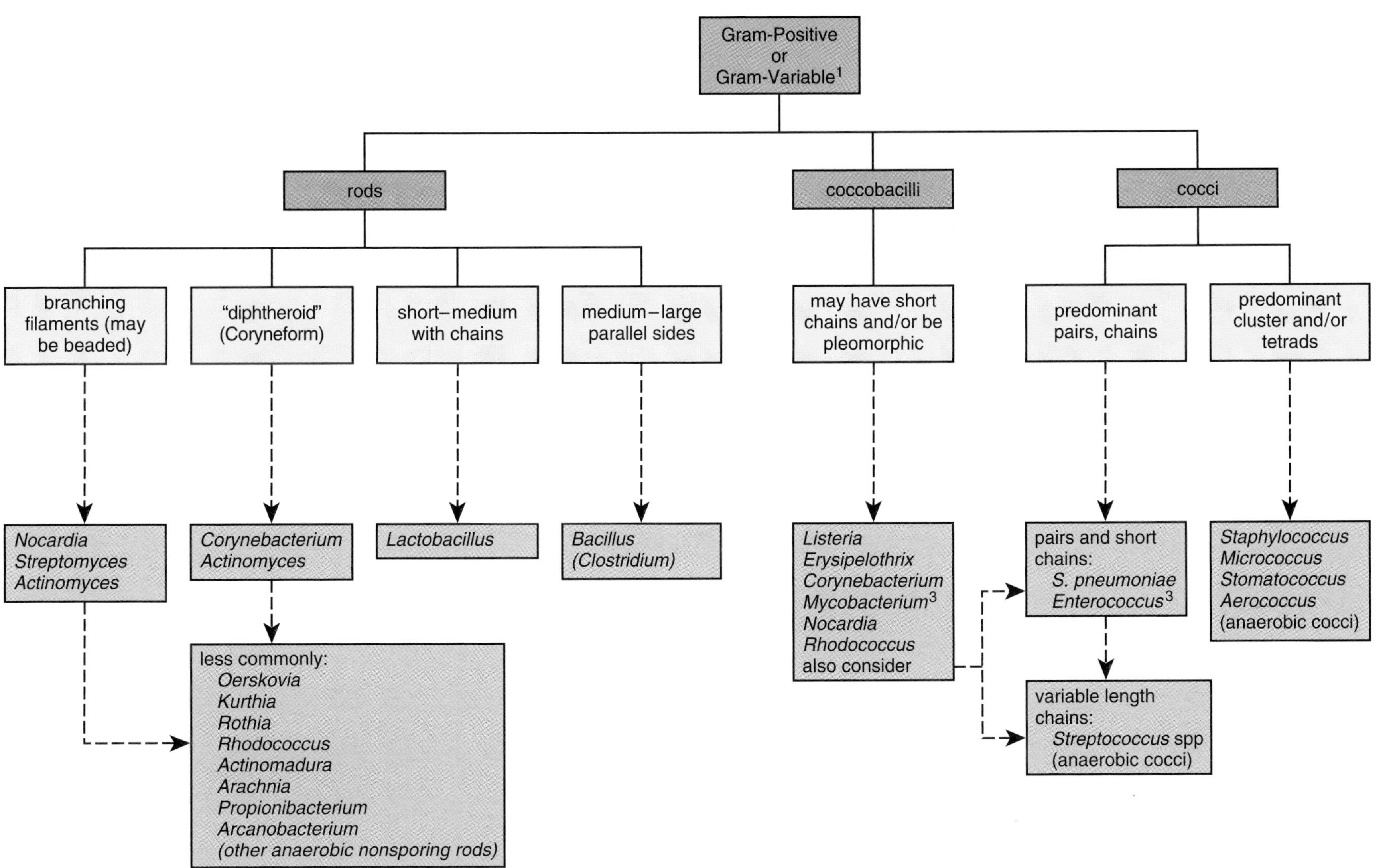

[1] Most gram-positive species can appear gram-variable or even gram-negative due to over-decolorization, phagocytosis, antibiotic-effect, age, etc.
[2] *Mycobacterium* species may stain gram-neutral and appear as "ghost" forms; they may also appear beaded, resembling chains of streptococci.
[3] Individual cells in chain vary in size.

A

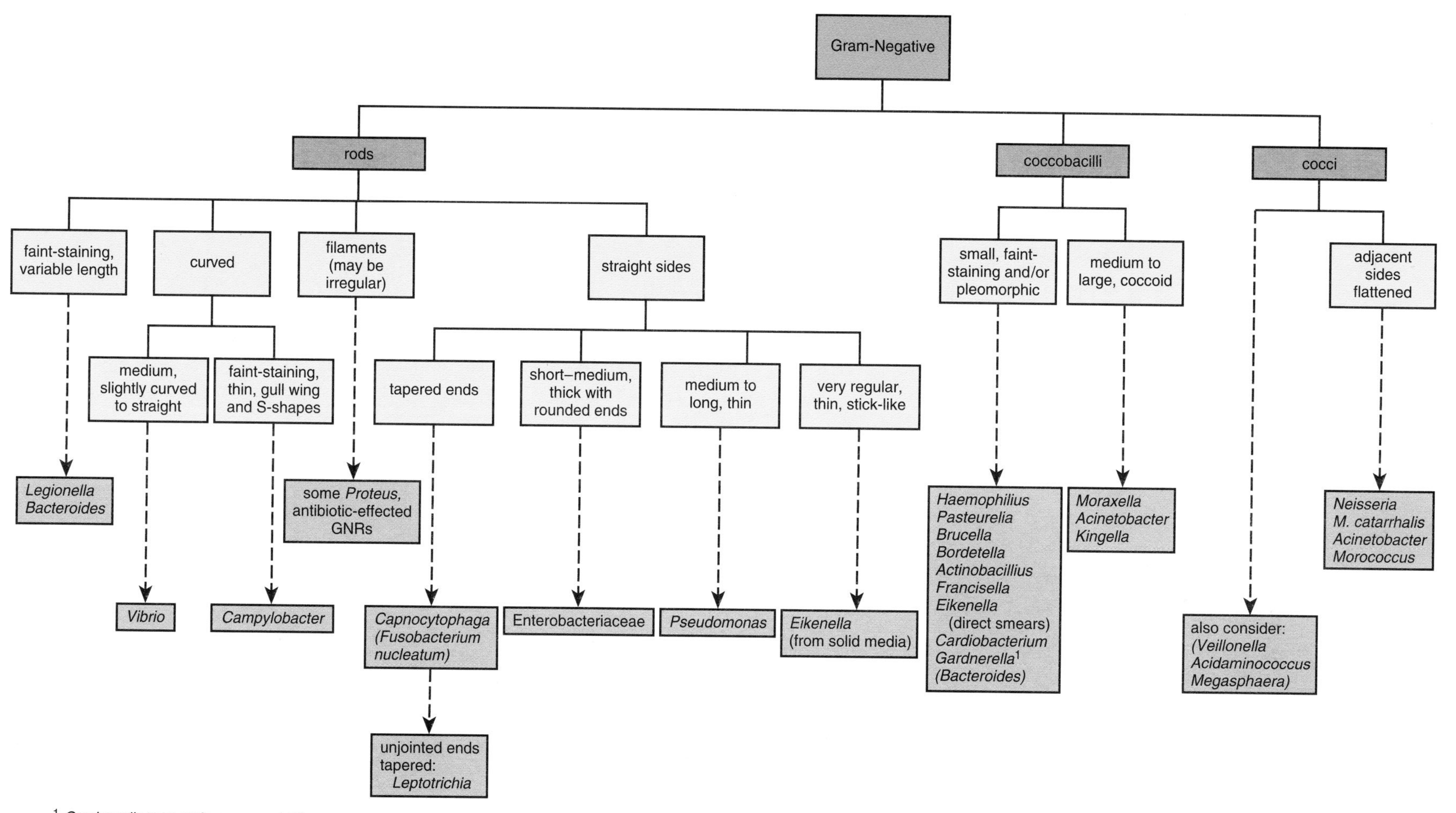

[1] *Gardnerella* may stain gram-variable.

B

Figure 26–1. *Morphology of organisms staining gram-positive or gram-variable* (A) *and gram-negative* (B). *GNRs, gram-negative rods.*

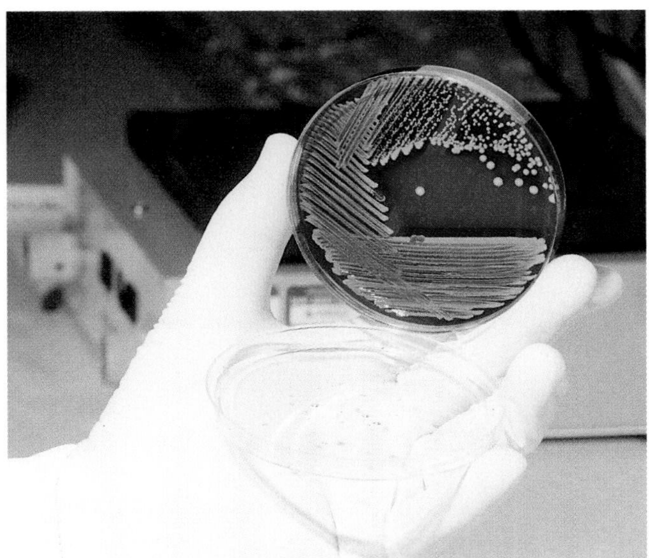

Figure 26–2. *Blood agar plate with pure culture of* Staphylococcus aureus.

bronchopneumonia, enterocolitis, and osteomyelitis. This organism is the second-leading cause of **nosocomial** infections.

Streptococci

Streptococci comprise another large genus of gram-positive organisms. They tend to grow in chains, and can be identified by Gram stain morphology, biochemical testing, and the type of colony produced on blood agar.

Streptococcus viridans (alpha-hemolytic streptococci) turns a greenish color and has a poorly defined, narrow zone of partial hemolysis around each colony grown on blood agar. *S. viridans* causes infections of the respiratory and circulatory systems, the most lethal of which is bacterial endocarditis.

S. pyogenes (a group A streptococcus) is a beta-hemolytic streptococcal organism that produces a very clear, easy-to-identify zone of complete hemolysis on blood agar. It is the most common human pathogen, accounting for approximately 90% of all streptococcal infections. *S. pyogenes* is often the pathogenic agent in **cellulitis, tonsillitis,** and **pharyngitis.** It can also spread to other parts of the body, causing **otitis media,** bronchopneumonia, rheumatic fever, or acute glomerulonephritis. When infections are left untreated, septicemia and **meningitis** may develop in the host.

Streptococcus agalactiae (a group B streptococcus) is a beta-hemolytic streptococci that produces CAMP factor. CAMP factor is a compound that acts in concert with the beta-toxin produced by certain strains of *S. aureus* to enhance beta-hemolysis. Many women carry this streptococci as genital flora. When transmitted during parturition, the organisms can cause serious systemic diseases in the neonate.

Enterococcus faecalis and *E. faecium* (nonhemolytic streptococci) are the most common enterococcal species encountered in humans. Enterococci are differentiated from streptococcal species by their ability to grow in 6.5% sodium chloride and 40% bile. They are part of the normal flora of the intestine, but they can also cause peritonitis, wound sepsis, urinary tract infections, and bacterial endocarditis. Enterococci are typically resistant to numerous antibiotics, making treatment difficult.

Pneumococci

Streptococcus pneumoniae is a diplococcus that can be differentiated from other streptococci on the basis of its lancet shape, its occurrence in pairs, and its well-defined capsule, all of which can be seen on Gram staining. It is commonly found in the throat of healthy individuals. Only a few virulent strains can penetrate the respiratory system defenses and invade the lung, causing lobar pneumonia. This most frequently occurs in people with a weakened or compromised respiratory system.

Gonococci

Neisseria gonorrhoeae is a gram-negative diplococcus whose only host is the human. Preliminary identification of this bacterial species is based on the presence of kidney-bean–shaped, gram-negative diplococci within the cytoplasm of intact white blood cells on a gram-stained smear prepared directly from a clinical specimen. Identification is further facilitated by growth of the organism on selective media, such as Thayer-Martin or modified Thayer-Martin. Definitive identification is based on the results of biochemical and serologic testing. This pathogen is generally spread through sexual intercourse and causes the venereal disease **gonorrhea.** If ignored and left untreated, gonococcal septicemia becomes a significant and severe complication. Penicillin-resistant *N. gonorrhoeae* now occurs with such frequency that penicillin is no longer the drug of choice for the treatment of gonorrhea.

Meningococci

Neisseria meningitidis is a gram-negative diplococcus that normally inhabits the nasopharynx. Identification is aided by a positive oxidase test and a smear that exhibits typical gram-negative diplococcal growth on selected media. Definitive identification requires biochemical and serologic testing. Occasionally, this organism can spread, producing septicemia and eventually settling in the **subarachnoid** space. This infection is then known as meningitis.

Enterobacteriaceae

The Enterobacteriaceae family comprises a large group of rod-shaped bacteria commonly referred to as enteric gram-negative bacilli. The Enterobacteriaceae family has expanded to include more than 100 species. Bacteria, such as *E. coli, Enterobacter* species, and *Klebsiella* species, are normal flora within the second half of the small intestine and the colon. Once outside this area, though, these normally **commensal** bacteria can become pus-producing, infectious agents. Pathogens, such as *Yersinia pestis, Shigella dysenteriae,* and *Salmonella* species, are among the most frequently isolated enterobacteriaceae in humans. Enterobacteriaceae are troublesome causes of wound infection and disease in every system of the human body. As a group, they are the most common cause of nosocomial infections, including urinary tract infections, pneumonia, and skin infections (Table 26–3).

Hemolytic-Uremic Syndrome

E. coli, serotype 0157:H7, is associated with hemolytic-uremic syndrome (HUS) in institutionalized older adults and young children. In 1993, an outbreak of HUS was found to be associated with the eating of hamburgers at a fast-food chain. The severe diarrhea associated with this outbreak of HUS caused several deaths, and hundreds of individuals became ill. An investigation revealed that the undercooked hamburger meat contained pathogenic *E. coli.* Following this documented episode, the Food and Drug Administration (FDA) adopted new guidelines for the preparation of ground meat sandwiches.

Table 26–3
Diseases and Conditions Associated With Enterobacteriaceae

URINARY TRACT INFECTION
Escherichia coli
Citrobacter
Klebsiella
Enterobacter
Serratia
Proteus
Providencia
Morganella

NEONATAL MENINGITIS
Escherichia coli
Edwardsiella
Citrobacter

DYSENTERY
Shigella

ENTERIC FEVER
Edwardsiella
Salmonella typhi
Salmonella arizonae

OPPORTUNISTIC AND NOSOCOMIAL INFECTION
Citrobacter
Enterbacter
Serratia
Providencia
Morganella

SEPTICEMIA
Escherichia coli
Edwardsiella
Salmonella choleraesuis
Klebsiella
Serratia
Proteus

DIARRHEA
Escherichia coli
Shigella
Edwardsiella
Salmonella arizonae
Salmonella enteritidis
Yersinia pseudotuberculosis
Yersinia enterocolitica

WOUND INFECTION
Edwardsiella
Citrobacter
Enterobacter
Serratia
Providencia
Morganella

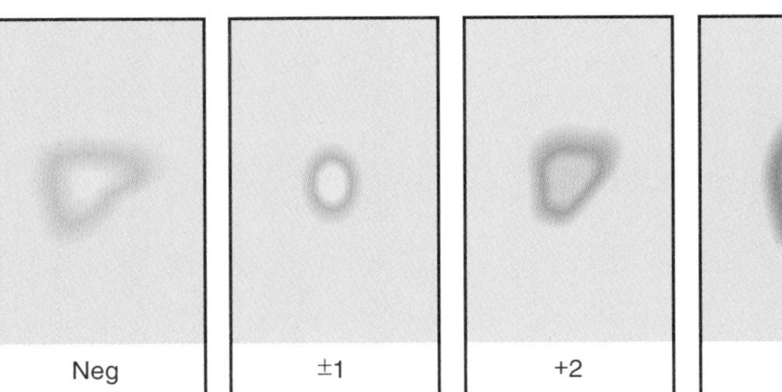

Degree of sensitivity measured by area of erythema and a wheal

Neg= no sensitivity or <5mm
±1= 5-9mm erythema; further testing needed
+2= >20mm erythema; with <10mm palpable wheal
+3= >30mm erythema with <10mm wheal
+4= >40mm erythema with <15mm wheal

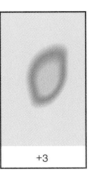

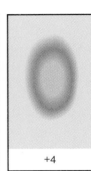

Figure 26–3. *The tuberculin tine test involves injecting a small amount of antigen into the superficial layer of the skin and observing any surface reaction. A numerical scale is used to measure the patient's degree of sensitivity. For example, a +4 rating indicates an area of redness (erythema) larger than 40 mm in diameter and a wheal (the mosquito-bite–like lesion) larger than 15 mm in diameter.*

Mycobacterium

The Mycobacterium species is also on the rise. The increase in infections secondary to Mycobacterium is related to the influx of immigrants and refugees from underdeveloped nations and the acquired immunodeficiency syndrome (AIDS) epidemic. One well-known source of mycobacterial infection is *Mycobacterium tuberculosis,* which causes the disease we know as tuberculosis.

Mycobacterium tuberculosis

M. tuberculosis infections account for a significant number of deaths worldwide. The organism is spread from person to person through the inhalation of airborne droplets containing mycobacterial organisms. The disease is most prevalent in developing nations; however, there has been a significant increase in tuberculosis infections in the United States recently. The development of antibiotic-resistant strains *of M. tuberculosis* is creating serious problems for public health agencies. The disease seems to be spreading most quickly in large cities, and elderly persons, non-Caucasians, alcoholics, and patients with AIDS are at increased risk for contracting the disease.

As stated earlier, tuberculosis is transmitted by airborne droplets, making health care workers particularly susceptible to the disease, especially before it is diagnosed in a patient. Because of the ease of transmission, all health care personnel should be thoroughly trained and have proper safety equipment available for preventing disease transmission once it has been diagnosed. All tuberculin-negative health care workers should undergo a skin test annually. In tuberculin-positive health care workers, a chest x-ray study should be performed annually (Fig. 26–3).

M. tuberculosis, also called acid-fast bacilli or MTB, may infect almost any tissue or organ, although the respiratory system is the one most commonly affected. The infection is confirmed by culturing expectorated **exudate** or **phlegm** for *M. tuberculosis.*

Identification of *M. tuberculosis* is accomplished by the use of specific staining techniques, such as the Ziehl-Neelsen, Kinyoun, or auramine-rhodamine fluorochrome stain. Specialized culture media, such as Löwenstein-Jensen medium, are preferred for culture examination. For safety reasons, the culture media used for the isolation and growth of Mycobacterium species are contained in glass tubes or jars with screw-top caps (Fig. 26–4).

Figure 26–4. *Screw-top slants used for culturing* Mycobacterium *and fungus.*

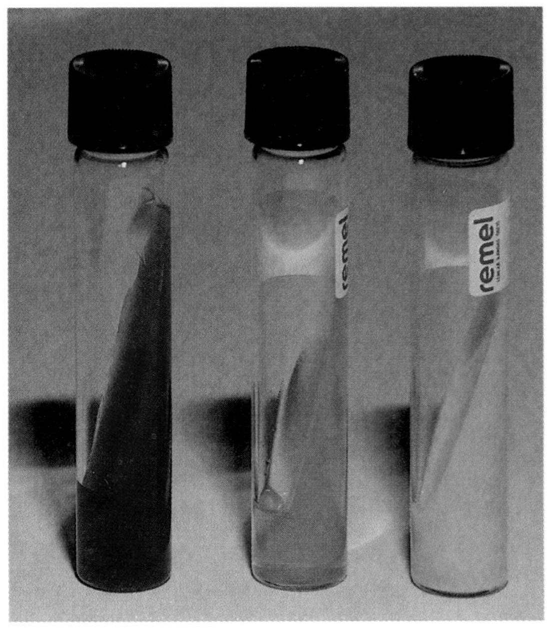

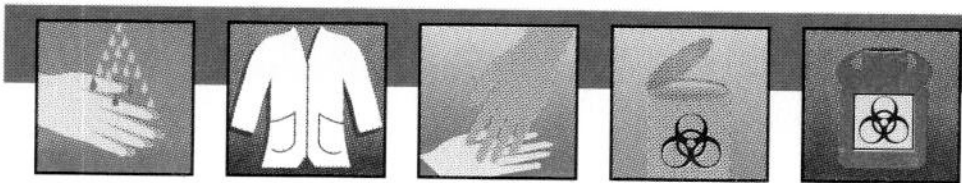

PROCEDURE 26–1

Administering and Reading a Tuberculin Tine Test

Principle

To embed a premeasured dose of old tuberculin into the epidermis and to ascertain the degree of response (induration)

Equipment and Supplies

alcohol prep pads
tine test disk
patient instruction leaflet

Procedural Steps

1. Explain the procedure to the patient.
2. Select an appropriate test site. The usual site is the anterior surface of the forearm, midway between the antecubital space and the wrist. The testing site must be free of all signs of trauma, as traumatized areas make it difficult to interpret test results.
3. Wash hands and put on gloves.
4. Cleanse the site with an alcohol prep pad to remove surface organisms.

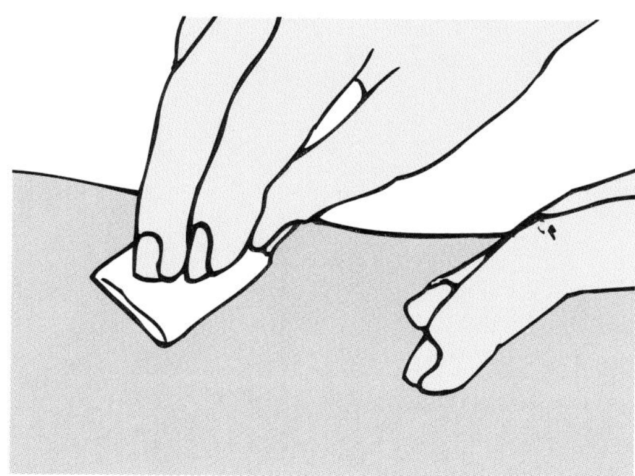

5. Remove the protective cap from the testing disk.

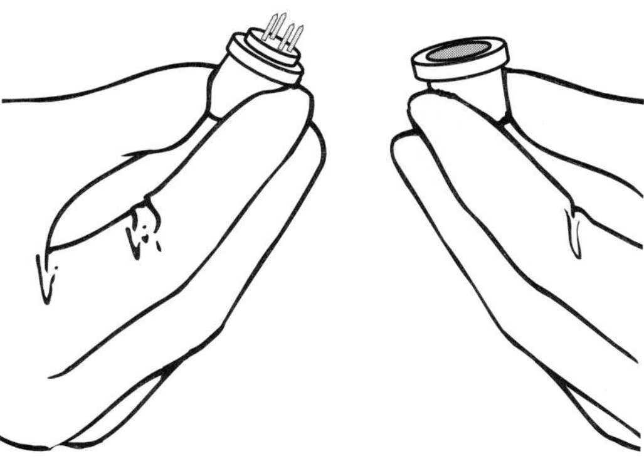

6. Stretch the skin tightly by grasping the forearm immediately beneath the testing site. This will create a smooth site for the puncture.
7. Gently but firmly place the tine tips into the skin and hold in place for 2 seconds. The tines must puncture the skin.

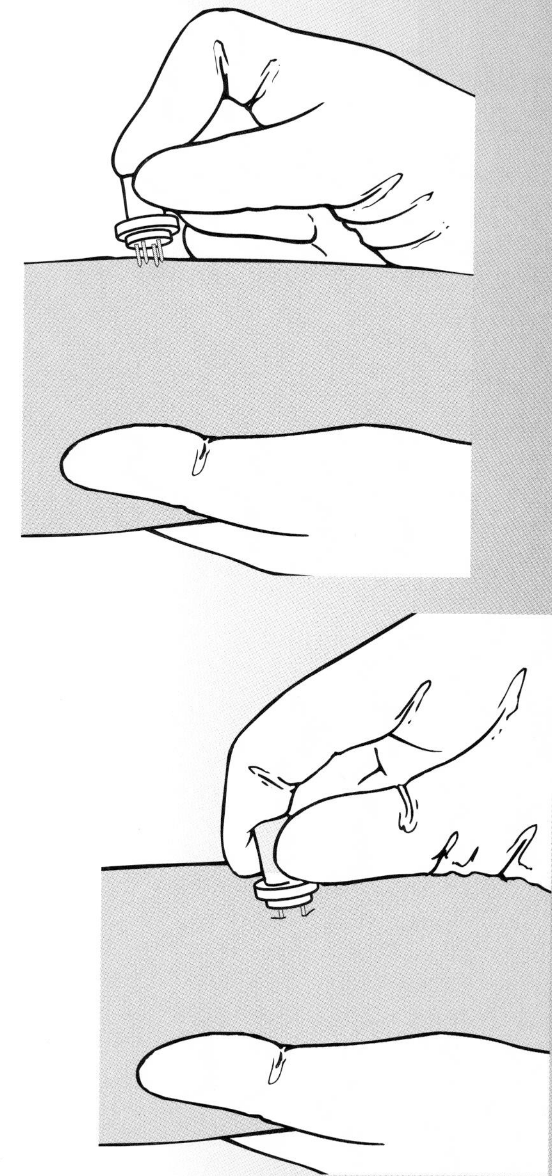

8. Relax your grasp. DO NOT rub the site.
9. Dispose of used testing material according to laboratory protocols.

(continued)

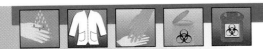

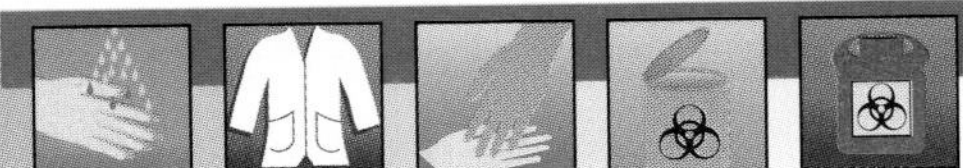

PROCEDURE 26–1

Administering and Reading a Tuberculin Tine Test (Continued)

10. Explain the procedure for reading the test site to the patient and provide them with an informational leaflet. The test must be read within 48 to 72 hours.
11. Record the test in the laboratory logbook.

Interpretation of Results

12. Using the millimeter rule provided in the testing container, measure the area of induration created by the test.
13. Palpate the test site and observe it for redness.
    Positive reaction: an area of induration measuring 2 mm or more in diameter
    Indeterminate reaction: an area of induration measuring less than 2 mm in diameter
    Negative reaction: no induration visible or palpable

Leprosy (Hansen's Disease)

Next to tuberculosis, leprosy is probably the most significant worldwide disease caused by the Mycobacterium species. The causative agent is *Mycobacterium leprae*.

Leprosy is a chronic disease affecting the skin, mucous membranes, and nerve tissue. There is a strong immunologic component to its etiology. The disease passes through various clinical stages, with the early stages characterized by leprotic bacilli multiplying in the skin. As the disease progresses, nerve tissue becomes involved.

The diagnosis of leprosy is established by examination of material obtained from the skin lesions or the earlobe of the infected person.

Identification of Bacterial Pathogens

Specimens for bacterial culture are inoculated onto selected and differential agars. The preliminary identification of bacteria is based on the examination of colonies growing on solid media. Isolation of bacteria is aided by the colony morphology on a specific media (Fig. 26–5). For example, Columbia colistin-nalidixic acid (CNA) agar contains antibacterial agents that completely suppress the growth of the Enterobacteriaceae and *Pseudomonas* species while allowing staphylococci, streptococci, enterococci and *Candida albicans* to grow.

MacConkey agar has the opposite effect. It inhibits the growth of gram-positive organisms, such as staphylococci and streptococci, and is selective for the growth

Figure 26–5. A, *Culture set-up area in a microbiology laboratory. Note the variety of plates used.* B, *Biosafety cabinet in a culture set-up area. Note the sharps container, incinerator, heat block, and culture loops.*

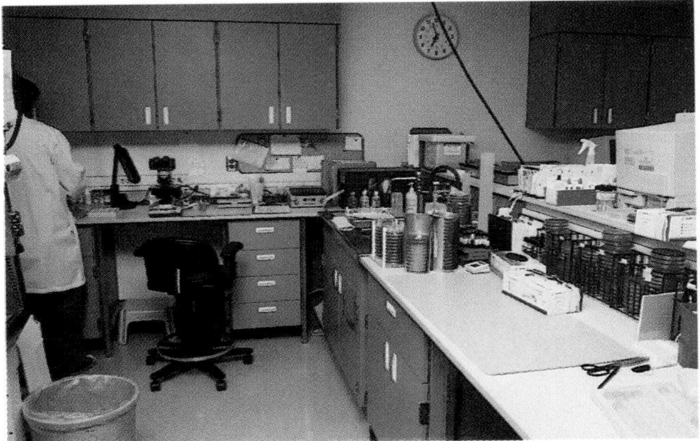

A

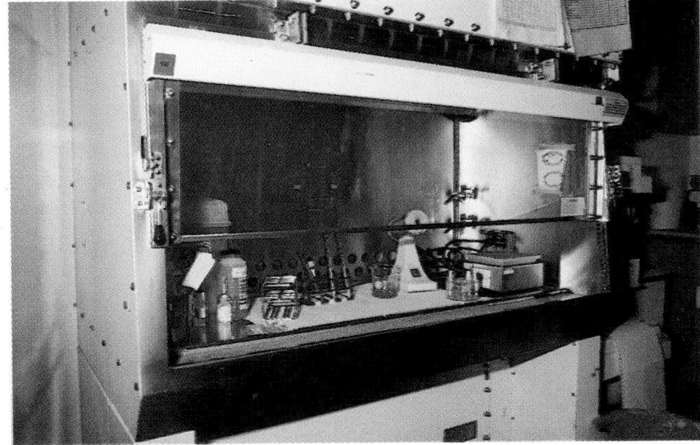

B

of gram-negative organisms, such as Enterobacteriaceae and *Pseudomonas* species.

Rapid Chemical Tests

Rapid tests can be performed on isolated bacterial colonies in the laboratory to aid in the rapid, preliminary identification of bacteria. This preliminary information may provide information that is helpful to the physician in determining the appropriate antibiotic or other treatment that would be effective against the suspected pathogenic agent.

Catalase Test

The catalase test is a rapid enzyme test used to distinguish members of the genus *Streptococcus* from those of the genus *Staphylococcus.* Staphylococcal organisms are catalase-positive, whereas streptococcal organisms are catalase-negative. The catalase reaction is based on the liberation of water and oxygen from hydrogen peroxide, which is a metabolic end-product that is toxic to bacteria.

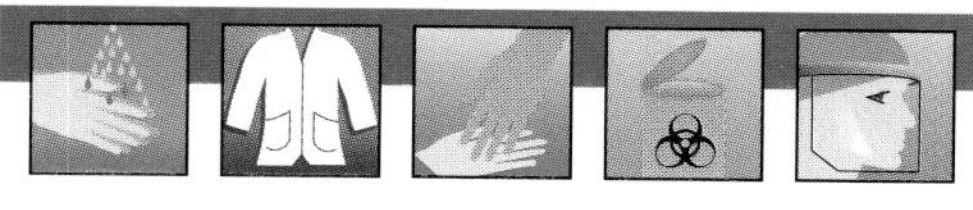

PROCEDURE 26–2

Performing a Catalase Rapid Enzyme Test

Principle

To distinguish members of the genus *Streptococcus* from those of the genus *Staphylococcus*

NOTE: This test should be performed only on bacteria grown on non–blood-containing media.

Equipment and Supplies

biohazard waste container
wire loop
loop incinerator
2 glass slides
pure culture of *Staphylococcus aureus* and *Streptococcus pyogenes*
3% hydrogen peroxide
small disposable pipettor

Procedural Steps

1. Wash hands and don appropriate safety attire.
2. Gather all needed equipment and supplies.
3. Turn on the loop incinerator.
4. Sterilize the wire loop.
5. Using the sterile loop, transfer a small amount of a pure colony of *S. aureus* to a dry glass slide.
6. **Immediately** place a drop of 3% hydrogen peroxide onto a portion of the colony on the slide.
7. Observe the slide for the production of gas bubbles, which will indicate a catalase-positive reaction.

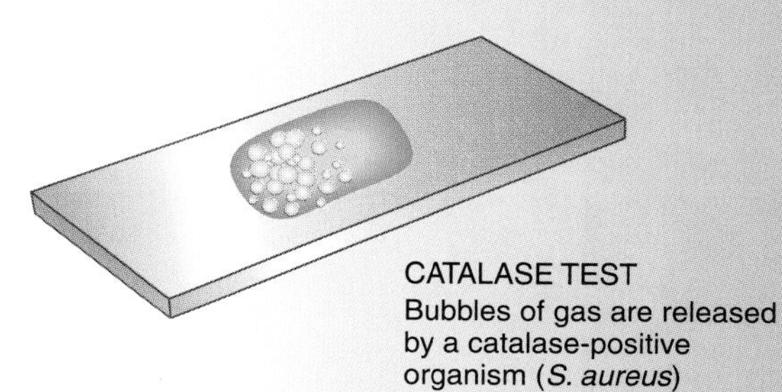

CATALASE TEST
Bubbles of gas are released by a catalase-positive organism (*S. aureus*)

8. Resterilize the wire loop.
9. Again using the sterile wire loop, transfer a small amount of a pure colony *of S. pyogenes* to a dry glass slide.
10. **Immediately** place a drop of 3% hydrogen peroxide onto a portion of the colony on the slide.
11. Observe the reaction. No visible bubbling indicates that the bacteria is catalase-negative.
12. Record and/or report the test reaction.
13. Clean the work area, disposing of biohazardous waste according to laboratory protocol.
14. Remove gloves and wash hands.

Interpretation of Results

Positive reaction: copious bubbles, indicating the presence of catalase-positive staphylococci

Negative reaction: no visible bubbling, indicating the presence of catalase-negative streptococci

NOTE: When determining the test results, do not confuse a weak positive reaction with the normal breakdown (bubbling) action of hydrogen peroxide.

Coagulase Test

Another test that helps to differentiate gram-positive from gram-negative bacteria is the coagulase test. Coagulase-positive cocci belong to the family Micrococcaceae, which includes the genus *Staphylococcus*. *S. aureus,* an important pathogen in humans, and *Staphylococcus intermedius,* which is rarely a human pathogen, are both coagulase-positive. Other staphylococci are coagulase-negative. Coagulase-negative staphylococci, such as *Staphylococcus epidermidis,* can be either pathogenic or nonpathogenic in humans (Fig. 26–6).

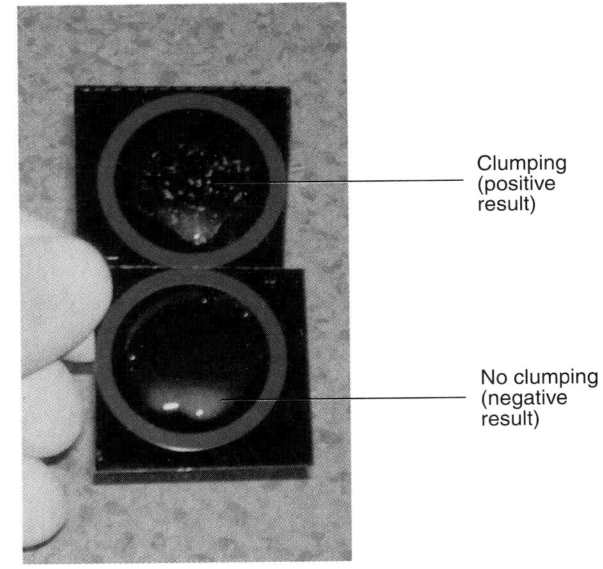

Figure 26–6. *Coagulase test results.*

Oxidase Test

When testing for gram-negative bacilli, two rapid tests are important: the oxidase test and the spot-indole test. The oxidase test is an important factor in the preliminary identification of *Pseudomonas* and *Neisseria* species. The oxidase test, when positive, yields a purple color. The purple color appears when a small sample of a colony of oxidase-positive organisms is applied to filter paper containing the oxidase reagent.

PROCEDURE 26–3

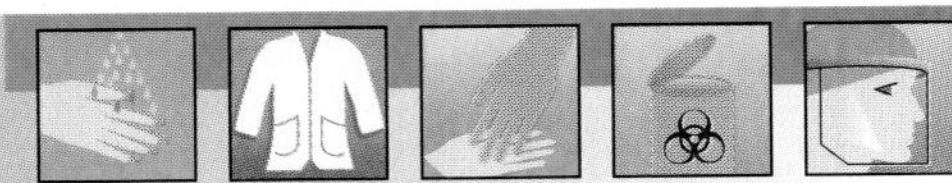

Performing an Oxidase Test (Kovác's Method)

Principle

To perform a test for the preliminary identification of *Pseudomonas* and *Neisseria* species

Equipment and Supplies

sterile disposable Petri dish
filter paper
Kovác's oxidase reagent
disposable pipette
wooden applicator stick
watch or timing device
pure culture of *Escherichia coli* and *Pseudomonas aeruginosa*

Procedural Steps

1. Wash hands and put on all safety equipment.
2. Gather supplies.
3. Place filter paper in the bottom of the Petri dish.
4. Moisten the filter paper with several drops of fresh Kovác's oxidase reagent.
5. Remove a small portion of an *E. coli* colony using the wooden applicator stick.
6. Rub the bacterial growth on the moistened filter paper.
7. Observe the paper for a color change to dark bluish purple within 10 seconds. **Timing is critical.**

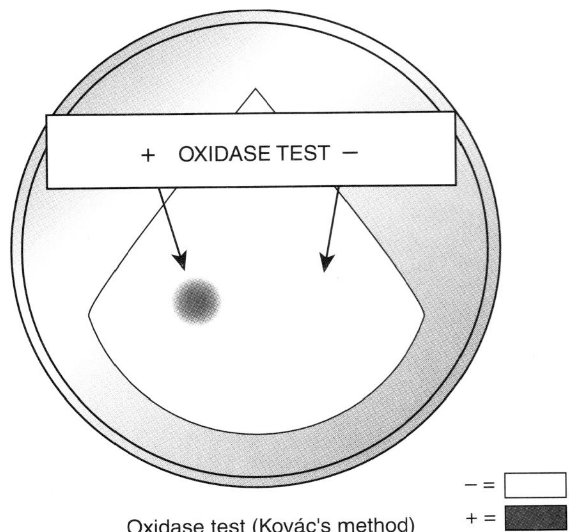

Oxidase test (Kovác's method)

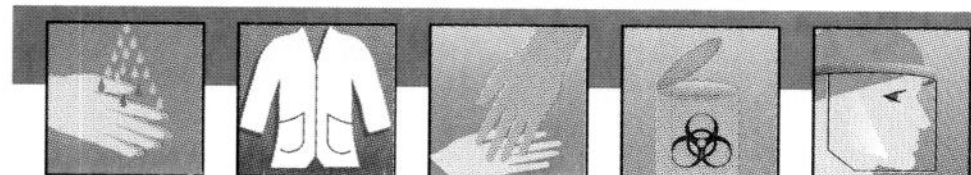

PROCEDURE 26–3

Performing an Oxidase Test (Kovác's Method) (Continued)

8. Repeat steps 5, 6, and 7 using a *P. aeruginosa* colony.
9. Record and/or report the results.
10. Dispose of all waste in appropriate containers according to laboratory protocol.
11. Remove gloves and wash hands.

Interpretation of Results

Positive result: Organisms such as Pseudomonas species will turn the filter paper dark bluish purple within 10 seconds.

Negative result: Organisms such as E. coli remain colorless or retain the color of the colony within 10 seconds.

Spot-Indole Test

The spot-indole test is used to characterize *E. coli* and to differentiate between indole-positive and non–indole-positive *Proteus* species. A blue-green color results when a portion of a colony of an indole-positive organism is rubbed on filter paper saturated with indole reagent.

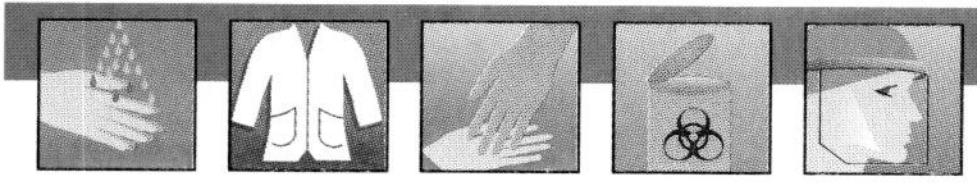

PROCEDURE 26–4

Performing a Spot-Indole Test for Escherichia Coli

Principle

To characterize *E. coli* and to differentiate between indole-positive and non–indole-positive (negative) *Proteus* species

Equipment and Supplies

indole reagent
No. 1 filter paper
Petri dish
wire loop
E. coli culture
loop incinerator

Procedural Steps

1. Wash hands and put on safety attire.
2. Gather all supplies.
3. Turn on the loop incinerator.
4. Fold the filter paper into a quarter circle.
5. Place it in the bottom of the Petri dish.
6. Saturate the filter paper with indole reagent.
7. Sterilize the wire loop using the incinerator.
8. Using the sterile loop, carefully remove a colony of *E. coli* from the culture plate.
9. Rub the colony on the filter paper.
10. Observe the filter paper for reaction. Rapid development indicates a positive test. Most indole-positive organisms turn blue within 30 seconds.

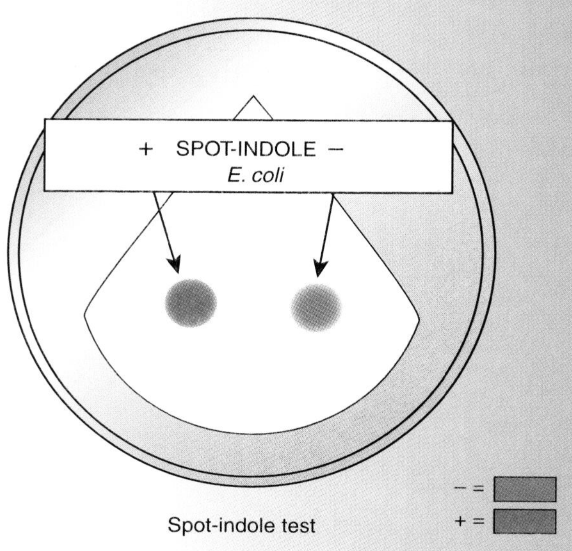

Spot-indole test

(continued)

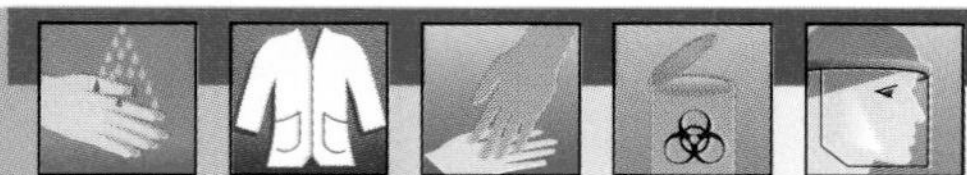

PROCEDURE 26–4

Performing a Spot-Indole Test for Escherichia Coli *(Continued)*

11. Record and/or report the test results.
12. Dispose of all waste in appropriate containers according to laboratory protocol.
13. Remove gloves and wash hands.

Interpretation of Results

Positive result: Organisms such as *E. coli* will turn the filter paper blue-green.

Negative result: Organisms that are nonreactive to indole will remain colorless or turn slightly pink.

Bile Solubility Test

The bile solubility test is useful in identifying *S. pneumoniae.* Bile solubility reagent (sodium desoxycholate) dissolves colonies of *S. pneumoniae* on blood agar plates. In contrast, colonies of other alpha-hemolytic streptococci are not dissolved by the reagent. For this test to be accurate, it must be performed on newly grown colonies.

L-Pyrrolidonyl-B-Naphthalamide Hydrolysis (PYR) Test

The L-pyrrolidonyl-B-naphthalamide hydrolysis (PYR) test is useful in identifying *Streptococcus pyogenes* and *Enterococcus* species. *S. pyogenes* and *Enterococcus* species produce an enzyme that hydrolyzes PYR. When a PYR-positive organism is applied to filter paper saturated with PYR reagent, a bright red color reaction occurs within 5 minutes. PYR-negative organisms produce an orange color, or no color change, during the reaction.

Biochemical Testing

Definitive identification of bacteria is accomplished by biochemical testing. Traditionally, biochemical testing is performed using an assortment of tubed media that have been inoculated. The reactions are then observed and compared with the reactions of known organisms to aid in the identification of bacteria. Today, most microbiology laboratories use miniaturized or micro-identification methods and compact, self-contained kits or panels containing numerous biochemicals and antibiotics.

Rapid Commercial Identification Kits

Multi-test commercial identification systems have provided laboratories with a simple, convenient, systematic method for species identification of most gram-negative bacteria. Many kits require only 4 hours of incubation, which facilitates a rapid diagnosis. All commercial kits occasionally require supplemental confirmatory tests for species identification of isolates that do not exhibit a pattern that can be clearly differentiated.

Rapid biochemical identification methods, such as the Rapid-NH, API Rapid E, Gonochek II, and MICRO-ID, are available for differentiating *Neisseria* species and *Haemophilus* species (Fig. 26–7). The Rapid-ANA panel is useful in the rapid identification of anaerobes.

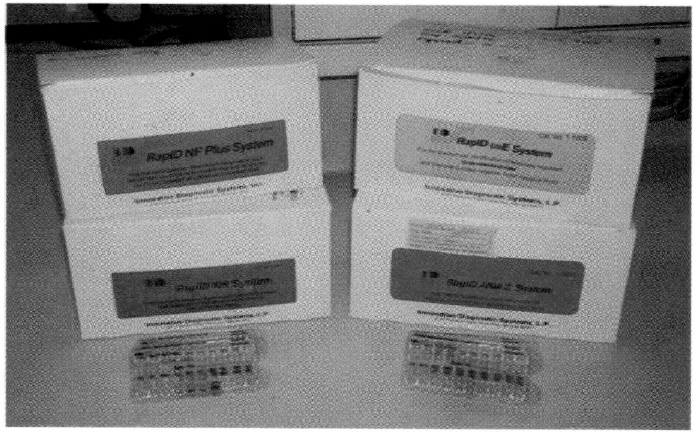

Figure 26–7. *Rapid biochemical test kits may be used to detect/identify anaerobes,* Neisseria, Haemophilus, *and other species of bacteria.*

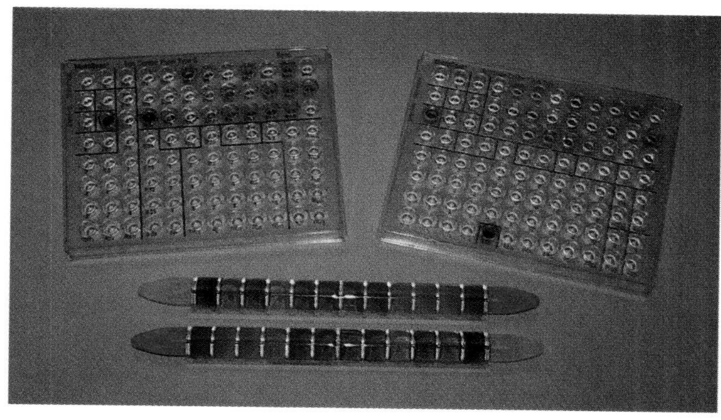

Figure 26–8. *Enterotube II and Microscan identification tests.*

Each system is self-contained and requires storage at 2° to 8°C.

Commercial Identification Kits

Commercial bacterial identification systems are designed to measure 23 standard biochemical tests. Certain organisms can be identified within 5 hours, whereas others require overnight incubation. All tests can be completed in less than 24 hours. Originally, these tests were designed to identify members of the Enterobacteriaceae family, but now they can identify a wide range of aerobic, gram-negative bacteria. The API 20E, Enterotube II, OXI/FERM Tube, N/F SYSTEM, and the r/b system are some of the kits that are used (Fig. 26–8).

Semi-Automated and Automated Microtiter Testing Systems

Numerous microtiter systems are available for biochemical identification alone, or biochemical identification in combination with quantitative and/or qualitative antimicrobial susceptibility testing. The methodology varies from manual to semi-automated to fully automated "walk-away" systems. Depending on the manufacturer, the substrates and antimicrobial agents are available in frozen, lyophilized, or dehydrated form. Most systems offer a computer program with reporting and epidemiologic analysis capabilities. Among these are the ARX Advantage Microbiology Center, Autobac II, Microscan System (Fig. 26–9, *A–C*), and the Septor System.

Major Microorganisms of the Body Systems

To some extent, the body system that is the source of the specimen material dictates the type of bacteria that will be isolated. Certain bacteria are often associated with specific body tissues and fluids (Table 26–4).

Blood

Sometimes, during the course of an infectious disease, blood is drawn for culture and organisms are grown. The presence of these organisms in the blood is termed **bacteremia.** Bacteremia signifies the presence of a positive blood culture in the absence of any marked classical symptoms. When immunity is low or the body's normal defenses are impaired, these organisms reproduce in the cytoplasm of healthy cells. As the once healthy cells become necrotic, the organisms, along with their waste products (known as toxins), are released into the blood. The blood culture will again be positive, but this time, the person will also become extremely ill. The condition is known as septicemia and indicates a complete breakdown of the body's defense system. This condition is so dramatic that it frequently causes death.

Identification of bacteria in the blood requires special advanced culture techniques that use whole blood collected into vials of liquid media containing nutrients and anticoagulants. Automated methods, such as the Bac-T Alert, aid in the rapid identification of bacteria in the blood (Fig. 26–10, *A–C*).

Frequent etiologic agents detected in the blood include *E. coli, Pseudomonas* species, *Enterobacter* species, *Proteus* species, *Staph. aureus, Strep. viridans, Enterococcus* species, *Strep. pneumoniae*, beta-hemolytic streptococci (e.g., *Strep. pyogenes*), and anaerobic bacteria, such as *Bacteroides* species, *Peptostreptococcus* species, and *Clostridium* species. Two significant fungal pathogens found in the blood are *C. albicans* and *Cryptococcus* species.

Respiratory System

The respiratory tract may be host to many bacteria. The upper respiratory tract has normal indigenous bacteria that are found in healthy individuals and do not commonly cause disease. Only under certain circumstances will these become pathogenic.

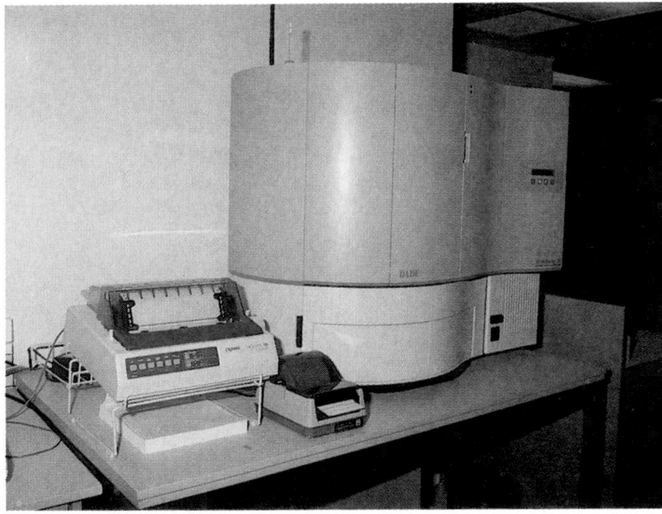

A

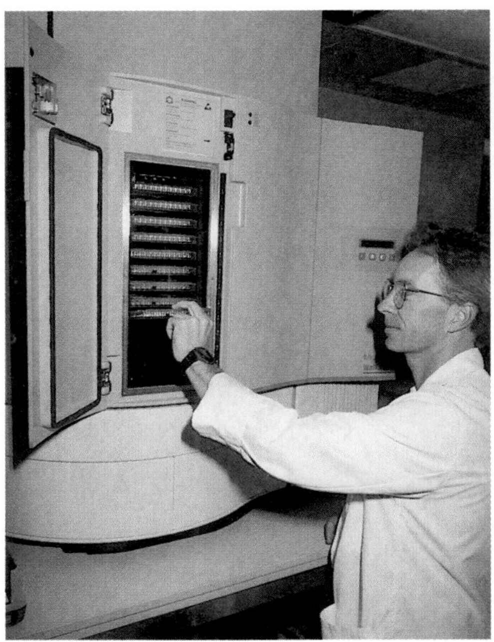

B

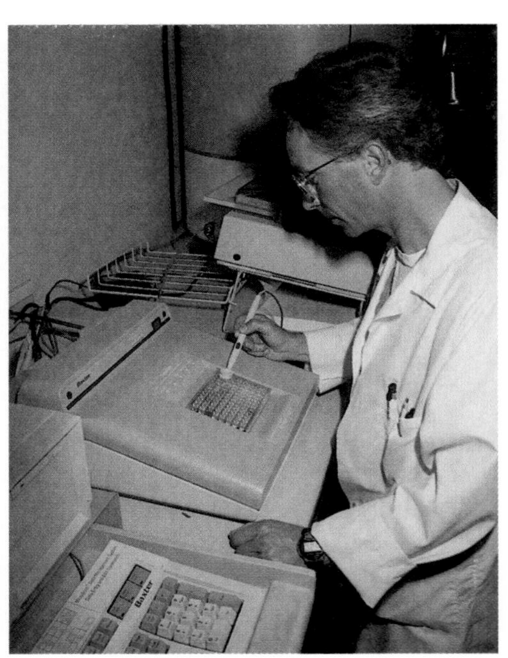

C

Figure 26–9. A, *Microscan instrument.* B, *Unloading of Microscan panels.* C, *Manual technique for reading Microscan panels.*

Organisms or other bacteria that are common pathogens in the upper respiratory tract are beta-hemolytic streptococci (Fig. 26–11), *S. viridans, S. pneumoniae, S. aureus, Corynebacterium diphtheriae, N. meningitidis, Acinetobacter* species, *Haemophilus influenzae,* Enterobacteriacae, and anaerobes, such as the *Bacteroides* species and *Peptostreptococcus* species. In addition, other organisms, such as *Cryptococcus neoformans, C. albicans,* and the herpes simplex virus are pathogens of the upper respiratory system.

Urinary System

In the urinary system, the urethra is the area that most frequently hosts bacteria. The bladder, ureters, and kidneys are usually sterile. Bacteriologic cultures are important diagnostic tools in the diagnosis and treatment of urinary tract infections (UTIs). The two most common types of urinary tract infections are cystitis and pylonephritis. Urinary tract disorders are seen more frequently in women than in men owing to the anatomic location and length of the urethra.

Table 26–4
Disease-Causing Organisms

Bacterial Species	***Description***	***Specimen***	***Tests***
Staphylococcus aureus \	Gram (+) cocci in clusters	Deep swab; aspirate of drainage	Culture and sensitivity
Streptococcus pyogenes (Group A streptococcus)	Gram (+) cocci in chains	Direct swab	Direct agglutination; culture; WBC and diff.
Streptococcus pneumoniae	Gram (+) cocci in pairs	Sputum; brochoscopic secretions	Culture; Gram stain
Neisseria gonorrhoeae	Gram (–) cocci in pairs Intracellular in WBC	Swab of cervix, urethra; rectal and pharyngeal swabs in homosexuals	Gram stain; culture
Neisseria meningitidis	Gram (–) diplococci	Nasopharyngeal swabs, CSF, blood	Gram stain; culture; cell counts and chemistry studies
Mycobacterium tuberculosis	Acid-fast beaded bacilli	Sputum	Culture; x-ray study; skin test
Mycobacterium leprae	Acid-fast bacilli	Skin scrapings	Skin smear; biopsy; serologic test
Escherichia coli *Proteus* sp. *Klebsiella* sp. *Pseudomonas aeruginosa*	Gram (–) bacilli	Clean-catch urine	Culture; urinalysis
Treponema pallidum	Spirochete	Blood	VDRL, RPR, FTA-ABS
Clostridium tetani	Gram (+) spore-forming bacilli; anaerobic	Blood; wound swab	Wound smear; culture
Clostridium perfringens	Gram (+) spore-forming bacilli; anaerobic	Swab; wound aspiration	Culture
Gardnerella vaginalis	Gram-variable bacilli	Vaginal swab	Wet prep; microanalysis
Listeria monocytogenes	Gram (+) bacilli	Stool, blood, CSF; amniotic fluid, placenta, vagina	Smear and culture; serologic test (CRP)
Chlamydia trachomatis		Genital swab; conjunctival swab	Culture; serologic immunofluorescent test

(+), positive; (–), negative; *WBC,* white blood cell count; *CSF,* cerebrospinal fluid; *Diff.,* differential blood count; *VDRL,* Venereal Disease Research Laboratory; *RPR,* rapid plasma reagin; *FTA-ABS,* fluorescent treponemal antibody absorption; *CRP,* C-reactive protein.

There are numerous species of normal flora in the urinary system, including coagulase-negative staphylococci, non-hemolytic streptococci, *S. viridans, Lactobacillus* species, *Corynebacterium* species, and the anaerobic *Propionibacterium* species.

Common pathogens include the Enterobacteriaceae family, such as *E. coli,* and *Pseudomonas* species, *S. aureus, Enterococcus* species, and beta-hemolytic streptococci.

Gastrointestinal System

The gastrointestinal tract is a tube that is open at both ends and connects us to our external environment. It is inhabited by a multitude of indigenous flora that aid in the function and protection of the system. Interference with the functioning of the normal flora may result in the introduction of potentially pathogenic organisms.

The gastrointestinal system contains numerous bacteria that cause infection. These bacteria produce disease by:

1. Producing a toxin
2. Causing loss of function through the destruction of the intestinal mucosa
3. Invading and destroying the mucosal epithelium, causing septicemia
4. Invading the intestinal mucosa, thereby interfering with absorption and secretion

Major gastrointestinal pathogens include *E. coli; Shigella* species (including *Shigella dysenteriae*), *Clostridium difficile, Clostridium perfringens, S. aureus, Vibrio*

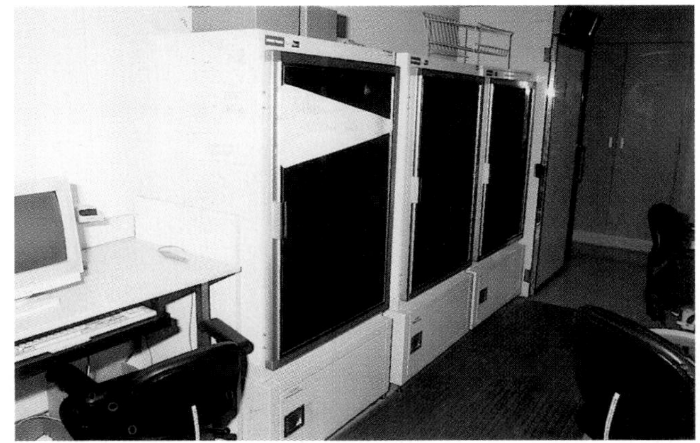

A

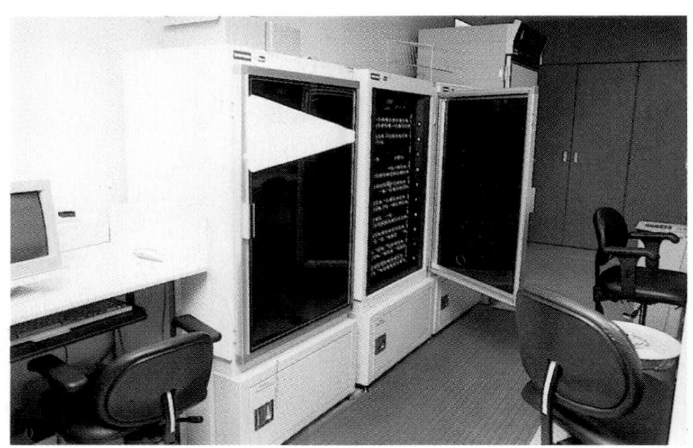

B

C

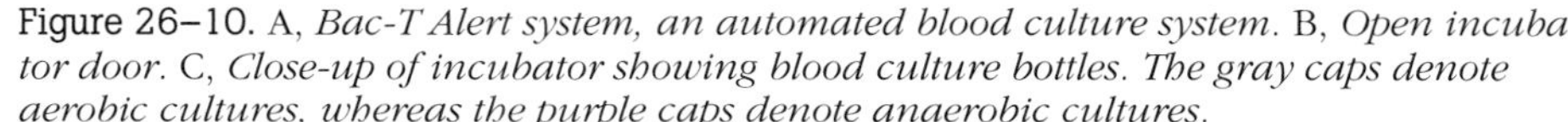

Figure 26–10. A, *Bac-T Alert system, an automated blood culture system.* B, *Open incubator door.* C, *Close-up of incubator showing blood culture bottles. The gray caps denote aerobic cultures, whereas the purple caps denote anaerobic cultures.*

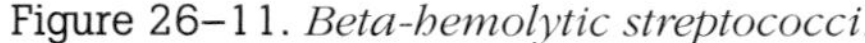

Figure 26–11. *Beta-hemolytic streptococci.*

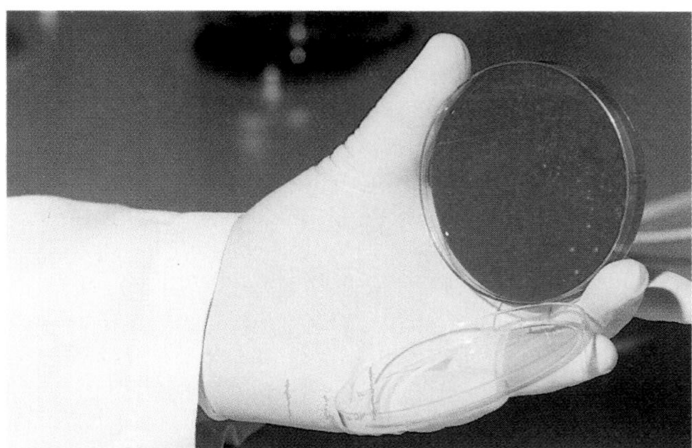

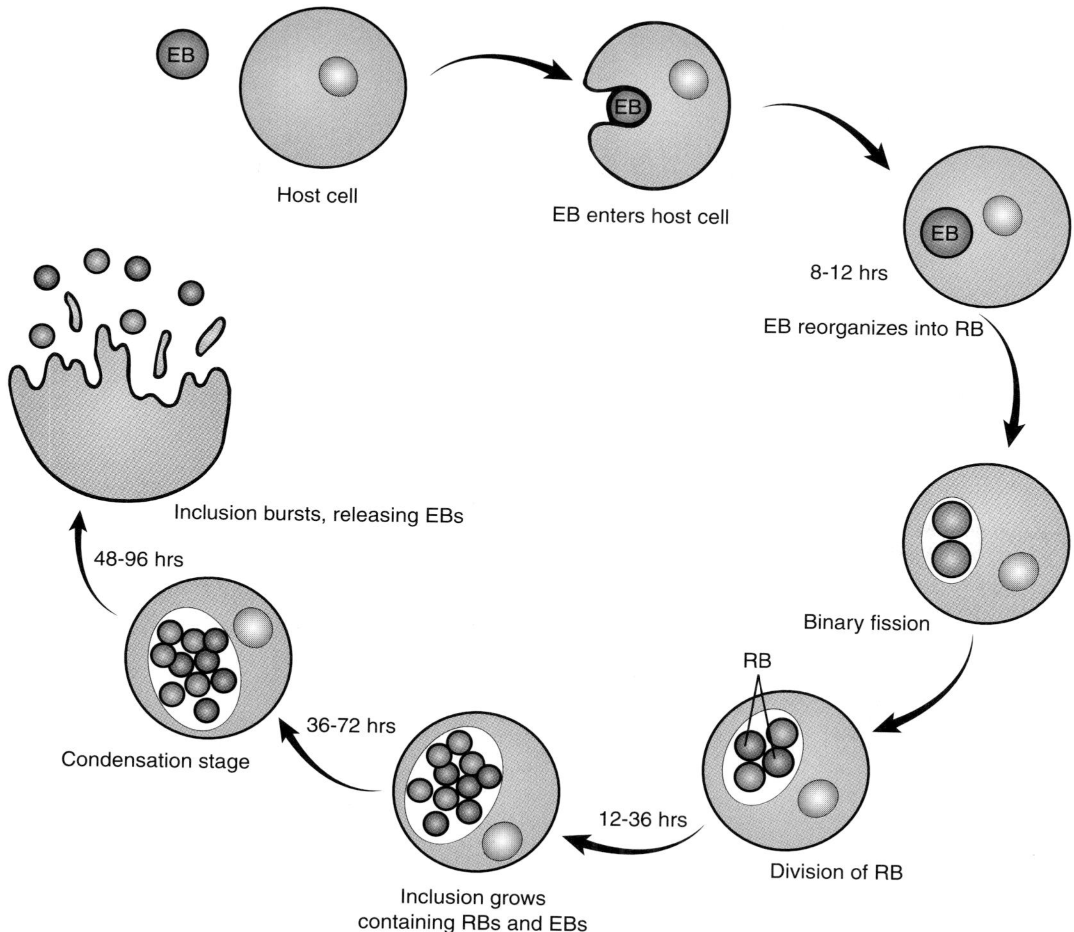

Figure 26–12. *Developmental cycle of Chlamydia. EB, elementary body; RB, reticulate body.*

species, *Campylobacter jejuni, Salmonella* species, *Vibrio cholerae,* and *Aeromonas* species.

Reproductive System

The normal human genital tract may contain both normal and pathogenic flora. Common microorganisms and sexually transmitted pathogens include *N. gonorrhoeae, Treponema pallidum, Chlamydia trachomatis, Gardnerella vaginalis,* and *Mycoplasma* species, in addition to viruses, such as herpes simplex, human immunodeficiency virus (HIV), cytomegalovirus, and the yeast *C. albicans*. Protozoans, such as *Trichomonas vaginalis,* are also common parasitic pathogens of the reproductive system.

Diagnosis of genital pathogens may be made by direct microscopic examination, cultural techniques, biochemical testing, or serologic procedures.

C. trachomatis belongs to a group of bacteria that differ from most bacteria. This species can reproduce only within the living cells of a host (Fig. 26–12). In the United States, chlamydial infection of the genitourinary tract has become the number one sexually transmitted disease, with an estimated 4 million new cases every year. In addition, *C. trachomatis* is the leading cause of blindness throughout the world.

In female patients, a chlamydial infection is suspected when the cervix bleeds when it is touched. In male patients it is frequently the pathogen involved in **urethritis.** The infection can be detected by cell culture, DNA probes, and immunoassay.

PROCEDURE 26–5

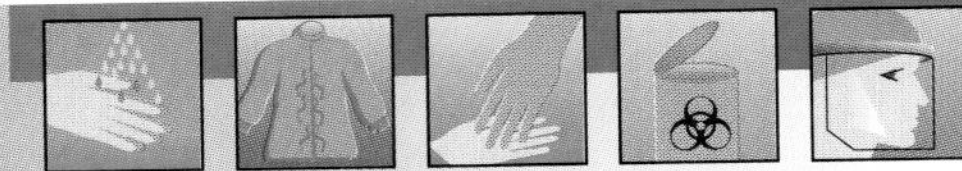

Assisting With Specimen Collection of and Testing for Chlamydia trachomatis

Principle

To assist with the collection and processing of *Chlamydia trachomatis* in order to detect chlamydial infection of the genitourinary tract, which has become the most prevalent sexually transmitted disease. The infection can be detected by immunoassay.

NOTE: This specimen collection is usually performed by the physician, with the assistance of a medical/laboratory assistant. In this procedure, you will assist with the collection of the specimen from the site and then you will prepare the sample for transport to and processing by the reference laboratory.

Equipment and Supplies

small specimen mailing container
Syva MicroTrak *Chlamydia trachomatis* Specimen Collection Kit
laboratory marking pen
ink pen
Dacron swabs

Procedural Steps

Specimen Collection

Urethral samples (Male)

NOTE: It is preferable that the patient refrain from urinating for 1 hour prior to sampling.

1. Wash hands thoroughly and don safety apparel.
2. Insert a small Dacron swab into the urethra to a depth of 2 to 4 cm.

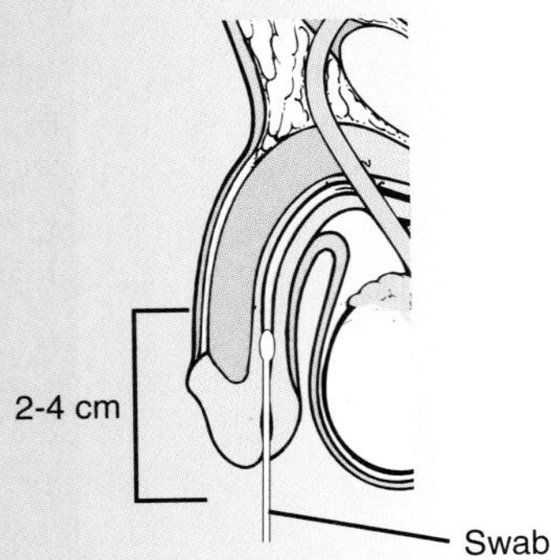

3. Rotate the swab and withdraw it.

Cervical samples (Cytology Brush)

1. Wash hands thoroughly and don safety apparel.
2. Wipe the exocervix with a cotton or Dacron swab to remove excess mucus. Dispose of the swab in a biohazardous waste container.
3. Gently insert the cytology brush into the endocervical canal, past the squamocolumnar junction.

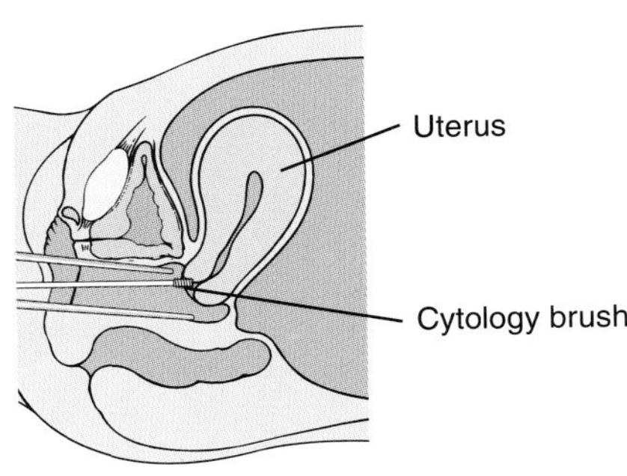

4. Leave the brush in place for 2 to 3 seconds.
5. Rotate the cytology brush 360 degrees.
6. Withdraw the cytology brush without touching any vaginal surfaces.

Cervical Samples (Swab)

1. Wash hands thoroughly and don safety apparel.
2. Wipe the exocervix with a cotton or Dacron swab to remove excess mucus. Dispose of the swab in a biohazardous waste container.
3. Insert a large Dacron swab into the endocervical canal until most of the Dacron tip is not visible.

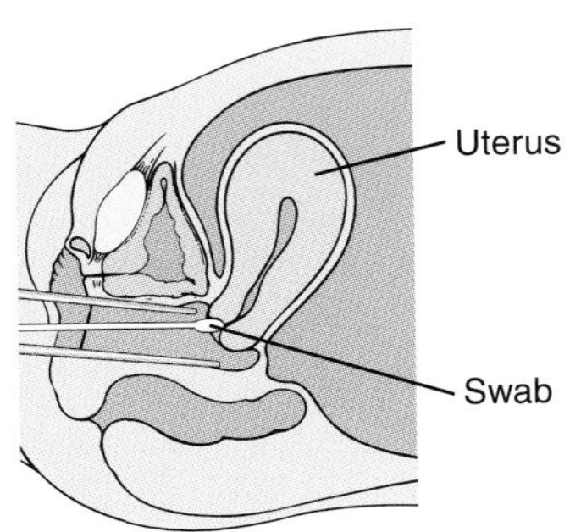

4. Rotate the swab inside the endocervical canal for 5 to 10 seconds.
5. Withdraw the swab without touching any vaginal surfaces.

Conjunctival Samples

1. Wash hands thoroughly and don safety apparel.

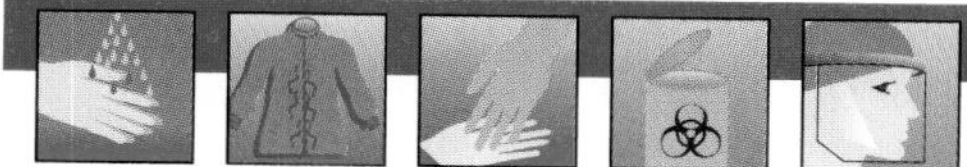

PROCEDURE 26–5

Assisting With Specimen Collection of and Testing for Chlamydia trachomatis *(Continued)*

2. Apply a topical, opthalmologic proparacaine-based anesthetic solution to the eye(s).
3. Using a small swab, thoroughly swab the inner surface of the lower eyelid, then do the same for the upper eyelid. If samples are taken from both eyes, swab the least affected eye first to avoid further contamination of that eye.

Slide Preparation

Immediately after the physician hands you the sample:

Swab Samples

1. Role the swab over the top half of the slide well, then roll the other side of the swab over the bottom half of the well.

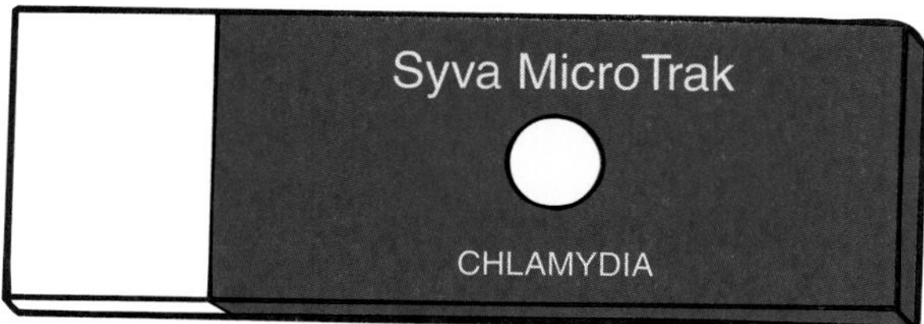

Cytology Brush Samples

1. Place the brush across the center of the slide well. Rotate and twist the brush, moving it back and forth across the well.
2. Check for adequate coverage.
3. Lay the slide flat.

Fixative Instructions

1. Do not remove the nozzle from the fixative container.
2. Hold the fixative container with the nozzle directed at the slide well.
3. Squeeze the container in the middle just until the glass inside breaks and fixative flows through the nozzle tip. Keep the plastic vial crusher ring on the vial while squeezing.
4. Flood the sample with the entire amount (0.5 mL) of fixative and let it evaporate completely. To speed evaporation, after 5 minutes, tip the slide to drain excess fixative.
5. Write the patient's name, the date and time the specimen was collected, the physician's name, and the collection site on the white end of the sample slide.
6. Place the properly labeled slide in the pack provided. Fold the pack.
7. Complete the label on the sample pack with the same information as on the slide.

Syva*MicroTrak*® ***Chlamydia trachomatis***

Patient's Name____________________

Physician____________________

Date____________ Site____________

8. Prepare the slide for transport according to the specifications of the reference laboratory.
9. Dispose of all hazardous waste according to laboratory protocol and clean and disinfect the work area with 10% bleach solution.
10. Record the procedure in the laboratory logbook and on the patient's record.
11. Remove gloves and wash hands.

Kit tests, such as Kodak's SureCell and Wampole Laboratories' Clearview are commonly used immunoassays. These tests are quick and easy to use and contain all the necessary controls. When the test yields a positive result, confirmation of test results by another form of testing is required before a definitive diagnosis can be ascertained.

Integumentary System

The skin and its accessory structures, hair, nails, **sebaceous** glands, and **sudoriferous** glands make up the integumentary system. The skin is the largest organ in the body, covering more than 3000 square inches and weighing more than 6 pounds. A major function of the skin is to protect the body against microorganisms, toxins, and poisons. It also regulates body temperature and contains the sensory receptors. Waste is secreted by the sudoriferous glands, and the sebaceous glands help protect against dehydration and the absorption of harmful substances. Infections of the integumentary systems may be localized or extensive.

Fungal infections caused by *Mucor, Rhizopus,* and *Aspergillus* species may occur in patients receiving cytotoxic or corticosteroid therapy or those with diabetic ketoacidosis. Mucormycosis is rare, but it is often fatal. Infection begins in the nasal or oral mucous membranes and then spreads to the brain.

Necrotizing fasciitis is usually caused by group A streptococci or *S. aureus.* Fortunately, necrotizing fasciitis does not occur frequently. When it does, it is very serious and often fatal. The infection starts in the **fascia** covering the skeletal muscle and the associated soft tissue. The infection then spreads rapidly, involving large areas of tissue. Often, amputation, or the surgical removal of infected tissue, is the only way to stop the spread of infection.

Cellulitis may be caused by mixed aerobic and anaerobic bacteria, such as *E. coli, S. aureus, Bacteroides fragilis,* and *Peptostreptococcus* species. Postoperative gangrene may also involve mixed aerobic and anaerobic bacteria.

Commonly encountered skin infections involve bites and burns. Human bites typically involve alpha-hemolytic streptococci, *S. aureus,* and group A streptococci. Any microorganism found in the human oral cavity may be the cause of an infection. Cat and dog bites have similar oral flora to those of humans and other animals. Mixed cultures of *Enterobacter cloacae, Pasteurella* species, *S. intermedius, Pseudomonas* species, *E. coli, Klebsiella* species, and *Proteus* species are frequently found in infected bites from animals.

Burn wound infections are essentially universal and may be associated with bacteremia. There are many organisms that are capable of infecting the burned area, and these may also interfere with the acceptance of skin grafts. Those most often encountered are various streptococci, *S. aureus, S. epidermidis,* Enterobacteriaceae, *Pseudomonas* species, and other gram-negative bacilli. Severe burns also cause excessive damage to the red blood cells (RBCs). The RBCs may undergo premature fragmentation and destruction. The presence of fragmented, bizarre-shaped RBCs (schistocytes) in the peripheral blood is characteristic.

Wounds and Abscesses

Disease, trauma, or surgical complications may produce abscesses or infections in wounds. Almost any bacteria may be involved. Normal flora, aerobes, anaerobes, and gram-positive or gram-negative organisms, either singly or mixed, can all cause infections.

Postoperative wounds may be infected by nosocomial pathogens like *Pseudomonas aeruginosa* or *S. aureus.* Normal intestinal flora may become pathogenic when disease, trauma, or surgery involves the abdominopelvic region. Anaerobic bacteria, such as *Clostridium* species and *Bacteroides* species, may also be involved in deep tissue abscesses and wounds.

Any sore, ulcer, laceration, abscess, lesion, fistula, or injury to the skin may be susceptible to an invading organism, which, in turn, may cause infection.

Musculoskeletal System

Infections involving solid tissue and bone pose special problems for specimen collection and processing. Solid tissue may be collected by surgical biopsy or excision, or during autopsy. This tissue must then be ground or minced, using aseptic technique and observing universal precautions. This procedure should be performed inside a biosafety cabinet.

Osteomyelitis is usually caused by *S. aureus,* but almost any bacteria may be the pathogenic agent. Solid tissue infections may be caused by bacteria, fungi, viruses, mycobacteria, or parasites. A well-documented patient history and clinical examination are very useful in determining which microorganism is the likely pathogen. Many microorganisms that produce infection in solid tissue or bone require special procedures for identification. Certain bacteria, such as *Listeria* species or *Legionella* species, require special media for growth. Fungi and viruses also require special collection procedures and processing techniques. Specimens may be sent to public health, reference, or university-affiliated laboratories for analysis.

Eye, Ear, Nose, and Throat

Infections involving the eye, ear, nose, and throat are always serious. These areas are highly vascularized and closely associated with the blood, lymphatic, nervous, and respiratory systems.

Conjunctivitis is the most common bacterial infection of the eye. Trachoma is one of the leading causes of blindness. It is caused by *Chlamydia trachomatis.* This organism infects the conjunctiva of neonates, who acquire it at birth from their mother's infected vaginal canal. The Syva MicroTrak kit is frequently used for direct specimen collection of cytologic samples of *C. trachomatis* (Fig. 26–13). The leading cause of conjunctivitis in children *is H. influenzae.* In adults it is *S. pneumoniae.*

Otitis externa and otitis media are the most frequently encountered bacterial infections of the ear. Oti-

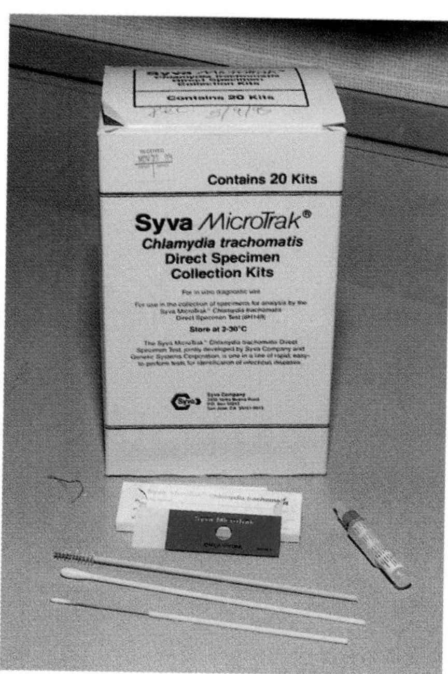

Figure 26–13. *Syva MicroTrak direct specimen collection kit.*

tis media in children is caused by *S. pneumoniae* and *H. influenzae*. Other bacteria, such as *S. aureus, P. aeruginosa*, or group A streptococci, may also cause otitis media. *M. tuberculosis* can sometimes cause **mastoiditis** and otitis media. Otitis externa may result from chronic suppurative otitis media. Swimmer's ear is a form of otitis externa that may be associated with swimming, hot tubs, spas, or even hot, humid weather. *P. aeruginosa* is the usual pathogen. Localized infections, in the form of pustules or furuncles, are often associated with *S. aureus*.

Sinusitis may be caused by *H. influenzae, S. pneumoniae, Moraxella catarrhalis, P. aeruginosa, or S. aureus*. Other bacteria, such as *Propionibacterium acnes*, may be involved less frequently.

Pharyngitis and tonsillitis are typically caused by *S. pyogenes*, group A streptococci, but other types of beta-hemolytic streptococci (Group B, C, or G) are less frequently involved. *C. diphtheriae* (diphtheria) and non–membrane-producing *Corynebacterium* species may be cultured from specimens collected in patients with pharyngitis. Other etiologic agents of pharyngitis and tonsillitis include *N. meningitidis, N. gonorrhoeae* (usually associated with oral genital sexual practices), *H. influenzae, S. pneumoniae*, and *S. aureus*.

Sterile Body Fluids

Cerebrospinal fluid (CSF), precordial fluid, peritoneal fluid, pleural fluid, and synovial (joint) fluid are normally sterile. However, these fluids may become infected by microorganisms. In cases of suspected infection, these body fluids are centrifuged to concentrate any microorganism present before culturing.

Cerebrospinal Fluid

Infection involving the central nervous system (CNS) is considered to be a medical emergency. CSF, which surrounds and protects the brain and the spinal cord, may become infected, resulting in a bacterial meningitis. When the inflammation caused by the bacteria is in the brain, it is called encephalitis. Encephalitis is most commonly caused by viruses. Organisms, such as *S. pneumoniae, H. influenzae, E. coli, N. meningitidis*, and *Listeria monocytogenes*, are important etiologic agents of meningitis (Fig. 26–14). *M. tuberculosis*, the yeast *C. neoformans*, and the fungi *Coccidioides immitis*, and *Histoplasma capsulatum* are among the other microorganisms that are clinically important agents of meningitis.

Pericardial Fluid

The heart is surrounded by a protective covering called the pericardium. Pericardial fluid, found between the pericardium and the epicardium, helps to protect and lubricate the heart. When this normally sterile fluid becomes infected, the pericardium becomes inflamed, and this can interfere with cardiac function. Viruses,

Figure 26–14. *Serologic test for* Haemophilus influenzae.

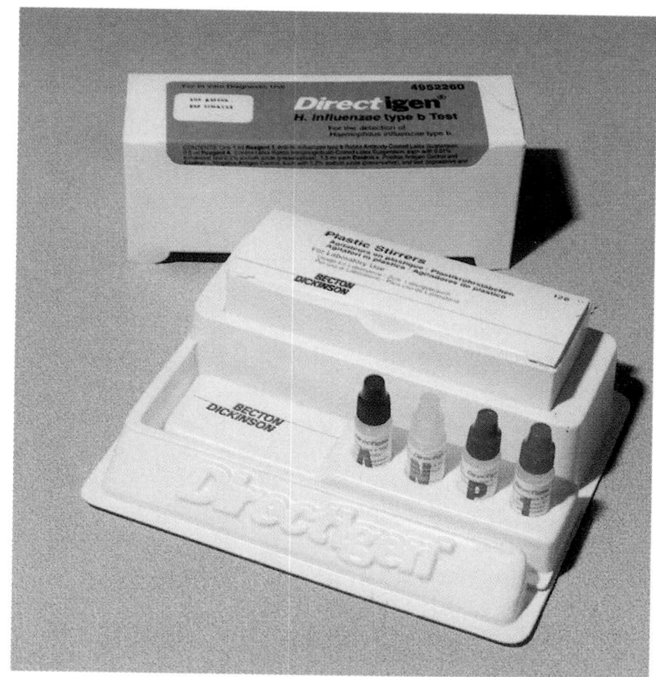

Mycoplasma species, *M. tuberculosis, S. pneumoniae, S. aureus*, and Enterobacteriaceae are the most prevalent causative agents of pericarditis.

Peritoneal Fluid

The peritoneal cavity contains a small amount of fluid that keeps the peritoneum moist. Microorganisms can infect the peritoneal fluid by way of surgery, trauma, or disease of the abdominopelvic cavity. During an infection, the volume of fluid increases; this is often referred to as ascites or ascitic fluid. *E. coli, S. pneumoniae,* and group A streptococci are the primary pathogenic agents.

Pleural Fluid

The pleural membranes are the serous membranes of the thoracic cavity. The parietal pleura lines the chest wall, whereas the visceral pleura covers the lungs. The pleural membranes secrete a serous fluid (pleural fluid) that prevents friction between the membranes as the lungs expand and contract. When this fluid becomes infected, it increases in volume and forms an exudate. Bacteria, such as *H. influenzae, S. aureus, S. pneumoniae, P. aeruginosa*, and Enterobacteriaceae, are the usual organisms involved.

Synovial Fluid

S. aureus, N. gonorrhoeae, and *H. influenzae* are the most frequently isolated bacteria in infectious arthritis. These bacteria infect the synovial fluid, which lubricates the body's movable joints. Synovial fluid can become infected in artificial as well as natural joints. Normal skin contaminants, such as *S. epidermidis,* may cause infection in artificial joints as a result of contamination during replacement surgery.

Susceptible Patients

Some patients develop infectious diseases because of increased susceptibility, which is usually related to an existing disease or condition. Moreover, the very young and the very old are also at increased risk for infection. Patients whose immune systems are suppressed by disease or as a result of treatment (e.g., chemotherapy), or those with certain diseases, such as diabetes mellitus, cystic fibrosis, or immunodeficiency syndrome, are at increased risk for infection. Hospitalized patients, particularly those with indwelling lines, shunts, and catheters, also have an increased likelihood of becoming infected.

Patients with AIDS develop infections to many microorganisms owing to the destruction of their immune system by HIV. Some of the most frequently encountered pathogens in patients with AIDS are *Mycobacterium* species, *C. albicans, Cryptosporidium* species, *Pneumocystic carinii,* cytomegalovirus, and herpes simplex.

Summary

Quality control of diagnostic microbiologic techniques requires the same attention as do other areas of the laboratory. Decontamination procedures should be of particular concern, as the accuracy and reliability of these procedures will determine whether or not microorganisms are isolated from specimens. Safety measures must be strictly observed, and any possible problem must be brought to the attention of the physician or laboratory technologist in charge. Immediately report any suspected organisms to the physician or the laboratory technologist for examination and confirmation.

Chapter Review

True or False

Circle T or F to indicate the correct answers to the following:

T F 1. Protocols for definitive identification of bacteria and antibiotic sensitivity are based on bacterial cell morphology.

T F 2. *Streptococcus viridans* causes bacterial endocarditis.

T F 3. The CAMP factor is a compound that acts within the lungs and causes pneumonia.

T F 4. *Streptococcus pneumoniae* is commonly found in the bones of healthy children.

T F 5. Tuberculosis is transmitted by airborne droplets.

T F 6. The presence of bacilli in the blood is termed bacteremia.

T F 7. *Chlamydia trachomatis* can only reproduce within living cells of a host.

Fill in the Blanks

Complete the following statements:

8. MacConkey agar inhibits the growth of gram-

    ______________ organisms.

9. Normal flora that become pathogenic are referred to as

    ______________ .

10. When referring to bacteria, the first name is the

_______________ and the second is the _______________ .

11. *Streptococcus pyogenes* is the pathogen in

_______________ , _______________ , and

_______________ .

12. Two significant fungal pathogens found in the blood are

_______________ _______________ and _______________

_______________ .

Multiple Choice

Circle the letter that represents the single best answer:

13. Staphylococci usually grow in:
    a. Chains
    b. Pairs
    c. Clusters
    d. Singles

14. In 1993, an outbreak of HUS was found to be associated with:
    a. Hospitalization
    b. Tuberculosis
    c. Leprosy
    d. Hamburger consumption

15. The catalase test is a rapid enzyme test used to distinguish between:
    a. *Streptococcus* and *Staphylococcus*
    b. Gram-positive bacteria and gram-negative bacteria
    c. Coagulase-positive *Staphylococcus* and coagulase-negative *Staphylococcus*
    d. Cocci and bacilli

16. In the urinary system, the structure that most frequently hosts bacteria is the:
    a. Ureter
    b. Bladder
    c. Urethra
    d. Kidney

Vocabulary

arthropod: a phylum of the animal kingdom that includes the arachnids, crustaceans, and insects

cecum: first portion of the large intestine

cosmopolitan: not limited to any one country; widespread

cysts: closed epithelium-lined sacs or capsules containing a liquid or semisolid substance

dermatophytid: a secondary skin eruption occurring on an area remote from the site of infection

endemic: present in a community at all times

enterocolitis: inflammation of the small intestine and colon

gastroenteritis: inflammation of the stomach and small intestinal lining

guaiac: a substance derived from the resin or sap from the *Guaiacum* tree and made into a chemical used in the testing of feces for occult blood

host: an animal or plant that houses and provides food for another organism (parasite)

hyphae: filaments or threads composing the mycelium of a fungus

ileum: the distal portion of the small intestine

jaundice: yellowness of the skin caused by excess bilirubin in the blood

larvae: the immature stage of the life cycle of a parasite

malaise: a vague feeling of uneasiness or body discomfort

malabsorption: impaired intestinal absorption of nutrients

morbidity: the ratio of sick to well persons in a given community or area

mycobacterium: a slender, acid-fast microorganism resembling the bacillus; refers to many species, including the one that causes tuberculosis

oocyst: the encapsulated stage in the development of any sporozoan

protozoan: a subkingdom of unicellular organisms that are frequently ingested and transmitted through contaminated feces

spore: a refractile, oval body formed within bacteria, which is regarded as a resting stage during the life of the cell

trophozoite: the active, motile feeding stage of a sporozoan parasite

urethral: pertaining to the tube leading from the urinary bladder to the outside of the body

vector: an arthropod carrier that transfers an infective agent from one host to another

virion: the complete viral particle that infects a living cell

Chapter Objectives

After reading this chapter, you should be able to:

1. Identify three disease-producing organisms other than bacteria.
2. Name three viruses that have caused a resurgence in the study of medically important viruses.
3. List seven signs and symptoms of a fungal infection.
4. Explain the temperature range in which molds and yeasts can grow.
5. List four common fungal infections.
6. Define deuteromycete and give examples of two forms of this class of fungus.
7. List three modes of parasitic transmission.
8. Identify four species of disease-causing parasites.
9. Name the three groups of parasitic worms and describe the characteristics of each group.
10. Explain why viruses are difficult to treat.

Chapter 27
Basic Mycology, Parasitology, and Virology

Bacteria are not the only microorganisms of concern in the clinical microbiological laboratory. In addition to bacteria, important disease-producing fungi, viruses, and parasites are also analyzed in the laboratory. Relatively few of the more than 50,000 species of fungi are important human pathogens. Mycology and parasitology have become increasingly important in recent years. Parasites that are **endemic** to other countries have gained access to the United States via people traveling and living in those areas. An increase in natural immigration and in refugee populations has caused an increase in the sources of transmission for parasites throughout the United States. Other sources of infection include those individuals who have compromised immune systems, particularly those with acquired immunodeficiency syndrome (AIDS) (Table 27–1).

Mycology

Medical mycology is the study of a group of primitive microorganisms that produce a variety of superficial and systemic diseases in humans. These primitive microorganisms, collectively called fungi, include molds and yeast. Signs and symptoms of a fungal infection are usually vague and nonspecific. Low-grade fever, night sweats, weight loss, tiredness, **malaise,** cough, and chest pain are often the presenting symptoms. In this regard, disseminated fungal diseases may mimic other infections, such as tuberculosis.

Common Fungal Infections

Dimorphic Fungi (Molds and Yeast)

Dimorphic fungi have the ability to grow in two forms, depending upon environmental conditions. When these fungi grow at room temperature

Table 27–1
Common Infectious Agents Associated With AIDS

FUNGAL	PARASITIC
Aspergillus	*Cryptosporidium*
Candida	*Pneumocystis carinii*
Cryptococcus	*Strongyloides*
Histoplasma	*Toxoplasma*
VIRAL	**BACTERIAL**
Cytomegalovirus	***Mycobacterium*** *avium-intracellulare*
Herpes simplex virus	*Mycobacterium tuberculosis*
Adenovirus	Other *Mycobacterium* species

(25° to 30°C), they are called molds. Examples of mold include athlete's foot and ringworm.

Fungi that grow at body temperature (35° to 37°C) are classified as yeasts. Examples of the yeast form include thrush and *Crytpococcus neoformans.*

Coccidioides immitis *(San Joaquin Valley Fever)*

San Joaquin Valley fever is caused by *Coccidioides immitis* (Fig. 27–1, *A* and *B*). It is endemic in hot, dry areas, with alkaline soil, such as the lower Sonora in Mexico and the western and southwestern desert regions of the United States. A part of the fungus, the conidium or **spore,** needs the intense heat of the subsurface desert sand to mature and become wind-borne. These conidia are small, very light in weight, and highly infectious for humans. They primarily produce pulmonary disease. A highly prevalent, acute, self-limiting, pulmonary disease in Kern County, California is now known to be caused by *Coccidioides immitis.* This is why coccidioidomycosis has been called San Joaquin Valley fever.

Sporotrichosis (Rose Gardener's Disease)

Sporotrichosis, caused by *Sporothrix schenchii* (Fig. 27–2), is primarily a subcutaneous mycosis found mostly in the midwestern United States, particularly in the states bordering the Missouri and Mississippi River valleys. It is also known as the rose gardener's disease because the primary lesion is often a nonhealing ulcer of the skin of the fingers, hand, or forearm, developing 1 to 2 weeks after having been punctured by a rose thorn or other spore-contaminated vegetation (sphagnum moss, for example). Masonry workers handling old bricks, miners, and others coming in contact with plant material are highly susceptible.

Histoplasmosis

Histoplasmosis (Fig. 27–3) is a frequently diagnosed systemic fungal disease in the United States. It is present in bird or bat droppings and in soil contaminated with these droppings. Bird roosts, chicken houses, caves, or buildings containing bats can be highly infective areas. Cleaning these areas may expose humans to large numbers of airborne spores causing pulmonary infection. The major endemic areas in the United States are the drainage basins of the Ohio and Mississippi River valleys, where virtually all of the native population tests positive to skin testing, indicating past infections or exposure to the causative organism, *Histoplasma capsulatum.*

Figure 27–1. A, Coccidioides immitis *fungi.* B, *Barrel arthrospores.*

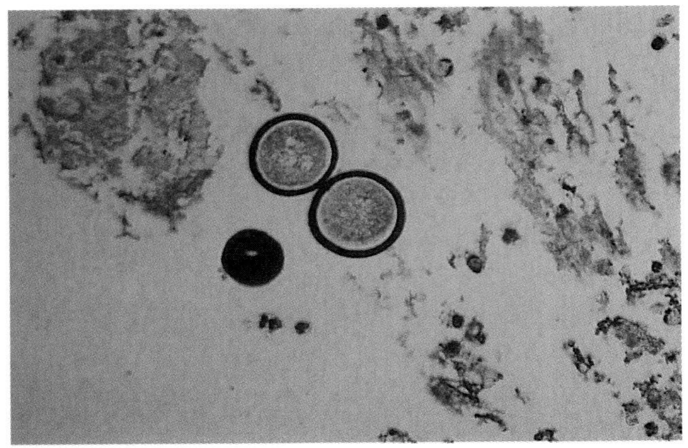

A

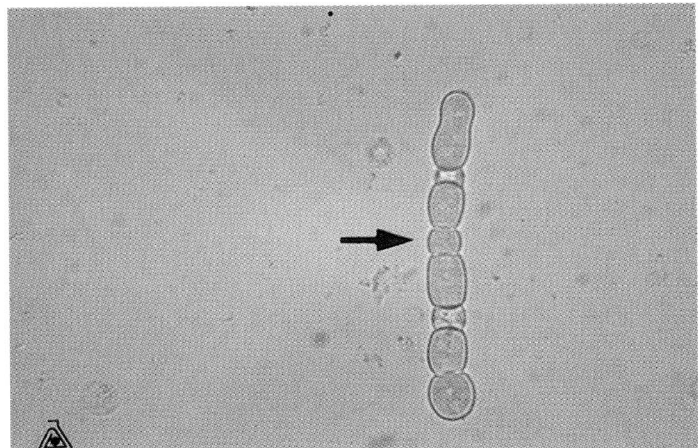

B

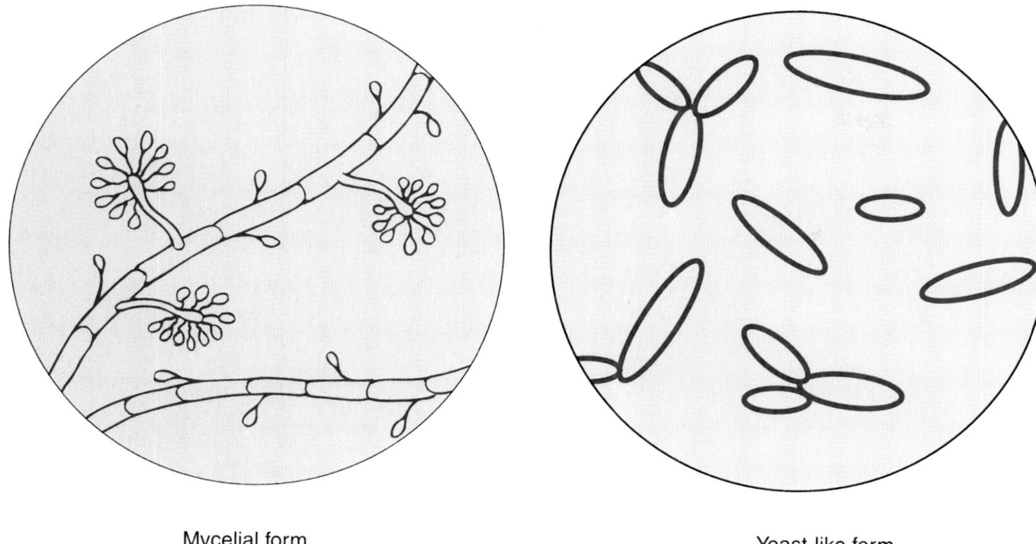

Figure 27–2. *Sporotrichosis*

Clinical symptoms of histoplasmosis vary from mild respiratory illness to temporary incapacity with general malaise, weakness, fever, chest pains, and a dry or productive cough. Without treatment, the disease may be fatal.

Dermatophytosis

The **dermatophytid** molds are a distinct group of fungi that infect the skin, nails, and hair of humans and animals. The genera *Epidermophyton, Microsporum,* and *Trichophyton* are the only fungi associated with cutaneous infections. The cutaneous mycoses are referred to as *tinea,* the Latin word for worm or ringworm. This group of mycoses is more common now than in the past owing to the increased number of antibacterial and immunosuppressive drugs available. *Tricophyton rubrum* is the most common dermatophyte to infect human skin and nails, and in rare cases, it infects the hair and scalp.

Prolonged use of antibiotics can result in a fungal superinfection. Dermatophytid mold is classified according to the type of tissue involved (Table 27–2). Three of the most common are tinea corporis, tinea pedis, and tinea cruris.

Tinea Corporis (Ringworm). Tinea corporis is commonly known as ringworm of the body because of the symmetrical pattern formed on the skin. The fungus is usually identified on the basis of the round, itching, scaling patches of skin affected by the mold. This may be caused by *Trichophyton tonsurans* (Fig. 27–4).

Tinea Pedis (Athlete's Foot). Athlete's foot is scientifically known as tinea pedis. Typical clinical symptoms include itching, scaling, or blisters containing a thin, watery fluid on the soles of the feet or between the toes. This occurs most often during the warm and humid times of the year. The fungal spore *Trichophyton mentagrophytes* is introduced into the tissue through a break in the skin. Walking on public swimming pool decks and using shower areas are simple ways humans become accidental hosts.

Tinea Cruris (Jock Itch). Tinea cruris is also known as jock itch. Clinical manifestations are seen in the inguinal and axillary regions. The clinical symptoms are

Figure 27–3. *Histoplasmosis.*

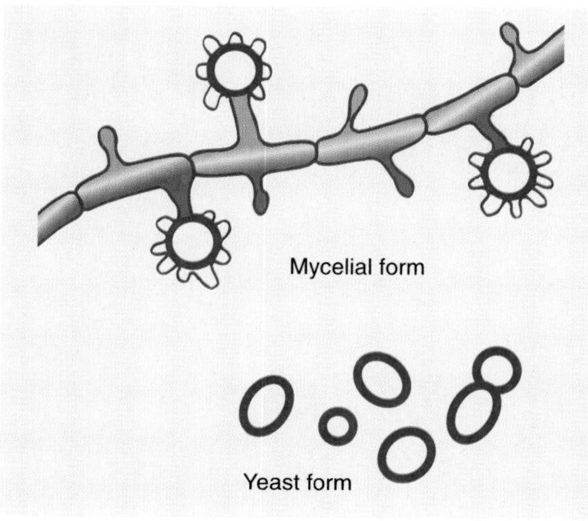

Table 27–2
Cutaneous Mycoses

Organism	***Hair***	***Skin***	***Nails***
TRICHOPHYTON			
T. rubrum (1)	×	× (tinea pedis)	× (tinea unguium)
T. mentagrophytes (2)	×	× (tinea pedis)	× (tinea unguium)
T. tonsurans (4)	× (tinea capitis in children)	×	×
T. verrucosum (6)	× (tinea barbae in men)	× (tinea corporis in men)	×
T. violaceum	× (most prevalent in Mediterranean, Middle East, Africa)	× (most prevalent in Mediterranean, Middle East, Africa)	×
T. schoenleinii	× (tinea capitis, favus)	×	×
MICROSPORUM			
M. audouinii	× (tinea capitis)	×	
M. canis (5)	× (tinea capitis, dogs and cats)	× × ×	
M. gypseum	×	×	
EPIDERMOPHYTON			
E. floccosum	× (tinea cruris, tinea pedis)	×	

Figure 27–4. Trichophyton tonsurans.

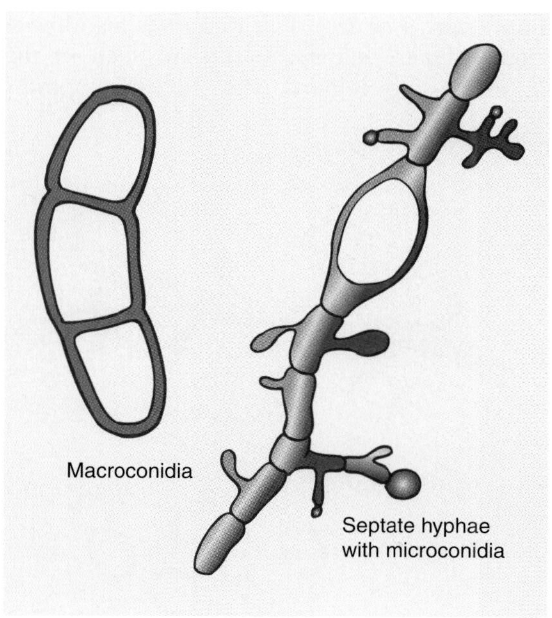

the same as those of ringworm of the body. The lesions appear as flat and ring-shaped. The periphery is reddish, vesicular, or pustular, and may be dry and scaly or moist and crusted.

Treatment and Diagnosis

Griseofulvin and similar topical antifungal compounds, available as over-the-counter preparations, are simple modes of treatment for tinea.

ANALYZE

Three Common Diagnostic Methods for Identifying Fungal Disease

- Direct microscopic examination of tissue scrapings
- Use of a Wood's light (ultraviolet light), which will cause infected hair to fluoresce a bright yellow-green
- A potassium hydroxide (KOH) test that detects spores or budding yeast cells

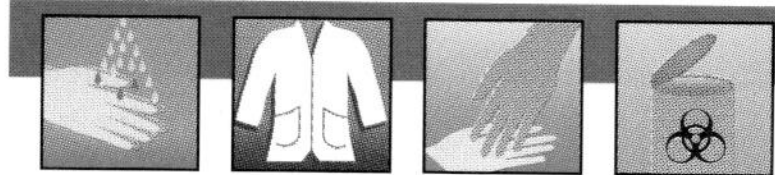

PROCEDURE 27–1

Performing a KOH Test to Determine the Presence or Absence of Nail Fungus

Principle

To determine the presence or absence of spores or budding yeast cells

Equipment and Supplies

sterile nail nippers
sterile scalpel with blade
70% alcohol prep pads
glass slides
10% potassium hydroxide (KOH)
heat source/incinerator
microscope

Procedural Steps

1. Explain the procedure to the patient.
2. Wash hands thoroughly and put on gloves and other protective gear.
3. Cleanse the infected nail area with 70% alcohol to remove bacteria.
4. Using a sterile nail nipper or scalpel, CAREFULLY collect a nail specimen from beneath the nail plate to obtain softened material from the nail bed. If this is not possible, collect shavings from the deeper portions of the nail.
5. Place the nail clipping(s)/shavings in a covered, sterile container.
6. Mix the specimen with one or two drops of KOH on a glass slide.
7. Spread out the specimen, covering the entire slide.
8. Expose the slide to gentle heat and allow it to dry.
9. Place the slide under the microscope's low-power objective and examine it, using low light, for mycelial fragments and/or budding yeast cells.
10. Report your findings and record the test procedure in the laboratory logbook.
11. Clean the work area and dispose of any biohazardous waste.
12. Remove gloves and wash hands.

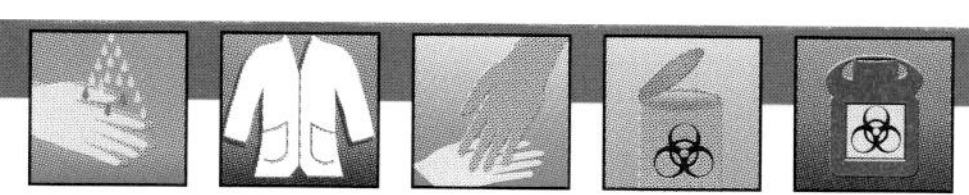

PROCEDURE 27–2

Using Calcofluor White Stain to Diagnose Tinea Pedis (Athlete's Foot)

Principle

To detect tinea pedis or the presence of other fungal species using fluorescent microscopy

Equipment and Supplies

SpotTest Calcofluor White Reagent (Difco Laboratories)
70% alcohol prep pads
sterile scalpel or wooden spatula
glass slides and coverslips
10% potassium hydroxide (SpotTest KOH 10%)
inoculating loop/needle
quality control cultures
fluorescent microscope

Procedural Steps

1. **Before beginning the testing procedure, first check the expiration date on the SpotTest kit. Then open the kit and read the enclosed instructions carefully.**

(continued)

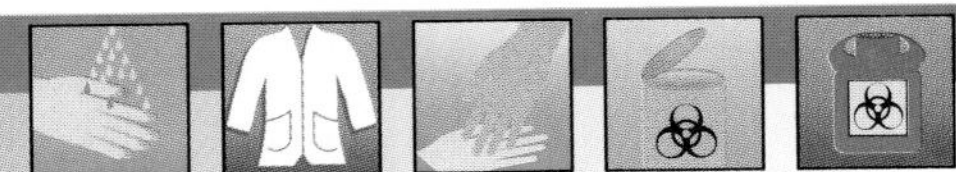

PROCEDURE 27–2

Using Calcofluor White Stain to Diagnose Tinea Pedis (Athlete's Foot) (Continued)

Collection of the Specimen

2. Explain the procedure to the patient.
3. Wash hands thoroughly and put on gloves and other protective gear.
4. Cleanse the test site with 70% alcohol to remove bacteria.
5. Scrape the peripheral erythematous margin of the lesions with a sterile scalpel or wooden spatula.
6. Place the scrapings into a covered, sterile container.

Testing Procedure

7. Place the specimen on a clean slide.
8. Add 1 to 2 drops of 10% KOH to the specimen and gently mix.
9. Holding the calcofluor dispenser upright and with the tip pointing away from you, squeeze the dispenser gently to crush the glass ampule inside it.
10. Invert the dispenser and squeeze it slightly to dispense the reagent on a per drop basis.
11. Dispense an equal volume of the SpotTest Calcofluor White Reagent onto the slide and mix with the specimen.
12. Mount the specimen with a coverslip.
13. Examine the specimen slide using a fluorescent microscope. If fungal elements are present, a brilliant apple-green fluorescence will be noted.
14. Check the reagent by testing it with the positive and negative control cultures. Remember that the positive culture should turn bright apple-green.
15. Report your findings.
16. Enter the test in the laboratory logbook.
17. Clean the work area and dispose of all biohazardous waste.
18. Remove gloves and wash hands.

Deuteromycetes

Most disease-producing fungi in humans are of the Deuteromycetes group of fungi. *Candida albicans* and *Cryptococcus neoformans* are examples of yeasts in this group.

Candida albicans *(Thrush)*

Candida albicans is an opportunistic yeast that causes oral thrush in infants and vaginal yeast infections in women. Thrush is an infection of the oral mucous membranes that is characterized by white patches on a

Figure 27–5. A, *Culture of* Candida albicans. *B,* Candida albicans *in tissue.*

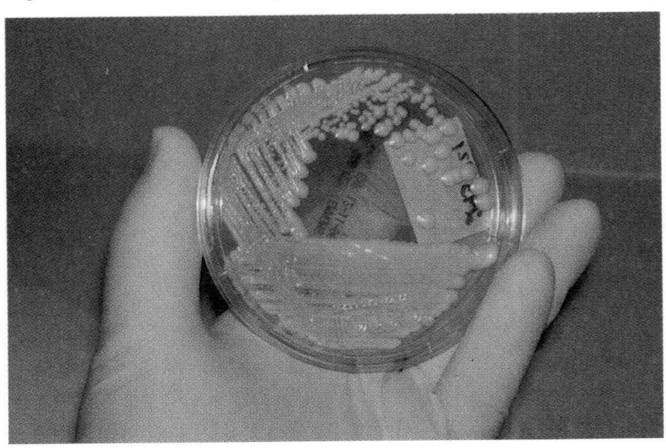

A

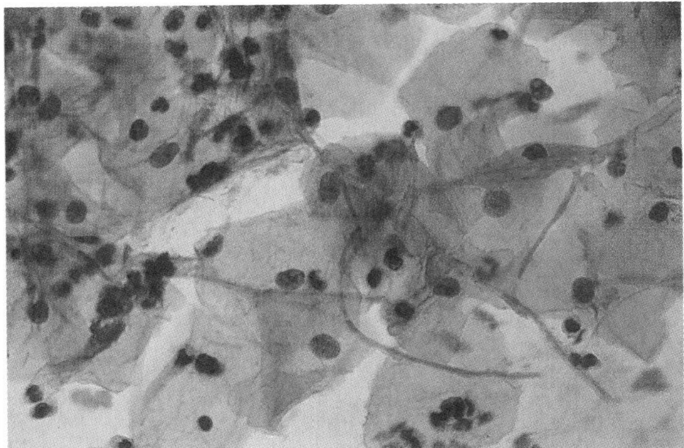

B

red, moist, inflamed surface. It can occur anywhere in the mouth, including the tongue, but usually involves the inner cheeks (Fig. 27–5, *A* and *B*). These patches are occasionally accompanied by pain and fever. Clinical symptoms include discomfort while nursing and a sore throat.

Cryptococcus neoformans *(Cryptococcal Meningitis)*

Cryptococcus neoformans produces a chronic severe disease in humans, occurring either as meningitis or meningoencephalitis. This organism is usually associated with bird droppings, especially on window ledges in aviaries, roosts, and nests. Humans and animals acquire the yeast by inhaling dust containing the spores. It is most frequently diagnosed on the basis of pulmonary lesions, subcutaneous tumor-like masses, acute pneumonitis, and/or generalized infection involving the organs of the body.

Cryptococcal meningitis is confirmed by microscopic examination of spinal fluid or pus. The fungus is then cultured, and is found to be able to grow at 37°C. Serologic tests are not reliable.

An India ink preparation was used for many years to identify the organism in spinal fluid. In this test, a suspension of the specimen was mixed with an equal amount of ink. The capsule would not absorb the ink, becoming visible under the microscope as a wide, clear halo. Today, many laboratories use the latex agglutination test for identification of *Cryptococcus neoformans* (Figs. 27–6 and 27–7, *A* and *B*).

Parasitology

Parasitic diseases are important causes of **morbidity** and mortality. Parasites have also retarded economic development in many parts of the world. Individuals with weakened immune systems, such as those with human immunodeficiency virus (HIV), are at increased risk for parasitic infections. Because of expanded international travel, a new interest in parasitology has recently developed.

Parasites are transmitted by several means:

- ingestion during the infective stage
- direct penetration of the skin by infective larvae
- inoculation by an **arthropod vector**

There are about 70 species of parasites that commonly infect the human body. It is not possible to identify a parasite accurately on the basis of a single specimen, and in humans, most are identified by blood or fecal tests. In addition to these common identification media, urine, sputum, tissue fluids, or tissue biopsy may also be used.

Parasites are organisms that live on or in a **host** organism. Some types may cause little or no injury to the host, whereas other parasites can cause serious illness, even death, if left untreated. Parasites seldom cause noticeable symptoms in a healthy host, but if the host's immune system has been compromised, serious harm may occur.

Parasitic Life Cycle

An understanding of parasitic life cycles is important in the diagnosis and treatment of parasite infections. This cycle consists of a host phase and a no-host phase. Sometimes a parasite will require an intermediate host or vector to complete its life cycle. Vectors are organisms, usually insects, that transmit the parasite to an uninfected host.

The parasite invades the host during the infective stage of the life cycle. Diagnosis is made when the parasite can be detected in the appropriate specimen. The diagnostic stage and infective stage may coincide in certain parasites, such as *Giardia lamblia*.

Intestinal parasites are usually diagnosed by the detection of parasitic cysts or trophozoites in the host's feces (Fig. 27–8, *A* and *B*). Blood parasites, such as malaria, are diagnosed by the presence of the parasite in blood smears. Other parasites, such as *Leishmania*, can be detected in aspirations or tissue samples.

Figure 27–6. Cryptococcus neoformans.

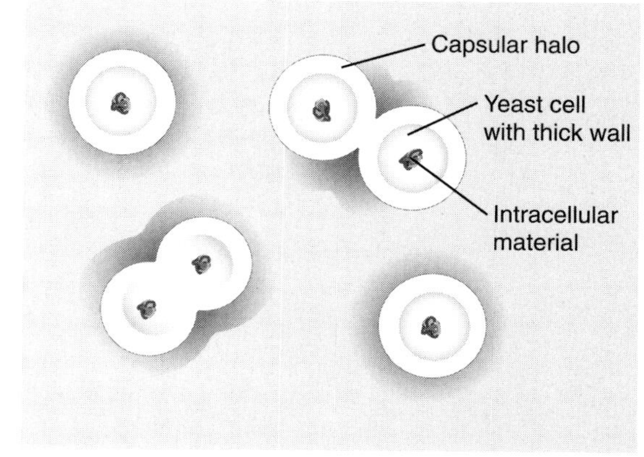

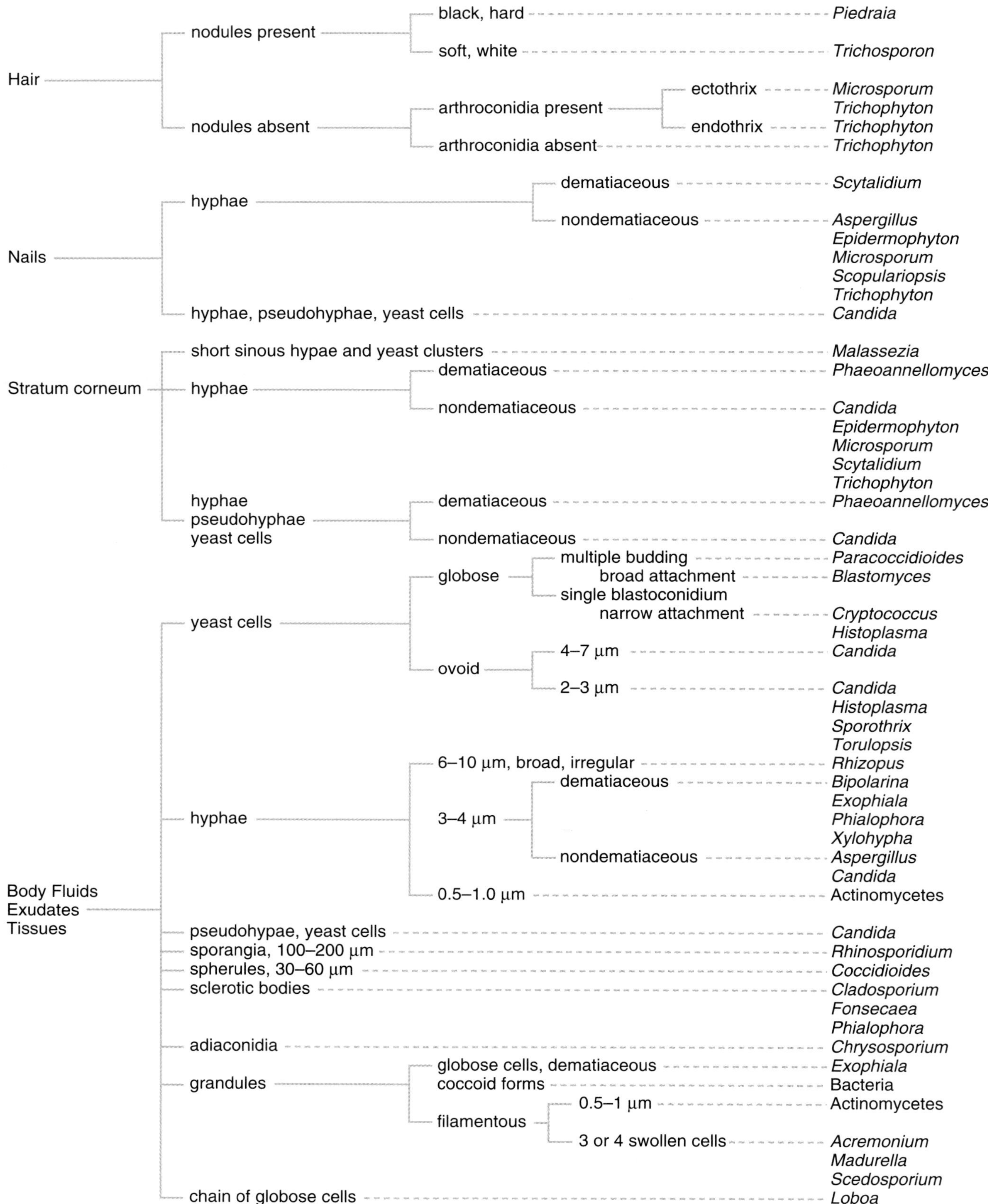

Figure 27–7. *Basic morphology of fungi by source.*

Commonly Identified Parasites

Entamoeba hystolytica

Entamoeba hystolytica (Fig. 27–9) is the **protozoan** that causes amoebic dysentery. Common symptoms are diarrhea, fatigue, and intestinal bleeding. This condition is often found in third world countries, but is rarely seen in the United States. It is spread by contaminated water and food, by flies, and by soiled hands of food handlers. The primary site of infection is the colon; thus, diagnosis is confirmed by examination of stool specimens or biopsy sections of the lesions on the colon.

Figure 27–8. *Stool processing.* A, *Fresh specimen.* B, *Preserved specimen.* C, *Processing and staining of stool for ova and parasites using a preserved specimen.*

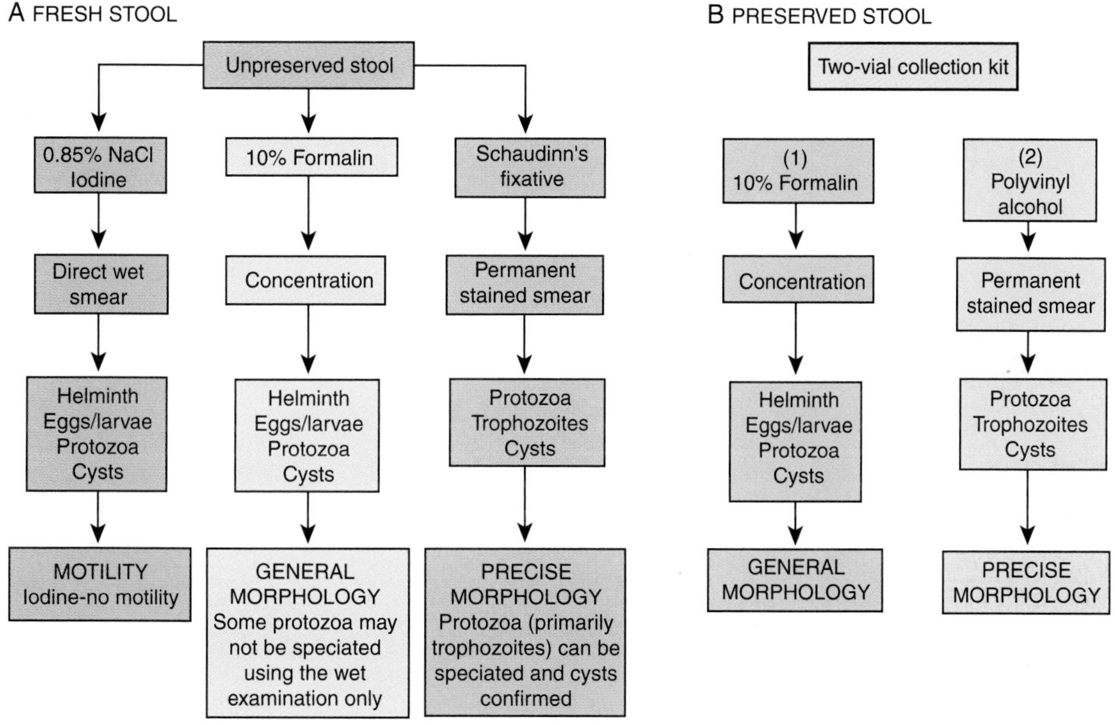

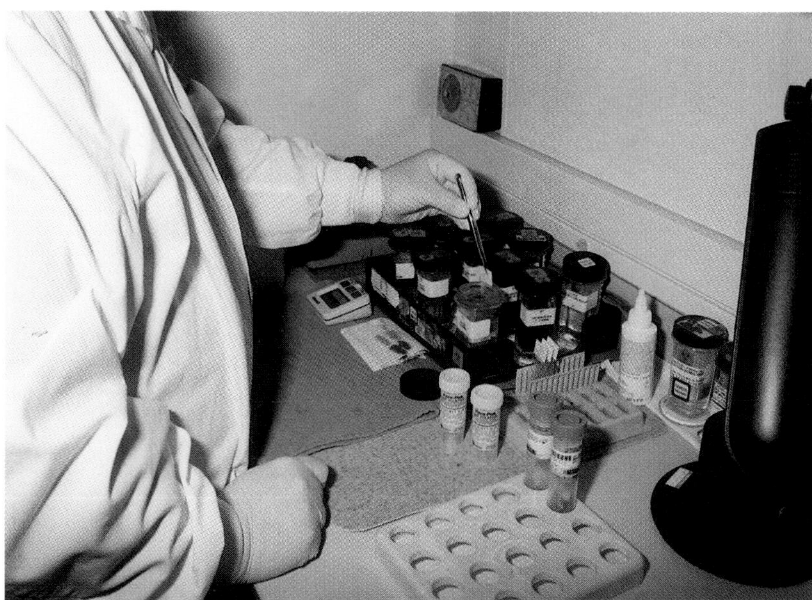

C

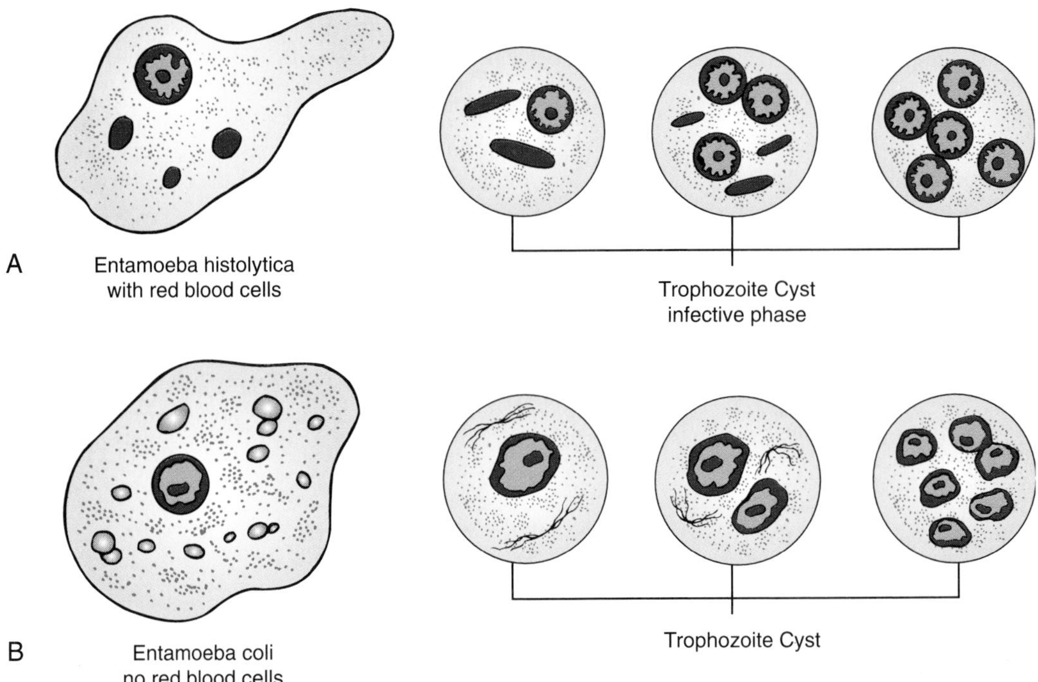

Figure 27–9. Entamoeba histolytica *and* Entamoeba coli.

Figure 27–10. Giardia lamblia.

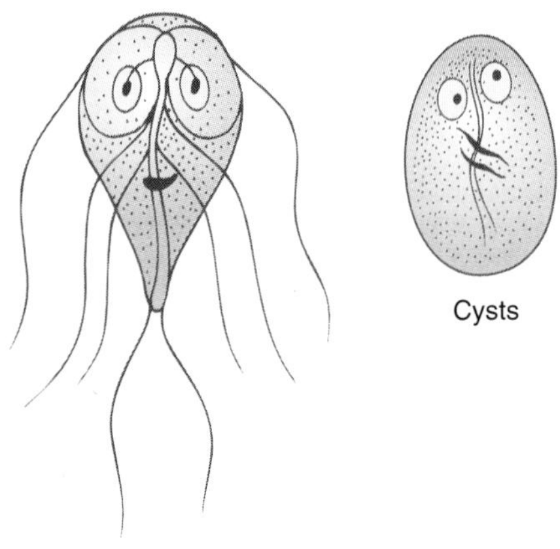

Giardia lamblia

Giardia lamblia is a common intestinal protozoic pathogen in the United States (Fig. 27–10). In the United States, outbreaks related to drinking water contaminated by infected human or animal feces are common, and infections among campers, homosexuals, and clients or caregivers in day care centers are frequent. Weight loss, diarrhea, gastrointestinal discomfort, and malabsorption are all symptoms of giardiasis. Diagnosis is confirmed by the presence of **cysts** and **trophozoites** of *Giardia lamblia* in stool specimens.

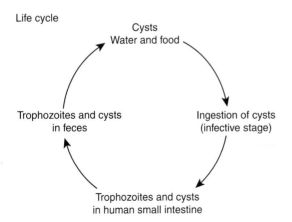

Figure 27–11. Trichomonas vaginalis.

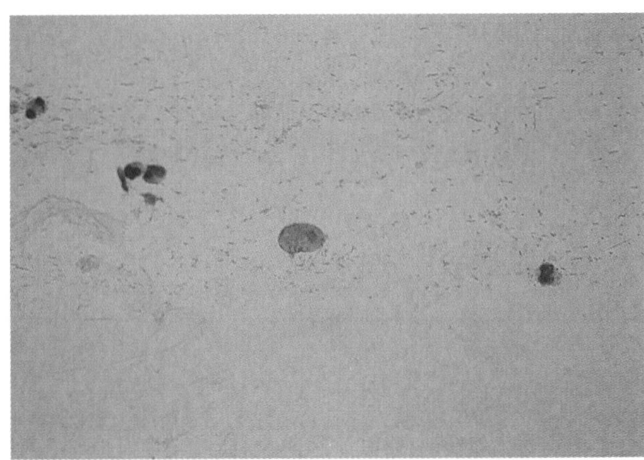

Trichomonas vaginalis

Trichomonas vaginalis causes an infection called trichomoniasis. It is a common, sexually transmitted infection in female and male adults. Diagnosis is confirmed by the detection of trophozoites in vaginal secretions or **urethral** specimens on direct saline (wet mount) microscopic examinations (Fig. 27–11). Slides can be prepared from a variety of specimens, such as vaginal, urethral, or penile discharges, scrapings of the urethral mucosa, or first-voided urine, which can then be examined microscopically under low- and high-power for the presence of actively moving organisms. Direct saline mount specimens must be examined within 1 hour of collection, as the trophozoites quickly lose their motility and dry out, after which they resemble white blood cells (WBCs).

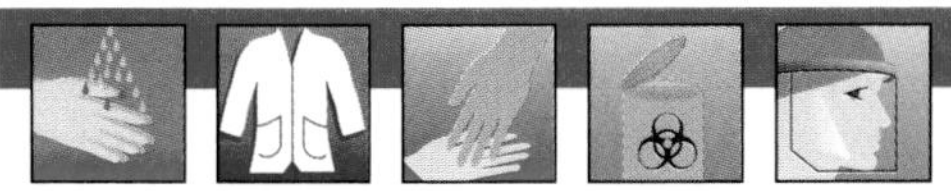

PROCEDURE 27–3

Preparing a Direct Saline Mount for Detection of Trichomonas vaginalis

Principle

To prepare a specimen for microscopic examination in order to confirm or rule out *Trichomonas vaginalis* infection

Equipment and Supplies

glass slide
coverslip
disposable pipette
specimen
normal saline solution
microscope

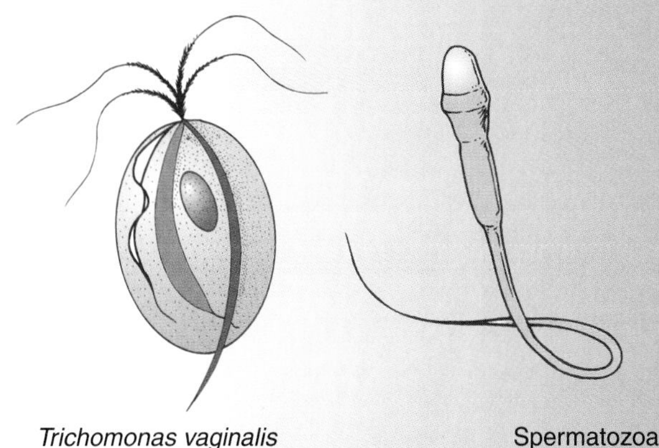

Comparison of size at 2000

Procedural Steps

1. Wash hands and put on gloves and safety gear.
2. Place a drop of the specimen onto a clean slide.
3. Immediately add 1 or 2 drops of saline.
   NOTE: If urine sediment is the specimen used, omit this step.
4. Mix the saline and specimen together with the tip of a pipette or the corner of the coverslip.
5. Cover the specimen with a No. 1 coverslip.
6. Examine the wet mount under the microscope's low-power (10) objective using low light.
7. Motile objects that are suspect can be examined using the high-power (40) objective.

NOTE: *T. vaginalis* is usually larger than a typical WBC and will exhibit flagellar movement. It is possible to confuse *T. vaginalis* with sperm, as both have flagellar movement. However, bear in mind that sperm are much smaller than WBCs, and are thus smaller than *T. vaginalis*.

8. The slide should be left in place so that the physician or technologist can confirm the findings.

NOTE: It is important to remember that the intense heat from the light of the microscope can immobilize the organism, so the specimen must be examined quickly by the physician or technologist.

9. Record the test results and enter the test in the laboratory logbook.
10. Clean the work area according to biohazard guidelines and laboratory protocols.
11. Remove gloves and wash hands thoroughly.

Interpretation of Results

Positive result: If the specimen contains motile flagellates, report the test result as positive for *T. vaginalis.*

Negative result: If flagellates are not seen, report the test result as negative for *T. vaginalis.*

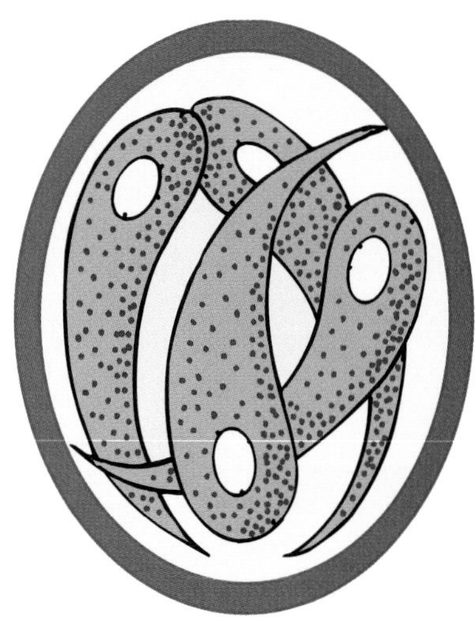

Figure 27–12. Cryptosporidium *oocyst.*

Cryptosporidium

Cryptosporidium is a genus of tiny, coccidian protozoa that are known to cause **enterocolitis** in domestic animals. This microorganism is now known to cause diarrheal disease in immunodeficient individuals, especially patients with HIV. In humans, the clinical symptoms are low-grade fever, watery or mucous diarrhea, persistent **gastroenteritis** with vomiting and abdominal cramping, and **malabsorption.** Diagnosis can be made by identifying an **oocyst** in fecal specimens (Fig. 27–12).

Parasitic Worms/Helminths

Parasitic worms comprise three groups:

1. Nematodes or roundworms
2. Cestodes or tapeworms (flatworms)
3. Trematodes or flukes (flatworms)

All of these parasitic worms are usually diagnosed by detection of eggs in feces. The characteristics that help to identify the eggs are size, shape, shell thickness, special structures of the shell, and the developmental stage of the egg contents. Occasionally, an adult worm may be obtained for identification. The number of worms harbored is the most important factor in the diagnosis of parasitic worms.

Nematodes

The species of nematodes that infect man include *Ascaris lumbricoides, Trichuris trichiura, Enterobius vermicularis,* the hookworms, and *Strongyloides stercoralis. Enterobius vermicularis,* commonly known as pinworm, has a **cosmopolitan** distribution. The organism is primarily a parasite of young children. Humans are infected by ingestion of mature eggs via hand-to-mouth transfers, by feces-contaminated fingers, by feces-contaminated food or fluids, or by inhaling eggs in air currents from infected areas. The eggs hatch in the small intestine, with the females migrating out of the anus, usually at night, to deposit the eggs. The eggs adhere to the skin, perianal hairs, sleeping garments, and other cloth items. This results in itching of the anus, whereby eggs come in contact with the hands and fingernails of the host. Parasitic ova may then be carried to the mouth and swallowed, reinfecting the host. Other family members may be infected through contact with contaminated clothing and bedding.

In children, specimens are best collected late at night or early in the morning, before a bowel movement, urination, or bathing. Petroleum jelly–impregnated paraffin swabs or cellulose tape patches may be used to collect eggs deposited by worms during sleep; the latter may then be attached to a glass slide for microscopic viewing. To identify adult worms, samples of feces are placed in special collection vials provided by the laboratory for amebiasis. The bottle label and the laboratory slip should be marked "rule out pinworm." Diagnosis is based on laboratory detection of the eggs in fecal smears (Fig. 27–13).

Figure 27–13. *Pinworm ova in fecal smear.*

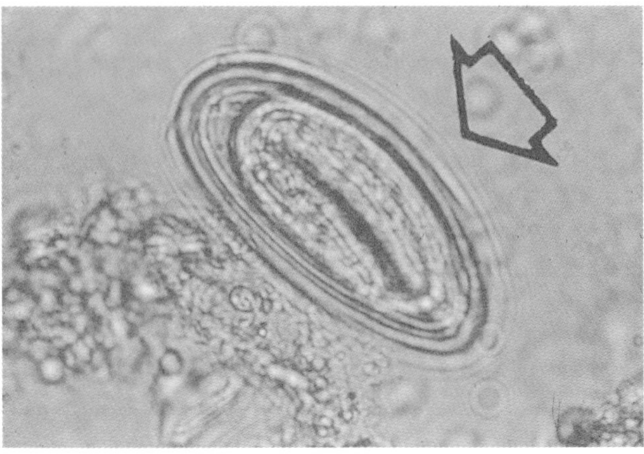

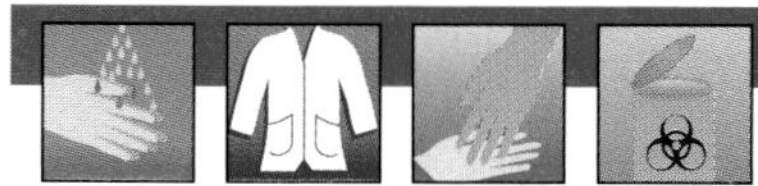

PROCEDURE 27–4

Performing a Cellulose Tape Test for the Collection and Microscopic Examination of Pinworms

Principle:

To obtain a rectal sample using cellulose tape for the purpose of testing for pinworm (*E. vermicularis*) eggs

Equipment and Supplies

glass slide
clear cellulose tape
wooden tongue depressor
toluene
microscope
gauze or cotton balls

Procedural Steps

NOTE: Specimens should be obtained first thing in the morning, before the child bathes or goes to the bathroom. If the parent prefers to bring the child to the lab for assistance with obtaining the specimen, ask the parent to assist you in holding the child.

1. Place a strip of cellulose tape on a glass slide, starting ½ inch from one end and, running toward the same end, continuing around this end lengthwise. Tear off the strip so that it is even with the other end.

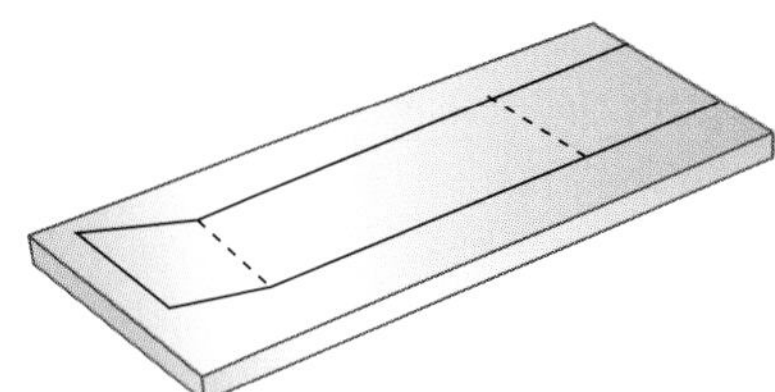

NOTE: Do not use Magic transparent tape; use regular clear cellulose tape.

2. Place a strip of paper measuring ½ × 1 inch between the slide and the tape at the end where the tape is torn flush. This will be the specimen label.
3. Wash hands thoroughly and put on gloves.
4. Remove the underwear of the patient and lay the child in a prone position, over parent's lap, with buttocks exposed.
5. To obtain a perianal sample, first peel back the tape on the slide by gripping the label. With the tape looped (adhesive side outward) over a wooden tongue depressor that is held against the slide and extended about 1 inch beyond it, press the tape firmly against the right and left anal folds.

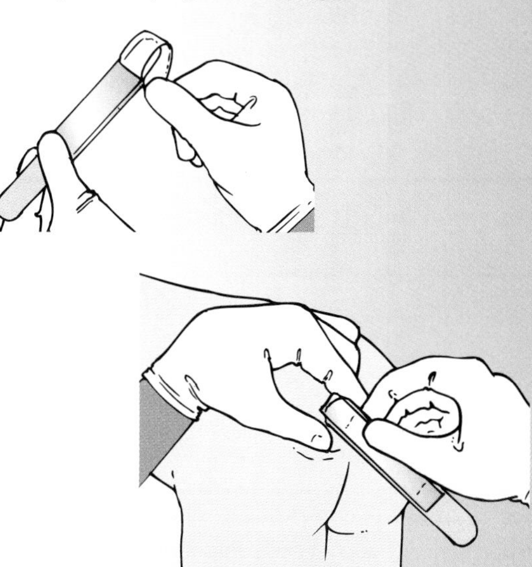

6. Spread the tape back on the slide, adhesive side down.

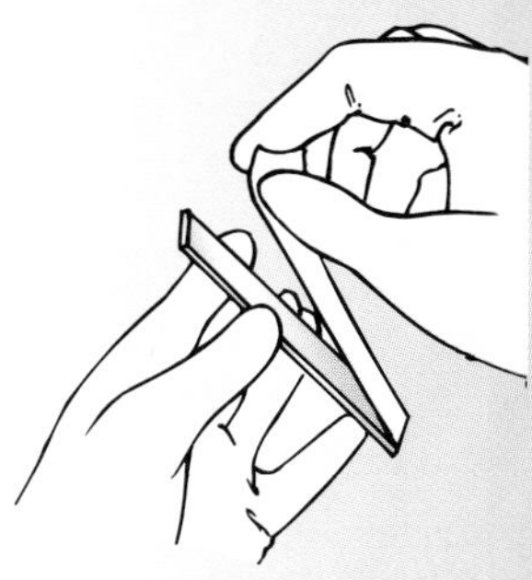

7. Smooth the tape using a cotton ball or gauze.

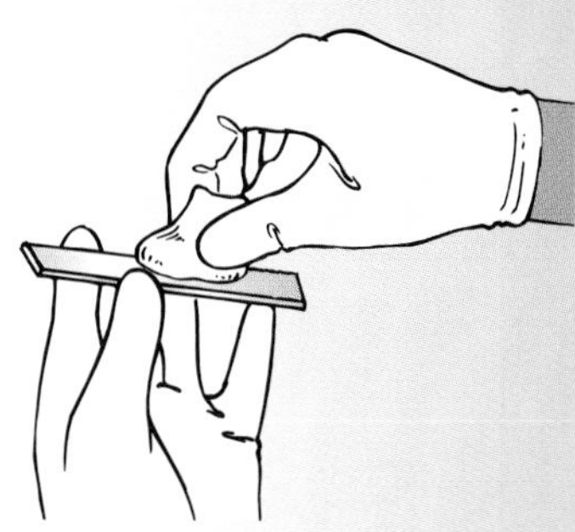

(continued)

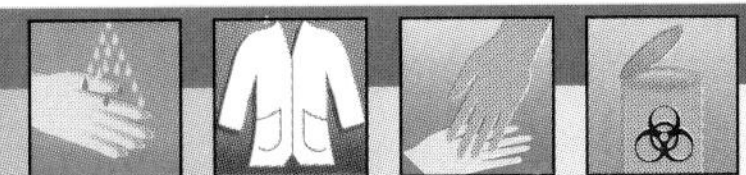

PROCEDURE 27–4

Performing a Cellulose Tape Test for the Collection and Microscopic Examination of Pinworms (Continued)

8. Place the patient's name and date on the label.
9. Replace the child's underwear and release the child to the accompanying adult.
10. Lift one side of the tape and apply 1 drop of toluene before pressing the tape back down on the glass slide. The specimen will then be cleared so that any eggs will be visible.
11. Place the prepared slide under the microscope's low-power objective and examine it under low illumination.
12. Report your findings. Enter the test in the laboratory logbook.
13. Clean the work area and dispose of all contaminated materials in designated containers.

Interpretation of Results

Positive result: Visualization of pinworm eggs
Negative result: No pinworm eggs visible

NOTE: At least four negative specimens should be obtained and examined before the patient is declared free of infection.

Roundworms

Ascaris lumbricoides is the largest worm, and is probably the cause of the most prevalent of human roundworm infestations. It has worldwide distribution. Eggs are usually passed in the feces of infected hosts and, as a result of improper hygiene, are ingested by the new host. Alternatively, they may incubate in the soil, get on the skin of the new host, and travel through the skin as larvae, thereby entering the system of the new host. The eggs hatch in the intestine, after which the **larvae** migrate through the liver to the lungs. The adult form then returns to the small intestine to live. Symptoms include cough, abdominal pain, vomiting, eosinophilia, and sometimes intestinal blockage. The diagnosis is established by observing fertile eggs in feces or, occasionally, the adult worm (Fig. 27–14).

Whipworms

Trichuriasis, or whipworm infestation, is caused by *Trichuris trichiura.* This worm has a worldwide distribution in warm, moist regions. In the United States, whipworm occurs primarily in the Southeast. Adult worms live on the wall of the **cecum** and, occasionally, on the walls of the large intestine, appendix, and lower part of the **ileum.** These worms commonly live for up to 10 years, sometimes, even longer. The life cycle of the infective egg is very similar to that of the roundworm (*A. lumbricoides*) in that both have soil require-

Figure 27–14. *Roundworms.*

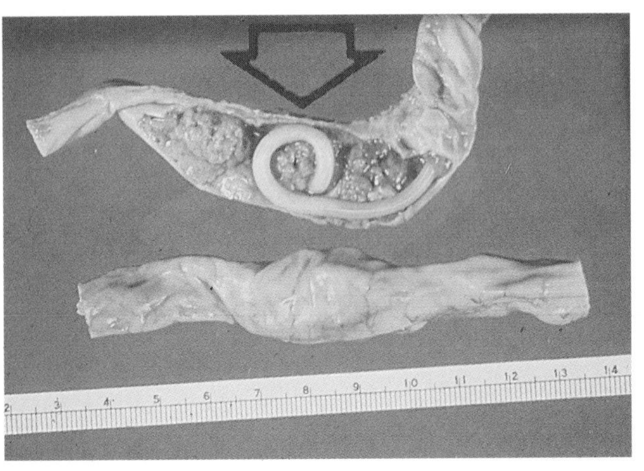

Figure 27–15. *Whipworms.*

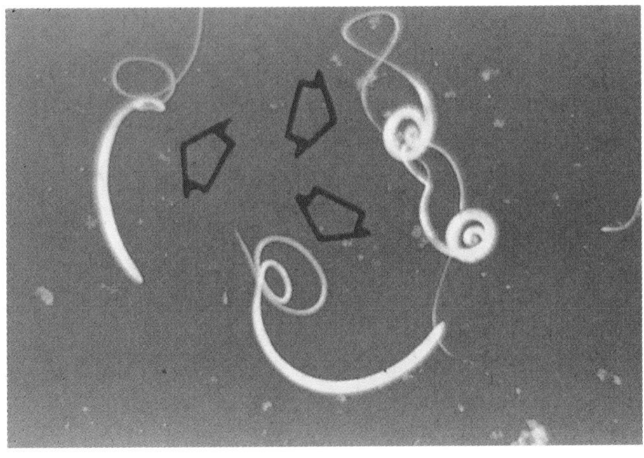

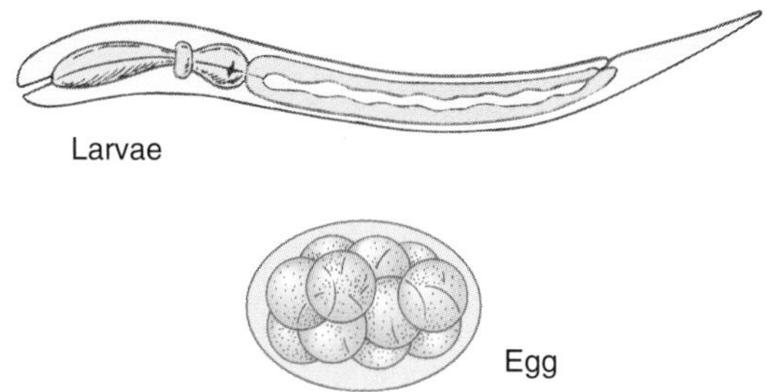

Figure 27–16. *Hookworms.*

ments. Heavy infestation with whipworms may be associated with diarrhea, abdominal cramping, rectal prolapse, dehydration, weight loss, and anemia. Diagnosis is confirmed by detecting the eggs on direct wet mounts of feces or fecal concentration procedures (Fig. 27–15).

Hookworms

Hookworm infestations have a wide distribution in the tropics, subtropics, and in areas with moist, temperate climates. The eggs hatch larvae in the soil. These larvae enter the body via the skin, usually the feet, and migrate to the lungs. There, they are coughed up in sputum and swallowed. In the intestines, they attach to the intestinal wall and ingest blood for nourishment. Characteristic symptoms include fatigue, weakness, abdominal pain, bloody diarrhea, iron deficiency anemia, pallor, and retarded development in infected children. The diagnosis is established by demonstrating the characteristic eggs in feces (Fig. 27–16).

Strongyloides

Strongyloides stercoralis is found predominantly in the tropics, subtropics, and moist, temperate regions. The eggs are hatched in the soil, and larvae can initiate infection by direct penetration of the skin. Once inside the body, they migrate into all tissues and organs. Infestation can lead to extensive hemorrhage and even death if left untreated. Symptoms are the same as for hookworm infestation. Diagnosis is based on the identification of larvae in a fecal specimen (Fig. 27–17).

Cestodes/Tapeworms

Cestode or tapeworm infestations are of importance in humans. Humans can become infected by eating raw

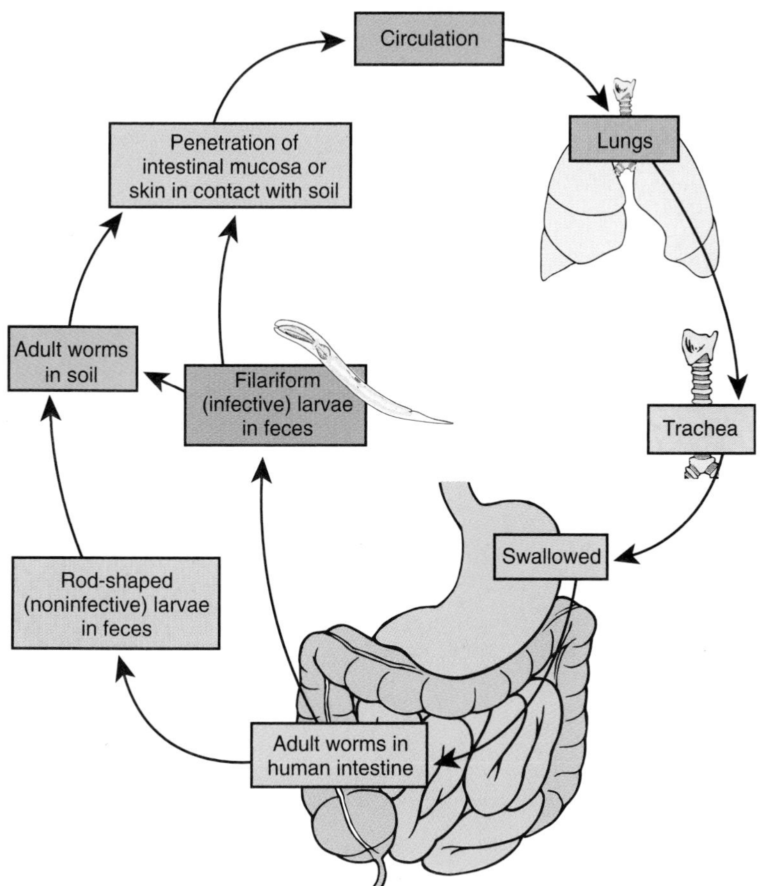

Figure 27–17. Strongyloides.

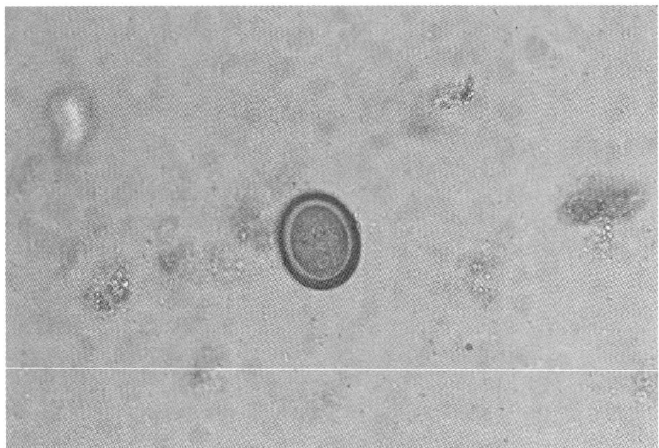

Figure 27–18. *Pork tapeworm* (Taenia solium).

or poorly cooked infected beef, pork, or fish. Adult tapeworms live in the intestinal wall, absorbing food from their host. Symptoms can range from headaches, nausea, vomiting, and vague hunger pains, to various nervous manifestations. The diagnosis is established by finding the eggs in a fecal specimen (Fig. 27–18).

Trematodes or Flukes

Trematodes or flukes infect humans who wade or swim in infected waters, who ingest uncooked water chestnuts or watercress, or who eat raw or uncooked freshwater fish. The diagnosis is confirmed by detection of eggs or by tissue biopsy (Fig. 27–19).

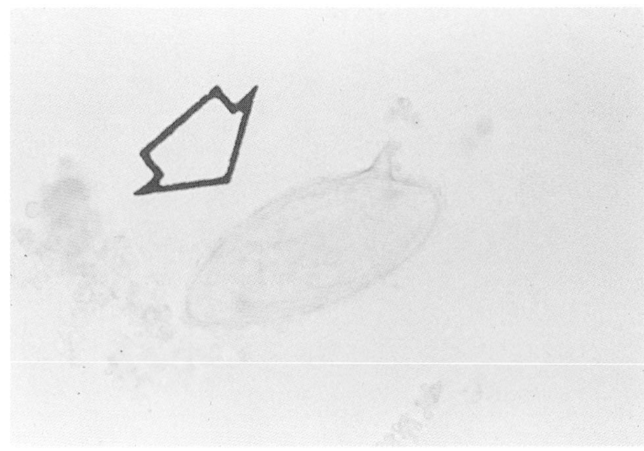

A

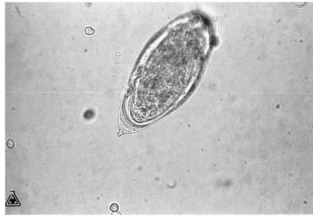

B

Figure 27–19. Schistosoma mansoni. A, *Trematode cyst.* B, *Hematologic findings.*

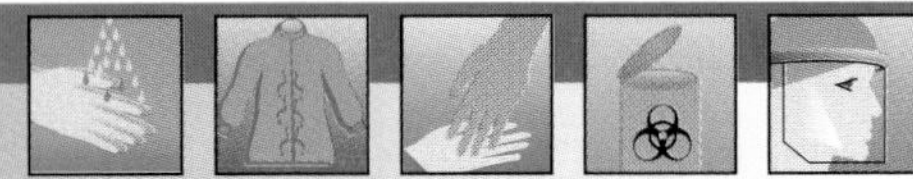

PROCEDURE 27–5

Performing a Rapid Clostridium difficile *Test (CDT) on a Stool Specimen*

Principle

To collect an uncontaminated fecal specimen and perform a test to detect parasites according to manufacturer's guidelines

NOTE: This is a bacterial study that is often performed in conjunction with stool studies for parasites. Check your laboratory procedure manual or contact the testing laboratory for detailed instructions concerning the disposition of the fecal specimen.

Equipment and Supplies

bedpan
specimen collection signs
tongue blades
specimen container with cover (as specified)
CDT kit
centrifuge
centrifuge tubes
vortex mixer
high-intensity light
wooden applicator sticks

PROCEDURE 27–5

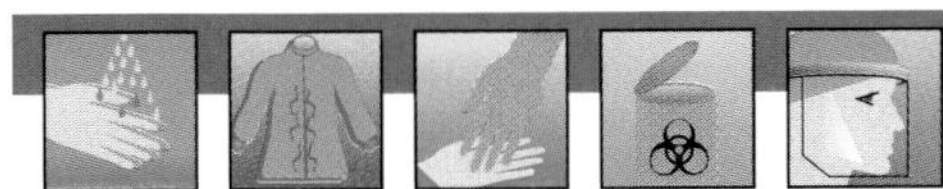

Performing a Rapid Clostridium difficile *Test (CDT) on a Stool Specimen (Continued)*

Procedural Steps

Collection of Stool Specimen

1. Observe universal precautions when handling the specimen. Treat the specimen as potentially infectious throughout the entire procedure.
2. Place a bedpan on top of the closed toilet for the patient's use.
3. Explain the procedure to the patient.
4. Post signs in the bathroom and on the bathroom door that state "DO NOT DISCARD STOOL" or "SAVE STOOL" as reminders that fecal specimen collection is in progress.
5. Wash hands thoroughly and don gloves and other safety apparel.
6. Using a clean tongue blade or similar device, collect the entire stool specimen in a dry, clean container with a properly fitting lid, as specified/provided by the testing laboratory. The specimen should be uncontaminated with urine or menstrual blood.
7. For best results, deliver the specimen to the testing laboratory immediately after collection (or follow laboratory protocols for specimen storage and transport).

Testing Procedure

8. Remove reagents from the refrigerator and allow them to warm to room temperature. Check the expiration date for each.
9. Mix the contents of the reagent bottles by gently inverting each several times before using.
10. Mix 0.5 gm of stool (or 0.5 mL of liquid stool) with 0.5 mL of Reagent 4 in a clean centrifuge tube.
11. Process the mixture, using the vortex device, for 30 seconds.
12. Centrifuge the mixture for 15 minutes at a minimum of 1500 × rpm.
13. Using a micropipette, place 1 drop of supernatant in the TEST circle and 1 drop in the NEGATIVE circle of a clean test card.
14. Add 1 drop of Reagent 1 to both the TEST circle and the POSITIVE circle.
15. Add 1 drop of Reagent 2 to the NEGATIVE circle.
16. Add 1 drop of Reagent 3 to the POSITIVE circle.

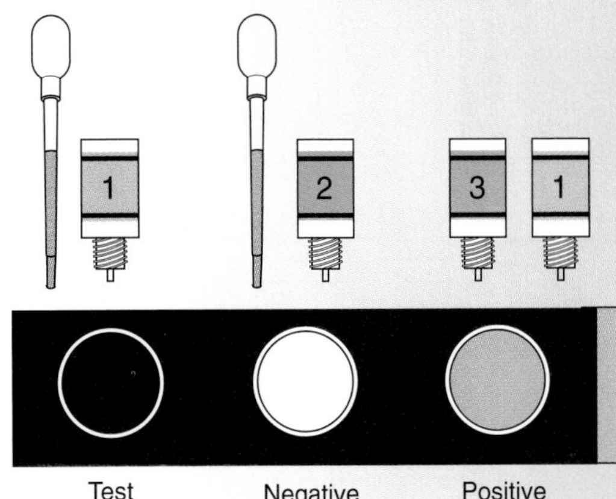

17. Mix the contents of each circle using a separate, clean applicator stick for each. Spread the contents over the surface of each circle.
18. Rock the test card for EXACTLY 3 minutes, using a timer to ensure accuracy. Alternatively, a mechanical rotator may be used to rotate the card for 3 minutes at 90 to 140 rpm.
19. Immediately read the test results by examining the test card macroscopically under a high-intensity, incandescent light.
20. Report your results.
21. Enter the test in the laboratory logbook.
22. Clean and disinfect the work area with antimicrobial disinfectant. Dispose of all biohazardous waste.
23. Remove gloves and wash hands.

Interpretation of Results

Positive result: Greater agglutination in the TEST circle than in the NEGATIVE circles indicates that antigen is present.

Negative result: No agglutination in either the TEST circle or the NEGATIVE circles indicates the absence of antigen.

Nonspecific result: An equal degree of agglutination in both the TEST and NEGATIVE circles indicates that repeat testing is warranted.

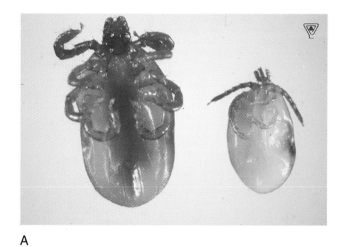

A

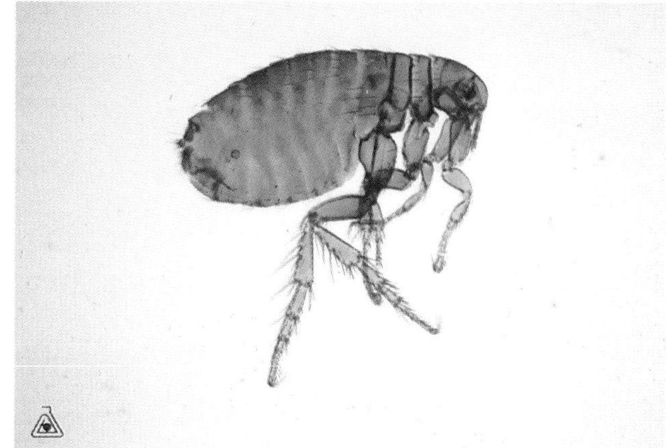

B

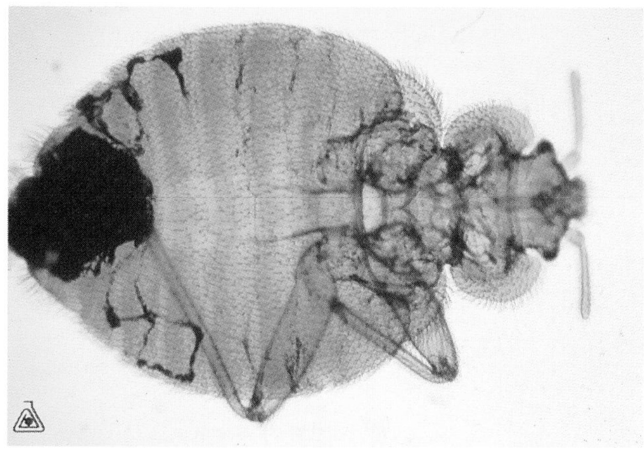

C

Figure 27–20. *Examples of insect vectors.* A, *Tick.* B, *Flea.* C, *Louse.*

Table 27–3
Important Human DNA and RNA Viruses

Virus	*Viral Appearance*	*Viral Members*
Adenovirus	Double DNA, icosahedral,* enveloped	Respiratory infections, pneumonia, conjunctivitis
Hepadnavirus	Double DNA, enveloped	Hepatitis B
Herpesvirus	Double DNA, multiple sides, enveloped	Cold sores, fever blisters, sexually transmitted herpes virus II, shingles, chickenpox
Polyomavirus/ papillomavirus	Double DNA, multiple sides	Warts, some cancerous tumors
Poxvirus	Double DNA, large, brick-shaped, enveloped	Smallpox
Arbovirus	RNA, cube-shaped, parasitic/vector	Colorado tick fever, encephalitis, yellow fever
Coxsackievirus	Single RNA, tiny, icosahedral*	Upper respiratory infections, meningitis, pneumonia
Orthomyxovirus	Enveloped, RNA, helix with envelope	Influenza A, B, and C; mumps; rubeola; rabies
Picornavirus	Single RNA, tiny, icosahedral,* enveloped	Colds, poliomyelitis, hepatitis
Reovirus	Double RNA, icosahedral,* enveloped	Intestinal infections
Retrovirus	Double RNA, helix, enveloped	Tumors, leukemia, HIV 1 and 2

*Having 20 sides.

Arthropods

Arthropods are insect vectors and parasites. Ticks (Fig. 27–20*A*), mosquitoes, and flies are insect vectors that transmit a variety of parasites, including, respectively, *Babesia, Plasmodium* (a malarial parasite), and *Leishmania* and *Trypanosoma*. In addition, lice and fleas (Fig. 27–20, *B* and *C*) can be directly parasitic to humans. The destruction of insect vectors has an important role in the control of insect-borne parasites.

Virology

With new and increasingly destructive viruses being constantly discovered, virology is becoming an important area of clinical microbiology. HIV, the Hantavirus, and the Ebola virus have caused a resurgence in the study of medically important viruses.

Viruses are the smallest of microorganisms but, unlike cellular organisms, they do not contain the biochemical mechanisms for their own replication. Viruses replicate by using the biochemical mechanisms of a host cell to synthesize and assemble their separate components. They are the most common of all human infections. An individual virus, or **virion,** is nothing more than a protein coat of RNA or DNA (Table 27–3). Viruses do not have a metabolism. They must invade cells of other living organisms for shelter, food, and missing nucleic acids. Within the host cell, viruses take over the metabolic machinery, thrive, and reproduce (Fig. 27–21). Their replication is directed by the viral nucleic acid within the host cell. They do not divide by mitosis or binary fission. When the host cell dies, usually from the virus, they spread to other cells. Some viruses, such as hepatitis B, can survive for a short period of time outside the environment, before infecting a new host (Fig. 27–22).

Viral infections are difficult to treat because antiviral drugs are toxic to the cells of the host. Antibiotics are useless against viruses, and are prescribed only to treat the secondary infections that often occur when the body is weakened by viral infection.

Some viruses produce a self-limiting infection, as occurs with the common cold. Others are responsible

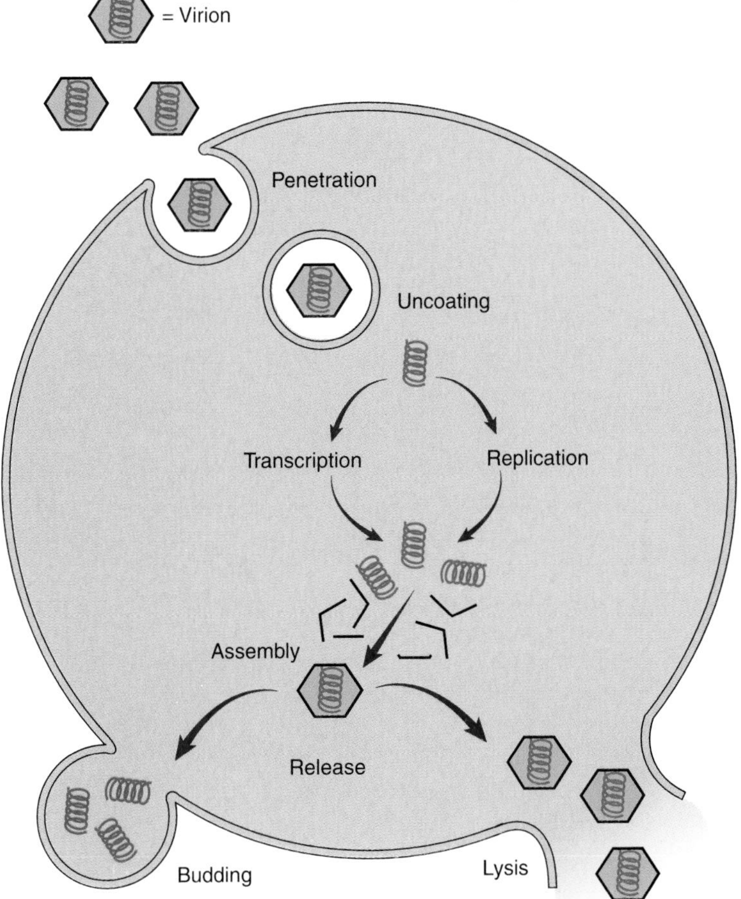

Figure 27–21. *Viral invasion of a cell.*

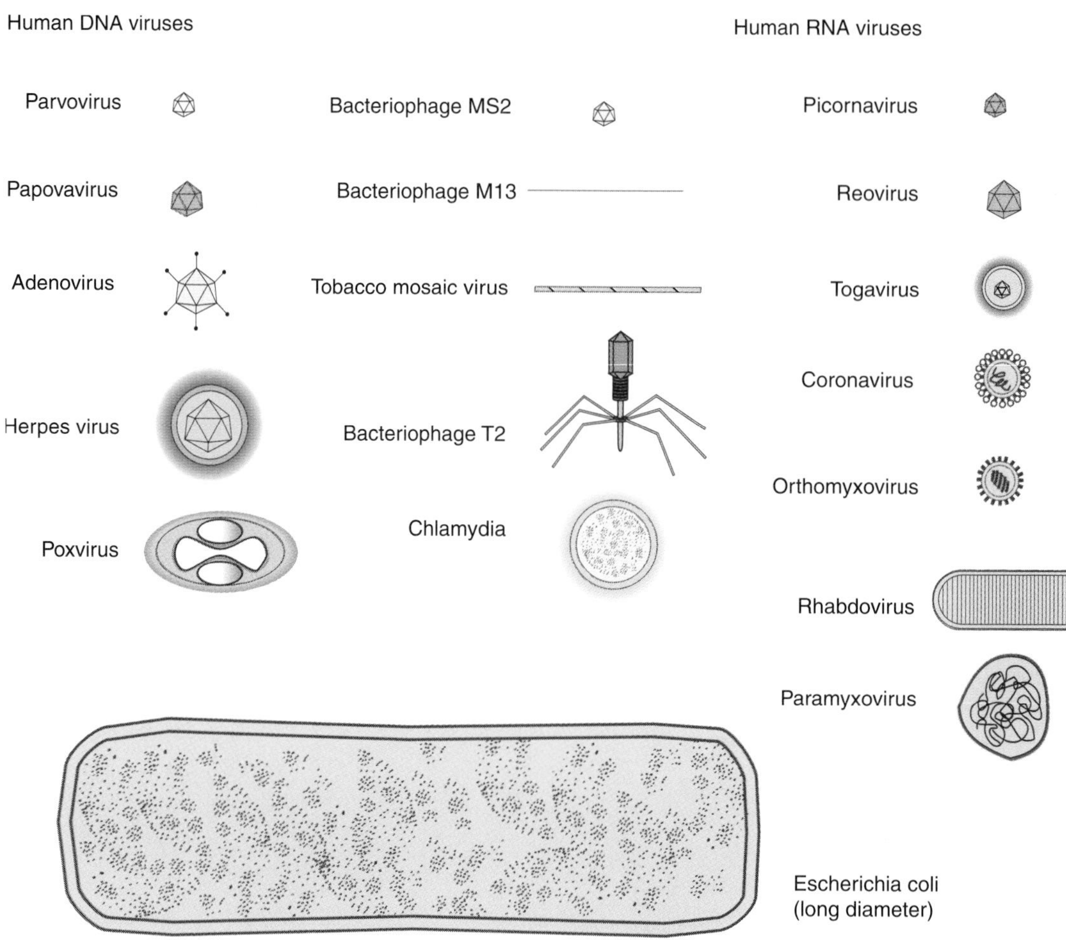

Figure 27–22. *Viral morphology.*

for such infectious diseases as hepatitis, AIDS, and other sexually transmitted diseases. Viruses are being considered as possible causative agents for cancer, and they can depress the immune system by making the individual susceptible to invading microorganisms. The varicella virus causes chickenpox in childhood; later in life, it can resurface as *Herpes zoster,* or shingles. The most common viruses are associated with measles, herpes, mononucleosis, mumps, warts, influenza, colds, chickenpox, HIV/AIDS, and hepatitis.

Specimen Collection

Correct specimen collection and processing is required for the detection of a suspected virus. Specimens for the detection of viruses should be collected as close to the onset of the disease as possible, as the virus may disappear shortly after disease onset (Fig. 27–23). The specimen should be processed immediately after collection to ensure viability. Procedures for mailing viral specimens must reflect the laboratory's biohazard protocols, including proper identification of the specimen on the container label. Most samples are mailed to large reference laboratories for testing.

AIDS

As the name suggests, AIDS is a complex of symptoms that develops when severe immunodepression is caused by HIV infection. HIVs are small RNA viruses related to, but distinct from, the immunodeficiency virus that affects animals. This virus cannot survive outside of human cells, and humans are the only source of infection transmission. The most common modes of transmission are blood transfusions or contact that involves a transfer of blood from one person to another. Typical symptoms are nonspecific and may include fever, night sweats, nausea, muscle pain, headache, sore throat, skin rash, and mild lymph node enlargement. These symptoms may disappear, only to reappear weeks or months later. The diagnosis of HIV infection and AIDS is based on clinical findings and laboratory tests. Laboratory tests include antibodies to HIV and lymphocyte counts. Approximately 50% of

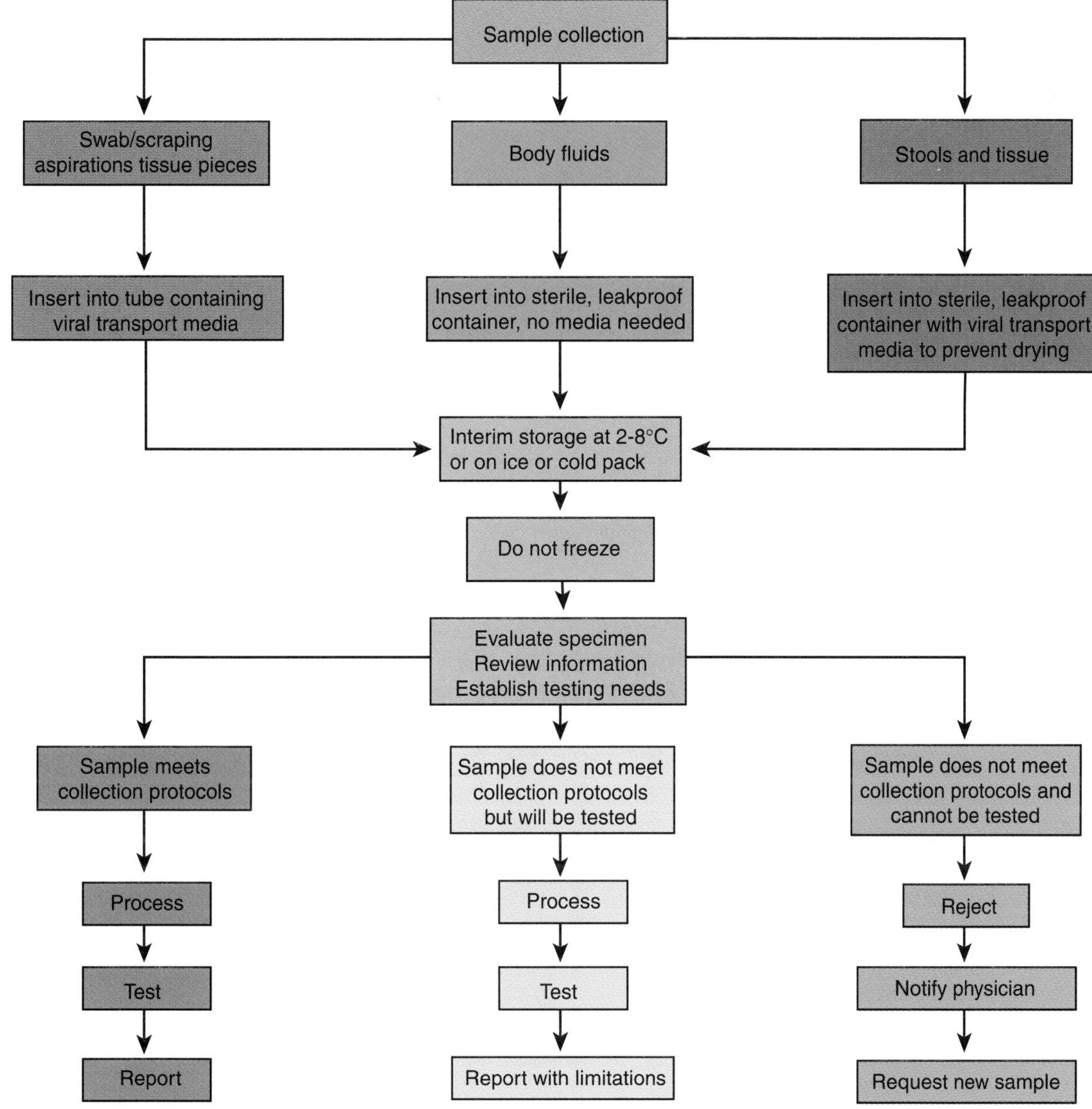

Figure 27–23. *Viral specimen collection.*

HIV-infected patients develop AIDS within 10 years of initial diagnosis.

Herpes

Herpes simplex virus is the virus most frequently isolated/diagnosed in the laboratory. This virus is referred to as herpes labialis when it affects the mucous membrane of the mouth and lips, causing cold sores and blisters. Herpes zoster, also known as shingles, affects a neural junction within the body, whereas genital herpes affects the adult genitalia. These viral skin diseases produce painful blisters, slight fever, malaise, and sometimes, psychological irritability. Laboratory diagnosis can be established by viral culture, microscopic viewing of affected cells from the vesicles, or serologic testing of acute viral titers. Permanent cure is not possible, although antiviral drugs, such as acyclovir, provide symptomatic relief.

Viral Hepatitis

Viral hepatitis is the most prevalent liver disease in the world. Particularly in the health care field, observance of proper procedures is critical in preventing transmission of the disease by blood or blood products from an infected blood donor or by the use of improperly sterilized syringes, needles, or instruments.

Many cases of viral hepatitis are mild, especially in children, but all patients with viral hepatitis exhibit similar hepatic changes. The liver becomes damaged, and its normal functions are interrupted and impaired. The

Table 27–4
Characteristics of Viral Hepatitis

Type	*Etiologic Agent*	*Mode of Transmission*	*Viral Site(s)*	*Frequency/ Virulence*	*Target Population*
Hepatitis A (infectious hepatitis)	Hepatitis A virus	Fecal-oral route Improper hygiene Ingestion of contaminated food	Saliva Stool	Very common in U.S.	Pandemic society
Hepatitis B (serum hepatitis)	Hepatitis B virus	Infected blood or blood products Sexual contact Illicit IV drug use Sharing of razors or toothbrushes	Blood, urine, tears, semen, vaginal secretions, saliva, breast milk	Very serious; may be fatal	Patients receiving transfusions or dialysis and IV drug users
Hepatitis C	Hepatitis C virus	Contaminated blood Contact with infected person in household Sexual contact	Blood, body fluids, B-virus persons		
Hepatitis D	Delta virus			Extremely pathogenic	Individuals with hepatitis B virus
Hepatitis E	Non-A, non-B hepatitis	Ingestion of contaminated food or water	Contaminated food/water	Not found in U.S.	Travelers to Asia and Africa

disease is divided into five categories known as hepatitis A, B, C, D, and E (Table 27–4). Each form of the disease has slightly different features, but all forms are most prevalent in children and young adults, and less common in the elderly. Symptoms include fever, anorexia, nausea, malaise, and abdominal discomfort associated with **jaundice.** The main source of infection is contact with the feces, urine, or blood of an infected person. Diagnosing the specific virus is difficult because the symptoms of each viral type are similar.

Of the known types of hepatitis, hepatitis B seems to be one of the most serious forms because of the many ways that it can be acquired and its potential for complications. Many people are infected with hepatitis B but never experience symptoms. When symptoms do occur, they may include a flu-like illness, fatigue, mild fever, muscle and joint aches, nausea, vomiting, loss of appetite, dull abdominal pain, and occasional diarrhea. Some people also become jaundiced and report dark urine, light-colored stools, and itching of the skin.

Most patients with viral hepatitis recover. However, up to 10% of adults who become infected with the hepatitis B virus become chronic carriers, capable of spreading the disease to others for an indefinite period of time. Infants and children who are infected with the hepatitis B virus are more likely than adults to develop the chronic-carrier state of the disease. Chronic carriers usually have no symptoms but have the greatest potential for developing long-term complications, such as chronic active hepatitis, cirrhosis, and primary cancer of the liver. Approximately 1 million persons in the United States are chronic carriers of hepatitis B (see accompanying chart).

Populations at Greatest Risk for Hepatitis B

Medical and dental office personnel
Hospital and ambulatory care personnel
Nursing home/residential care employees
Dialysis and drug-treatment center personnel
Personnel involved in blood collection and processing
Health care personnel in industrial facilities
Medical and dental equipment maintenance/repair personnel
Law enforcement/fire and rescue/life-saving personnel
Employees of correctional institutions
Employees of schools for the mentally handicapped
Regulated waste handlers
Morticians and/or embalmers
Users of illicit IV drugs
Individuals with numerous sex partners
Individuals requiring frequent blood transfusions

Table 27–5
Normal Characteristics of Feces

Parameter	*Normal Findings*
Color	Brown
Consistency	Soft/formed
Mucus	Absent
Occult blood	Negative

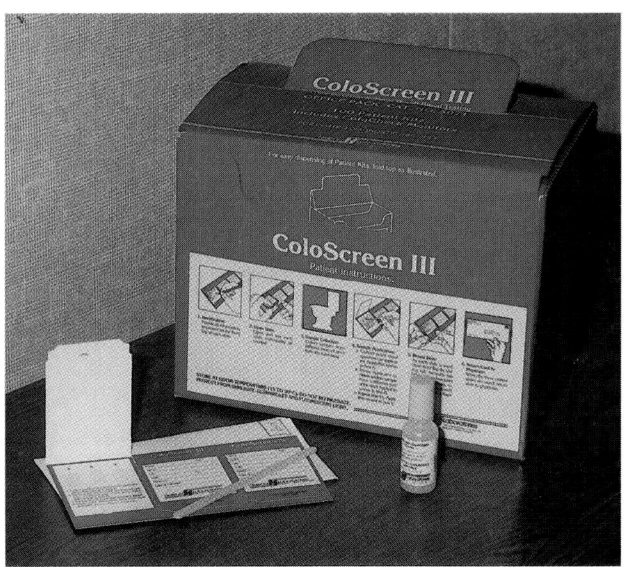

A

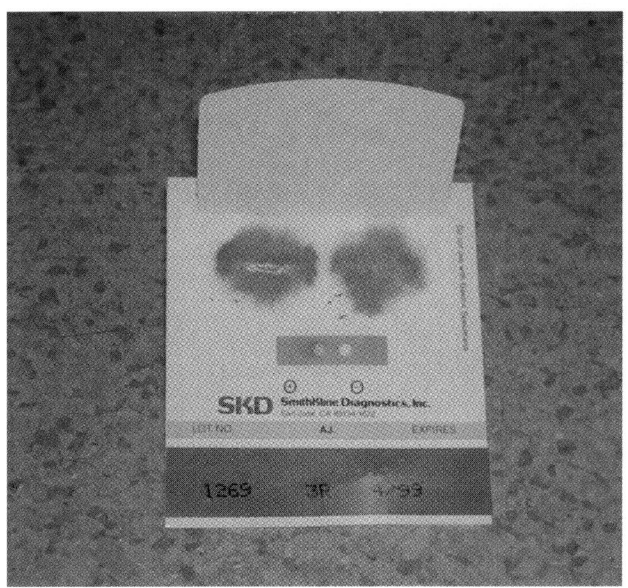

B

Figure 27–24. A, *ColoScreen III occult blood testing kit.* B, *Hemoccult II testing card showing positive results.*

Serologic tests for specific viral markers have made it easier to diagnose the specific type of hepatitis. Testing methods include radioimmunoassay (RIA) and enzyme-linked immunosorbent assay (ELISA).

Occult Blood

The elimination of digestive waste products from the body is necessary to health. The excreted waste from the gastrointestinal system is known as feces or stool. Fecal examination is one means of evaluating patients with gastrointestinal bleeding, obstruction, parasites, dysentery, colitis, or increased fat excretion.

The output of feces depends on a series of body functions. Most adults excrete 100 to 300 gm of fecal matter every 24 hours. This mass is made up of approximately 70% water. The balance is a collection of indigestible material, bile, bacteria, intestinal secretions, inorganic material, and unabsorbed food (Table 27–5).

Blood is not found in stool obtained from healthy adults. If the person is experiencing bleeding of the intestinal wall, the blood is likely to be occult or hidden. This means it cannot be seen with the naked eye. This condition may remain relatively painless for some time. For this reason, the American Cancer Society recommends that a fecal occult blood test be a routine part of the physical examination of adults.

The most frequently performed fecal test is a chemical screening for occult blood. The primary purpose of the test is to detect pathologic lesions that may be cancerous. Cancer of the colon is one of the leading causes of death in the United States. Recent mass screening programs for colorectal cancer have resulted in the early detection of a remarkable number of colon cancers that are still localized and curable.

Occult Blood Testing (Guaiac Testing)

A number of easy-to-perform testing kits are available for the detection of occult blood. Most of these kits consist of a test card containing paper squares coated with **guaiac.** Guaiac or guaiac-based indicators react with the hemoglobin in blood when in the presence of hydrogen peroxide, which is used in the development process. This reaction produces a blue color on the paper squares of the test card. Two commonly used testing kits are ColoScreen (Helena Laboratories) and Hemoccult II (SmithKline Diagnostics) (Fig. 27–24, *A* and *B*).

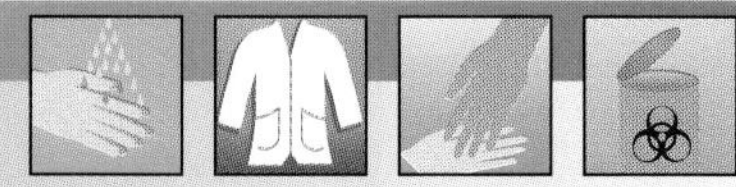

PROCEDURE 27-6

Testing for Fecal Occult Blood

Principle

To detect the presence of occult blood in a fecal specimen as a screening test for primary colorectal cancer

Equipment and Supplies

ColoScreen Fecal Occult Blood Testing Kit
three prepared specimen slides

Preparation of the Patient

NOTE: If the samples are to be obtained by the patient at home, the patient will need the following instructions. It is always advisable to review the instructions verbally with the patient and then give them a copy of the instructions to refer to at home. Be sure to explain the purpose of the test and the collection procedure.

Instructions to the Patient

1. For at least 2 days prior to the testing period and during the testing time, eat a high-fiber diet. The diet may include:
   - Well-cooked poultry and fish
   - Cooked fruits and vegetables
   - Bran cereals
   - Raw lettuce, carrots, and celery
   - Moderate amounts of peanuts and popcorn

   AVOID:
   - Red and partially cooked meats
   - Turnips, cauliflower, broccoli, parsnips, and melons (especially cantaloupe)
   - Alcohol, aspirin, and vitamin C.

Specimen Collection

2. Write your name, age, and address on the front of each slide.

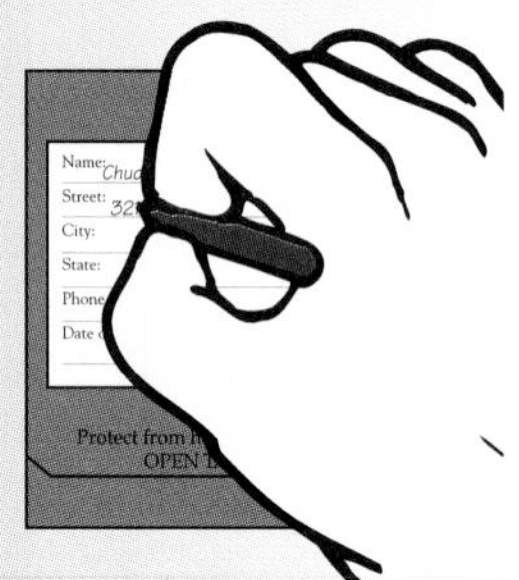

Identification

3. After a bowel movement, open the front of one slide and, using one of the wooden applicators, collect a small sample of feces from the toilet bowl.
4. Spread the sample in Box A.

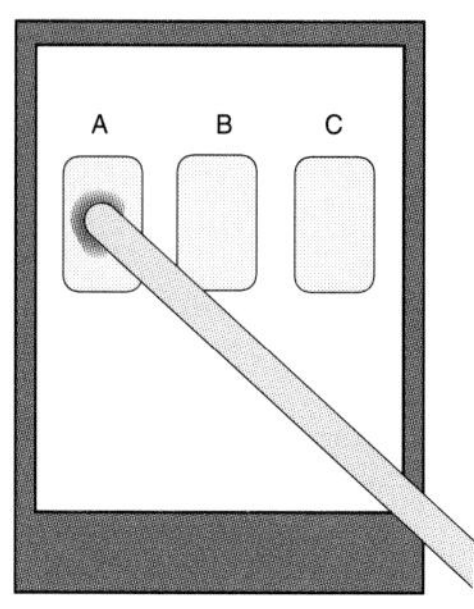

Preparation

5. Using the same wooden applicator, collect a second sample from a different part of the stool.
6. Spread this sample in Box B.
7. Discard the wooden applicator in a biohazardous waste container. DO NOT flush the wooden applicator.
8. Reseal the cover of the slide and complete the information requested on the outside of the cover.
9. Repeat steps 3 through 8 for your next two bowel movements.
10. Place all three slides in the envelope provided and transport it to your doctor or laboratory immediately.

Procedural Steps

Performing the Occult Blood Test

1. When the slides arrive at the laboratory, confirm that all the necessary information is written on the slide cover.
2. Observe universal precautions during testing. Don appropriate safety attire.
3. Open the back sides of all three slides.
4. Place two drops of ColoScreen Developer on each specimen.

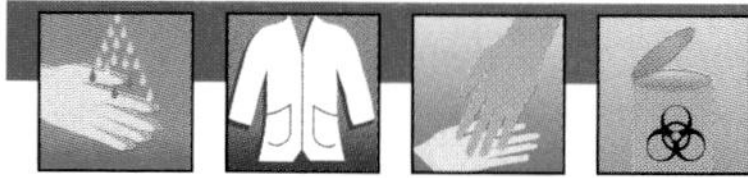

PROCEDURE 27-6

Testing for Fecal Occult Blood (Continued)

5. Wait 30 seconds.

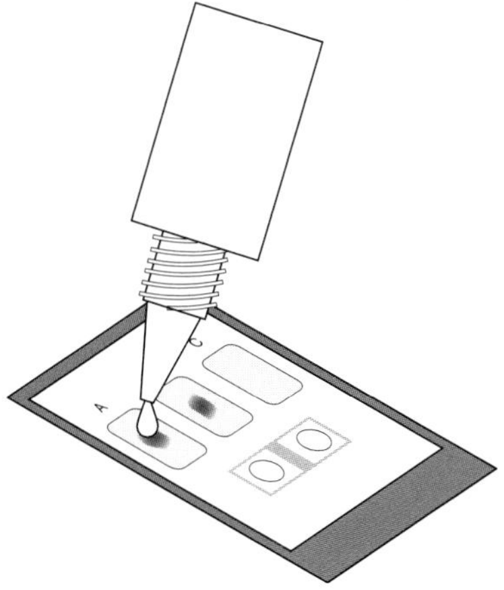

Development of test

6. Read the test results within 2 minutes. Any blue color visible around the fecal smears indicates a positive result.

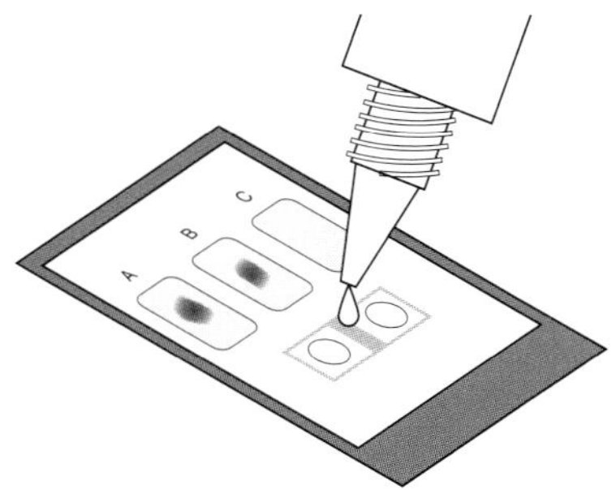

Development of preformance monitors

7. To develop the ColoCheck Monitor, place one drop of developer between the monitor boxes (red area). Wait 30 seconds and read the test results within 2 minutes.
8. Compare your results with the color photos (indicating positive and negative results) located in the informational folder included in the test box.
9. Record and report the test results.
10. Clean the work area according to laboratory protocol.
11. Remove gloves and wash hands.

False-Positive Test Results

One of the main problems encountered in testing feces for occult blood is the number of false-positive results that are obtained. A diet that is high in red meat, turnips, horseradish, and/or bananas can cause falsely positive results. Likewise, bleeding, such as that which occurs during a nosebleed, can also produce a false-positive result. Certain therapeutic drug regimens may also lead to positive findings owing to the effects of the pharmacologic agents on the gastrointestinal tract. Nonsteroidal anti-inflammatory drugs, aspirin, iron preparations, anticoagulants, adrenocorticocosteroids, and colchicine are examples of such drugs. Ascorbic acid intake can produce the opposite result, a false-negative reading.

Summary

Throughout this chapter, you have studied and learned about a variety of superficial and systemic diseases in humans. Many of these diseases are cosmopolitan in nature. The need for continuous observance of safety measures/protocols cannot be overemphasized. A quality control program is necessary in any laboratory, regardless of size, to monitor the reliability and the quality of the work performed. Constant surveillance and frequent checking are crucial. All media reagents and staining solutions should be evaluated frequently for effectiveness. Incubators should be checked for temperature control accuracy. Whenever in doubt, wash your hands. Be careful not to put your hands to your mouth or rub your eyes while you are in the laboratory area. Remember how tiny many of these organisms are, and how easily they can be transported out of the laboratory area to patients, fellow employees, and family members.

Chapter Review

True or False

Circle T or F to indicate the correct answers to the following:

T F 1. Molds and yeast are types of fungi.

T F 2. Amoebic dysentery is caused by a protozoan.

T F 3. *Giardia lamblia* is diagnosed by throat culture.

T F 4. Nematodes and cestodes are forms of parasitic worms.

Fill in the Blanks

Complete the following statements:

5. Cryptococcal meningitis is confirmed by microscopic examination of ______________ ______________, or ______________.
6. *Candida albicans* is an opportunistic fungus that causes ______________ in infants.
7. Dermatophytid molds infect human ______________, ______________, and ______________.

Multiple Choice

Circle the letter that represents the single best answer:

8. The most common systemic fungal disease in the United States is:
   a. Trichomonas
   b. *Coccidioides immitis*
   c. Sporotrichosis
   d. Histoplasmosis
   e. Hepatitis
9. The most prevalent liver disease in the world is:
   a. AIDS
   b. Thrush
   c. Viral hepatitis
   d. Histoplasmosis
   e. *Candida albicans*
10. The immature stage in the life of a bacterium is called:
    a. Larva
    b. Spore
    c. Oocyst
    d. Arthropod
    e. Trophozoite

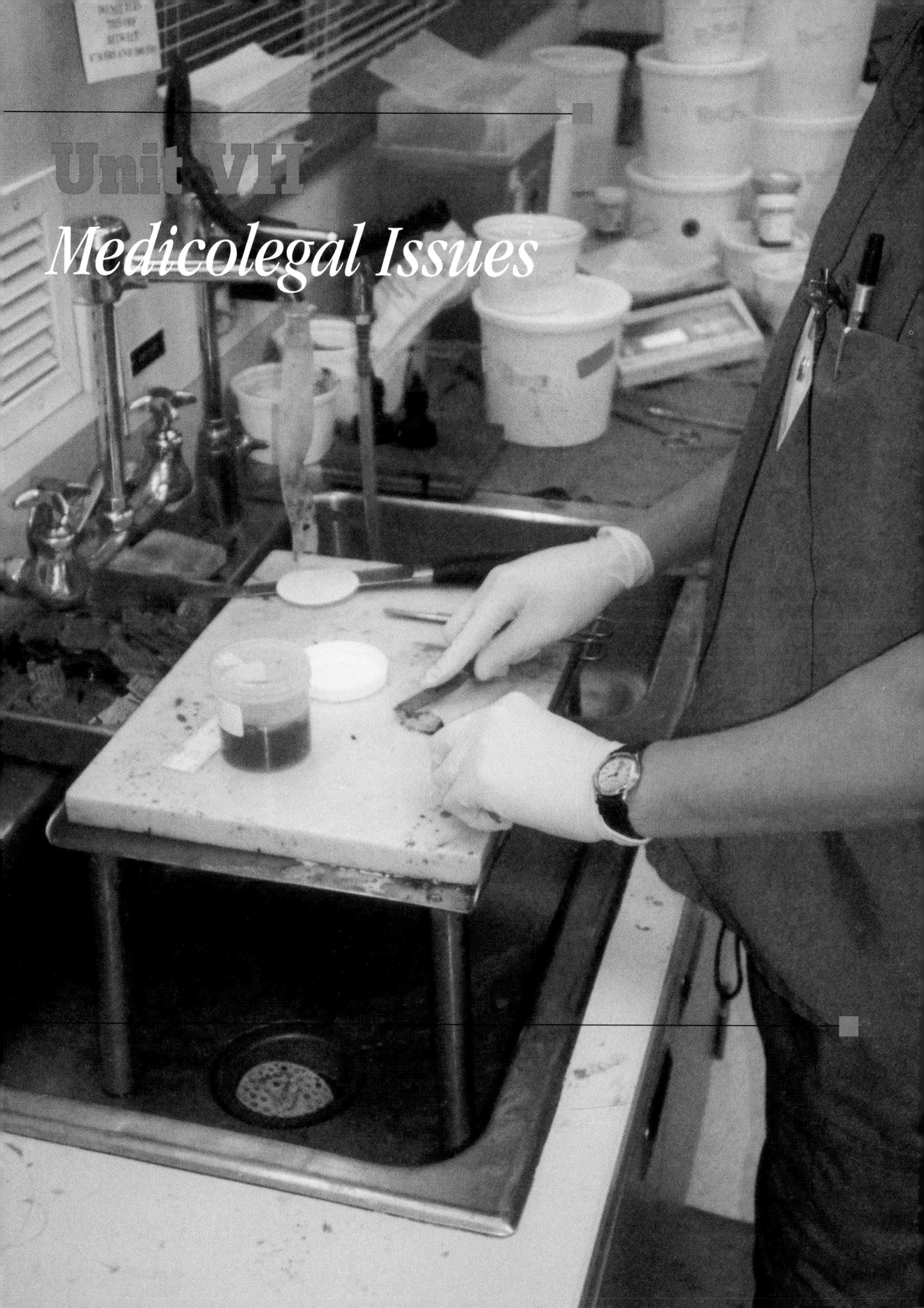

Unit VII
Medicolegal Issues

Vocabulary

anatomic pathology: the science dealing with the nature of and changes in human body cells and tissue that are caused by disease

endometrium: the mucous membrane lining the uterus

epidemic: a disease that affects many people in a region at the same time; widely diffused and rapidly spreading

etiology: an assigned cause of disease

meiosis: the process whereby two cells fuse into one cell, which may result in the formation of a zygote

mitosis: the process of cell division that results in the formation of two daughter cells and the replacement of dead cells

microtome: an instrument used to cut thin sections of tissue for microscopic study

phospholipid: an oily, waxy compound that contains phosphorus and that is found in cell membranes

zygote: the cell that results from the union of the male sperm and the female ova

Chapter Objectives

After reading this chapter, you should be able to:

1. Describe the laboratory's role in disease prevention.
2. Identify the two major types of infections.
3. List the ways the laboratory can assist in identifying possible epidemic areas.
4. Differentiate between the terms cytology and histology.
5. Understand mitosis and meiosis.
6. List types of samples that may be used for cytologic study.
7. Describe the method used to prepare a tissue sample for microscopic examination.
8. Identify the two stains used for most histologic studies.

Chapter 28
Ancillary Responsibilities

Epidemiology, histology, and cytology are not part of the daily work procedures in the physician's office laboratory (POL). Yet histology and cytology are important parts of anatomic pathology. Epidemiology involves all areas within a medical institution, as well as all individuals working within that setting. When a patient comes into the medical office for a Papanicolaou (PAP) test and the specimen is prepared for cytologic testing, you tend to overlook the department that will be responsible for performing the test. Requests are made daily for laboratory testing that must be performed by the cytology and histology departments. We rely on these results to aid in our health and well-being.

Epidemiology is part of our everyday lives. Whenever you read about a "flu bug attack", an *Escherichia coli* outbreak, or the dangers of Ebola virus, you are reading about the work of some very busy epidemiology departments.

Epidemiology

Epidemiology refers to the study of the factors influencing or determining the distribution, causes, and frequency of disease or health alterations in a defined population. When studying epidemiology, there are two facts that can be accepted as fundamental:

1. Diseases do not occur by chance.
2. Diseases are not randomly distributed in a population.

The major role of all laboratories is to assist in the diagnosis and treatment of patients. However, the laboratory can also serve as a valuable public resource by recognizing and reporting infections of public health importance. The infections that are spread from one person to another, such as tuberculosis, sexually transmitted diseases, and some forms of diarrhea, are among the diseases that need to be reported. In addition to infections, data obtained from the laboratory logbook may suggest an impending epidemic outbreak within the community.

The laboratory can assist the infection control team in the investigation of disease outbreaks in the hope of avoiding an **epidemic** or helping with corrective measures. Epidemiology is concerned with two general types of infections: nosocomial and community-acquired infections.

Nosocomial Infections

Nosocomial infections are those that are acquired in an institutional setting, particularly hospitals, convalescent facilities, and prisons. Many of these infections first appear after a patient has been discharged from the hospital, depending on the incubation period. Thus these infections are frequently identified during follow-up care in the doctor's office and POL.

The National Nosocomial Infections Study (NNIS), conducted by the Centers for Disease Control (CDC), indicated that 5% to 6% of all hospitalized patients develop nosocomial infection. These infections add direct charges of at least $1800 per patient. Thus, for the United States, nosocomial infections cost far in excess of $4 billion per year in direct charges to patients. As a result of the findings of the NNIS, all hospitals and convalescent facilities are required to institute an active infection control program.

Epidemiologic Factors

Have you ever asked yourself the question, "Why did patient A get the infection when patient B did not?" The answer lies in one of three factors:

1. The susceptibility of the patient
2. The virulence of the infecting organism
3. The nature of exposure

Generally speaking, hospitalized persons have an increased susceptibility to infection owing to their weakened condition. Moreover, people with serious, community-based infections are admitted to hospitals for treatment. Given these unalterable circumstances, the only solution to these concerns is early identification and control of the elements of exposure.

The most important means of transmission of nosocomial infections is by direct contact with infected persons. Handwashing by all personnel, both before and after each patient contact, remains the most important means of preventing the spread of nosocomial infections.

Community-Acquired Infections

Until 1900, community-acquired infectious disease was the leading cause of death. These deaths occurred following exposure to disease-producing organisms such as those causing smallpox, tuberculosis, influenza, whooping cough, typhoid fever, diphtheria, and tetanus. During the 20th century, however, improvements in public sanitation, antibiotic drugs, and vaccination programs resulted in substantial disease control.

Transmission

Community-acquired infections (communicable diseases) can be transferred directly from one person to another, although direct transmission is not always a prerequisite. Colds, measles, mumps, and gonorrhea are all examples of communicable diseases. Pathogenic organisms may also be transferred to people from other animals, in which case the animal is referred to as the *vector.* Diseases caused by vectors include malaria, which is caused by parasitic protozoa; rabies, which is caused by the bite of an infected animal; and typhus, which is caused by the microorganism *Rickettsia prowazaki* and which is spread from person to person by body lice and poor sanitation.

Every few years, a new strain of influenza virus appears. Carried from country to country by travelers, these new viral strains cause outbreaks of influenza that often reach epidemic proportions. In the United States, hygiene, sanitation, and antibiotics have been very effective in eliminating many infectious diseases caused by bacteria, parasites, and worms, but diseases caused by viruses still cannot be treated effectively.

Prevention

The old adage, "An ounce of prevention is worth a pound of cure," could be the hallmark of epidemiology. Many of the infectious diseases that killed millions of people in the past have been practically eliminated, partially as a result of the efforts of public health officials. However, new infectious agents continue to arise, and some of them are spread rapidly throughout the world. These infectious diseases arise for several reasons. Three primary reasons are:

1. Changing lifestyles of people
2. Travel of people carrying communicable diseases
3. Biologic emergence of new infectious bacteria and viruses

As a result of the jet age, we have become a global (one-world) society; because of this, disease is easily transmitted from group to group.

Disease Control

Few diseases have a single **etiology.** Most are the result of the interaction of genetic, physical, emotional, and environmental factors. However, it has always been convenient to describe diseases by the principle causative factor, which may include heredity, infectious organism, lifestyle, accident, poison, or toxic chemical.

Control mechanisms can also be grouped into categories: sanitation, hygiene, and medical care, which encompasses nutrition, immunizations, and antibiotics. Infectious diseases have largely been controlled through these means, but such control is an ongoing battle. New diseases, such as Lyme disease, acquired immunodeficiency syndrome (AIDS), and Legionnaire's disease, are present-day reminders of this continual struggle.

All health care personnel must serve as medical "watchdogs." In the laboratory, we can watch for and monitor tests showing similar bacterial or parasitic results, or a greater-than-usual number of requests for communicable disease screening (e.g., strep throat cultures). When either is seen, the situation should be recognized and appropriate action taken.

Anatomic Pathology

Pathology is the study of disease. Specifically, it is the study of the structural and functional changes occurring in cells, tissues, and organs in the human body which lead to, or are caused by, disease. Forensic pathology is a specialized area of study associated with anatomic and clinical pathology. This specialized area is discussed in detail in Chapter 29.

Most of this text has focused on the clinical aspects of pathology. You have undoubtedly spent endless hours processing and testing samples of urine and blood for clinical values. You have seen that great advances have been made in the technology available in the clinical pathology department. **Anatomic pathology** is equally important in advancing the physician's goals of the diagnosis, treatment, and prevention of disease. In anatomic pathology, though, the focus is primarily on cells and tissues.

Anatomic pathology involves the study of cells and tissues of the body using cytologic and histologic techniques and procedures. Cytologists and histologists are the highly skilled laboratory professionals who perform this specialized work. In the clinical laboratory, the medical technologist is the primary professional, whereas in the anatomic area, the cytologist and histologist are the principal professionals. As discussed in Unit I, all work is performed under the direction of a pathologist, all of whom are specially trained and licensed.

Table 28–1
The Human Body—Levels of Organization

Body Unit	***Definition/Function***
Cell	Basic structural unit of living organisms Cells differentiate during development into specialized cell types charged with specific tasks.
Tissue	A group of similar cells that together perform a specialized function
Organ	Two or more specific tissues that perform a specific function or group of functions
System	A set or group of organs that act or work together in a common purpose to produce specific results
Organism	A collection of systems working in harmony to promote and sustain life

Cytology

The study of the formation, structure, function, biochemistry, and pathology of cells is called *cytology.* Cells are the body's building blocks (Table 28–1). All cells living in the human body come from other cells. When one cell divides to make two new cells, the process is called **mitosis.** In **meiosis,** two cells fuse into one new cell. The formation of a **zygote** from the fusion of the sperm and ovum in sexual reproduction results from meiosis.

The basic cell consists of a cell wall or cell membrane made of **phospholipids.** Contained within the cell membrane is the nucleoplasm. Cytoplasm is the protoplasm found outside the cell nucleus, whereas nucleoplasm is the protoplasm found within the cell nucleus. The nucleus is surrounded by the nuclear membrane or nuclear envelope, and it contains the cell's genetic material. Chromosomes containing long strands of deoxyribonucleic acid (DNA) and proteins make up the genetic structure. The cytoplasm contains cellular structures and organelles, such as mitochondria, Golgi apparatus, lysosomes, endoplasmic reticulum, and ribosomes (Fig. 28–1). Cells differentiate as they develop into various types of cells, each with a specific function and purpose.

Cytologic Testing

Cytologic testing is a means of examining or screening cells to detect precancerous or malignant cells. Exfoliated or shed cells in body fluids and tissue are studied

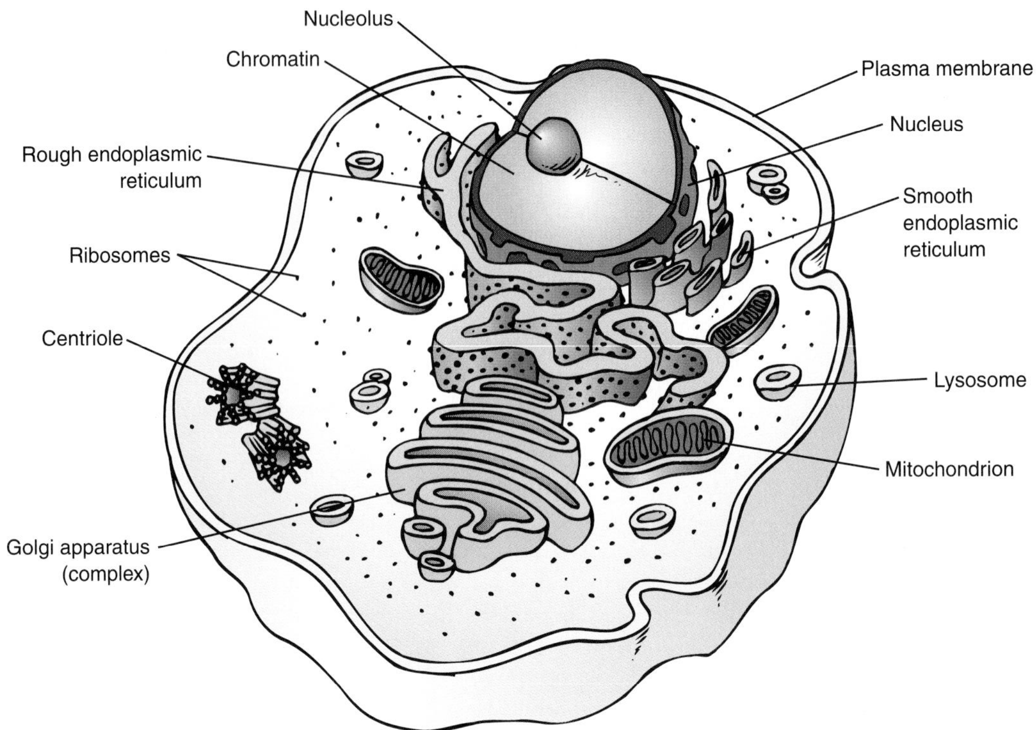

Figure 28–1. *Basic components of a human cell.*

microscopically after specialized staining procedures (Fig. 28–2). George Papanicolaou developed the most commonly used cytologic staining technique, the PAP smear. The PAP smear is primarily used to diagnose precancerous and cancerous conditions involving the female reproductive tract, including the cervix, uterus, and **endometrium.** PAP smears are of great importance in the early detection of cervical cancer, and it is recommended that all sexually active women and/or women older than 20 years of age undergo the test once a year. The best time to have a PAP smear done is 2 weeks after the first day of the last menstrual period. PAP smears should definitely not be performed when the patient is menstruating. In addition to diagnosing cancer, the PAP smear technique can be used to determine female sexual chromosomes and the presence of certain fungal and viral infections.

Specimen Collection

Samples from any body fluid or tissue can be used for cytologic studies. Specimens from sputum, bronchial washings, and cerebrospinal fluid (CSF), as well as other sterile body fluids, gastric aspirations, and urine sediment, are routinely collected for cytologic testing. Specimens are typically collected by means of aspira-

Figure 28–2. *Automated cytology stainer.*

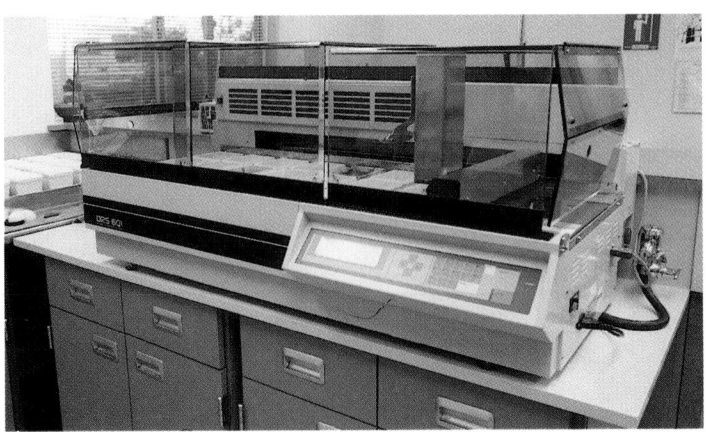

tion, brushings, lavage, and swabs. Many specimens, such as gynecologic specimens, are collected in the physician's office. Other specimens, such as bronchial washings/brushings, may require anesthesia for collection, and so are obtained in a hospital setting.

Gynecologic samples are smeared on a labeled slide and fixed in 95% alcohol. Several types of spray fixatives are also available. Nongynecologic specimens are usually collected without preservative. This type of sample must be handled very carefully to avoid specimen degeneration or drying. It is important to check the laboratory procedure manual or to consult with the referral laboratory for the exact collection requirements. Regardless of the body site from which the sample is obtained, all specimens should be sent to the testing laboratory as soon as they are obtained to prevent any process or condition that would alter the specimen material prior to study.

Results of cytologic studies are more easily obtained and available sooner than those of histologic studies, but they are not always diagnostically conclusive. Positive cytologic results are usually confirmed by surgical biopsy.

PROCEDURE 28–1

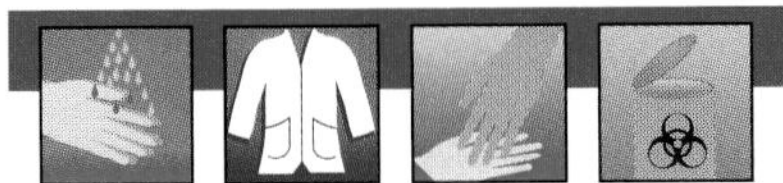

Preparing a PAP Smear

Principle

To accommodate the needs of the patient and to assist the physician in securing and preparing a specimen for cytologic (PAP) testing

Equipment and Supplies

vaginal speculum
glass slides
marking pen for labeling
wooden spatulas or cotton-tipped applicators
lubricant
preservative or spray fixative
cytology request forms

Procedural Steps

1. Explain the procedure and the purpose of the test to the patient.
2. Ask the patient to remove all clothing below the waist and to don an examination gown. If they prefer, they may keep their shoes and/or socks on.
3. Assemble all needed equipment and supplies.
4. Wash hands thoroughly and put on gloves.
5. Position and drape the patient in the lithotomy position on a gynecologic examination table.

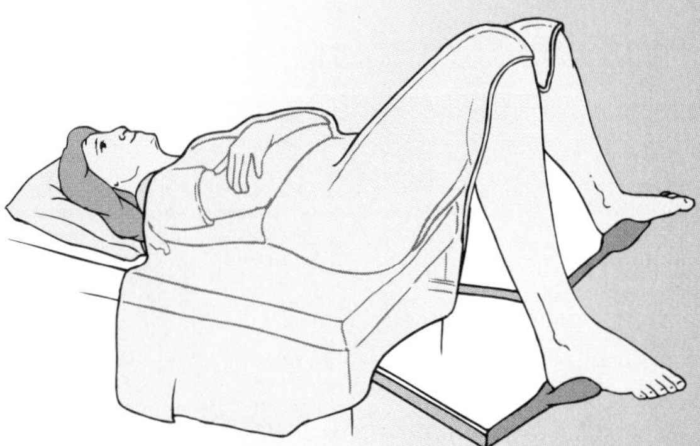

6. Lubricate a warmed vaginal speculum using warm water ONLY and hand it to the physician.
7. The physician will then obtain vaginal and cervical samples while the speculum is in position.
8. When the physician hands you the spatulas or applicators containing the samples, prepare one slide with the cervical scrapings and a second slide with the vaginal secretion.

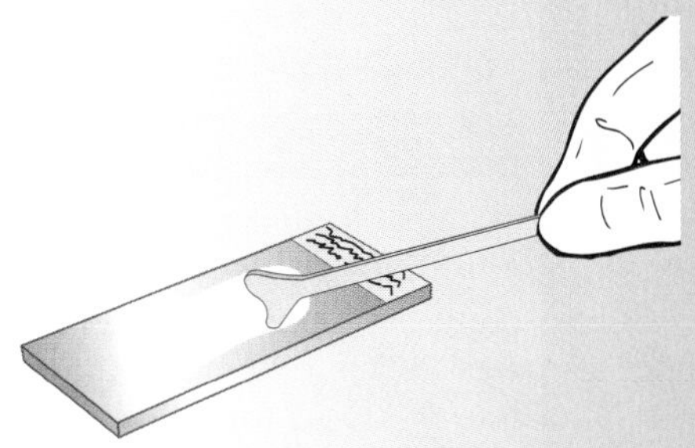

(continued)

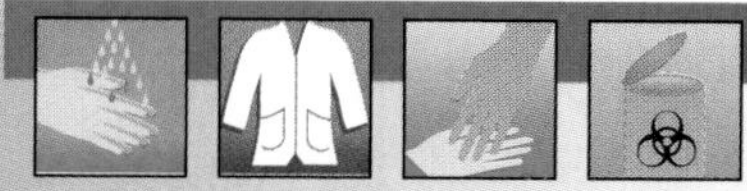

PROCEDURE 28–1

Preparing a PAP Smear (Continued)

9. Label the slides with the correct patient information.
10. Spray fixative on the slides, or place them in preservative.

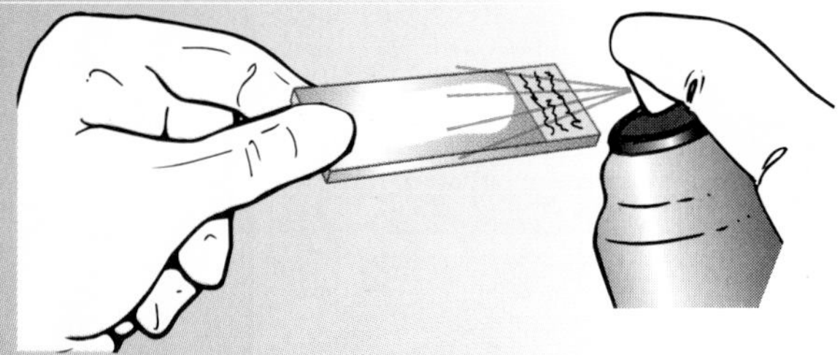

11. When the physician has completed the examination, assist the patient to sit up and instruct her to get dressed.
12. Place the slides in a labeled specimen folder. Then place the folder into a secure mailing container.
13. Be sure the mailing container is appropriate for cytologic samples.
14. Prepare the reusable speculum for sterilization, or if it is disposable, discard it in a biohazard container.
15. Return all supplies to the proper storage area.
16. Remove gloves and wash hands.
17. Record the procedure in the laboratory logbook.

Interpretation of Results

PAP smear results are reported in various ways, depending on the laboratory's preference. The traditional method for reporting is as follows:

Class I: Normal cells/typical cell formation
Class II: Atypical cells, but not malignant; mild cervical dysplasia
Class III: Atypical cells, suggestive of malignancy; mild cervical dysplasia
Class IV: Atypical cells, suggestive of malignancy; severe cervical dysplasia
Class V: Cancer cells present; conclusive for malignancy/cancer

NOTE: Abnormal results warrant a repeat PAP smear or cervical biopsy.

Histology

A group of cells that perform a specific or specialized function is called a *tissue* (Table 28–2). The study of the origin, structure, function, and pathology of tissue is termed *histology*. Histologic techniques are used to confirm the diagnosis of malignant disease based on positive screening test results.

Specimen Collection

Specimens for histologic examination are collected by surgical biopsy. Histologic studies are also performed on tissue removed during surgery or at autopsy. Tissue collected during surgery may be frozen and examined while the patient is still undergoing surgery. This rapid procedure can provide a diagnosis within minutes, allowing the surgeon to decide the optimal approach to and extent of the surgical procedure while the patient is still under anesthesia. This valuable and timely information may eliminate the need for a second surgery at a later date (Fig. 28–3).

Tissue biopsies are performed using different types

Table 28–2
Basic Tissues of the Human Body

Tissue Type	*Characteristics/Function*
Epithelial	Forms the outer and inner layer of the external and internal surfaces of the body and all its structures
	Functions in absorption, excretion, protection, and secretion
Connective	The most abundant tissue in the body; found in bones, tendons, ligaments, cartilage, fat, and blood
	Functions in body support, shape of body structures, and body maintenance
Muscle	Includes three types of muscle: (1) cardiac (heart); (2) smooth or visceral, involuntary muscle (internal organs), and (3) striated or skeletal muscle, which is under voluntary control of the host
	Functions to create and sustain movement
Nervous	Has properties of excitability and conductivity, which allow it to control and coordinate the activities of the body
	Acts as the body's communication network

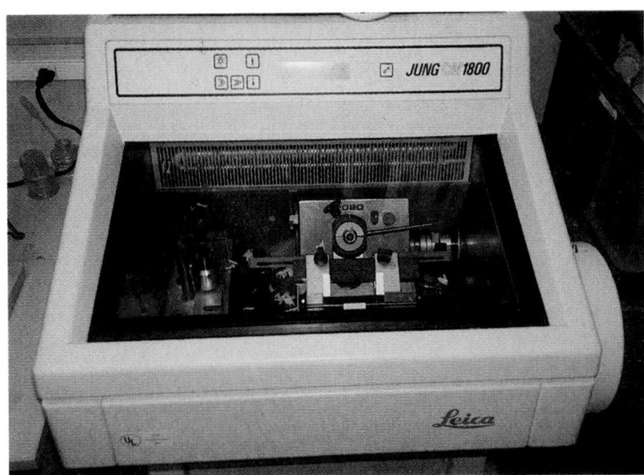

Figure 28–3. *A cryostat instrument used in the preparation of tissue for rapid examination during surgery.*

of specialized needles (Fig. 28–4). Biopsies are routinely performed on the breast, liver, lymph nodes, lung, and muscles. Biopsies may be surgical procedures involving the excision of an entire lesion, or they may involve only aspiration of a small sample of the lesion. Malignant disease can be confirmed only by biopsy study.

Tissue Processing and Analysis

The proper collection, handling, and processing of tissue for histologic testing are crucial to ensure accurate and reliable results. The definitive diagnosis of diseases, such as cancer, is dependent on meticulous technique.

Specimens for histologic study arrive in the laboratory, where they are first examined by a pathologist. This visual (gross) examination includes a complete description of the tissue. The tissue is then dissected and sectioned into blocks for processing (Fig. 28–5).

Figure 28–4. *Various types of biopsy needles.*

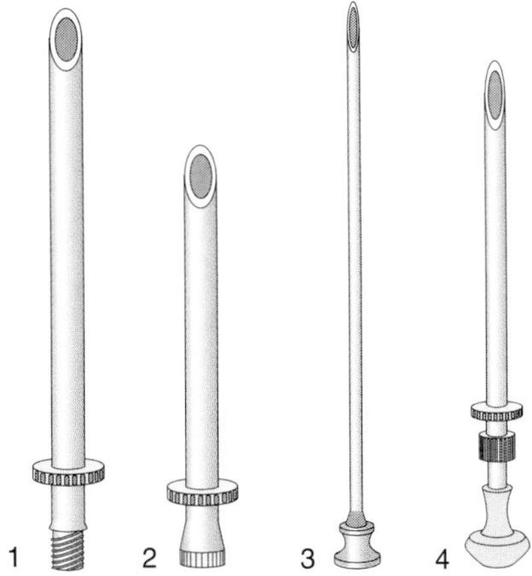

1 Menghini liver biopsy needle
2 University of Illinois bone marrow biopsy needle
3 Franklin-Silverman tissue biopsy needle
4 Menghini kidney biopsy needle

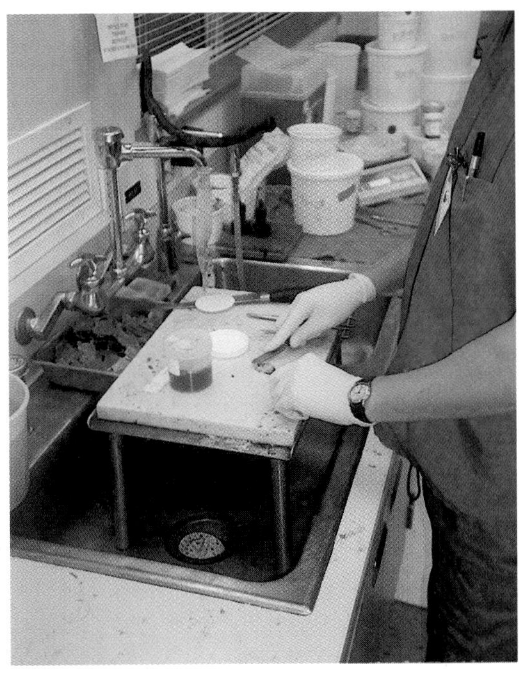

Figure 28–5. *Dissection and sectioning of tissue into blocks for processing.*

Tissue processing involves fixation, washing, dehydration, clearing, and infiltration. Processing may take 18 to 24 hours, and is done by a special tissue processing machine (Fig. 28–6). Once the tissue is processed, it is embedded in a melted paraffin-based compound. Once this hardens, the tissue block can then be sectioned or cut using a special instrument called a **microtome.** A microtome contains a blade that will cut tissue into sections that are one cell layer thick (Fig.

Figure 28–6. *Automated tissue processor.*

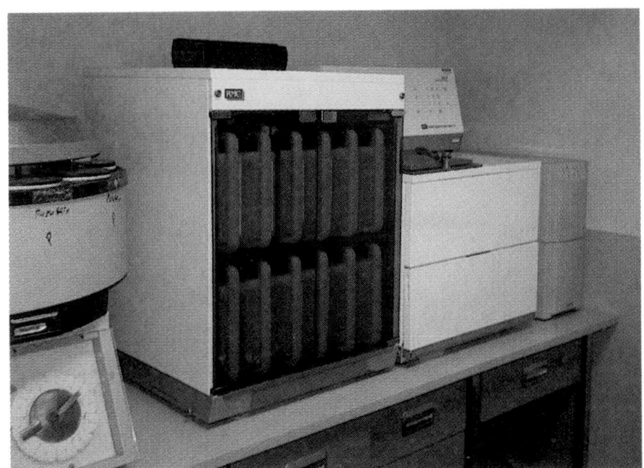

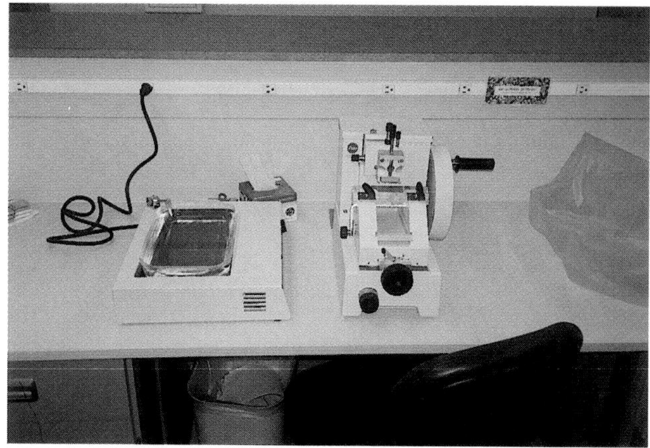

A

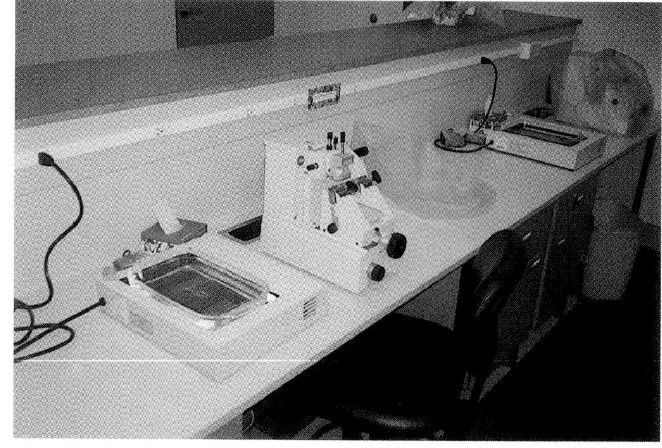

B

Figure 28–7. *Microtome.* A, *Frontal view.* B, *Lateral view with blade in cutting position.*

28–7, *A* and *B*). These sections are then fixed to glass slides, which can be stained. Special stains are used to make specific structures visible during the microscopic examination. The basic stain for most histologic studies is hematoxylin-eosin (H & E) stain. This stain is used to determine the general relationship between cells and tissues. Special stains, such as the Feulgen staining method that is used in DNA testing, are frequently used in conjunction with the H & E stain. Such histologic examinations are performed by a pathologist.

Summary

This chapter presented an overview of several areas of laboratory medicine that are not usually covered in basic laboratory textbooks. As you familiarized yourself with the base philosophy of epidemiology, you learned that disease does not occur by chance, and continuing your reading you saw how laboratory science serves a valuable purpose in establishing the cause, the path of transmission, and the method of treatment. Knowledge of all areas of the laboratory will assist you in providing better care to the patients you serve. Indeed, your professional satisfaction and achievement in the working world have a direct correlation to your level of knowledge and understanding.

Chapter Review

True or False

Circle T or F to indicate the correct answers to the following:

T F 1. Epidemiology refers to the study of the factors influencing the distribution, causes, and frequency of diseases in a defined population.

T F 2. The major role of all laboratories is to assist in the diagnosis and treatment of patients.

T F 3. Tuberculosis is a vector-transmitted disease.

T F 4. The medical technologist is the primary professional in the anatomic laboratory area.

Fill in the Blanks

Complete the following statements:

5. Epidemiology is concerned with two general types of infections: ______________ - ______________, and ______________.

6. Nosocomial infections are those that are acquired in a ______________, ______________ ______________, or ______________.

7. Diseases caused by vectors include ______________, ______________, and ______________.

8. When one cell divides to make two new cells, the process is called ______________.

9. The purpose of cytologic testing is to examine or screen cells for ______________ or ______________ cells.

Multiple Choice

Circle the letter that represents the single best answer:

10. Hospitalized persons have an increased susceptibility to infection owing to:
    a. Their age
    b. Their susceptibility
    c. Their weakened condition
    d. The virulence of their disease

11. The PAP smear is used to diagnose:
    a. Cancer
    b. Sexual chromosomes
    c. Fungal and viral infections
    d. All of the above

12. A special instrument used to cut tissue into sections that are one cell layer in thickness is the:
    a. Scalpel
    b. Dermatome
    c. Lance
    d. Microtome

Vocabulary

asphyxia: a condition in which there is a deficiency of oxygen in the blood and an increase in carbon dioxide in the blood and tissues

autopsy: an examination of the body after death to determine the manner and cause of death

blebs: anatomical, elevated structures of the skin that usually measure more than 5 mm in diameter

homicide: any killing of a person by another person

lividity: discoloration as a result of pooling of blood

natural: occurring in the ordinary course of events

suicide: the act of killing oneself deliberately

unnatural: not in accordance with the expected or ordinary course of events

Chapter Objectives

After reading this chapter, you should be able to:

1. Define forensic pathology.
2. Compare forensic medicine with clinical medicine.
3. List the types of deaths that are subject to forensic medicine studies.
4. Explain the guidelines followed in postmortem investigations.
5. Describe the role of the pathology staff in establishing the cause and manner of death.
6. Outline the findings that establish the time of death.
7. List the usual order of body decomposition.
8. Discuss some of the concerns of the immediate family of the deceased.

Chapter 29
Forensic Pathology

The relationship of forensic pathology to medicine is illustrated by the following saying of Hippocrates: "The Physician must know what his predecessors have known, if he does not wish to deceive both himself and his patients."

The word *forensic* means pertaining to legal proceedings and elements of law. *Pathology* is the branch of medicine dealing with the essential nature of disease and the changes in body tissues and organs that cause or are caused by disease or death. Pathology also applies to the resolution of clinical problems, especially through the use of laboratory methods of clinical diagnosis.

Forensic or legal medicine is the speciality of medicine dealing with *postmortem* study. Postmortem involves scientific observation and gathering of evidence and the construction of reasonable inferences based on this observation and evidence. These inferences, and their relationship to the law, are the bases of forensic medicine.

Forensic Medicine

Forensic medicine involves the investigation of death as part of a legal proceeding. Evidence is produced in informal or formal settings. Types of evidence used in an investigation would include witnesses, dying declarations, phenomena and signs of death, causes of death, medical and law enforcement investigative findings, findings on postmortem examination, and the identity of the victim.

Deaths that are subject to forensic medicine are unnatural deaths, such as those resulting from **asphyxia,** suffocation, strangulation, hanging, drowning, lightning, heat or cold, starvation, poisoning, **suicide, homicide,** and accidents.

Death Certificate

A death certificate is a legal document that gives the vital information, including the time and cause of the person's death. This document is signed

Table 29–1
Factors Associated With Natural and Unnatural Deaths

Natural Death	*Unnatural Death*
Cessation of breathing	Unexpected event
Cessation of heart beat	Unusual circumstances
Cessation of urinary output	Suspicious circumstances
Progression of life's events (old age)	Accidental cause
Medical disease process	Homicide
	Suicide
	Involvement of law enforcement officials

by the county coroner or the patient's attending physician. After it is signed, it is filed in the county hall of records. Before a death certificate may be issued, the cause and manner of death must be determined. This is true whether the death is considered to be **natural** or **unnatural** (Table 29–1).

Postmortem Study

Any death has possible civil, criminal, and/or economic ramifications for the family of the deceased and for society as a whole. It is a basic civil right of every person for a professional, competency-based investigation to be conducted to determine the cause of the person's death. Knowing the actual cause of a family member's death often provides the family with a sense of closure. In addition to the family, society needs to understand the circumstances surrounding certain types of death (e.g., homicide).

Death investigations are handled by the coroner's office or a medical examiner. When a death occurs outside of an established medical facility, the first contact with the deceased is by law enforcement officials, who, in turn, contact the coroner's or medical examiner's office. How deaths are handled depends on the circumstances, and may vary from state to state. Deaths in medical facilities are typically treated differently than deaths that occur outside of the hospital.

The guidelines for a postmortem examination are the same as for an investigation into any health problem during life. The investigation begins with a history of the deceased and then proceeds to a physical examination (autopsy) and clinical laboratory tests. It is common practice to perform x-ray studies, in addition to clinical and anatomic laboratory studies. All of the information is then examined and a diagnosis (cause of death) is determined.

History

The investigation of an unnatural death begins at the scene of the body's location. Law enforcement officials play a vital role in this part of the study. Physical evidence is collected, such as blood stains, photographs, and fingerprints. The position of the body of the de-

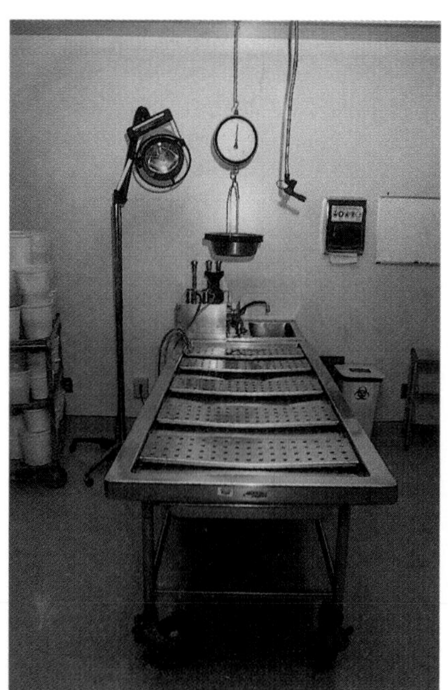
A

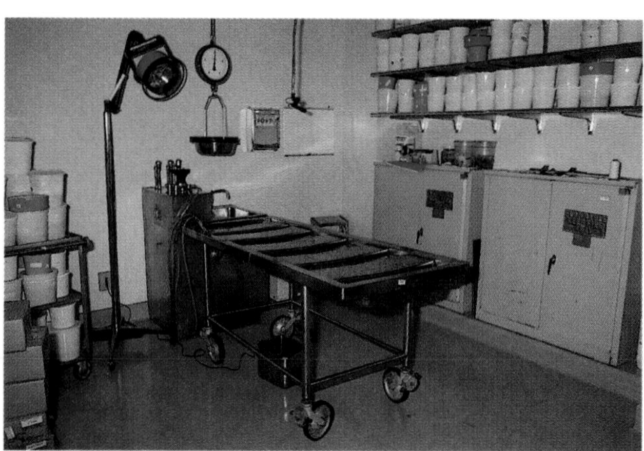
B

Figure 29–1. *Postmortem examining table* (A) *and forensic laboratory* (B).

Table 29–2
Forensic Postmortem Procedures

GUNSHOT WOUNDS

Obtain radiographs of all entrance and exit wounds.
Locate bullets and fragments.
Photograph entrance/exit sites.

SHARP WOUNDS

Obtain radiographs of all wound sites.
Photograph wound sites without altering original condition.
Photograph wound sites after cleansing.
Check hands and arms for defense wounds.
Photograph severed cartilage.

BLUNT FORCE INJURIES

Obtain radiographs of hands and arms for defense wounds.
Obtain radiographs of all affected areas.
Photograph wounds before and after cleaning.
Check for possible rape using a rape kit.

SPECIAL BATTERY

If sexual assault is suspected, perform the following in order:

With the body in the supine position, secure the following samples:

- Scalp and pubic hair
- Oral fluid samples
- Semen from inner thighs

With the body in the prone position, secure the following samples:

- Anal specimen
- Vaginal specimen
- Material from fingernails and under fingernails
- Pubic hairs, 25 from entire area
- Head hair, 25 from affected area

Obtain samples from any body area suspected of containing the assailant's tissue or semen.

DRUG OVERDOSE

Photograph injection sites; residue on lips, teeth, tongue, and oral membranes; nose; and hands.
Assess the mouth area and body for bite marks that suggest seizure activity.
Palpate the lymph nodes, spleen, and liver (abnormal in IV drug users).

CHILD ABUSE

Obtain radiographs of and photograph the entire body.
Perform an external examination, noting in particular the presence or appearance of the following:

- Conjunctival petechiae
- Fingertip bruises
- Torso and shoulders
- Frenulum
- Back, posterior thighs, and buttocks

Perform an internal examination, noting in particular the following:

- Hematomas
- Appearance of the retina upon removal of the eyes (distinctive in sudden infant death syndrome [SIDS])
- Recent or healed fractures

ceased, the type of injuries sustained, the possible means (instruments) by which those injuries may have been inflicted, and any other crime scene paraphernalia that may have some implication are carefully noted and/or photographed, collected, and marked. It is important that evidence be carefully preserved in the event that a civil or criminal legal proceeding follows. After all available evidence is secured, the body is then removed from the scene and transported to a designated establishment for **autopsy** (Fig. 29–1).

Physical Examination of the Deceased (Autopsy)

An autopsy involves both an external and an internal examination. The external examination includes an overall investigation of the condition of the physical body, and involves the classification of any wounds, injuries, and/or traumatized areas. Photographs, radiographs, blood samples, and external tissue and fluid specimens may be obtained. The external examination also includes an investigation to rule out sexual assault and/or molestation.

The internal investigation includes an examination of the internal organs. When organs are examined for forensic reasons, each must be weighed and measured; additionally, a gross description of each is provided, and samples are taken for tissue analysis. Further investigation of wounds, traumatized areas, and body fluids, such as gastric, lung, and bowel contents, may be warranted, with samples taken for laboratory testing and examination (Table 29–2).

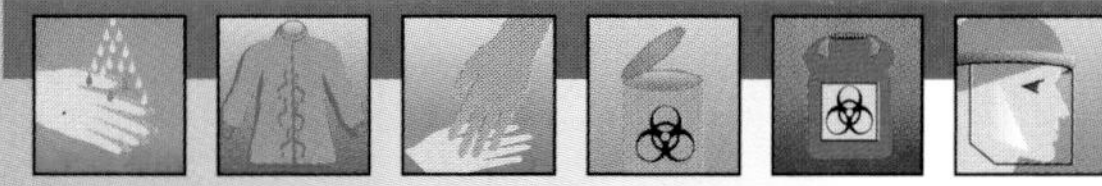

PROCEDURE 29–1

Assisting With Autopsy

Principle

To observe and assist (if allowed) a pathologist during postmortem examination so as to gain a deeper understanding of the physiology of the human body and the relationship between diseases and laboratory testing and analysis

Equipment and Supplies

OSHA safety equipment
other safety equipment as requested by the pathologist

Procedural Steps

NOTE: You will only be observing and assisting the pathologist as needed. Before entering the autopsy area, you will need to wash your hands and don a gown, gloves, and goggles. Adhere strictly to OSHA regulations and observe universal precautions.

1. Identify the body and tag the great toe with the person's name, sex, age, and case number.
2. Weigh and measure the body.
3. Describe and record information about the deceased's clothing and any valuables. Remove and give these items to the family or to law enforcement officials.
4. Fingerprint all 10 digits.
5. Cleanse the body of all blood, dirt, or other materials. If the face was bloody or dirty, rephotograph after cleaning.
6. Perform an external examination. Using a body diagram, mark all identifying marks and describe each one.
7. Photograph all injuries from at least two different views.
8. X-ray studies may now be done to verify gross anatomical deformities, or for the purpose of identifying the deceased through dental or bone films.
9. Beginning with the head and continuing to the feet, describe by color and feature all anatomical features, injuries, wounds, bruises, and lacerations.
10. The internal investigation includes complete head-to-pelvic dissection, with removal of every organ. When removed, each organ is described, weighed, measured, and grossly examined. Organ samples are obtained and prepared for microscopic investigation.
11. Blood specimens are withdrawn by syringe from the heart and aorta. Vitreous humor is withdrawn from the eyes, bile from the gallbladder, and urine from the bladder. These samples are labeled and placed in the refrigerator until examination.
12. If cultures of body tissues/fluids are needed, use sterile instruments to obtain specimens. The area to be cultured must be scrubbed with betadine for 5 minutes before the culture is obtained.
13. When the autopsy is completed, the organs are returned to the body and the incisions are closed by suturing.
14. Remove protective gear and dispose of it properly.
15. Wash hands and dry them thoroughly.

Laboratory Studies

Blood and other body fluids are examined for alcohol level, over-the-counter (OTC) and prescription drug levels, and controlled substance levels. Other chemical constituents, such as glucose or enzymes, may also be tested. There are specified procedures that must be completed when the death is suspected to have occurred under criminal circumstances. Many such cases are classified as deaths by violence (see Table 29–2).

Determination of the Cause and Manner of Death

Based on evidence assembled during scene investigation, the findings at autopsy, and laboratory results, the cause and manner of death are determined. This information is then placed on a death certificate and the body is readied to be released to the family.

Time of Death

Determination of the time of death may be an issue in both natural and unnatural deaths. Time of death is useful when determining death benefits for insurance proceeds, in cases of unwitnessed deaths, or when body parts have been altered to conceal an individual's identity.

When death occurs, breathing, circulation, and voluntary movement cease. Occasionally, several hours after the determined time of death, voluntary muscles may flicker when pinched, and spasms of both skeletal and visceral muscles may occur.

The time of death is an estimate of the time range within which a person's death may have occurred. It is important to remember that there is no single, accurate marker for time of death. The time of death estimate is based on several factors, described in the following sections.

Cadaveric Spasm

Cadaveric spasm is an uncommon event consisting of a violent spasm of the muscles at the moment of death. This phenomenon most frequently involves the hands, which may remain gripping a weapon, a steering wheel, or a piece of clothing.

Rigor Mortis

Rigor mortis is a condition that results from the stiffening of the fibers of all muscles due to pH changes and the lack of adenosine triphosphate (ATP) in the muscle tissues. The fibers shorten and stiffen, and all groups of muscles become prominent and rigid, fixing the limbs. Rigor mortis can be observed in the faces of some people within the first 5 to 7 hours after death. It then spreads to the shoulders and arms, eventually extending down to the trunk to involve the legs within about 12 hours. At this point, the process has reached its peak; during the next 12 hours, it will resolve, leaving the body muscles in their original state. No close estimate of the time of death can be established from observation of rigor mortis alone.

A skin change, called "goose fleshing," commonly occurs during rigor mortis as a result of contraction of the erector muscles of the hairs. Freezing temperatures may confound estimates of time of death, as they, too, cause stiffening of the muscles, effectively postponing rigor mortis until the body is thawed.

Algor Mortis

During the first 18 hours after death, cooling of the body is the only real benchmark for determining the time elapsed since death. Its early measurement is important in establishing an approximate time of death. At room temperature, the clothed body will cool in air at the rate of about 2½ degrees per hour for the first 6 hours. The body will lose heat more slowly as the temperature comes nearer to that of its surroundings. The body will feel cool in about 12 hours, and will be cold in about 18 to 24 hours.

The internal organs should be the same temperature as the environment within 18 to 24 hours. The most accurate temperature readings come from the rectum. Factors that may play a role in the rate of cooling include environmental temperature, clothing and bedding, obesity, and amount of ventilation (Fig. 29–2).

Livor Mortis

Lividity is a deep staining of the skin and organs of the body. This results from the settling of blood in dependent body parts as a result of gravity. Lividity begins to develop within about 1 to 2 hours after death, as the body begins to cool, becoming marked or fixed within 3 to 12 hours. Fixed lividity remains even if the body is moved or turned to a new position. Livid stains cannot develop in areas where the pressure of clothing cushions the weight of the body, as this pressure prevents the vessels from filling. The color of livid areas bears a direct relationship to the color of the blood at the time of death. For example, those dying of carbon monoxide poisoning have blood that is a bright cherry red, and the areas marked by lividity will mimic this color. It is not difficult to distinguish livid stains from bruises, as the appearance and the color are noticeably different.

Decomposition

Within 48 hours after death, a greenish staining of the skin develops in both flanks of the abdomen. Soon, a reddish discoloration of the veins, beginning at the base of the neck, continuing over the shoulders, and then proceeding into the groins, brings them into prominence, often producing a "marbled effect." This is

Figure 29–2. *Postmortem changes according to time and temperature*

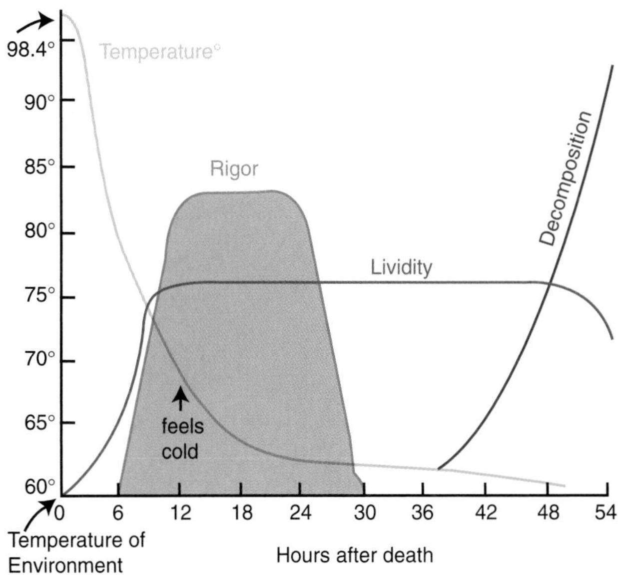

due to the chemical breakdown of cells and organs by intracellular enzymes and putrefaction resulting from bacterial action. Anaerobic gas-forming organisms, growing in the intestines, move into the systemic veins, staining the tissues first red and then green as hemolysis occurs. Small bubbles disrupt the tissue, creating **blebs** on the skin. This phenomenon is linked to climate. Warm weather speeds the process, whereas cool weather slows it down.

Insect Activity

Flies and other flesh-eating insects are associated with decomposition of the body. This process is accelerated by airborne bacteria and hindered by immersion in water or by burial. When a body is discovered partially decomposed and there is overwhelming fly activity, an *entomologist* (an expert on insects) may be called in to aid in the investigation and to help establish the time of death.

Putrefaction

Changes in the chemistry of body tissues, combined with the decomposition of the body, produce a "rotting" tissue odor. This becomes increasingly strong as flies and bacteria fill the body; the former lay eggs, and the larvae hatch and feed. Moreover, as the time elapsed since death increases, the potassium level in the vitreous humor of the eye changes. The longer the time since death, the greater the concentration of potassium.

These findings may vary when the time interval between actual death and the initial death investigation is months or years. Additionally, climatic conditions may influence body changes. For example, dry heat, especially when aided by currents of air, as in the tropics or inside a chimney, will prevent bacterial decomposition and putrefaction (Table 29–3).

The usual order of body decomposition is as follows:

1. Intestines, stomach, liver, blood, and heart muscle
2. Lungs
3. Brain
4. Kidneys, bladder, and testes
5. Voluntary muscles
6. Uterus, prostate

Family Concerns

The human response to death varies among societal groups. Societal responses are strongly influenced by culture, religion, race, and habits. For these reasons, a family may find decisions regarding autopsy to be very difficult. Explaining the need for the procedure and the questions that can be resolved by such an examination may help them to accept it. Showing concern and respect for the deceased and for the family of the deceased can help to reduce the family's anxiety about and objections to after-death testing, and can help avoid misinterpretations. The family should be assured that nothing will be done to the body without their

Table 29–3
Time Table for and Signs of Decomposition in Land and Water

Parameter	*Time Elapsed (hr)*	*Land*	*Water*
Cooling	0–12	1.5–2° F/hour	3° F/hour
	12–24	0.75–1° F/hour	1.5° F/hour
		The body feels cool to touch within 10–12 hours.	Within 5–6 hours after death, the body feels cool to touch.
		The body is cold to touch within 20–24 hours.	Within 8–10 hours after death, the body is cold to touch.
Lividity	3–5	Developing lividity	Whitening of skin; no lividity
Chemical Changes	12–72	Rise in potassium level of the vitreous humor	Slight decline in the potassium level of the vitreous humor

permission except as required by law. If the family expresses concern about mutilation of the body or the possibility of a delay in the release of the body for burial, provide clear and concise information to facilitate the decision-making process. If there is a religious concern, encourage them to contact their clergy for counseling and information. Remember **ALWAYS** to obtain a signed, witnessed consent form prior to autopsy and laboratory testing of the deceased's body tissue and fluids.

Summary

Forensic pathology provides for both mandatory and routine procedures, especially if the death is sudden, suspicious, or unexplained. This field of inquiry has established a set of guidelines for our legal system that provides a matrix for responsible, comprehensive investigation. The findings of a postmortem examination may help the family of the deceased to cope with the loss of their loved one. When an autopsy is performed, the information gathered also provides a framework for developing improved and increasingly sophisticated treatments for disease and illness. One example of a new development in forensic pathology involves the use of molecular biology techniques to match the DNA (genetic material) "fingerprints" left at a crime scene with the DNA of criminal suspects. As autopsy is performed only in designated facilities, it is very unlikely that you will ever have to assist with this procedure. However, there is a strong likelihood that a family to whom you provide care will have to make a decision regarding autopsy. With knowledge comes understanding; with understanding, you can provide support to those families facing issues relating to the death of a loved one.

Chapter Review

True or False

Circle T or F to indicate the correct answers to the following:

T F 1. Accidental death is considered to be a form of natural death.

T F 2. Society needs to understand the circumstances surrounding a homicide.

T F 3. Investigation of a health problem and postmortem investigation follow the same general guidelines.

T F 4. The physical evidence surrounding a death can include blood stains, photography, and fingerprints.

Fill in the Blanks

Complete the following statements:

5. Before issuing a death certificate, the ______________ and ______________ of death must be determined.
6. Death investigations are handled by the ______________ ______________ or a ______________ ______________.
7. Autopsy involves both an ______________ and an ______________ examination.
8. The ______________ ___ ______________ is an estimate of the time range within which death may have occurred.

Multiple Choice

Circle the letter that represents the single best answer:

9. The investigation of an unnatural death begins:
   a. At the scene of the crime
   b. At the scene of the body's location
   c. With an autopsy
   d. With location of the weapon
10. Algor mortis refers to:
    a. Stiffening of all body muscles
    b. Cooling of the body
    c. Staining of the skin
    d. Decomposition of the body
11. Lividity is related to the:
    a. Temperature of the body
    b. Location of the body
    c. Color of the blood
    d. Insect activity and odor
12. Family concerns regarding postmortem examination:
    a. Are ignored by law enforcement
    b. Can delay an investigation
    c. Vary depending on whether the death was natural or unnatural
    d. Are always the same

Vocabulary

cause of action: the fact or facts that give a person a right to judicial relief
foreseeable: able to be seen or known in advance; that which can be reasonably anticipated (e.g., the expectation that harm or injury is likely to result from certain acts or omissions)
intentional act: an action or state of mind that denotes the desire to cause the consequences of an act, or the belief that the consequences are substantially certain to occur
respondeat superior: a doctrine meaning "Let the master answer." This doctrine applies only when the relationship between the "master" and the "servant" existed at the time of the wrongdoing and arose out of the master/servant (employer/employee) relationship.
strictly liable: having direct legal responsibility, as, for example, a person who sells a defective product that is dangerous to the user/consumer and that ultimately causes harm to the user/consumer
tort: a civil wrong or injury, other than a breach of contract, for which the court will provide a remedy in the form of an action for damages
trespasser: a person who intentionally and without consent or privilege enters another's property
vicariously liable: having indirect legal responsibility, as, for example, an employer deemed to be responsible for the act of an employee, or a principle for the act of an agent

Chapter Objectives

After reading this chapter, you should be able to:

1. Discuss the legal ramifications for negligent conduct.
2. Define "standard of care" and give examples of its application.
3. List the elements necessary for a cause of action for negligence.
4. Describe the four conditions that must be satisfied when invoking the doctrine of *res ipsa loquitur.*
5. Explain how intentional acts differ from negligent acts.
6. Discuss premises liability.
7. Describe the federal legislation that is directly concerned with employment.
8. Identify the federal legislation that deals with laboratory safety.
9. List the elements that constitute sexual harassment.

Chapter 30
Legal Issues

Health care is a business, whether or not we choose to acknowledge it as such. Unlike most businesses, health care is highly regulated. Therefore, it is important that all health care professionals have a basic understanding of how the law relates to their work. The *law* is a compilation of rules of action or conduct established by an authority, such as the state, which has binding legal force.

Economics, advances in technology, and new and ballooning regulatory schemes are changing health care dramatically. As a result, legal issues are arising that tend to challenge and bewilder us.

There are available entire texts devoted to medical law. It is beyond the scope of this chapter to discuss, in depth, all of the many legal issues you may encounter as a health care worker. Instead, this chapter focuses on several of the issues that apply to all laboratories, including physicians' office laboratories (POLs). Keep in mind, as you study this material, that the term laboratory refers to any facility performing clinical laboratory specimen collection and testing.

Laboratories are subject to federal, state, and local regulations. Examples of regulating agencies include the Occupational Safety and Health Administration (OSHA and the ADA, as well as their state counterparts. In addition, local government may regulate laboratories through zoning regulations, construction requirements, business licensing regulations, and taxation policies.

Conduct

Laboratories must provide for the safety and protection of their employees and patients. They must employ reasonably skilled and competent personnel and must maintain the same degree of care, diligence, and skill provided by other, comparable institutions. This level of competency is based on the circumstances (the location and purpose of the lab) or through any implied or expressed agreement with patients and employees (for example, in cooperative laboratories or Health Management Organization laboratories). Laboratories may be legally responsible for the negligent or intentional conduct of its employees.

Negligence

A person is *negligent* when he or she does or does not do something that a reasonably prudent person would have done or not done under the same or similar circumstances. The universally accepted definition for "standard of care" is based on an ordinary, reasonable, and prudent person acting under the same circumstances. The term "ordinary" is, in this instance, accorded its true meaning; that is, not requiring the conduct of an extraordinary, extremely careful person. The reasonable and prudent person upon whose actions "standard of care" is based is a fictitious person who would take the appropriate action in a given set of circumstances.

In its objective aspect, the standard of care measures the negligent party's conduct against the appropriate conduct of an average person. An adult's mental ability and experience are not taken into account. The subjective aspect of the standard of care considers the physical characteristics or disabilities of the negligent party. However, it is expected that that person would know his or her personal physical limitations/disabilities and would exercise appropriate care in light of those limitations/disabilities, as would another person with such knowledge. For example, if you were blind, your conduct would be measured against that of a reasonable and prudent blind person under the same circumstances.

A professional must exercise the knowledge and skill that a member of his/her profession in good standing in the same or similar localities would exercise (see chart). Specialists are held to a higher standard of care than are professionals. For example, a cardiac surgeon would be held to a higher standard in cardiac surgery than a cardiologist.

A legal remedy or **cause of action** for negligence requires more than negligent conduct. The traditional elements necessary for a cause of action for negligence are:

- A duty to use reasonable care
- Breach of this duty by failure to comply with the required standard of care
- A reasonably close factual and legal connection (causation) between the negligent conduct and the resulting injury
- Actual injury, damages, or loss to another

A laboratory may be liable, under the doctrine of **respondeat superior,** for an injury caused by the negligence of anyone employed by the laboratory.

Res ipsa loquitur means "the thing speaks for itself." The doctrine of *res ipsa loquitur* shifts the burden to the defendant to present evidence of the lack of negligence. Four conditions must be satisfied before the plaintiff can rely on this doctrine:

1. The event does not normally occur unless someone is negligent.
2. The event is caused by an agent or instrument totally within the defendant's control.
3. The event is not attributable to any voluntary action or contribution by the plaintiff.
4. Evidence of the true explanation of the event is more readily accessible to the defendant than to the plaintiff.

Historically, this doctrine has been applied more often in surgical settings than in laboratories. However, the doctrine of *res ipsa loquitur* can be applied in the laboratory setting in certain cases, such as those involving injuries to a nerve secondary to routine injection or venipuncture.

Intentional Acts

Under **tort** law, an employer's legal responsibility for an employee's **intentional act** is determined in a different manner than is the employer's liability for negligent con-

Scope of Practice for Medical Laboratory Assistants

With the authorization of a licensed physician or podiatrist who is physically present in the facility, the medical laboratory assistant **MAY:**

- Perform electrocardiograms (ECGs), electroencephalograms (EEGs), and plethysomography tests (except full-body).
- Collect specimens for testing, such as urine, sputum, semen, and stool, by noninvasive techniques.
- Assist patients in obtaining a specimen for testing.
- Provide information and instructions to the patient, as directed by the physician or podiatrist.
- Collect and record basic information about present and previous tests.
- Perform simple laboratory and screening tests, but without interpreting testing results.
- After successful completion of specified training, perform venipuncture or skin puncture to withdraw blood.

The medical laboratory assistant **MAY NOT:**

- Perform arterial punctures.
- Administer intravenous medications.
- Insert urinary catheters.
- Analyze test results.
- Advise patients about their condition.

NOTE: Check with your state scope of practice regulations. This list is a guideline that most states follow but it is not official.

duct. The laboratory may be **vicariously liable** for an intentional act of its personnel when the intentional act was incidental to, or arose out of, the duties of employment. For example, a laboratory would NOT be vicariously liable for the sexual assault of a patient by an employee, but it may be liable for negligent hiring or supervision. Neither would a laboratory be liable for an injury resulting from a phlebotomist's attempt to train a friend to draw blood while at the friend's home. However, a laboratory could be held legally responsible if a patient is forced to submit to a procedure against his/her wishes. Common intentional torts include assault, battery, false imprisonment, trespass, conversion, invasion of privacy, and emotional distress.

Laboratories may also be liable for failing to provide supplies, equipment, and facilities that are appropriate, reasonable, safe, and adequate for use in patient care. Laboratories have a further obligation to provide a reasonably safe work environment for their employees.

PROCEDURE 30–1

Completing an Incident Report

Principle

To become familiar with the state requirements and time lines for filing an incident report and to gain an understanding of what constitutes an incident, and the need to report ONLY what was directly seen or said

Read the following case report. After completing the reading, answer the questions based on the information presented in Chapter 30. You may use outside reference books to assist you in the answers. Be prepared to discuss and defend your conclusions in class.

> Immediately following open heart surgery, a burn was discovered on a patient's chest, approximately 5 cm to the left of the incision and in line with the patient's left nipple. During surgery, this area was covered with sterile drapes. No lasers, heat, caustic chemicals, or cauterization were used during the procedure. No one present during the surgery noticed anything unusual. The surgeon could not explain how the patient had been burned.
>
> The burn was examined by a plastic surgeon while the patient was in the recovery unit. The burn appeared to be a severe, first-degree burn. The burned area was approximately 5 cm wide and 11 cm long, much larger than when first discovered. During examination of the burn on the morning after surgery, the burned area was upgraded as follows: center of burn, third degree; area immediately around the center, second degree; outer rim, first degree.
>
> The burn did not affect the outcome of the primary surgery nor the patient's recovery. However, surgery would be required to remove scar tissue after the burned area healed. Some permanent scarring would remain, even after cosmetic surgery was completed.
>
> Shortly after surgery, one of the high-intensity lamps in the surgery room was found to have a missing heat shield. During surgery, this lamp had been positioned over the patient, directly over the area that had been burned. An investigation by the hospital revealed that the heat shield had been removed by a hospital employee during a bulb change. The employee had forgotten to replace the heat shield.

Answer the following questions:

1. What type of damages is the patient entitled to recover?

   ____

   ____

   ____

2. How might the following categories of patients affect the damages awarded?
   a. 60-year-old male:

      ____

   b. 70-year-old female:

      ____

   c. 20-year-old male model:

      ____

   d. 18-year-old female beauty pageant contestant:

      ____

3. Explain how the *res ipsa loquitur* doctrine applies to this incident.

   ____

Premises Liability

Laboratories are responsible for maintaining the premises in a reasonably safe manner. The general rule is that an owner of real property is legally responsible for failing to use ordinary care and skill in the management of his or her person or property so as to avoid injuring those on or near it. Owners include those who control the property, such as lessees and occupiers. This duty applies to all visitors, whether they are invitees (on the premises for a business purpose), licensees (on the premises for a social purpose), or **trespassers.**

Generally, a clinical laboratory must exercise ordinary care to ensure the safety of everyone he knows or should expect to be on the property. There may also be an affirmative duty to protect visitors and employees from the wrongful conduct of others (including other employees and/or visitors). The owner must also protect against **foreseeable** criminal acts.

The scope of the duty to protect is partially determined by balancing the burden of the duty against the ability to foresee harm. This duty extends to all areas that visitors are implicitly or expressly intended to use, and over which the laboratory exercises apparent or actual control (e.g., a parking lot used by laboratory visitors that is separately owned).

Employment

Employment law is important to all industries, including the health care field. The health care industry in general, and laboratories in particular, have unique aspects that make this area particularly complex. One example that can be cited is the strict regulations regarding exposure to blood and body fluids.

Factored into the employer-employee equation is the concern for providing safe, competent, economical, and continuous health care. Employment issues of concern in laboratories are safety, discrimination, and sexual harassment.

Preserving the safety and well-being of employees has been an issue of national concern for decades. Guided by federal regulations, state and local governments have enacted regulations governing workplace safety (see chart).

In 1970, Congress passed the Occupational Safety and Health Act. This legislation created OSHA, an agency responsible for establishing and enforcing compulsory, uniform standards for health and safety in the workplace. Laboratories and other health care institutions are covered by the Act. Additionally, many states have enacted their own safety and health standards.

Laboratories must know and comply with all OSHA standards that apply to them and must make this information available to all employees. OSHA conducts periodic inspections to ensure compliance with these standards.

The Act imposes two fundamental obligations on employers. The first requires that employers provide all employees with employment that is free from recognized hazards that cause or are likely to cause serious injury and/or death. Second, the employer must comply with the safety and health standards set forth in the Act. Enforcement is provided for in the form of abatement orders and penalties, primarily consisting of fines.

State laws must be at least as strict as the federal law. Many states have enacted "right-to-know laws" for employees. Right-to-know laws provide for access to information about employer and employee duties and rights relating to safety and health issues.

The Centers for Disease Control (CDC) have established proposed guidelines for Universal Precautions (discussed in detail in Chapters 2 and 3). OSHA enforces these guidelines under the Bloodborne Pathogen Standards Act.

Laboratory workers face biological, chemical, and physical hazards on a daily basis. Educational training on all hazards must be a constant process.

Laboratory personnel use the tools of technology daily. Hazards associated with the use of such technology include musculoskeletal problems, such as carpal tunnel syndrome, and vision problems associated with computer monitors and video display terminals. Additionally, stress-related illnesses are increasing among health care workers. In particular, stress-related workers' compensation claims caused by job loss or fear of job loss as a result of downsizing, implementation of managed care, and increases in the pace and volume of work are becoming more common (Fig. 30–1).

Important Federal Legislation Pertaining to Employment

1935	Wagner Act
	Social Security Act
1938	Fair Labor Standards Act
1963	The Equal Pay Act
1964	Civil Rights Act
1967	Age Discrimination in Employment Act
1970	Occupational Safety and Health Act
1973	Rehabilitation Act
1974	The Employee Retirement Income Security Act
1976	Pregnancy Discrimination Act
1992	The Americans with Disabilities Act

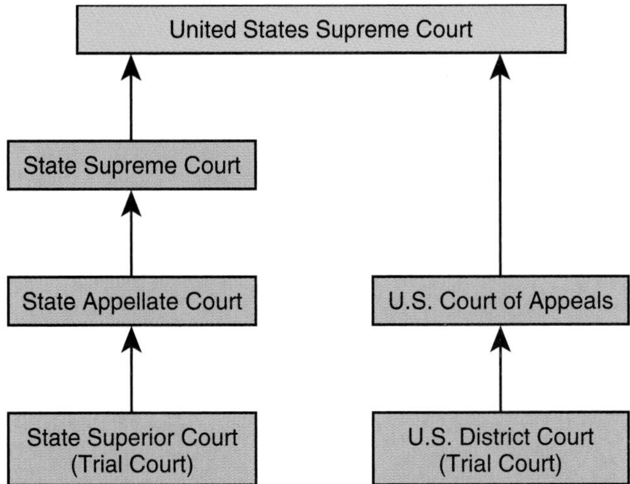

Figure 30–1. *The American state and federal court system.*

Workers' Compensation

State and federal workers' compensation laws have been enacted to compensate employees who are injured at work. Workers' compensation regulations usually provide for fixed awards to employees or their dependents for work-related injuries and diseases. Some states provide for an insurance system, which may be administered by the state or by an independent agency.

The purpose of workers' compensation laws is to dispense with proof of negligence and make employers **strictly liable** for injuries or diseases that arise out of and during employment. When workers' compensation laws apply, they are usually the employee's exclusive remedy. In some states, however, exceptions may be made, and employees may be awarded further compensation if the employer is found to have behaved in a reckless or wanton manner. Most states require that all employers inform employees of their workers' compensation rights.

It benefits both employers and employees when all on-the-job injuries or illnesses are reported immediately under the proper guidelines. Immediate reporting allows time for the appropriate agencies to open a "case folder." Once this folder is open, for medical services and disability as well as insurance, notification can be executed. This step can greatly aid the emotional and physical wellness of the injured employee. The employer is also seen as a more caring and understanding person for the manner in which the claim was handled.

As a laboratory employee, you are affected by workers' compensation laws in two ways. First, as an employee, you have coverage in the event of work-related injury/illness, and second, you may be in a position to provide treatment to an injured worker.

Discrimination

Federal legislation regarding employment was first enacted many years ago. Title VII of the Civil Rights Act of 1964 made discrimination in the workplace illegal. Many states have enacted similar regulations, and these laws often have more rigorous requirements and provide for more classifications of coverage than does the federal law.

Employers must not discriminate in connection with employment. Targeted classifications for discrimination include age, sex, race, color, creed, marital status, national origin, or disabilities.

The prohibition against discrimination applies to interviewing and hiring practices, compensation, benefits, working conditions, privileges, and opportunities of employment. It also applies to discharge and termination practices.

The Americans with Disabilities Act prohibits discrimination against disabled persons in employment and mandates equal access for disabled persons to specified public places. In addition to the discrimination provisions, the ADA requires that employers take action to reasonably accommodate disabled persons provided the accommodation does not cause undue hardship on the employer.

Laboratories and other health care facilities are covered under the federal and state laws regarding discrimination. Most of these laws apply only to employers who employ at least 15 employees, the qualified minimum number established by the law.

Sexual Harassment

Title VII of the Civil Rights Act prohibits sex-based discrimination. Sexual harassment is treated by the courts as a type of sex-based discrimination.

The United States Equal Employment Opportunity Commission (EEOC) was established under Title VII of the Civil Rights Act. Many states have established their own offices of Equal Employment Opportunity.

The U.S. EEOC has defined sexual harassment as follows:

> Unwelcome sexual advances, requests for sexual favors and other verbal or physical conduct of a sexual nature constitute sexual harassment when (1) submission to such conduct is made either explicitly or implicitly a term or condition of an individual's employment; (2) submission to or rejection of such conduct by an individual is used as a basis for employment decisions affecting such individuals; or (3) such conduct has the purpose or effect of unreasonably interfering with an individual's work performance or creating an intimidating, hostile, or offensive working environment.

Laboratories, as employers, may be held liable in certain cases when an employee engages in sexual harassment. When the person violating the prohibitions is a manager or supervisor, the employer is usually liable. When the violating employee is not a manager or supervisor, the employer is liable if the employer knew or should have known about the employee's actions and did nothing to stop the behavior.

Education and training are the most important steps an employer can take to prevent sexual harassment. When a claim of harassment is made, it should be investigated thoroughly and all actions well documented.

Summary

Laboratories are affected by a multitude of laws and regulations. These laws cover all facets of laboratory operation, from day-to-day business functions, to upkeep of the laboratory premises, to the conduct of the laboratory and its employees. When working in a laboratory, you must understand the basic concepts of laboratory testing and the legal ramifications of your work. Too often, tasks can become so routine or mundane that "shortcuts" become a habit. This compromises the accuracy and safety of techniques and protocols, and may lead to negligent or intentional acts of misconduct. Once such an act is committed and an injury occurs, the "I'm so sorry" comments invoked cannot reverse the outcome. Wishing you had the chance to "do it over differently" is a wonderful wish, but it cannot be granted. The answer is never to get yourself into a situation in which you are on the receiving end of a summons and complaint.

Chapter Review

True or False

Circle T or F to indicate the correct answers to the following:

T F 1. All health care professionals have a basic understanding of how the law relates to their work.

T F 2. Laboratories are not legally responsible for the intentional conduct of their employees.

T F 3. A legal remedy or cause of action for negligence requires more than negligent conduct.

T F 4. The laboratory owner is not responsible for foreseeable criminal acts unless he/she witnesses the act in question.

Fill in the Blanks

Complete the following statements:

5. The ____________ is a compilation of rules of action or conduct established by an authority.
6. Laboratories are subject to ____________, ____________, and ____________ regulations.
7. A laboratory would NOT be ____________ liable for an employee's sexual assault on a patient.
8. Employment issues of concern in laboratories include ____________, ____________, and ____________ ____________.

Multiple Choice

Circle the letter that represents the single best answer:

9. Laboratories must provide for their employees both:
   a. Safety and protection
   b. Education and training
   c. Health and welfare
   d. Retirement and health insurance
10. In 1970, Congress passed the:
    a. American Civil Liberties Act
    b. Centers for Disease Control Act
    c. Occupational Safety and Health Act
    d. Bloodborne Pathogen Standards Act
11. Stress-related illness is ____________ in health care workers.
    a. Insignificant
    b. Seldom diagnosed
    c. Decreasing
    d. Increasing
12. Laboratories and other health care facilities are covered under the federal and state laws regarding:
    a. Workers' compensation
    b. Vacations and sick leave
    c. Disability benefits
    d. Work involving injury

Glossary

abjure: to reject or renounce formally

absorption: the method or movement by which a substance reaches and enters the blood

accuracy: an indication of how close the obtained answer or test result is to the true value

acidosis: an abnormal increase in the body's hydrogen ion concentration yielding a pH value of less than 7.4

ADP: adenosine diphosphate; a product of the hydrolysis of adenosine triphosphate (ATP)

aerobic: requiring oxygen for the maintenance of life

aerosols: nebulized particles suspended in a gas or air

agglutination: the clumping together of cells as a result of interaction with specific antibodies called agglutinins; the antigen-antibody reaction

aggregation: the clustering or clumping of blood cells

AIDS: acquired immunodeficiency syndrome

albumin: a water-soluble, heat-coagulable protein

algae: primitive plants capable of producing their own food

aliquot: a sample that is representative of the whole

anaerobe: an organism that lives, grows, and functions in the absence of molecular oxygen

anaerobic: able to grow and function without air or oxygen

analytes: any component in blood or other body fluid that can be measured

anatomic pathology: the science dealing with the nature and changes in human body cells and tissue that are caused by disease

ankylosing: characterized by immobility or stiffening of a joint

antecubital space: the area in front of and at the bend of the elbow

antibodies: protein substances manufactured by lymphocytes when there is an antigen invasion

anticoagulant: an agent that prevents or delays the clotting mechanism of the blood

antidiuretic hormone (ADH): a hormone secreted by the posterior lobe of the pituitary gland that suppresses the secretion of urine

antigen: a foreign or natural material in the body that causes antibodies to be produced

arthropod: a phylum of the animal kingdom that includes the arachnids, crustaceans, and insects

asepsis: the absence of viable pathogenic organisms

aseptic: free of infection and/or infectious materials

asphyxia: a condition in which there is a deficiency of oxygen in the blood and an increase in carbon dioxide in the blood and tissues

assay: an analysis of the purity or effectiveness of any biological substance, including drugs

asymmetric: characterized by a lack of similarity of size, shape, or position

asymptomatic: without signs or symptoms

atherosclerosis: a common condition in which deposits

of yellowing plaques containing cholesterol and lipid material form on the inside walls of the arteries

authorized person: an individual authorized under state law to order tests or receive test results, or both

autoclave: an instrument that uses steam, dry heat, or chemicals at high pressure to kill possible contagious or infectious agents

autoimmune: pertaining to an immune response to one's own tissues

autologous: related to or belonging to self

automated testing: laboratory testing in which a series of steps performed by a preprogrammed analyzer

autopsy: an examination of the body after death to determine the manner and cause of death

autotrophs: organisms that are capable of producing needed nutrients as long as water, carbon dioxide, inorganic salts, and a source of energy are available

B cells: lymphocytes that change into plasma cells and secrete antibodies

bacitracin: an antibacterial substance, obtained from a strain of Bacillus, which is useful in the treatment of a wide range of infections

bacteremia: the presence of bacteria in the blood

bacteria: unicellular microorganisms that do not have membrane-enclosed nuclei

bacteriostatic: pertaining to a substance that inhibits or retards bacterial growth

bacteriuria: the presence of bacteria in the urine

benign: noncancerous; not life-threatening

bifurcation: the point of forking or separating into two branches

bilayered: split, or with two distinct layers present

bilirubin: the orange-yellow pigment of bile formed by the breakdown of heme in hemoglobin

bioluminescence: a reaction, found in nature, between an enzyme and oxygen, producing cold light

biopsy: excision of a small sample of tissue from the body for diagnostic or therapeutic purposes

blebs: anatomical elevated structures of the skin that usually measure more than 5 mm in diameter

bone marrow: specialized soft tissue located in the cancellous bone of the epiphyses

Bowman's capsule: a cup-shaped membrane surrounding the glomerulus

brucellosis: a disease (also known as undulant fever) caused by coccal bacteria (brucella)

calibration: the testing and adjusting of test systems to provide a known relationship between the measurement response and the substance value measured by the test

calibration verification: the assaying of calibration materials to confirm that the calibration has remained stable throughout the laboratory's reportable range for patient test results

catalyze: to cause an increase in the rate of a chemical reaction

catheterization: the insertion of a small tube into the bladder through the urethra for the purpose of removing urine

cause of action: the fact or facts that give a person a right to judicial relief

caustic: any substance that is destructive to living tissue

cecum: first portion of the large intestine

cellulitis: a diffuse inflammatory process within solid tissues

centrifuge: a laboratory machine used to separate particles of different densities within a liquid by spinning them at very high speeds

chemoluminescence: light generated as a result of a chemical reaction

Chlamydia: a genus of microorganisms that live as intracellular parasites and are pathogenic in humans

cholinesterase: an enzyme that is present throughout the body and is released when a nerve impulse reaches the myoneural junction

chronic: recurring; developing slowly and persisting over a long period of time

CK (CPK): abbreviation for creatine kinase (creatine phosphokinase)

coagulase: an enzyme that causes coagulation of citrated plasma

coagulation: the process of transforming a liquid into a solid

cold light: light produced in the absence of heat

commensal: living on or within an organism without causing harm to the host

complement: blood protein that aids antibodies in destroying antigens

control: a serum solution with a known range for the serum being tested

convalescent: pertaining to the period of recovery after an illness

cortex: the outer layer of an organ

cosmopolitan: not limited to any one country; widespread

crenation: the formation of notches or leaf-like edges in red blood cells, as well as a shriveled surface

critical measurement: a measurement in which accuracy is vitally important

cyanotic: pertaining to a bluish discoloration of the skin and mucous membranes

cysts: closed, epithelium-lined sacs or capsules containing a liquid or semisolid substance

cytology: the study of cells and their formation

cytopenia: cellular deficiency in the blood

cytoplasmic: pertaining to all of the substances of a cell other than the nucleus

cytotoxin: a substance produced by the killer cells that destroys invading foreign cells

decongestant: an agent that reduces swelling

dehydration: a condition that results from undue loss of water from the body or body tissues

dermatophytid: a secondary skin eruption occurring on an area remote from the site of infection

diabetes mellitus: a disturbance in the oxidation and utilization of glucose caused by malfunction of pancreatic beta cells, which are responsible for the secretion of insulin

diastema: a congenital defect characterized by dwarfing, or changes in bone spacing and clefting

differential white cell count: a count based on observation of the different kinds of white cells and reported as percentages of the total number examined. (Usually, 100 cells are examined to determine the percentage of each type.)

diurnal variation: normal variation in blood cells in the body throughout a 24-hour period

drug sensitivity: the body's susceptibility to a drug or an antigen

dyscrasia: a morbid condition, usually referring to an imbalance of the components of blood or bone marrow

edema: an interstitial collection of fluid

edematous: pertaining to an abnormal collection of interstitial fluid that causes swelling

EDTA: ethylenediaminetetra-acetic acid; an anticoagulant used in hematologic studies

electrolyte: an element or compound which, when dissolved, turns into ions that are able to conduct an electricity

embolus: a foreign object obstructing the flow of blood

emulsify: to combine two liquids that are not mutually soluble

endemic: present in a community at all times

endocarditis: inflammation of the lining of the heart and heart valves

endometrium: the mucous membrane lining the uterus

enterocolitis: inflammation of the small intestine and colon

enumeration: a listing or counting

enzyme: a protein produced by living cells, which acts as a catalyst, increasing the rate at which a chemical reaction occurs

epidemic: rapid, widespread occurrence of a disease among many people in a given region at the same time

estradiol: the most potent naturally occurring estrogen hormone in humans

etiology: an assigned cause of disease

eukaryotic: pertaining to organisms with a true nucleus, such as fungi, protozoa, and most algae

exotoxins: poisonous substances secreted externally

exudate: a fluid with a high concentration of protein and cellular debris that has escaped the blood vessels, usually as a result of inflammation

fascia: a sheet of fibrous connective tissue deep in the body that supports and separates muscles

fast: abstinence from food

feces: the end product of digestion discharged from the large intestine; bowel movement

fibrinolysis: the continuous process of fibrin decomposition by fibrinolysin; the normal mechanism for the removal of small fibrin clots

fibrometer: an instrument used to perform coagulation tests, such as prothrombin time, that involve detection of the formation of a fibrin clot in plasma

flagellate: any microorganism having a long, whip-like, mobile appendage

flocculus: small tuft or mass of fibrous material containing downy or flaky sheds

forensic: pertaining to the legal aspects of a given test or health care procedure

foreseeable: able to be seen or known in advance; that which can be reasonably anticipated (e.g., the expectation that harm or injury is likely to result from certain acts or omissions)

fungi: microorganisms that live on decaying organic material

gastric: pertaining to the stomach

gastroenteritis: inflammation of the stomach and small intestinal lining

genetic: inherited; relating to birth or origin

germicidal agent: a drug that kills pathogenic microorganisms

gestation: the period of time between conception and birth *glans:* the cone-shaped enlargement at the end of the penis which, in the uncircumcised male, is covered by the foreskin

glaucoma: disease of the eye resulting in pathologic changes in the optic nerve

glomerulonephritis: inflammation of the glomerulus located in the nephron of the kidney

glomerulus: a mass of capillaries surrounded by Bowman's capsule

glycosuria: the presence of glucose (sugar) in the urine

gonorrhea: a sexually transmitted infection characterized by inflammation of the mucous membranes of the reproductive and urinary tracts

gout: a hereditary form of arthritis characterized by excessive quantities of uric acid in the blood

guaiac: a substance derived from the resin or sap from the *Guaiacum* tree and made into a chemical used in the testing of feces for occult blood

HBV: hepatitis B virus

HIV: human immunodeficiency virus; a virus that causes AIDS and that is transmitted through sexual contact and exposure to infected blood or blood components

hematology: the study of the characteristics, formation, and effects of blood

hematuria: the presence of red blood cells in urine

heme: the nonprotein, insoluble, iron protoporphyrin constituent of hemoglobin

hemin: nutrients present in lysed red blood cells

hemoglobinuria: the presence of hemoglobin in urine

hemolytic: pertaining to the breakdown of red blood cells and the release of hemoglobin-into the plasma

hemophilia: a hereditary disorder resulting from deficiency or absence of factor VIII or factor IX in the blood

hemostasis: the termination of bleeding by mechanical or chemical means

heparin: a naturally occurring antithrombin factor that prevents intravascular clotting

heterophil: an antibody that reacts with antigens other than the one it is expected to react with

hilum: a notch in the medial border of the kidney

histology: the science dealing with the microscopic identification of cells and tissue

homeostasis: the maintenance of relatively constant conditions in the body's internal environment

homicide: any killing of a person by another person

hormone: a chemical substance secreted by an endocrine gland and carried through the blood to its designated target

host: an animal or plant that houses and provides food for another organism (parasite)

hydrational: relating to the absorption of water or combination with water

hyperlipidemia: an abnormally high level of fat in the blood

hypersplenism: exaggeration of the hemolytic function of the spleen, resulting in deficiency of peripheral blood elements

hypersthenuria: the production of urine having a high specific gravity

hyphae: filaments or threads composing the mycelium of a fungus

hyposthenuria: the production of urine with low specific gravity

icterus: jaundice caused by a high level of bilirubin

idiosyncrasy: an abnormal susceptibility to a drug or other agent that is peculiar to the individual

ileum: the distal portion of the small intestine

immunoglobulins: major components of the humoral immune response

immunology: the study of the reaction of tissues of the immune system of the body to antigenic stimulation

index: the numerical ratio produced when measuring any part in comparison with a fixed standard

indices: plural of index

infectious mononucleosis: an acute infection caused by the Epstein-Barr virus

infectious organisms: pathogenic microorganisms that invade the body, causing disease by local cellular injury

inoculum: serum or other substances introduced onto culture media

intentional act: an action or state of mind that denotes the desire to cause the consequences of an act, or the belief that the consequences are substantially certain to occur

interferon: an antiviral protein secreted by T cells, that can stimulate macrophages to engulf bacteria

interleukins: proteins that activate immune responses and stimulate the growth of T-cell lymphocytes

invasive procedure: a diagnostic or therapeutic technique that requires entering a body cavity

inversion: reversal of the normal position of a specimen

in vitro: pertaining to a biological reaction that occurs in an artificial environment, usually within a test tube

in vivo: pertaining to a biological reaction that occurs within the living body

isoenzymes: forms of enzymes that catalyze the same reaction but do so at different reaction rates

isoimmunization: development of antibodies in response to an antigen derived from a genetically dissimilar individual of the same species

isosthenuria: the production of urine with consistently low specific gravity, regardless of fluid intake

jaundice: yellowish color of the skin and mucous membranes secondary to hyperbilirubinemia

ketoacidosis: the accumulation of fatty acids, called ketone bodies, in the blood

ketonuria: the presence of ketone (acetone) in the urine

labia majora: the two folds of adipose tissue that extend from the mons pubis to the perineum in females

labia minora: the two thin folds of epithelial tissue that are situated between the labia majora and the opening of the vagina

laboratory: a facility for the biological, microbiological, serologic, chemical, immunohematologic, hematologic, biophysical, cytologic, pathological, or other examination of materials derived from the human body for the purpose of providing information for the diagnosis, prevention, treatment of any disease or condition affecting the health of human beings

larvae: the immature stage of the life cycle of a parasite

LDH: abbreviation for low-density lipoprotein

leaching: separating soluble from insoluble matter by slowly running water through the material

legionella: a small, rod-shaped bacterium that is the causative agent in legionnaires' disease

leukopenia: abnormal deficiency in the white blood cell count

liberation: the release of a prescribed drug from its dosage

lipids: the free fatty acids in the blood

lipiduria: the presence of fat in the urine

lividity: discoloration (black and blue) as a result of pooling of blood

Luer-Lok: the syringe mechanism that securely holds a needle in place

luminol: an organic compound with luminescent qualities

lymphocytes: white blood cells that control the immune system response and produce antibodies to destroy antigens

lymphokines: chemicals produced by T-cell lymphocytes

lyophilization: the creation of a stable preparation of a biologic substance by rapid freezing and dehydration of the frozen product under high vacuum

lysis: destruction of a cell caused by a lysin

macrophages: large phagocytes that destroy worn-out red blood cells

malabsorption: impaired intestinal absorption of nutrients

malaise: a vague feeling of uneasiness or body discomfort

manual testing: a method for obtaining laboratory test results that involves performing a series of steps by hand or by personal physical means

mastoiditis: inflammation of the air cells of the portion of the temporal bone lying behind the external opening of the ear

mean: the average of all values in a set of numbers that are distributed equally on both sides of a symmetrical curve

medium: a nutritive substance upon which bacteria are placed for growth

medulla: the inmost portion of an organ

meiosis: the process whereby two cells fuse into one cell, which may result in the formation of a zygote

meningitis: an inflammation of the meninges causing edema of the brain's covering, which, in turn, causes pressure on brain tissue

meniscus: convex surface of a liquid in a tube or pipette

metabolism: the sum of all body processes involved in the disposition of substances absorbed into the blood

metabolite: a substance produced by the metabolism of a drug in the body

microbe: a microscopic organism

microtome: an instrument used to cut thin sections of tissue for microscopic study

micturition: urination

mitosis: the process of cell division that results in the formation of two daughter cells and the replacement of dead cells

MN blood group: a blood grouping system discovered by Landsteiner and Levine that is based on M and N antigens, which are products of paired genes; it is helpful in paternity testing, but rarely clinically significant

morbidity: the ratio of sick to well persons in a given community or area

mordant: a substance that fixes or intensifies a stain or dye

morphology: the study of the form, structure, and size of organisms, organs, tissues, or cells

mortality: the ratio of the total number of deaths occurring to the total or given population

myasthenia gravis: an autoimmune disease manifested by fatigue and exhaustion of the muscles

mycobacterium: a slender, acid-fast microorganism resembling the bacillus; refers to many species, including the one that causes tuberculosis

myocardial infarction: death of all or part of the heart muscle

natural: occurring in the ordinary course of events

necrosis: morphologic changes indicative of cell death caused by enzymatic degradation

nephron: the basic unit of the kidney

nephrotic: pertaining to the nephron, which is the fundamental unit of the kidney

neurotransmitter: a substance that is released from a nerve when it is excited by an impulse

nomenclature: a classified system of technical names, such as for organisms or structures

noncritical measurement: a measurement in which estimated accuracy is acceptable

nonfastidious: easy to please; hard to disguise

normal flora: microorganisms that live on or within a body and compete with disease-producing microorganisms, thereby providing a natural immunity against certain infections

nosocomial: pertaining to the spread of infection among patients, staff, and visitors inside a hospital

occult: hidden or difficult to observe directly

ocular micrometer: a small ruler on a glass disk used in measuring microorganisms under the microscope

oocyst: the encapsulated stage in the development of any sporozoan

opaque: neither translucent nor transparent; impervious to light

opportunistic: pertaining to a normally harmless species of bacteria that becomes pathogenic under specific circumstances

otitis media: inflammation of the middle ear

paronychia: inflammation involving the folds of tissue surrounding the nail

pathogenic: pertaining to an agent that causes or is capable of causing disease

pathogens: any disease-producing agent or microorganism

pathology: the scientific study of the characteristics, causes, and effects of disease

peptidoglycan: a polysaccharide attached to short, cross-linked peptides found in bacterial cell walls

peripheral: pertaining to an outside surface or the area surrounding a body part

Petri dish: a round, shallow, flat-bottomed transparent glass or plastic dish with vertical sides and a cover that is similar and slightly larger

phagocytes: a white blood cell that is able to surround, engulf, and digest microorganisms and debris

phagocytosis: the process by which certain cells surround, engulf, and ingest microorganisms and cellular debris

pharyngitis: inflammation of the throat (pharynx)

phlegm: a viscid mucus excreted from the respiratory tract

phospholipid: an oily, waxy compound that contains phosphorus and that is found in cell membranes

plaque: a yellowish area within an artery that causes the internal surface to bulge into the lumen

plasma cell: a cell originating from B-cell lymphocytes that secretes antibodies

polycythemia vera: a condition of unknown origin that is characterized by a marked increase in total blood volume, RBCs, WBCs, platelets, and hemoglobin

polymorphonuclear: having a multilobed nucleus (e.g., the neutrophil)

polymorphs: leukocytes appearing in different forms in different developmental stages

polyuria: the excretion of urinary volume exceeding 2000 mL in 24 hours

precision: the extent to which a measurement yields the same results when repeated under identical conditions

prenatal: pertaining to the gestational time preceding birth

prokaryotic: pertaining to organisms without a true (membrane-bound) nucleus, such as bacteria and viruses

proteinaceous: pertaining to any protein, that is a large organic compound made up of one or more chains of amino acids

proteinuria: the presence of an excess of serum proteins in the urine, are usually albumin

protozoa: single-celled microorganisms; the lowest class of life

protozoan: a subkingdom of unicellular organisms that

are frequently ingested and transmitted through contaminated feces

psychosis: a state in which a person's mental capacity to recognize reality is impaired

pyuria: pus in the urine

qualitative: pertaining to a precise measurement that determines the amount of a substance that is present or absent

qualitative test: a test that determines the presence or absence of a substance

quality assurance: a set of policies and procedures that are followed to ensure that every test performed is valid

quality control: the process by which final results are validated and variations are quantified

quantitate: to measure or determine the quality of mass

quantitative: pertaining to a precise physical measurement that determines the amount of energy or mass that is present or absent

quantitative test: a test that determines the amount of a substance per unit volume or unit weight

radiant: capable of emitting rays, such as light or heat

reference value: the range of test values expected for a designated population of individuals (e.g., 95% of individuals presumed to be healthy)

reliability: an indication of the reproducibility of a measurement

renal corpuscles: bodies forming the beginnings of nephrons and consisting of a glomerulus and Bowman's capsule

renal pelvis: a funnel-shaped basin located at the distal end of the tubules that drain urine from the kidney into the ureter

reportable range: the range of test values over which the relationship between the instrument, kit, or system's measurement response is shown to be valid

reservoir host: a host that harbors infectious organisms, without sustaining injury or illness to self, and that may serve as a carrier of disease to others

respondent superior: a doctrine meaning "Let the master answer." This doctrine applies only when the relationship between the "master" and the "servant" existed at the time of the wrongdoing and arose out of the master/servant (employer/employee) relationship.

reticulocyte: a nonnucleated immature red blood cell

retroperitoneal: lying behind the peritoneum

rouleaux: a roll of red blood cells resembling a pile of coins

salmonellosis: a disease caused by rod-shaped bacteria (salmonellae)

sclerosis: abnormal hardening of tissue

sebaceous: an oil-secreting gland in the skin

sediment: a deposit of relatively insoluble material that settles to the bottom of a container of liquid; the solid (bottom) portion of a centrifuged urine specimen

sensitivity: the ability of a test to identify the condition or disease being tested for; susceptibility to a drug or an antigen

septicemia: disease associated with toxins in the blood; blood poisoning

serology: laboratory medicine that studies blood serum for evidence of infection by evaluating antigen-antibody reactions in vitro

serum: the liquid portion of blood that remains after the clotting proteins and cells have been removed

solute: the substance dissolved in a solution

solvent: a substance capable of dissolving another material

specific gravity: a measure that reflects the ratio of waste products to fluid in the urine

specificity: the ability of a test to distinguish between the specific antibody or antigen being tested for from others not being tested for

splenectomy: surgical removal of the spleen

spondylitis: inflammation of the vertebrae

spores: refractile, oval bodies formed within bacteria; regarded as a resting stage during the life cycle of the cell

standard: a solution with an exact known value for the constituent being tested

STAT: immediately

sterile: free of all forms of microbial life

strictly liable: having strict liability for having sold a product in a defective condition that is unreasonably dangerous to the user or consumer and that ultimately causes harm to the user/consumer

subarachnoid: between the surface layer and the pia mater layer of the skull

sudoriferous: glands in the skin that produce sweat

suicide: the act of killing oneself deliberately

supernatant: the liquid portion of a centrifuged urine specimen lying above the insoluble cell layer

suppressant: an agent that stops secretion, excretion, or normal discharge

suppuration: the production of pus and purulent matter

systemic lupus erythematosus: an autoimmune connective tissue disease, affecting more women than men, that produces a high level of autoantibodies, indicating a defect in regulatory mechanisms

syndrome: a group of signs and symptoms resulting from a common cause or appearing in combinations

synovial fluid: the transparent viscid fluid found in joint cavities, bursae, and tendon sheaths

TC: a pipette marking indicating *to contain*

T cells: lymphocytes that act directly on antigens to destroy them

TD: a pipette marking indicating *to deliver*

thalassemia: an anemia in which the different types of hemoglobin are present that are normally found only in the fetus

thrombocytopenia: a condition in which there is an abnormal decrease in the number of platelets circulating in the blood

thrombocytosis: a condition in which there is an abnormal increase in the number of platelets circulating in the blood

titer: the quantity of a substance required to react with or to a given amount of another substance

tonsillitis: inflammation of the palatine tonsil in the throat

tort: a civil wrong or injury, other than a breach of contract, for which the court will provide a remedy in the form of an action for damages

toxicity: the level at which a drug becomes poisonous in the body

toxicology: the scientific study of poisons, their detection, their effects, and methods of treatment for the conditions they produce

toxins: poisons, usually proteins, that cause antitoxins to form in the body, thus establishing immunity to a disease

trespasser: a person who intentionally and without consent or privilege enters another's property

trophozoite: the active, motile feeding stage of a sporozoan parasite

tubule: a small canal forming the last part of the nephron unit that the glomerular filtration passes through before entering the renal pelvis

turbid: clouded, or obscured, as in solids in suspension in a solution

typing of blood: laboratory testing to determine ABO grouping

UL: Underwriters' Laboratory

unnatural: not in accordance with the expected or ordinary course of events

urea: the end product of protein metabolism after ammonia is broken down by the liver; a systemic osmotic diuretic found in urine

urethra: the canal connecting the urinary bladder to the exterior of the body through which urine and sperm (in males) are discharged

urethral: pertaining to the small tube connecting the bladder to the outside of the body through which urine and sperm (in males) are discharged

urethritis: inflammation of the canal that extends from the bladder to the outside of the body

urinary meatus: external opening of the urethra

urination: the discharge or passage of liquid out of the body from the urinary meatus

urobilinogen: the presence of bilirubin in the urine

urochrome: the color spectrum of urine

vasculitis: inflammation of a vessel

VDRL: a serologic flocculation test for syphilis

vector: an arthropod carrier that transfers an infective agent from one host to another

vibrio: an organism of the genus *Vibrio,* or other motile spirillum organism

vicariously liable: having indirect legal responsibility, as, for example, an employer deemed responsible for the act of an employee, or a principal for the act of an agent

virion: the complete viral particle that infects a living cell

virus: an infective agent smaller than bacteria

void: urinate

voiding: the process of urinating

volatile: capable of boiling at a low temperature or evaporating quickly at room temperature

zygote: the cell that results from the union of the male sperm and the female ova

Appendix A
Test Values

Specimen Rejection Policy and Procedure

When using this policy/procedure, remember that this is only a sample. Every laboratory must develop a policy, but these policies frequently differ slightly. Be sure to check the Policy/Procedure document from the laboratory that will be processing your institution's specimens.

Establishing Standards for Acceptance or Rejection of Specimens

Every laboratory establishes standards for the suitability of specimens received for testing, recognizing the necessity to address situations in which specimens cannot easily be recollected in the proper manner. The purpose of establishing standard criteria is to ensure that only appropriately collected and labeled specimens are used for laboratory testing purposes, and that criteria are established for handling and processing different types of outpatient specimens.

Criteria

Specimen Labeling/Patient Identification

Specimen Labeling/Identification Requirements

1. Patient identification information should be written on the label of the container (i.e., name and medical records number [usually a Social Security number], date of birth).
2. The date and time the specimen was obtained should be noted on the requisition form and the specimen container.
3. The sampling site from which the specimen was obtained should be written on the requisition form and on the container if more than one sample of specimen is submitted for the same patient.
4. The test(s) requested should be specified on the requisition form.

Improperly labeled specimens are held for testing until the necessary information can be obtained from the physician's office or the draw station staff.

Circumstances Resulting in Specimen Rejection or Delay in Testing

1. No patient's name written on the specimen container or carrier for the specimen container
2. Name on the specimen container does not match that on the associated collection label or test requisition form
3. Absence of a date and/or time of specimen collection, or conflicting dates/times noted on two or more samples from the same patient
4. Missing, conflicting, or inappropriate test results
5. No specimen source noted on container or on requisition form
6. Specimen container inappropriate for specimen

Whenever possible, problems associated with improper or inadequate labeling should be resolved by obtaining another specimen. When this is not possible, it is the responsibility of the assistant or the receptionist at the physician's office or draw station to confirm the identity of the patient, the specimen type and/or site of sampling, and/or the test requested before it will be accepted for testing.

When such problems are discovered after normal working hours, the laboratory pathologist on duty will determine which tests are to be performed in the absence of adequate information on the requisition form or the specimen container.

Specimens for which a collection date and/or time is necessary but not specified will be processed. However, a disclaimer will be added to the reported test results indicating the questionable nature of the results obtained.

Rejected Specimens That Must Be Processed

When specimens must be tested that would normally be rejected, a disclaimer should be included in the test report to advise the physician that the results may or may not be accurate owing to the compromised nature of the test sample.

Examples of Disclaimer Statements

1. No date and/or time of specimen collection was specified. Test results may be clinically invalid.
2. The specimen was received in an inappropriate collection device. Test results may be clinically invalid.
3. The specimen received for analysis was not received within an acceptable time period. Test results may be clinically invalid.
4. Storage/transport of the specimen was inappropriate. Test results may not be clinically valid.

Criteria for Specimen Rejection

Specimens for all departments in the laboratory should be submitted in sterile containers that have been appropriately labeled with patient/specimen identification information. Transport containers should be sealed properly to prevent leakage of contents and to avoid contaminating the specimen or endangering the personnel handling the specimen.

Certain specimens may be considered unsuitable for testing by specific departments within the laboratory. Various criteria for specimen rejection are presented in the charts that follow, organized by the type of test or the specific laboratory department affected.

GUIDELINES

Handling Rejected Specimens or "Quantity Not Sufficient" (QNS) Specimens

NEVER discard rejected specimens or those that are of insufficient quantity (QNS) for any department in the laboratory. Rather, hold all specimens that are rejected or deemed to be QNS in designated areas within the respective department until a physician or supervisor states that they can be discarded along with the other routinely processed specimens.

Rejection Criteria for Urinalysis Specimens

1. Unrefrigerated, random urine specimens collected more than 2 hours before testing
2. Refrigerated urine specimens collected more than 24 hours before testing

Rejection Criteria for Hematologic Specimens

1. Grossly hemolyzed specimens
2. Anticoagulated test tubes containing clots
3. Specimens containing an incorrect anticoagulant
4. Improperly filled or mixed anticoagulant tubes
5. Westergren sedimentation rate samples collected in Vacu-Tek tubes more than 2 hours prior to testing if stored at room temperature, or more than 12 hours prior to testing if stored at 2° to 8°C
6. Westergren sedimentation rate samples collected in Vacu-Tek tubes that were filled to less than 12 mm below the fill line or more than 5 mm above the fill line
7. An arterial line specimen from which questionable results were obtained, possibly as a result of inadequate clearing of the arterial line prior to specimen collection
8. A specimen yielding questionable test results that was obtained from an arm with an IV line in place, suggesting possible contamination with IV or other fluid
9. An ethylenediaminetetra-acetic acid (EDTA)–anticoagulated specimen collected more than 24 hours prior to performing a complete blood count (CBC), hemogram, or differential testing
10. An EDTA-anticoagulated specimen, collected for reticulocyte testing, that was obtained more than 24 hours prior to testing if stored at 2° to 6°C, or more than 8 hours prior to testing if stored at room temperature

Rejection Criteria for Coagulation Test Specimens

1. A specimen with a hematocrit of less than 20% or greater than 55% that was *not* collected in specially prepared tubes. The amount of citrate must be adjusted depending on the hematocrit. These tubes are prepared by Hematology laboratory personnel.
2. Specimens for Protime, fibrinogen, and thrombin time testing that were obtained from citrate tubes filled to less than 75% of capacity
3. Specimens for partial thromboplastin time (PTT), including circulating anicoagulant and factor VIII samples, that were obtained from citrate tubes filled to less than 90% of capacity
4. Specimens containing an incorrect anticoagulant
5. Moderately to grossly hemolyzed specimens (unless collection of another specimen is not feasible)
6. Specimens containing clots
7. Specimens for Protime analysis that were collected more than 4 hours prior to testing if unspun and stored at room temperature, or if separated and stored at 2° to 8°C; frozen samples (–20°C) that are not tested within 2 weeks of specimen collection

Rejection Criteria for Blood Chemistry Specimens

1. Grossly hemolyzed samples obtained for potassium, serum glutamic-oxgloacetic transminase (SGOT), low-density lipoprotein (LDL), lipase, alkaline phosphate, or bilirubin testing
2. Blood ammonia testing
   a. A sample that was not kept on ice, or that was received more than 1 hour after it was drawn (even if kept on ice)
   b. A blood specimen that has not been anticoagulated (with EDTA or heparin)
3. Arterial blood gas determination
   a. A clotted sample
   b. A sample not kept on ice (although a sample delivered for testing within 10 minutes is acceptable without ice)
   c. Use of an anticoagulant other than sodium or lithium heparin
   d. An improperly sealed sample (i.e., a capped needle or a needle in a stopper)
4. A lactic acid tube (sodium fluoride-potassium oxalate) that was not kept on ice and/or was not delivered to the laboratory immediately
   (NOTE: The specimen must be separated within 15 minutes of collection.)
5. Prolonged exposure of a bilirubin test sample to light, as the sample is stable for only 4 to 8 hours
6. A urine sample that does not contain the proper preservative for the test requested
7. Specimens drawn from an improperly cleared heparin lock or arterial line. (NOTE: This can often be determined only after the test is performed.)

Rejection Criteria for Serologic Specimens

1. Grossly hemolyzed or lipemic specimens

Rejection Criteria for Immunohematologic Blood Bank Specimens

1. Grossly hemolyzed specimens
2. Obviously contaminated specimens
3. A sample that was drawn into a tube other than a clot tube (red top, NO gel)
4. Serum and cell specimens that are transported to the Blood Bank in separate tubes if crossmatch and/or ABO/Rh determinations are requested. (Iso-filters in clot tubes are acceptable.)
5. Incorrect or missing information, such as a misspelled patient name, no date or time of draw specified, and/or no initials of the person drawing the specimen noted

Rejection Criteria for Microbiologic Specimens

1. Specimens not collected in sterile containers, except in the case of stool specimens, which may be submitted in clean cardboard or plastic wide-mouthed containers, and specimens sent for stain/smear analysis, which may only be placed in clean, nonsterile containers
2. Specimens in containers whose exteriors have been contaminated by leakage of the sample
3. Specimens that are not labeled with the date and time of collection or the site of origin
4. Urine samples received more than 2 hours after collection when held at room temperature, more than 24 hours after collection if refrigerated, or more than 48 hours after collection when stored in a gray-top Vacutainer urine transport container
5. Sputum samples, tracheal aspirations, and stool specimens received more than 2 hours after collection when held at room temperature; stools submitted for culture that have been refrigerated; or stools that were collected more than 2 hours prior to testing and that were not placed in an authorized culture and sensitivity transport container
6. Swab specimens received more than 24 hours after collection; swabs for gonococcal culture or vaginal/cervical culture that are received more than 1 hour after collection or that are refrigerated
7. A disclaimer regarding the accuracy of test results (based on questionable specimen quality) is warranted if the transport capsule for a swab specimen is not crushed to help maintain viability of the organism(s) in the specimens being tested
8. Sputum specimens heavily contaminated with saliva, as determined by stain results
9. A duplicate specimen collected within less than 24 hours after the initial sampling

Summary of Urine Preservatives

Assay	*Collection Time (hr)*	*Refrigeration/ No Preservative*	*Boric Acid*	*6NHCl*	*Freezing*	*Other*
Aldosterone	24	—	A	—	P	pH=4
Amino acids	24	A	—	30 mL	P	pH=3–5
Aminolevulinic acid (ALA)	24	—	—	A	P	Protect from light
Amylase	2	P	—	—	—	—
Arsenic	24	—	—	20 mL	—	—
β_2=Microglobulin	Random/ high diuresis	—	—	—	P	pH=6–8
Cadmium	24	P	—	—	—	—
Calcium	24	—	—	30 mL	—	pH<3
Catecholamines	24	—	—	25 mL	P	pH=2–4
Chloride	24	P	—	—	—	—
Human chorionic gonadotropin (hCG) (qualitative)	Random	P	A	—	—	First AM specimen
Chromium	Random	P	—	—	—	Acid-washed container
Citric acid	24	A	10 gm	—	P	—
Creatinine	24	P	A	A	A	—
Glucose	24	—	1 gm	—	—	—
17-Ketosteroids	24	A	1 gm	—	—	—
Lipase	24	P	—	—	—	—
Magnesium	24	—	—	25 mL	—	pH<2
Microalbumin	24	P	—	—	—	—
Nitrogen	24	—	—	P	—	pH<4
Osmolality	Random	A	—	—	P	—
Oxalate	24	—	—	40 mL	—	pH=2–3
Porphyrins	24	—	—	—	—	Protect from light
Potassium	24	P	A	A	—	—
Protein	24	P	—	—	—	—
Sodium	24	P	A	A	—	—
Substance abuse panels	Random	P	—	—	A	—
Urea nitrogen	24	A	10 gm	A	—	—
Uric acid	24	A	—	—	—	Sodium carbonate (5 gm)
Urobilinogen	2	—	—	—	P	Protect from light

P, preferred method of storage and/or collection; *A*, acceptable method of storage and/or collection; —, unacceptable or unproven method.

Blood Collection Tube Information

Color	*Optimum Vol. (mL)*	*Minimum Vol. (mL)*	*Additive*
ADULT TUBES			
Blue	4.5	4.5	Sodium citrate; no additive (for trace metals)
Blue Navy	7	NA	Heparin (for trace metals)
FSP (fibrinogen split products; blue top)	2	2	Thrombin trypsin inhibitor
Gray	10	10	Potassium oxalate
			Sodium fluoride
Green	10	3.5	Heparin
Lavender	7	2	EDTA
Orange	10	NA	Thrombin
Red	10	NA	None
Red (for tissue typing)	10	NA	Heparin added
Red/gray (gel)	10	NA	Inert barrier clot activator
Yellow	5	NA	ACD solution
Yellow/black	7	NA	Thrombin
PEDIATRIC TUBES			
Blue	2.7	2.7	Sodium citrate
Yellow (culture)	3.3	3.3	SPS
Green	2	2	Heparin
	2	0.6	
Lavender	3	0.9	EDTA
	4	1	
	2	NA	
Red	3	NA	None
	4	NA	

NA, not applicable; *EDTA,* ethylenediaminetetra-acetic acid; *ACD,* acid citrate dextrose; *SPS,* sodium polyanethole sulfonate

Recommended Minimum Blood Draw Volumes for Blood Chemistry Tests

Assay	***Whole Blood Vol. (mL)***	***Minimum Serum/ Plasma Vol. (μL)***	***No. of Full Microtainers* (Green or Pink† unless otherwise noted)***
Albumin	0.75	0.5	1
Alkaline phosphatase	0.75	0.5	1
AST (SGOT)	0.75	0.5	1
Ammonia	0.75	0.5	1 Venous or arterial, EDTA‡/iced
Amylase	0.75	0.5	1
ALT (SGPT)	0.75	0.5	1
Bilirubin, direct	0.75	0.5	1
Bilirubin, total	0.75	0.5	1
Blood gas (capillary)	0.24	Whole blood	1 Full heparinized/iced
Blood gas (arterial)	1.0	1.0	Heparinized syringe/iced
BUN	0.75	0.5	1
Calcium	0.75	0.5	1
Chem 12	1.5	1.0	2
Chem 20 (Dacos)	1.5	1.0	2 Pink only (due to iron)
Cholesterol	0.75	0.5	1
CPK	3.0	1.5	4 Pink only (due to MB)
C-reactive protein	1.5	0.75	1½ Pink only
Electrolytes	0.75	0.5	1
Glucose	0.75	0.5	1
IgA, IgG, IgM	1.5	1.0	2 Pink only
Iron/binding capacity	1.5	1.0	2 Pink only
Lactic acid	1.5	0.5	Gray-top Vacutainer/iced
LDH	2.0	1.0	2½ Pink only (due to iso-enzymes)
Magnesium	0.75	0.5	1
Metabolic status panel	2.0	1.0	2½
Phosphorus	0.75	0.5	1
Protein (total)	0.75	0.5	1
Renal panel	2.0	1.0	2½
Triglyceride	0.75	0.5	1
Uric acid	0.75	0.5	1

*Microtainer tubes are color-coded according to the additive they contain.
†One full pink microtainer holds 0.75 mL.
‡Fill EDTA Microtainers only to the 500 μL mark.

Minimum Blood Draw Volumes for Drug Level Testing

Assay	*Whole Blood Vol. (mL)*	*Minimum Serum/ Plasma Vol. (mL)*	*No. and Type of Microtainers**
Acetaminophen	0.75	0.4	1 pink
Amikacin	0.75	0.4	1 pink
Carbamazepine (Tegretol)	0.75	0.4	1 pink
Chloramphenicol	0.75	0.3	1 pink or green (EDTA for plasma also)
Digoxin	2.0	1.0	2½ pink
Ethosuximide (Zarontin)	0.75	0.3	1 pink or green (EDTA for plasma also)
Gentamycin	0.75	0.4	1 pink
Lidocaine	0.75	0.3	1 pink or green (EDTA for plasma also)
Methotrexate	1.5	0.5	2 pink or green (EDTA for plasma also)
Phenobarbital	0.75	0.4	1 pink
Phenytoin (Dilantin)	0.75	0.4	1 pink
Primidone	0.75	0.3	1 pink or green (EDTA for plasma also)
Procainamide/*N*-acetylated procainamide (NAPA) (Pronestyl)	0.75	0.4	1 pink
Quinidine	0.75	0.3	1 pink
Salicylate	0.75	0.4	1 pink
Theophylline	0.75	0.4	1 pink
Tobramycin	0.75	0.4	1 pink
Valproic acid (Depakene)	0.75	0.3	1 pink or green (EDTA for plasma also)
Vancomycin	0.75	0.4	1 pink

*Do not use serum separator tubes.

Minimum Blood Draw Volumes for Blood Banking*

Assay	*Minimum Whole Blood Vol. (mL)*	*No. of Full Pink-Top Microtainers†*
Antibody identification	5–6	Amount too great for Microtainer use
Crossmatching	2.5	3–4
Direct Coombs' test	0.5	3–4
Elution	3–4	4–5
Type and screen	1.5	2

*The Blood Bank should be consulted to verify the necessity of the blood draw and the amount needed to be collected.
†One full Microtainer tube holds 0.75 mL. The Microtainer tubes are color-coded according to the additive they contain.

Guidelines for Selection of Routine Primary Plating Media for Bacteriologic Specimens

Type or Source of Specimen	ANA BBE/ CNA	ANA BRUC	ANA LKV	ANA CCFA	CHOC/ MTM	BAP	CHOC	CMG	CNA	CVA	HE	MAC	MAC/ SORB	SEL	SXT	XLD	Gram Stain
Abscess						****	****	****				****					****
Beta-Strep Screen						****									****		
Body Fluid						****	****	****				****					****
Bone						****	****	****				****					****
Cat Scratch Disease								****									****
Cervix					****	****						****					****
Clostridium Culture				****													
Conjunctiva						****	****	****				****					****
CSF						****	****	****									****
Cyst						****	****	****				****					****
Drainage						****	****	****				****					****
Ear						****	****	****				****					****
Eye						****	****	****				****					****
Feces—Routine Culture						****			****	****	***		****	****		****	
GC Culture					****	****			****	****	***		****	****		****	
Vibrio						****			****	****	***		****	****		****	
Yersinia						****			****	****	***		****	****		****	
GC Culture					****												****
Legionella Culture																	****
Lymph Node						****	****	*****				****					****
Mitral Valve						****	****	*****				****					****
Mouth						****	****					****					****
Nasal/Nares						****	****					****					****
Nasopharyngeal—Routine						****	****					****					****
Nasopharyngeal—Diphtheria						****	****		****			****					****
Neisseria gonorrhoeae (GC)					****												
Neisseria meningitidis					****												
Oral Cavity						****	****					****					****
Paracentesis						****	****	****				****					****
Pericardial						****	****	****				****					****
Peritonsillar Abscess						****	****	****				****					****
Pleural Fluid						****	****	****				****					****
Prostate					****	****		****				****					****

(continued)

Guidelines for Selection of Routine Primary Plating Media for Bacteriologic Specimens *(Continued)*

Type or Source of Specimen	ANA BBE/ CNA	ANA BRUC	ANA LKV	ANA CCFA	CHOC/ MTM	BAP	CHOC	CMG	CNA	CVA	HE	MAC	MAC/ SORB	SEL	SXT	XLD	Gram Stain
Pus						****	****	****				****					****
Rectal Abscess						****	****	****	****		***	****					****
Soft Tissue Aspirate						****	****	****				****					****
Sputum						****	****					****					****
Stool—Routine Culture						****			****	****	***		****	****		****	
GC Culture					****	****			****	****	***		****	****		****	
Vibrio						****			****	****	***		****	****		****	
Yersinia						****			****	****	***		****	****		****	
Synovial Fluid						****	****	****				****					****
Throat—Beta-Strep						****									****		
Screen																	
Diphtheria						****	****		****			****			****		****
GC–N. gonorrhoeae					****	****	****					****			****		
N. meningitidis					****	****	****					****			****		
Routine Culture						****	****					****			****		
Tissue						****	****	****				****					****
Urine—Use 0.001																	
mL loop																	
Clean-catch																	
Catheterized																	
Urine—Use 0.01						****	****	****				****					
mL loop																	
Bladder urine						****	****	****				****					
Cystoscopy/kidney						****	****	****				****					
Ileal conduit urine						****	****	****				****					
Suprapubic						****	****	****				****					
Wound—Deep						****	****	****				****					****
Postoperative						****	****	****				****					****
Superficial						****	****	****				****					****

Refer to Table 25–1 for explanation of abbreviations.

Appendix B
Sample Protocol for Treatment of Patients With High Blood Cholesterol Levels

Plasma Cholesterol Concentrations Risk Factor

	Total Cholesterol (mg/dL)		**LDL Cholesterol (mg/dL)**		**HDL Cholesterol (mg/dL)**
Age (yr)	***Moderate Risk***	***High Risk***	***Moderate Risk***	***High Risk***	***Increased Risk***
MEN					
0–14	173	190	106	120	38
15–19	165	183	109	123	30
20–29	194	216	128	148	30
30–39	218	244	149	171	29
40–49	231	254	160	180	29
≥50	230	258	166	188	29
WOMEN					
0–14	174	170	113	126	36
15–19	173	195	115	135	35
20–29	184	208	127	148	35
30–39	202	220	143	163	35
40–49	223	246	155	177	34
≥50	252	281	170	195	36

Recommendations for High Blood Cholesterol

	Recommended Intake	
Nutrient	***Step One Diet***	***Step Two Diet***
Total Fat	Less than 30% of total calories	
Saturated fat	<10% total calories	<7% total calories
Polyunsaturated fat	Up to 10% of total calories	
Monounsaturated fat	10–15% of total calories	
Carbohydrates	50–60% of total calories	
Protein	10–20% of total calories	
Cholesterol	**<300 mg/day**	**<200 mg/day**
Total calories	According to height and desired weight	

Appendix C
Abbreviations Pertinent to Laboratory Procedures

ABO	blood types: A, B, and O
ACT	activated clotting time
AFB	acid-fast bacillus
AIDS	acquired immunodeficiency syndrome
ALA	aminolevulinic acid
ALT	alanine aminotransferase
ANA	antinuclear antibody
Arb.	arbitrary units
ASAP	as soon as possible
AST	asparate aminotransferase
BUN	blood urea nitrogen
C	Celsius, centigrade
C&S	culture and sensitivity
CBC	complete blood count
CEA	carcinoembryonic antigen
Ci	curie
CIN	cervical intraepithelial neoplasia
CIS	carcinoma in situ
CK	creatine kinase
Cl	chloride
CML	chronic myologenous leukemia
CMV	cytomegalovirus
CPK	creatine phosphokinase
crit	hematocrit
CSF	cerebrospinal fluid
Diff	differential count of white blood cells
DNA	deoxyribonucleic acid
EBV	Epstein-Barr virus
ESR	erythrocyte sedimentation rate
F	Fahrenheit
FBS	fasting blood sugar
GC	gonorrhea; gonococcus
GGT	gamma glutamyltransferase
GI	gastrointestinal
gm	gram
GTT	glucose tolerance test
GU	genitourinary
Hb or Hgb	hemoglobin
HBV	hepatitis B virus
hCG	human chorionic gonadotropin hormone
HCl	hydrochloric acid
HDL	high-density lipoprotein
H&H	hemoglobin and hematocrit
HIB	hepatitis B
HIV	human immunodeficiency virus
hpf	high-power field
HSV	herpes simplex virus
IEP	immunoelectrophoresis
IgG, IgM, IgA, IgE, IgD	immunoglobulin G, M, A, E, and D
IM	intramuscular; infectious mononucleosis
IU	international units
J	joules
K	kelvin
K	potassium
KB	Kirby-Bauer sensitivity

KOH	potassium hydroxide
L	liter
LDH	lactate dehydrogenase
LDL	low-density lipoprotein
lpf	low-power field
L/S ratio	lecithin-sphingomyelin ratio
lytes	electrolytes
M	molar
MBC	minimum bacterial concentration
MCH	mean cell hemoglobin
MCHC	mean cell hemoglobin concentration
MCV	mean cell volume
mEq	milliequivalent
mg	milligram
MI	myocardial infarction
MIC	minimal inhibitory concentration
min	minute
mL, ml	milliliter
MLT	medical laboratory technologist
mm	millimeter
mmol	millimole
MT	medical technologist
MTB	mycobacterium tuberculosis
Na	sodium
NaCl	sodium chloride
nm	nanometer
O&P	ova and parasites
PBI	protein-bound iodine
PCV	packed cell volume
pH	hydrogen ion concentration
plts	platelets
PT	prothrombin time; pro-time
PTH	parathyroid hormone
PTT	partial thromboplastin time
RA	rheumatoid arthritis
RBC	red blood cell
RF	rheumatoid factor
Rh	Rh factor in the blood
RIA	radioimmunoassay
RPR	rapid plasma reagin
rout.	routine
SABE	subacute bacterial endocarditis
Sed rate	erythrocyte sedimentation rate
SGOT	serum glutamic-oxaloacetic transaminase
SGPT	serum glutamic-pyruvic transaminase
SI	Système International d'Unités
sp. gr.	specific gravity
spt	sputum
SST	serum separator tube
stat	immediately
STS	serologic test for syphilis
T_3	Tri-iodothyronine
T_4	thyroxine
T&C	type and crossmatch
TAT	turn-around time
TB	tuberculosis
TBG	thyroxine-binding globulin
U	unit
UTI	urinary tract infection
VDRL	Venereal Disease Research Laboratory
VLDL	very low-density lipoprotein
VMA	vanillylmandelic acid
WBC	white blood cell

Index

Page numbers in *italics* indicate figures; those with a t indicate tables; those with a b indicate boxed procedures.